Mass Gathering Medicine

Mass Gathering Medicine

A Guide to the Medical Management of Large Events

Edited by

William J. Brady
University of Virginia, Charlottesville, Virginia

Mark R. Sochor
University of Virginia, Charlottesville, Virginia

Paul E. Pepe
Metropolitan EMS Medical Directors Global Alliance, Fort Lauderdale, Florida

John C. Maino II
Emergency Physician, Jackson, Michigan

K. Sophia Dyer
Boston University Chobanian and Avedisian School of Medicine, Boston, Massachusetts

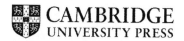
CAMBRIDGE
UNIVERSITY PRESS

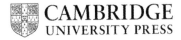

Shaftesbury Road, Cambridge CB2 8EA, United Kingdom

One Liberty Plaza, 20th Floor, New York, NY 10006, USA

477 Williamstown Road, Port Melbourne, VIC 3207, Australia

314–321, 3rd Floor, Plot 3, Splendor Forum, Jasola District Centre,
New Delhi – 110025, India

103 Penang Road, #05–06/07, Visioncrest Commercial, Singapore 238467

Cambridge University Press is part of Cambridge University Press & Assessment,
a department of the University of Cambridge.

We share the University's mission to contribute to society through the pursuit of education,
learning and research at the highest international levels of excellence.

www.cambridge.org
Information on this title: www.cambridge.org/9781009101950

DOI: 10.1017/9781009105156

First published 2024

A catalogue record for this publication is available from the British Library

Library of Congress Cataloging-in-Publication Data
Names: Brady, William, 1960– editor. | Sochor, Mark R., editor. | Pepe, Paul E., MD, editor. |
Maino John C., II, editor. | Dyer, K. Sophia, editor.
Title: Mass gathering medicine : a guide to the medical management of large events / edited
by William J. Brady, Mark R. Sochor, Paul E. Pepe, John C. Maino II, K. Sophia Dyer.
Description: Cambridge, United Kingdom ; New York, NY : Cambridge University Press,
2024. | Includes bibliographical references and index.
Identifiers: LCCN 2023027892 (print) | LCCN 2023027893 (ebook) | ISBN 9781009101950
(paperback) | ISBN 9781009105156 (ebook)
Subjects: MESH: Mass Gatherings | Disaster Planning – methods | Emergency Medical
Services – organization & administration | Risk Management – methods | Mass Casualty
Incidents – prevention & control | Disaster Medicine – methods
Classification: LCC HV553 (print) | LCC HV553 (ebook) | NLM WA 295 | DDC
363.34/8–dc23/eng/20231220
LC record available at https://lccn.loc.gov/2023027892
LC ebook record available at https://lccn.loc.gov/2023027893

ISBN 978-1-009-10195-0 Paperback

William J. Brady

I would like to dedicate this work to all the event medical providers of the world . . . for the long hours of work, frequently under challenging conditions, and usually with limited resources . . . all to ensure the safety and well-being of us all. I would also like to thank my colleagues in the University of Virginia (UVA) Emergency Department, UVA Special Event Medical Management, and Albemarle County Fire Rescue for their dedication in the expert care of our patients over the past three decades. And, of course, I dedicate this book to my wife and four adult children . . . three nurses, one doctor, and one firefighter-EMT . . . not only for who they are but also for what they do. And last, but certainly not the least, to my two grandsons, who are just plain awesome.

Mark R. Sochor

I dedicate this work to all those who make any event safe and fun for the participants and the audience. I want to thank these dedicated providers (often volunteers) who are away from their loved ones while working through the night, weekends, and with limited resources. The ingenuity and friendship I have enjoyed through the years working side by side with these dedicated individuals holds a special place in my heart. Lastly, I thank my wife Sara and my sons Keenan, MacLean, and Harrison for their sacrifices of so many weekends so that I may provide care for others.

Paul E. Pepe

This work is not only dedicated to the safety and fulfillment of audiences, spectators, fans, evacuees, and gatherers of all types in highly populated events, but also to the talented men and women behind the scenes optimizing their welfare and protection, especially in less fortunate mass gatherings. It is a salute to fellow public safety responders with whom I have witnessed and coendured many tragic events, but also to the gifted, resilient crew members and event security specialists, now treasured family, with whom I bonded, admired, cared for, and learned from, during many large-scale global tours managing mass audiences. Kudos to the brilliant authors here who shared their unmatched first-hand experiences and knowledge, but my deepest gratitude goes to my wife and children who encouraged and supported my time away to help and protect so many others.

John C. Maino II

I dedicate this work to the efforts, energy, and cooperation of the "behind the scenes" worldwide medical providers, EMS, fire and law enforcement personnel, who ensure that a mass gathering show/event is safe and successful. I would like to thank Penske Motor Sports, Michigan International Speedway (MIS), and NASCAR for the opportunities to plan, staff, and work their events as well as my colleagues and residents at Henry Ford Allegiance Health, Jackson Michigan, regional EMS, Michigan District 1 Regional Medical Coalition, and the EMS Fellows at the University of Michigan and Western Michigan University Schools of Medicine.

I would especially like to dedicate my efforts to my wife, five adult sons, their wives, four grandsons, and three granddaughters.

I dedicate this work to a special colleague and friend, who I helped mentor throughout his career and who passed away during the writing of this book: Christopher L. Krall, MD, FACEP. Chris was an emergency physician, working both in the ED and at mass gatherings. Chris frequently worked as a Medical/Rescue Team Physician or the Chief Physician at the APBA Gold Cup Hydroplane Races, Great Lakes Offshore Powerboat Racing Association as well as a "track physician" at Michigan International Speedway, Brooklyn, MI, from 1993 to 2022, staffing numerous NASCAR, CART, and IRL auto races. Through his expertise, hard work, and many hours of commitment, Chris was instrumental in developing this evolving emergency medicine specialty of mass gathering medicine.

K. Sophia Dyer

I would like to dedicate this work to the innumerable front-line providers who work tirelessly at their craft. From small to large events, this work you do is important to the world. To my colleagues at Boston EMS, from whom I continue to learn from and stand in awe of your commitment. With a special recognition of Captain Robert "Sarge" Y. Haley, Special Operations Division, who departed us too soon, but whose wisdom continues to guide us today. I am grateful for all the authors who shared their experience with us. Finally, to my husband for his continued support on this journey.

Contents

List of Contributors ix
Foreword xiii
Korin Hudson

Preface xv

1 **An Introduction to Mass Gathering Medicine** 1
Steven Garbin, William Brady, and Daniel Griffith

2 **Patient Care at Mass Gathering Events: Basic, Advanced, and Critical Care** 6
Erica Simon, Jonathan D. Trager, and Bryan Wilson

3 **Prediction of Medical Need and Event Risk Assessment at Mass Gathering Events** 21
Thomas Hartka and Matthew A. Hewitt

4 **Medical Logistics and Operational Planning for Patient Care at Mass Gathering Events** 41
Scott A. Goldberg, L. Scott Nichols, Michael S. Molloy, and Gerald W. (Jerry) Meltzer II

5 **Medical and Medical Support Staffing at Mass Gathering Events** 57
Lucian A. Mirra

6 **Mass Gathering Medicine: Equipment and Planning Considerations** 74
Robert Alexander, Tatum Lemly, Melanie Welcher, and Kostas Alibertis

7 **Incident Command System at Mass Gathering Events** 83
Lucian A. Mirra

8 **Security and Other Nonmedical Logistical Support Issues at Mass Gathering Events** 97
Mark Shank, Colleen Shank, Emily Wheeler, Amy Lowther, and Courtney Kirkland

9 **Understanding Local, State, and Federal Public Safety, Health Care, and Support Agencies** 105
William Fales and William Selde

10 **Common Themes and General Considerations across Mass Gathering Event Types** 120
Erica Simon, Jonathan D. Trager, and Bryan Wilson

11 **Mass Gathering Events: Youth, High School, Collegiate, Olympic, and Professional Sporting Events** 144
Korin Hudson, Matthew Sedgley, and Aaron J. Monseau

12 **Mass Gathering Events: Music Concerts and Festivals** 158
W. Michael Bogosian, Gerald W. (Jerry) Meltzer II, and Paul E. Pepe

13 **Mass Gathering Events: Motor Sport Events** 179
Paul A. Kozak, Jeff Grange, and John Aguilar

14 **VIP and Executive Medicine Considerations at Mass Gathering Events** 199
Asa M. Margolis, Glenn H. Asaeda, C. Crawford Mechem and Paul E. Pepe

15 **Mass Gathering Events: Community Events** 210
Ana M. Romero-Vasquez and K. Sophia Dyer

16 **Mass Gathering Events: Endurance Athletic Events** 221
Kristin Whitney and Pierre d'Hemecourt

17 **Mass Gathering Events: Extended Duration Events** 230
Sarah Kleinschmidt and Rebecca G. Breslow

18 **At-Risk Populations within Mass Gathering Events** 248
Megan C. Marino, Andrew L. Garrett, Aileen M. Marty, and Paul E. Pepe

19 **Crowd-Related Considerations at Mass Gathering Events: Management, Safety, and Dynamics** 268
Katie Klatt, Richard Serino, Edward Davis, and Jennifer O. Grimes

20 **Civil Unrest and Terrorism Involving Mass Gathering Events** 284
Pierre A. Carli, Debra G. Perina, and Paul E. Pepe

21 **Impact of Weather and Climate Change on Mass Gathering Events** 305
John W. Martel and J. Matthew Sholl

22 **Occurrence of the Mass Casualty Incident at a Mass Gathering Event** 320
Gregory A. Peters and Eric Goralnick

23 **Touring Medicine** 342
Paul E. Pepe, Gerald W. (Jerry) Meltzer II, L. Scott Nichols, Stephen E. (Jake) Berry, and Peter H. Hackett

24 **Infectious Disease and Mass Gathering Medicine** 372
Vivek Kak and Mehekmeet Bhatia

25 **Toxicology and Mass Gathering Medicine** 380
Abigail Kerns, Brian Nao, and John C. Maino II

26 **Medicolegal Considerations in Mass Gathering Medicine** 388
Bruce D. Gehle

27 **Business Considerations in Mass Gathering Medicine** 401
Andrew Matthews, L. Scott Nichols, and Kevin M. Ryan

Index 406

Contributors

John Aguilar
EMS Physician, Madison Emergency Physicians, MEP Health, Madison, WI, USA

Robert Alexander
Emergency Physician, Department of Emergency Medicine, University of Virginia Health System, Charlottesville, VA, USA

Kostas Alibertis
Chief, Western Albemarle Rescue Squad, Crozet, VA, USA

Glenn H. Asaeda
Chief Medical Director, Fire Department of New York, Brooklyn, NY, USA

Stephen E. (Jake) Berry
Founder and CEO, Jake Berry Productions, Scottsdale, AZ, USA

Mehekmeet Bhatia
Physician, Department of Internal Medicine, Henry Ford Allegiance Health, Detroit, MI, USA

W. Michael Bogosian
Senior Director, Global Security Operations, Live Nation Entertainment, Beverly Hills, CA, USA

William Brady
Professor, Vice Chair, & Medical Director of Emergency Medicine, University of Virginia; Professor of Medicine (Cardiovascular) & Nursing, University of Virginia; Medical Director, Special Event Medical Management, University of Virginia Health System, Charlottesville, VA, USA; Medical Director, Albemarle County Fire Rescue, Charlottesville, VA, USA

Rebecca G. Breslow
Sports Medicine Physician at Brigham and Women's Hospital, Instructor of Orthopaedic Surgery, Brigham and Women's Hospital, Harvard Medical School, Boston, MA, USA

Pierre A. Carli
Professor & Chair, Anesthesiology and Critical Care Department, Hospital Necker, Paris, France
Director, Service d'Aide Médicale Urgente (SAMU), Paris, France

Edward Davis
Police Commissioner (Former), Boston Police Department, Boston, MA, USA

Pierre d'Hemecourt
Assistant Professor, Sports Medicine Division, Department of Orthopedic Surgery & Director, Sports Medicine Ultrasound Clinic, Harvard Medical School Boston, MA, USA
Co-Medical Director, Boston Marathon, Boston, MA, USA
Team Physician, National Womens' Hockey League Boston Pride, Boston, MA, USA

K. Sophia Dyer
Professor, Department of Emergency Medicine, Boston University Chobanian and Avedisian School of Medicine, Boston, MA, USA

William Fales
Professor & Chief, Division of EMS and Disaster Medicine; EMS Medical Director, Department of Emergency Medicine, West Michigan University, Kalamazoo, MI, USA

Steve Garbin
Emergency Physician, Department of Emergency Medicine, Inova Fairfax Hospital, Falls Church, VA, USA

Andrew L. Garrett
Associate Professor, Medical Director, & Section Chief, Emergency Health Services, George Washington University School of Medicine, Washington, DC, USA

Bruce Gehle
Chief Operating Officer, Piedmont Liability Trust, University of Virginia, Charlottesville, VA, USA

Scott A. Goldberg

Director of EMS, Department of Emergency Medicine & Medical Director, Emergency Preparedness, Brigham and Women's Hospital, Harvard Medical School, Boston, MA, USA

Eric Goralnick

Medical Director, Gillette Stadium, Foxborough, MA, USA
Associate Professor, Department of Emergency Medicine, Brigham and Women's Hospital, Harvard Medical School, Boston, MA, USA

Jeff Grange

Associate Professor, Department of Emergency Medicine, Loma Linda University School of Medicine, Loma Linda, CA, USA

Daniel Griffith

Administrator of Operations, Department of Emergency Medicine, University of Virginia School of Medicine, Charlottesville, VA, USA

Jennifer O. Grimes

Emergency Physician, Harvard National Preparedness Leadership Initiative, Harvard University, Boston, MA, USA

Peter H. Hackett

Tour Physician and Clinical Professor, Division of Pulmonary Sciences & Critical Care Medicine, Department of Medicine and Altitude Research Center, University of Colorado, Denver, CO, USA

Thomas Hartka

Associate Professor, Department of Emergency Medicine, University of Virginia, Charlottesville, VA, USA

Matthew A. Hewitt

Emergency Physician, Department of Emergency Medicine, University of Virginia, Charlottesville, VA, USA

Korin Hudson

Professor of Emergency Medicine & Co-Head Team Physician, Georgetown University
Team Physician, Washington Wizards
Consulting Physician, Washington Capitals
MedStar Georgetown University Hospital & Washington Hospital Center

Vivek Kak

Physician & Specialist in Infectious Disease, Department of Internal Medicine, Henry Ford Allegiance Health, Detroit, MI, USA

Abigail Kerns

Senior Fellow, Division of Toxicology, Department of Emergency Medicine, University of Virginia Health System, Charlottesville, VA, USA

Courtney Kirkland

Emergency Physician & Clerkship Faculty, College of Medicine, Florida State University, Tallahassee, FL, USA

Katie Klatt

Public Health Senior Analyst, The Public Health Company, Palo Alto, CA, USA
Harvard T. H. Chan School of Public Health, Harvard University, Boston, MA, USA

Sarah Kleinschmidt

Assistant Professor & Assistant Fellowship Director in Wilderness Medicine, Department of Emergency Medicine University of Massachusetts Medical School-Baystate Medical Center, Springfield, MA, USA

Paul A. Kozak

Consultant, Department of Emergency Medicine, Mayo Clinic-Arizona, Phoenix, AZ, USA

Tatum Lemly

Emergency Physician, University of Maryland - Upper Chesapeake Medical Center, Bel Air, MD, USA

Amy Lowther

Emergency Physician, College of Medicine, Florida State University, Tallahassee, FL, USA

John C. Maino II

Medical Director, Michigan International Speedway, Brooklyn, MI, USA
Emergency Physician & Chief Medical Examiner, Jackson, MI, USA

Asa M. Margolis

Deputy Medical Director, United States Secret Service, Washington, DC, USA Associate Professor of Emergency Medicine, Johns Hopkins University, Baltimore, MD, USA

Megan C. Marino

Director & Medical Director, New Orleans Emergency Medical Services, New Orleans, LA, USA

John W. Martel
Emergency Physician, Department of Emergency Medicine, Maine Medical Center, Portland, ME, USA

Aileen M. Marty
Distinguished Professor of Infectious Diseases, Department of Medicine, Florida International University, Miami, FL, USA

Andrew Matthews
Emergency Physician, Department of Emergency Medicine & Boston Medical Center EMS Fellowship, Boston University, Boston, MA, USA

C. Crawford Mechem
Professor, Department of Emergency Medicine, Perelman School of Medicine at the University of Pennsylvania and Medical Director, Philadelphia Fire Department, Philadelphia, PA, USA

Gerald W. (Jerry) Meltzer II
Senior Partner, Sequel Tour Solutions and EventMed Live Event Medical Alliance, Bingham Farms, MI, USA

Lucian A. Mirra
EMS Training Officer & Emergency Medical Technician-Paramedic, Hanover County Fire-Rescue, Hanover, VA, USA
Paramedic, Special Event Medical Management, University of Virginia Health System, Charlottesville, VA, USA

Michael S. (Mick) Molloy
Consultant and Associate Professor in Emergency Medicine,
University College Dublin and Wexford General Hospital, Wexford, IE
Dean, Faculty of Sports and Exercise Medicine, Royal College of Surgeons in Ireland (RCSI), Dublin, IE

Aaron J. Monseau
Professor & Chief, Division of Sports Medicine & Program Director, Sports Medicine Fellowship, Department of Emergency Medicine, West Virginia University, Morgantown, WV, USA
Head Team Physician,
West Virginia University Athletics, West Virginia University, Morgantown, WV, USA

Brian Nao
Assistant Medical Director, Michigan International Speedway, Brooklyn, MI, USA

Paul E. Pepe
Professor (retired) of Medicine, Surgery, Pediatrics, Public Health & Chair, Emergency Medicine and Regional Director, Disaster/Event Preparedness, University of Texas Southwestern School of Medicine & Parkland Emergency-Trauma Center, Dallas, Texas; Division Lead, Health Security and Event Medicine, Sequel Tour Solutions; Director, Metro EMS Medical Directors ("Eagles") Global Alliance, Fort Lauderdale Florida, USA; Emergency Medical, Trauma and Health Security Consultant, National Basketball Association Trainers Association (NBATA), Atlanta, Georgia, USA

Debra G. Perina
Professor Emeritus Department of Emergency Medicine, University of Virginia, Charlottesville, VA, USA

Gregory A. Peters
Emergency Physician, Department of Emergency Medicine, Massachusetts General Hospital – Harvard University School of Medicine, Boston, MA, USA

Ana Romero-Vasquez
Emergency Physician, Department of Emergency Medicine, University of Virginia, Charlottesville, VA, USA

Kevin M. Ryan
Assistant Professor, Department of Emergency Medicine, Boston University Chobanian and Avedisian School of Medicine, Boston, MA, USA

L. Scott Nichols
Chief Executive Officer, Sequel Tour Solutions, Bingham Farms, MI and Senior Vice President for Business Development, Titan Health and Security Technologies, Newport Beach, CA, USA

Matthew Sedgley
Attending Physician-Family & Sports Medicine, MedStar Health, Washington, DC, USA
Team Physician, Baltimore Orioles, Baltimore, MD, USA

Will Selde
Assistant Professor, EMS Physician, & Medical Director, Department of Emergency Medicine, Western Michigan University, Kalamazoo, MI, USA

Richard Serino
Deputy Administrator (former) of Federal Emergency Management Agency, Washington, DC, USA

Colleen Shank
Emergency Physician, Sarasota Memorial Hospital, Sarasota, FL, USA

Mark Shank
Emergency Physician, Sarasota Memorial Hospital, Sarasota, FL, USA

J. Matthew Sholl
Emergency Physician, Maine Medical Center, Portland, ME, USA

Erica Simon
Assistant Professor, Department of Emergency Medicine, San Antonio Uniformed Services Health Education Consortium, San Antonio, TX, USA

Jonathan D. Trager
Emergency Physician, Medical Director, & Intensivist, Departments of Emergency Medicine & Critical Care Medicine, St. Luke's University Health Network, Bethlehem, PA, USA

Melanie Welcher
Emergency Medical Technician-Intermediate, Event Medicine Consultant, & Captain, Western Albemarle Rescue Squad, Crozet, VA, USA

Emily Wheeler
Emergency Physician, Sarasota Memorial Hospital, Sarasota, FL, USA

Kristin Whitney
Assist Professor of Orthopedics, Harvard Medical School, Boston, MA, USA
Sports Medicine Physician, Boston Childrens Hospital, Boston, MA, USA

Bryan Wilson
Emergency Physician & EMS Fellowship Director, Department of Emergency Medicine, St. Luke's University Health Network, Bethlehem, PA, USA

Foreword

Korin Hudson

It can be said that the physicians who practice Event Medicine have backgrounds and experiences as varied as the events that they organize and cover. My own career has borne that out as I have transitioned from athletic trainer to firefighter/paramedic to emergency physician and back to sports medicine again. Yet, in each of these roles, I managed to find myself on a sideline, at a finish line, in a first aid station, or backstage somewhere providing medical care for events large and small. All told, I have covered, or helped organize medical coverage for hundreds of mass gathering events including sporting events from Little League and local Special Olympics to the Stanley Cup Finals, and from "COVID bubbles" to the Boston Marathon. I have been a part of the coverage team for graduations, rallies, fairs, demonstrations, parades, speeches, and even once at a gathering of Nobel Laureates. And one time, years ago, in the middle of a Rolling Stones concert, in a 60,000-seat arena, I helped evacuate the band and thousands of spectators during a bomb threat.

Over the years, I have witnessed immense growth and evolution in the field of Event Medicine, so much so that it has become a subspecialty unto itself. No longer are events staffed by a couple of off-duty emergency medical technicians (EMTs) hoping to earn some overtime pay, or by an on-duty ambulance staged somewhere near – but not actually at – the event. Planning and preparation for large events now requires complex inter-agency coordination with months of pre-event planning, separate command centers, communications systems, equipment caches, adequate staffing, and disaster plans. Yet, before this text, we have arrived well into the 2020s without a definitive textbook on the topic of mass gathering and Event Medicine.

I've known Bill Brady for more than two decades. As an emergency medical services (EMS) medical director, he rode in the ambulance with me (then an EMT/ medic) teaching me nuances about electrocardiogram

(ECG) interpretation that I pass along to trainees to this day. As the event director, he gave me (then an emergency medicine resident) the prime position as the "backstage physician" for the infamous Rolling Stones concert, which, despite the brief interruption for an evacuation and explosives search, was an excellent show! Together we have staffed the aid stations and command centers for road races, concerts, sporting events, steeplechase races, and countless other mass gathering events. Bill is a mentor, a colleague, and a friend, and he has built a career as a true leader in the field of Emergency Medicine.

Alongside Dr. Brady are coeditors Drs. Paul Pepe, Sophia Dyer, Mark Sochor, and John Maino, who have likewise distinguished themselves in the field of Emergency Medicine with additional experience in EMS, Event Medicine, public safety, and disaster preparedness. No group could better bring together the depth and breadth of Event Medicine and the nuances that deserve special consideration before disaster strikes. Much of this text springs from their own vast experience and their many lessons learned.

Dr. Pepe has spent over forty years as a global leader in Emergency Medicine and EMS. Paul developed the National Disaster Life Support family of classes, created updated trauma triage guidelines for mass casualty incidents, and has been involved in the medical care of and as consultant for several high-profile groups and events including visiting heads of state, the White House medical unit, national presidential political conventions, and the NBA championships. Dr. Sophia Dyer is an emergency physician with experience in both toxicology and EMS. Sophie has been medical director for Boston EMS for over a decade and is co-medical director for the Boston marathon. Her experience in coordinating endurance events and managing disaster response is second to none. Dr. Mark Sochor brings a wealth of experience and was the inaugural chair of the Event Medicine section of American College of Emergency Physicians

(ACEP), which was an idea borne out of a conversation at a NASCAR track. Dr. Sochor brings a different perspective through his injury biomechanics background as well as years of experience in Event Medicine in motor sports. Mark brings what colleagues describe as a "common sense" approach to everything, including his approach to managing large events. Dr. John Maino is an emergency physician with approximately forty years of experience in mass gathering medicine. John's accolades are too numerous to list but among them are NASCAR track physician of the year and countless acknowledgments from the State of Michigan for all his efforts to keep spectators and participants safe. John's decades of experience providing care to the drivers and spectators at motorsports events (from snowmobile racing to NASCAR) brings unmatched experience and perspective regarding events.

Together, this group of physicians brings decades of remarkable experience from around the country, and in fact around the world, managing and providing medical care at events of all types and all sizes. In this volume they will discuss the foundations of Event Medicine from planning to execution to post-event analysis and review. They will guide us through the similarities and differences between a road race and a political rally, between a music festival and a college football game, how to handle dignitaries, weather events, civil unrest, and other unforeseen challenges. The experts recruited to contribute to this text will discuss the keys to integration between and across departments and agencies and will describe and define parts of the process often overlooked or forgotten.

This text will serve as a manual for anyone tasked with a first-time leadership role for a large-scale event. It will be a guide for those embarking on a career in Event Medicine and will be an ongoing resource for those of us who have been doing this for years. It is a reference that I will come back to again and again.

Preface

What is a mass gathering? Briefly stated, a mass gathering is a nonroutine activity within a community which brings together many people. A slightly more detailed response notes that the event typically involves a large number of people, defined as 1,000 or more persons in a defined geographic area, attending a "nonroutine" gathering; such a gathering potentially places a strain on community resources, including public safety, medical care, and other important infrastructure [1, 2]. This quantitative definition, however, is limited in that smaller venues with certain populations located in specific areas also regularly present challenges for a community. Beyond the gathering of a large number of persons, the event itself can also create additional needs and challenges for the local community, such as security precautions surrounding a dignitary visit or civil unrest resulting from a celebratory occasion. And, of course, the most appropriate approach of a community to such an event involves planning, preparation, and mitigation strategies, representing yet another set of challenges.

The next important question focuses on the delivery of medical care at the mass event: What is mass gathering medicine? This question has a much more involved answer, appropriately provided in the following pages of this textbook. In brief, however, mass gathering medicine is a coordinated deployment of healthcare providers at an event; furthermore, these healthcare providers are only one asset in an overall incident command structure of public safety providers and event officials, among others. And, importantly, mass gathering medicine is much more than an EMT, nurse, or physician with bandages, a blood pressure cuff, a defibrillator, and an ambulance.

The last important question to consider is where does mass gathering medicine belong in the healthcare world? Mass gathering medicine is not strictly emergency medical services nor emergency medicine; it is in fact a blend or composite of both areas of medical care with varying doses of sports medicine,

tactical medicine, wildness medicine, and expedition medicine blended in, depending upon the specific venue or event [3, 4]. The medical perspective of mass gathering medicine is also important to consider – the provision of care to spectators and participants of an event at the location of the event, thus optimizing outcomes and simultaneously reducing demands on local public safety and hospital resources.

This textbook was created with these questions and subsequent answers in mind. It is the first organized and collected discussion of mass gathering medicine in one concise collection. It was written and edited by a range of healthcare providers, venue organizers, law enforcement personnel, and risk managers, among many others, who work in the mass gathering medical space. We have created this work to not only recognize this emerging niche of the healthcare world but also to assist medical practitioners and planners in the development of rational, effective, and practical strategies for the management of mass gathering events.

The textbook, entitled *Mass Gathering Medicine: A Guide to the Medical Management of Large Events*, contains twenty-seven chapters. Approximately one-third of the book addresses the basics of mass gathering medicine, including its definition and history; staffing, supplies, and equipment; care delivery settings; operational response, incident command structure, and communication; prediction of medical needs; and the interface with local public safety and hospital-based authorities. Another large portion of the book considers the broad range of mass gathering events, ranging from athletic competitions, motorsports, and musical concerts to celebrations, dignitary visits, and touring medicine. The final sections of the book address crowd management, adverse weather, multiple casualty incident, civil unrest, terrorism, and infectious disease and toxicologic considerations; and lastly, medicolegal and risk management aspects of mass gathering medicine are discussed.

As noted, this book was created to recognize this emerging niche of the healthcare world, a fusion of emergency medicine and EMS … mass gathering medicine. We editors, along with the range of authors drawn from around the world, hope that you find it of value in your work as a mass gathering medical official, whether you are a healthcare provider, law enforcement personnel, or venue organizer or administrator.

References

1. Jaslow D., Yancy A. 2nd, Milsten A. Mass Gathering Medical Care. National Association of EMS Physicians Standards and Clinical Practice Committee. *Prehospital and Emergency Care*. 2000;4:359.

2. Milsten A. M., Maguire B. J., Bissell R. A., Seaman K.G. Mass-Gathering Medical Care: A Review of the Literature. *Prehospital and Disaster Medicine*. 2002;**17**:151.

3. Martin-Gill C., Brady W. J., Barlotta K., et al. Physician Integration into an EMS-Managed Mass Gathering Event. *American Journal of Emergency Medicine*. 2007;**25**:15–22.

4. Locoh-Donou S., Guofen Yan G., et al. Mass Gathering Medicine: Event Factors Predicting Patient Presentation Rates. *Internal and Emergency Medicine*. 2016;**11**:745–752.

An Introduction to Mass Gathering Medicine

Steven Garbin, William Brady, and Daniel Griffith

Until now, Mass Gathering Medicine has been largely defined by what it is not. Not Sports Medicine. Not Emergency Medicine. Not Emergency Medical Services (EMS). Not Urgent Care. Not Guerilla Medicine. Not Battlefield Medicine. The notion of Mass Gathering Medicine, though, becomes easier to define when thinking of it as something more than a field of medicine. Mass Gathering Medicine describes both a niche of expertise, and a way of thinking, organizing, and anticipating [1]. This book, therefore, aims to define and describe Mass Gathering Medicine as a means of planning and providing for the medical needs of communities in temporary communion.

Beginnings: The Development and Evolution of Prehospital Medical Care

The first consistent use of ambulances and field hospitals occurred in the Napoleonic wars, over 100 years before organized EMS systems emerged. Baron Dominique Jean Larrey, a French military surgeon, is credited with the invention of the battlefield ambulance, a horse-drawn cart which he termed a "flying ambulance." These flying ambulances were able to rapidly maneuver across the battlefield, pick up wounded soldiers, and transport them to field hospitals immediately adjacent to the zone of hostilities. The concept of triage, again attributed to Larrey, was practiced in these field hospitals, providing early stabilizing care prior to transfer to an established hospital, usually housed in a convent or monastery behind the lines. The ambulance and field hospital were developed further during the American Civil War. Subsequently, the invention and mass production of the automobile near the turn of the twentieth century provided for more rapid evacuation and transport of injured soldiers and civilians.

In World War II, jeeps moved injured soldiers to aid stations where basic care was rendered before evacuation to hospitals. The Korean Conflict, in the early 1950s, brought the next major development in emergency medical care and transport when the US military introduced the use of helicopters to rapidly evacuate wounded soldiers from the battlefield to a definitive care facility, termed a mobile army surgical hospital, or MASH unit. Further refinements of this model occurred during the Vietnam War.

As hostilities continued in southeast Asia and battlefield medicine advanced and evolved, the US civilian population was experiencing high rates of death and severe disability resulting from motor vehicle crashes. In 1966, the National Academy of Sciences delivered a report entitled *Accidental Death and Disability: The Neglected Disease of Modern Society* to President Lyndon B. Johnson. The report, termed "The White Paper" in EMS circles, identified accidental injuries as the "leading cause of death in the first half of life's span," and noted that more Americans died in motor vehicle crashes than were killed in recent military conflicts. Further, the report stated that a severely injured person would likely receive better care in a combat zone than on a civilian street in the United States. Finally, "The White Paper" documented a lack of consistent training, standards of operation, and so on, among existing ambulance and public safety services, and therefore recommended the standardization of emergency training for "rescue squad personnel, policemen, firemen and ambulance attendants." This standardization led to the first nationally recognized curriculum for the emergency medical technician-ambulance (EMT-A) in 1971. Two years later, the Emergency Medical Services Act provided federal guidelines and funding for the development of regional EMS systems. The modern EMS system was born.

The concept of advanced life support delivery via EMS was introduced several years later. Regional public services systems such as Los Angeles County in California, New York City, and Belfast in Northern Ireland, among other areas of the world, were experimenting with the concept of highly trained EMTs extending the capabilities of a physician into the prehospital setting and providing a high level of care before the patient arrived in the hospital. In the 1970s, the paramedic concept was popularized by the television program *Emergency* in the United States. This TV drama followed the daily career of a paramedic unit and engine company stationed in Los Angeles County Fire Station 51. These fictional paramedics worked closely with emergency physicians and nurses in an established emergency department at Rampart General Hospital where physicians provided medical guidance via radiotelephone and viewed cardiac telemetry and other mobile diagnostics. This TV series played a significant role in the further development of today's advanced life support EMS system, with an emphasis on communication and the importance of working closely with hospital-based, dedicated emergency healthcare providers, including physicians and nurses.

Emergence of a Philosophy: The Birth of Mass Gathering Medicine

As emergency medical services systems matured, various additional applications were developed beyond the traditional EMS response to medical and traumatic emergencies in the community. One application was the use of EMS resources at mass gathering events. An early example of EMS staffing of mass gathering situations included the traditional ambulance standby for the weekly high school football game, county fair, or municipal celebration [2, 3]. This was simple from a logistical and planning perspective. Essentially, an on-duty ambulance would be prepositioned at such an event and poised for response. However, these ambulances were also often responsible for emergency calls beyond the mass gathering venue.

As EMS systems grew and added medical capabilities, deployments at mass gathering events similarly increased in complexity. Based on early experiences, including notable stadium disasters associated with European football, EMS professionals in the mass gathering space realized that, while they were the natural medical personnel to staff such events, a direct translation of "traditional response"

emergency medical services philosophy, personnel, and equipment was not the most appropriate approach [4]. Altered strategies of medical care and mission were required to adapt existing approaches and create new systems of care. Medical guidelines required changes. New or altered equipment was needed. Additional personnel were often required [5].

Mission Goals of Mass Gathering Medicine

The underlying philosophy of mass gathering deployment focuses on the assumption that the responsibility for increased need for care created by the venue and/or event lies with the medical team staffing the event. Related to this philosophy, the medical deployment at a mass gathering event has several important goals, including:

(1) provision of medical care to spectators, ranging from routine care, allowing release back to the venue, up to and including resuscitation and stabilization of major illness or injury followed by evacuation to a definitive care facility;

(2) additional medical care delivery to venue VIPs and their staff;

(3) reduced burden on local EMS and hospital emergency departments; and

(4) venue-oriented risk management and reduction.

These goals are, of course, interrelated.

Scale and Specific Needs

The mode of forethought, preparation, and response that defines Mass Gathering Medicine is scalable and adaptable to the scope and specific needs of the gathering in question [6]. In the initial stages of planning, attention to the event type and duration is paramount. Political rallies, musical performances, and sporting events will draw different crowds with variable emotions and intentions. There may be notable celebrities at a rock concert or sporting event, but the security needs of a political event may surpass all other considerations if a sufficiently important dignitary is present (i.e., the President of the United States). Substance use may be more prevalent at a particular concert or music festival and may rouse or pacify a crowd. The planning, preparation, and logistical complexity of an event is also likely to expand with the length and scale of the gathering. Sporting events can be confined to a single afternoon or evening in a particular arena or stadium or they may engulf the resources and infrastructure of an entire city for weeks at a time – as is the case with the Olympic Games or the World Cup.

Attendees

Mass gatherings are defined chiefly by the sort of people who come together and their intentions in gathering. In some way or another, mass gatherings of all types draw a community [4, 7]. These groups may be united by their allegiance to a specific college or university, their adoration for a particular band, or their dedication to drinking alcohol while horses are racing. No matter the gathering, attention should be paid in preparation for the anticipated demographics of attendees. Is this going to be an event that draws older individuals who are likely to bring comorbidities and chronic medical conditions to the considerations of care, or can a younger, relatively healthy slice of the population be relied upon to attend? Is the presence of alcohol or other intoxicants anticipated (encouraged?) or are there other more pressing considerations [8, 9]? Will the attendees be sedentary or engaged in vigorous physical activity? Finally, it is important to consider the likely or possible influence of the event or act itself on the crowd. Mosh pits, court storming, and the toppling of goal posts may not be preventable, but they can be predicted and planned for in a manner that maximizes the safety of participants and thus reduces the burden on those triaging, transporting, and rendering care both at the event and potentially in local hospitals.

Space, Architecture, Infrastructure

Mass gatherings are impacted heavily by the physical space they occupy. The architecture and location of the space housing a given event will almost certainly influence planning for medical care that can feasibly be delivered on or near the premises. A modern stadium with state-of-the-art electronics and amenities is likely to pose different logistical challenges to the evaluation of patients and potential treatment pathways than a pop-up festival with little to no existing electrical infrastructure or plumbing. Triage and transportation needs are influenced by the location of the event relative to preexisting sites of care in the local community, and the safety and security of both patients and medical personnel are often reliant on the characteristics of the structure (or lack thereof) in which care is provided. Lastly, although it is not up to medical directors to ensure the structural integrity of the location or physical environment hosting a mass gathering, disaster planning and contingency worst-case-scenario protocols should always consider loss of/damage to the physical environment and communicating infrastructure in the event of force majeure, terrorism, or other potentially catastrophic occurrences.

Weather, Climate, Environment

A reasonable initial question related to the physical space containing a mass gathering is always: Will the event be outdoors? If so, specific attention to the regional climate, historic weather, and plans for unlikely extremes are warranted. Exposure-related conditions including heat stroke, heat exhaustion, dehydration, hypothermia, frostbite, sunburn, and so on should be anticipated. More recently, the COVID-19 pandemic has illustrated the importance of infectious disease precautions. In the case of droplet-transmitted viral illnesses, masking, distancing, airflow/outdoor events, and vaccine status of attendees should be considered. In much the same manner, common-sense public health measures to limit the spread of STIs via widespread availability of condoms is likely to beneficial if sexual activity is likely – as is the case in the Olympic Athletes Village.

Climate change necessitates the responsibility to consider human impact on the local environment and habitat of existing flora and fauna. Is the event likely to significantly disrupt local plant life, wildlife, waterways, or air quality? If so, mitigation procedures or reconsideration of the scale and/or location of the event are appropriate, if not mandatory.

Preservation of Local Resources

Caring for large groups in mass gathering necessarily requires attention to the variables previously described as well as the local and regional population not participating in the gathering – with the goal of delivering high-quality triage and care of event-goers while preserving the capacity of in-place resources to care for the preexisting local population [3, 10, 11, 12, 13]. Medical staff must also be familiar with the overall event command structure to both recognize and adapt to the ways centralized (usually nonmedical) command may affect triage and transport.

Delivering High-Quality Care

Fixed treatment locations, whether a specified room or rooms in a larger structure, portable tents, prefabricated structures, or trailers have been introduced to allow for enhanced delivery of treatment. Healthcare providers not only staff these fixed locations but can also be stationed throughout larger venues on foot, bicycles, or all-terrain vehicles. The traditional ambulance is also deployed, but largely for transport to a local hospital.

The provision of medical care for any person at an event is the responsibility of the deployment team. This care most often is delivered to patients with lower acuity medical and traumatic issues. This care, delivered by a team including an on-site physician, allows the patient to have their issue addressed and hopefully return to the event. A minority of patients may develop major medical or traumatic issues at the venue. In these cases, the event medical team will resuscitate the patient, with the aim of stabilization, and arrange for appropriate air or ground transport to a definitive care facility, such as a hospital-based emergency department. The location of any event relative to the nearest existing medical infrastructure must be considered with attention to transport logistics to the highest level of care available. Traditional triage is often employed with modifications for dignitaries, celebrities, and athletes. The type and magnitude of medical care delivered by the event medical team is a direct function of the specific mission goals, venue leadership desires, and related resource allocation (staffing numbers, personnel abilities, and equipment). Incorporated into these goals is a consideration of rational medical thought and planning. Certain deployment models are engineered to manage minor issues with the plan of transporting any medical event of significance to a local hospital. Other models are more robust, allowing for enhanced diagnostic and treatment modalities, an approach which requires significantly greater resource allocation. Regardless of the deployment model used, mass event medical care most often represents the first step, or phase, of treatment. Some patients will need follow-up at a later time with a nonevent healthcare provider for the lower acuity issues, while others with more significant medical needs will be transferred directly from the event to a regional hospital for an immediate escalation of care.

Command and Control

Another significant consideration in medical planning as well as the delivery of care to specific patients involves the reality that comprehensive medical care cannot be delivered to some patients and that the event medical authorities will almost certainly answer operationally to the overall venue command structure. Medical staff must be familiar with the overall event command structure to both recognize and adapt to the ways centralized (usually nonmedical) command may affect triage and transport [2, 12]. This command structure must be embraced by all event medical personnel and tends to be a relatively new concept for hospital-based providers.

Disaster Planning

Generally speaking, a distinction has been made in prior studies of Mass Gathering Medicine regarding care rendered as planned at mass gatherings and any emergency response to natural disasters, terrorist attacks, infrastructure failure, or other unforeseen catastrophic events. It is, however, within the purview of mass gathering medicine and prudent for strategic medical planning to create worst-case or disaster scenario plans [14]. Such plans should be revisited and refreshed periodically with attention to evolving local and geopolitics, climate concerns, and so on.

Research and Quality Improvement

As this book intends to define and describe an emerging approach to medical planning and provision of care, it is essential that research and statistical methods be tested and developed with the goals of mass gathering medicine in mind. Exploration, analysis, and application of novel statistical and computing languages to mass gathering medicine, in addition to the continued digitization of both ticketing, crowd surveillance, and the medical and public service record, is sure to push the field forward in addition to raising new ethical and legal questions both with regard to research and the provision of care at events. As researchers are better able to gather, analyze and interpret data from prior gatherings, we anticipate both exciting research and careful insights that will allow for the safest, most efficient delivery of care at mass gatherings.

As noted, until now, Mass Gathering Medicine has been an increasingly important – if ill-defined –

reality in the medical care of communities that continue to gather in increasingly large numbers. Humans will continue to gather in communities and will inevitably require medical care when they do so. With this book, the authors invite us to explore an emerging field of medicine as a means of planning and organizing while providing the highest quality care to communities as they gather in communion today and as our world – and inevitably our gatherings – continue to grow and evolve.

References

1. Hutton A., Ranse J., Zimmerman P. A. Rethinking Mass-Gathering Domains for Understanding Patient Presentations: A Discussion Paper. *Prehospital and Disaster Medicine*. 2021;36(1):121–124. doi: 10.1017/S1049023X20001454. Epub 2020 Dec 1. PMID: 33256882.

2. Glick J., Rixe J., Spurkeland N., Brady J., Silvis M., Olympia R. P. Medical and Disaster Preparedness of US Marathons. *Prehospital and Disaster Medicine*. 2015;30(4):344–350. doi:10.1017/S1049023X15004859.

3. Johnston A. N., Wadham J., Polong-Brown J., Aitken M., Ranse J., Hutton A., Richards B., Crilly J. Health Care Provision During a Sporting Mass Gathering: A Structure and Process Description of On-Site Care Delivery. *Prehospital and Disaster Medicine*. 2019;34(1):62–71. doi:10.1017/S1049023X18001206.

4. Still K., Papalexi M., Fan Y., Bamford D. Place Crowd Safety, Crowd Science? Case Studies and Application. *Journal of Place Management and Development*. 2020;13(4):385–407. doi:10.1108/JPMD-10-2019-0090.

5. Milsten A. M., Maguire B. J., Bissell R. A., Seaman K. G. Mass-Gathering Medical Care: A Review of the Literature. *Prehospital and Disaster Medicine*. 2002;17(3):151–162. doi: 10.1017/s1049023x00000388. PMID: 12627919.

6. Turris S., Rabb H., Munn M. B., Chasmar E., Callaghan C. W., Ranse J., Lund A. Measuring the Masses: The Current State of Mass-Gathering Medical Case Reporting (Paper 1). *Prehospital and Disaster Medicine*. 2021;36(2):202–210. doi:10.1017/s1049023x21000066.

7. Hartman N., Williamson A., Sojka B., Alibertis K., Sidebottom M., Berry T., Hamm J., O'Connor R. E., Brady W. J. Predicting Resource Use at Mass Gatherings Using a Simplified Stratification Scoring Model. *American Journal of Emergency Medicine*. 2009;27(3):337–343. doi:10.1016/j.ajem.2008.03.042.

8. Hutton A., Savage C., Ranse J., Finnell D., Kub J. The Use of Haddon's Matrix to Plan for Injury and Illness Prevention at Outdoor Music Festivals. *Prehospital and Disaster Medicine*. 2015;30(2):175–183. doi:10.1017/S1049023X15000187.

9. Hutton A., Ranse J., Munn M. B. Developing Public Health Initiatives Through Understanding Motivations of the Audience at Mass-Gathering Events. *Prehospital and Disaster Medicine*. 2018;33(2):191–196. doi:10.1017/s1049023x18000067.

10. Sanders A. B., Criss E., Steckl P., Meislin H. W., Raife J., Allen D. An Analysis of Medical Care at Mass Gatherings. *Annals of Emergency Medicine*. 1986;15(5):515–519. doi:10.1016/S0196-0644(86)80984-2.

11. Locoh-Donou S., Yan G., Berry T., O'Connor R., Sochor M., Charlton N., Brady W. Mass Gathering Medicine: Event Factors Predicting Patient Presentation Rates. *Internal and Emergency Medicine*. 2016;11(5):745–752. doi:10.1007/s11739-015-1387-1.

12. Koski A., Kouvonen A., Sumanen H. Preparedness for Mass Gatherings: Factors to Consider According to the Rescue Authorities. *International Journal of Environmental Research and Public Health*. 2020;17(4):1361. doi:10.3390/ijerph17041361.

13. Turris S. A., Lund A., Hutton A., Bowles R., Ellerson E., Steenkamp M., Ranse J., Arbon P. Mass-Gathering Health Research Foundational Theory: Part 2 – Event Modeling for Mass Gatherings. *Prehospital and Disaster Medicine*. 2014;29(6):655–663. doi:10.1017/S1049023X14001228.

14. Goralnick E., Gates J. We Fight Like We Train. *New England Journal of Medicine*. 2013;368(21):1960–1961. doi:10.1056/NEJMp1305359.

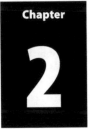

Chapter 2

Patient Care at Mass Gathering Events: Basic, Advanced, and Critical Care

Erica Simon, Jonathan D. Trager, and Bryan Wilson

Mass Gathering Medical Care and the Need for Healthcare Resources

Mass gathering medical care is defined as organized health services offered to participants and attendees at an event, for a limited duration [1]. Planning for mass gatherings presents several challenges. Factors such as crowd size, event duration, participant behavior, venue characteristics, and weather have been known to significantly impact the demand for healthcare resources [2–4]. Although mass gathering attendees tend to be in good health as compared to the general population, they are more likely to experience accidental, incidental, and deliberate health threats due to environmental exposure, behavioral factors often as a result of alcohol consumption or drug use, and the threat of terrorism [5, 6].

Previously, several conceptual models have detailed mechanisms by which to determine medical response requirements at mass gathering events. In 2001, Arbon et al. described psychosocial, biomedical, and environmental domains with which to guide stakeholders in the development of mass gathering medical plans; creating regression models to estimate patient presentation rates (PPRs) and transport-to-hospital rates (TTHRs) [7]. Years later Zeitz et al. performed a retrospective longitudinal study of agricultural events in South Australia, identifying historical event data as a valuable resource for the prediction of future PPRs [4].

Historically, data indicates that skin lesions, minor trauma, and neurologic symptoms (e.g., headache and dizziness) are the most common presenting complaints at mass gathering events [8–10]. Nearly 10 percent of individuals who access care at mass gatherings can be treated on site, while an estimated 1 percent will require transport by ambulance for definitive care [9]. Among mass gathering attendees, transport rates increase predictably with patient age [10]. As there is significant variability in PPRs at mass gathering events (ranging from 0.14 to 90 patients per 1,000 attendees) [1], event organizers are encouraged to consider the perspectives of Arbon et al. and Zeitz et al. when generating hypotheses regarding the demand for medical care [4, 7].

The Goals of Mass Gathering Medical Care and the Medical Plan

The goal of mass gathering medical care is to reduce the burden on community healthcare resources by delivering on-site care and/or stabilization with the goal of decreasing the volume or acuity of transports off-site [2–4, 11, 12]. The provision of care at a mass gathering event is detailed in the event medical plan; created by the Event Medical Director, in cooperation with event hosts, community stakeholders, and local emergency medical service (EMS) Medical Directors. The medical plan must address (1) research regarding the historic demand for event healthcare services; (2) physician medical oversight; (3) levels of care to be delivered; (4) human resources available for the provision of pre-hospital care; (5) on-site medical equipment; (6) patient treatment facilities; (7) patient transportation; (8) patient access to care; and (9) healthcare documentation [1]. Vital functions such as emergency operations, communications procedures, public health initiatives including public education, and continuous quality improvement processes are also included [1, 13]. The Incident Command System (ICS) Form 206 provides a useful template for the development of the medical plan (Figures 2.1A, 2.1B, and 2.1C) [14, 35]. Key medical leadership involved in preplanning these events should have completed basic level ICS training including NIMS-700, NIMS-800, ICS-100, and ICS-200. It is recommended that these individuals have completed

MEDICAL PLAN (ICS 206)

| 1. Incident Name: | 2. Operational Period: | Date From: | Date To: |
| | | Time From: | Time To: |

3. Medical Aid Stations:

Name	Location	Contact Number(s)/Frequency	Paramedics on Site?
			☐ Yes ☐ No
			☐ Yes ☐ No
			☐ Yes ☐ No
			☐ Yes ☐ No
			☐ Yes ☐ No
			☐ Yes ☐ No

4. Transportation (indicate air or ground):

Ambulance Service	Location	Contact Number(s)/Frequency	Level of Service
			☐ ALS ☐ BLS
			☐ ALS ☐ BLS
			☐ ALS ☐ BLS
			☐ ALS ☐ BLS

5. Hospitals:

Hospital Name	Address, Latitude & Longitude if Helipad	Contact Number(s)/ Frequency	Travel Time — Air	Travel Time — Ground	Trauma Center	Burn Center	Helipad
					☐ Yes Level:_____	☐ Yes ☐ No	☐ Yes ☐ No
					☐ Yes Level:_____	☐ Yes ☐ No	☐ Yes ☐ No
					☐ Yes Level:_____	☐ Yes ☐ No	☐ Yes ☐ No
					☐ Yes Level:_____	☐ Yes ☐ No	☐ Yes ☐ No
					☐ Yes Level:_____	☐ Yes ☐ No	☐ Yes ☐ No

6. Special Medical Emergency Procedures:

☐ Check box if aviation assets are utilized for rescue. If assets are used, coordinate with Air Operations.

7. Prepared by (Medical Unit Leader): Name: _____ Signature: _____

8. Approved by (Safety Officer): Name: _____ Signature: _____

| ICS 206 | IAP Page _____ | Date/Time: _____ |

Figure 2.1A Federal Emergency Management Agency ICS Form 206: Medical Plan [14, 35]

Federal Emergency Management Agency. (n.d.). Incident Command System Form 206: Medical Plan. Retrieved December 30, 2021, from https://emilms.fema.gov/IS201/assets/ICS%20Forms%20206.pdf

ICS 206
Medical Plan

Purpose. The Medical Plan (ICS 206) provides information on incident medical aid stations, transportation services, hospitals, and medical emergency procedures.

Preparation. The ICS 206 is prepared by the Medical Unit Leader and reviewed by the Safety Officer to ensure ICS coordination. If aviation assets are utilized for rescue, coordinate with Air Operations.

Distribution. The ICS 206 is duplicated and attached to the Incident Objectives (ICS 202) and given to all recipients as part of the Incident Action Plan (IAP). Information from the plan pertaining to incident medical aid stations and medical emergency procedures may be noted on the Assignment List (ICS 204). All completed original forms must be given to the Documentation Unit.

Notes:
- The ICS 206 serves as part of the IAP.
- This form can include multiple pages.

Block Number	Block Title	Instructions
1	**Incident Name**	Enter the name assigned to the incident.
2	**Operational Period** • Date and Time From • Date and Time To	Enter the start date (month/day/year) and time (using the 24-hour clock) and end date and time for the operational period to which the form applies.
3	**Medical Aid Stations**	Enter the following information on the incident medical aid station(s):
	• Name	Enter name of the medical aid station.
	• Location	Enter the location of the medical aid station (e.g., Staging Area, Camp Ground).
	• Contact Number(s)/Frequency	Enter the contact number(s) and frequency for the medical aid station(s).
	• Paramedics on Site? ☐ Yes ☐ No	Indicate (yes or no) if paramedics are at the site indicated.
4	**Transportation** (indicate air or ground)	Enter the following information for ambulance services available to the incident:
	• Ambulance Service	Enter name of ambulance service.
	• Location	Enter the location of the ambulance service.
	• Contact Number(s)/Frequency	Enter the contact number(s) and frequency for the ambulance service.
	• Level of Service ☐ ALS ☐ BLS	Indicate the level of service available for each ambulance, either ALS (Advanced Life Support) or BLS (Basic Life Support).

Figure 2.1B Federal Emergency Management Agency ICS Form 206: Medical Plan [14, 35]

Federal Emergency Management Agency. (n.d.). Incident Command System Form 206: Medical Plan. Retrieved December 30, 2021, from https://emilms.fema.gov/IS201/assets/ICS%20Forms%20206.pdf

ICS-300 and ICS-400 to ensure their familiarity with the incident action plan, ICS forms, and the overall function of the event.

Main Concerns in Planning Medical Care

Planning for the provision of medical care is essential, for both humanitarian and legal reasons and so medical care at the venue is equal to or greater than the standard of care currently provided in the community. This should be addressed in the permitting process. One of the main reasons for providing on-site medical care is to reduce the demand on local EMS and the emergency departments at local hospitals in the area of the event. Event organizers may choose to contract with a health service provider, who may not be associated with the usual local service provider [35].

Block Number	Block Title	Instructions
5	Hospitals	Enter the following information for hospital(s) that could serve this incident:
	• Hospital Name	Enter hospital name and identify any predesignated medivac aircraft by name a frequency.
	• Address, Latitude & Longitude if Helipad	Enter the physical address of the hospital and the latitude and longitude if the hospital has a helipad.
	• Contact Number(s)/ Frequency	Enter the contact number(s) and/or communications frequency(s) for the hospital.
	• Travel Time • Air • Ground	Enter the travel time by air and ground from the incident to the hospital.
	• Trauma Center ☐ Yes Level:_____	Indicate yes and the trauma level if the hospital has a trauma center.
	• Burn Center ☐ Yes ☐ No	Indicate (yes or no) if the hospital has a burn center.
	• Helipad ☐ Yes ☐ No	Indicate (yes or no) if the hospital has a helipad. Latitude and Longitude data format need to compliment Medical Evacuation Helicopters and Medical Air Resources
6	Special Medical Emergency Procedures	Note any special emergency instructions for use by incident personnel, including (1) who should be contacted, (2) how should they be contacted; and (3) who manages an incident within an incident due to a rescue, accident, etc. Include procedures for how to report medical emergencies.
	☐ Check box if aviation assets are utilized for rescue. If assets are used, coordinate with Air Operations.	Self explanatory. Incident assigned aviation assets should be included in ICS 220.
7	Prepared by (Medical Unit Leader) • Name • Signature	Enter the name and signature of the person preparing the form, typically the Medical Unit Leader. Enter date (month/day/year) and time prepared (24-hour clock).
8	Approved by (Safety Officer) • Name • Signature • Date/Time	Enter the name of the person who approved the plan, typically the Safety Officer. Enter date (month/day/year) and time reviewed (24-hour clock).

Figure 2.1C Federal Emergency Management Agency ICS Form 206: Medical Plan [14, 35]

Federal Emergency Management Agency. (n.d.). Incident Command System Form 206: Medical Plan. Retrieved December 30, 2021, from https://emilms.fema.gov/IS201/assets/ICS%20Forms%20206.pdf

Verification of the service provider credentials should ensure that they are appropriately licensed and regulated. The event medical provider must coordinate with the local health and emergency services to plan a response to any emergency or incident requiring further assistance. Prior to the event initiation, it is important to notify local health authorities of the details of the event and provide them with emergency plans for a major incident. Additionally, local hospitals should be notified of the event in writing at least thirty days in advance and this should also include the estimated number of attendees [35].

Question to ask regarding the logistical issues to address in medical care planning include [35]:

• How many medical stations will be required on-site?
• Will medical personnel operate in a facility to which the injured must make their way, or will clearly identified medical teams patrol spectator areas?
• How will spectators identify medical personnel on the site (uniforms, vests, etc.)?
• Will vehicles be available to transport spectators to the medical facility?
• Will medical vehicles be appropriate to the terrain? Four-wheel drive vehicles may be

- required for off-road areas and golf carts or similar vehicles required for high-density spectator areas.
- Where an ambulance is not required, will a "chauffeur system" be provided to transport persons from the on-site medical facility to their own transport vehicle?
- How will medical personnel be notified of, or summoned to, spectators requiring assistance in vast spectator areas?
- What means of communication will be available to permit attending medical personnel to communicate with offsite medical personnel, event organizers, security, and other support personnel?
- Are there any sponsorship conflicts between the event sponsor and any medical service operators?
- What level of on-site medical care, if any, do you expect to be required, given the nature of the event?
- What mix of medical personnel (first aid providers, paramedics, nurses, doctors) will you require on-site?
- Who will provide the personnel? How will the cost for their services be funded?
- Are the health service providers from the local area? If not, how will their services be integrated with the local services?
- How will security concerns for health care personnel on-site be addressed?
- Are the selected personnel appropriately skilled to respond to anticipated medical problems at the event? They may require additional training.
- Will medical personnel or vehicles need special credentials to allow them access to all parts of the venue, especially to any restricted areas?
- Are medical personnel assigned for public safety workers at the event?
- Are aero-medical services and landing zones available?
- Where is the closest trauma center?
- Have primary and secondary receiving hospitals been identified?
- Does the area hospital have adequate bed and personnel capacity to respond to the emergency requirements of an event of the size that is being planned?

Event organizers and the assigned medical teams should perform an Emergency Medical Services Venue Assessment (Figures 2.2A and 2.2B) which will assist in planning and resource allocation.

A multitude of tasks need to be addressed regarding the management and planning of event medical care and include the following [35]: (1) Determine which other organizations will be involved. Who will be the lead agency?; (2) conduct planning meetings involving health personnel, emergency services personnel, and event organizers; (3) determine what is expected of each organization involved in the provision of medical care; (3) determine likely levels of care that will be required; (4) determine any local laws, rules, or regulations governing emergency first aid; (5) determine the budget for the provision of medical care services; (6) establish liaison with other emergency services (police, fire, and security); (7) identify the equipment required and potential suppliers. Will the equipment be purchased, hired, or borrowed?; (8) will volunteers be used? What accreditation will they be required to possess? What benefits will they be offered?; (9) ensure the security of medical stations and the safety of the staff; (10) establish a patient information management system for patients who are treated, including patient care reporting, etc.; and (11) determine in advance the disposition of patient records after the event.

Physician Medical Oversight

A physician, possessing a valid medical license issued in the state in which the event is being held, should be appointed as the Event Medical Director. It is recommended that this individual be trained in emergency medicine, emergency medical services and/or sports medicine, and possess intimate knowledge of local EMS systems and prehospital provider skill-levels [2, 3, 15–28]. Medical oversight at a mass gathering should include elements of direct and indirect medical direction. The specific nature of the mass gathering event will dictate the structure of this oversight, but direct medical oversight may occur via online medical direction via telephone or radio, specific for the event or via on-scene medical direction with physicians integrating into the event's response plan. The elements of indirect medical oversight that are vital to the success of the event include: clinician credentialing, on-scene training and orientation to the site and equipment, and approving protocols or standing orders specific to the event – as permitted by local laws and regulations.

A topic worthy of discussion is that of the requirement for on-site medical oversight. Retrospective studies from Boyle et al. (United States Air Shows)

EMERGENCY MEDICAL SERVICES VENUE ASSESSMENT CHECKLIST

Event Type

Hazards: _____

Vulnerabilities: _____

Environment

Indoor/Outdoor: _____

Climate: _____

Alcohol/Drugs: _____

Demographics of Spectators and Participants

Age: _____

Mobility: _____

Numbers: _____

Attitude: _____

VIPs: _____

Transportation

Access/Egress: _____

Americans with Disabilities Act (ADA) Compliance: _____

Internal/External: _____

Facility

Visibility/Lighting: _____

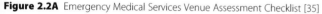

Figure 2.2A Emergency Medical Services Venue Assessment Checklist [35]

and Grange et al. (NASCAR event) demonstrated that the presence of an on-site physician dramatically decreased the utilization of community healthcare resources – on-site physicians were able to perform appropriate interventions, disposition patients without the need for further treatment, and address refusals of care [18, 21]. Grange et al. specifically noted an 89 percent decrease in their TTHR given physician presence [18].

As a counterpoint to the data presented by Grange et al., in their evaluation of 32 rock concerts in Illinois during which online medical oversight was provided by radio, McDonald et al. identified 438 patient encounters with no known adverse events (based upon the absence of inquiries or complaints to the EMS system, emergency department records, and venue patient care records). Notable concerns presented in the McDonald et al. study including poor

EMERGENCY MEDICAL SERVICES VENUE ASSESSMENT CHECKLIST (CONTINUED)

Fixed or Festival Seating: _____

Layout: _____

ADA Compliance: _____

Communications

Internal: _____

External: _____

Aid Station on Site   YES / NO

Number: _____

Staffed for event?   YES / NO

Mobile teams to be used   YES / NO

Foot: YES / NO   Number: _____

Bike: YES/ NO   Number: _____

Carts: YES / NO   Number: _____

Other: YES / NO   Number: _____

Figure 2.2B Emergency Medical Services Venue Assessment Checklist [35]

patient care documentation, failure to document all patient encounters (e.g., dispensing Band-Aids), failure to document medical decision-making capacity for patient refusals of care, and failure to obtain parental/guardian approval for the care of minors [22]. Given these significant medicolegal concerns, the presence of on-site medical oversight is advised [1–3].

In order to limit the need for on-site physician assessments, the Event Medical Directors may develop treat-and-release protocols for use at mass gathering events, when allowed by local laws and regulations [23]. Prehospital providers (i.e., emergency medical responders and emergency medical technicians) do not commonly make patient disposition decisions. Treat-and-release directives, however, may allow for scope expansion – reducing the need for physician assessment and the demand for advanced medical care. One prospective observational study of a twelve-hour outdoor concert in Toronto, Canada, utilized such a technique. During the event, 357 patients were provided acetaminophen, an anti-histamine, or an antibiotic salve as

indicated, and dispositioned to home [3, 23]. While the authors note the beneficial reduction in the demand for healthcare resources among patients with minor injuries and illnesses, this topic requires further evaluation for safety and efficacy [23].

The Event Medical Plan

The event medical plan must clearly delineate the levels of care to be provided, namely, basic life support (BLS), and advanced life support (ALS) capabilities. EMS providers at mass gatherings may serve as mobile medical first responders with or without transport capabilities to on-site medical facilities; primary or secondary medical responders performing transport outside of the venue; or as providers in on-site facilities [2, 3, 23]. The medical plan should address how assets and personnel will be deployed to provide emergency medical care, and include maps of the venue illustrating the locations of personnel and resources. While there are no widely accepted standards, when considering geographic placement, it is recommended that basic first aid be provided within four minutes of injury, ALS within five minutes, and transport to a medical care facility within thirty minutes [1, 13, 25]. The level of care provided at a mass gathering event should reflect, at a minimum, that which is available in the local community [1].

Mass Gathering Medical Care

Basic medical care at mass gatherings is provided by volunteers, emergency medical responders (EMRs) and emergency medical technicians (EMTs). Basic medical interventions range from simple wound care to hemorrhage control. EMTs are capable of assisting patients in administering their own medications and delivering physician-approved over-the-counter medications (oral glucose for hypoglycemia aspirin for chest pain, etc.) in accordance with event and local protocols. Refer to Table 2.3 for a description of a recommended framework delineating the roles of medical providers at mass gathering events. Initially developed by the American College of Emergency Physicians in 1995, this model has been adapted to include the National EMS Scope of Practice Model framework [28, 29].

Most mass gatherings will most likely not have the facilities or capabilities to provide critical care treatment. If the plan includes those resources, then the providers staffing must have the appropriate training and certification. It is also recommended that they have at least two years of full-time clinical experience in the management and care of critical care patients, preferably in a busy intensive care unit or critical care transport program. In the United States, education in critical care for paramedics is available from a variety of institutions, for example, the CCEMTP (Critical Care Emergency Medical Transport Program) course created by the University of Maryland Baltimore County in Maryland, USA [32]. Certification as a critical care paramedic and flight paramedic is attainable through the IBSC (International Board of Specialty Certifications) [33]. There are specific organizations in other countries that provide this training and certification. Nurses can obtain certification as Critical Care Registered Nurses (CCRN) through the American Association of Critical Care Nurses. The minimum requirements are [34]:

Practice as an RN or Advanced Practice Registered Nurse (APRN) for 1,750 hours in direct care of acutely/critically ill patients during the previous 2 years, with 875 of those hours accrued in the most

recent year preceding application. Alternatively, practice as an RN or APRN for at least 5 years with a minimum of 2,000 hours in direct care of acutely/critically ill patients, with 144 of those hours accrued in the most recent year preceding application.

Resource Management

Historic recommendations regarding event staffing models vary. In the late 1990s, football authorities published medical provider-to-attendee ratios, advising: one to two physicians per 50,000 attendees, one to two paramedics and one emergency medical technician per 10,000 attendees, and one basic first aid provider per 1,000 event participants [24]. In subsequent years, after reviewing fifty-five publications regarding the provision of care at mass gathering events, Hartman et al. developed a system (the University of Virginia model) to forecast the need for medically trained personnel at mass gathering events [24]. The Medical Resource Prediction Model (Table 2.1) proposed by Hartman et al. from the University of Virginia has yet to be prospectively validated, it once again highlights important concepts previously elucidated by Arbon [7] and Zeitz [4].

Today, experts recommend approximating PPR and TTHR from previous similar mass gathering events, and then multiplying these ratios by the expected maximal attendance figures for the planned event to determine the number of patient presentations and transports to be expected. Utilizing these numbers, staffing models can be matched with the demand for healthcare resources [1]. As human resources must be sources from the community in which the event is held, event planners must balance the risks to attendees and propensity for mass casualty scenarios with the strain placed upon the local EMS system. The medical plan should clearly delineate roles and responsibilities for personnel with advanced medical training [1].

On-Site Medical Personnel

Healthcare providers at mass gatherings must possess the ability to perform a targeted patient assessment, treat injuries and illnesses according to individual scopes of practice, and package patients for transport and evacuation [13]. The National Association of EMS Physicians (NAEMSP) recommends that Event Medical Directors publish protocols, and train all BLS and ALS providers to deliver care to address a range of emergency conditions [1], as noted in Table 2.2.

Table 2.1 Medical Resource Prediction Model [24]

	Resource Prediction Model				
Weather	Attendance	Ethanol	Crowd Age	Crowd Intention	Point Value
>90°F	>15,000	Significant	Older	Animated	2
<90°F	1,000–15,000	Limited	Mixed	Intermediate	1
Climate Controlled	<1,000	None	Younger	Calm	0
Event	**Definition**				
Major	Total score > 5, or scores of 2 in 2 categories				
Intermediate	Total score > 3 but < 5, or a score of 2 in any category				
Minor	Total score < 3				
Event	**Staffing Recommendation**				
Major	Multiple transport units with advanced care providers (physicians and nurses)				
Intermediate	2 Transport units staffed by 1–3 ALS and 1–6 BLS providers				
Minor	1 Transport unit staffed by an ALS provider and 1 BLS provider				

(ALS – Advanced Life Support; BLS – Basic Life Support)

Table 2.2 Emergency Conditions for Stabilization [1]

Patient Chief Complaint	
Abdominal pain	Hazardous materials
Airway obstruction	Headache
Anaphylaxis	Hemorrhage
Animal bites	Drowning and near-drowning
Back pain	Water-related trauma
Blast injury	Ophthalmologic illness/injury
Burns	Overdose/toxidromes
Cardiac arrest	Pregnancy problems/labor & delivery
Chest pain/cardiac symptoms	Psychiatric Emergencies
Cerebrovascular Accident	Respiratory distress
Diabetic Emergencies	Seizures
Electrocution	Syncope
Environmental emergencies	Traumatic Injuries

While there are likely to be limitations based upon the availability of local healthcare personnel, physicians, physician extenders, nurses, and EMS personnel are recommended to provide care at events in which there are a large number of attendees and there is a high propensity for life and limb-threatening injuries and illnesses (e.g., trauma, acute myocardial infarction, asthma exacerbations)

[1–3, 18, 20]. Physicians, physician extenders, and nurses most commonly deliver care from on-site treatment facilities. In accordance with the anticipated demand for healthcare services (PPR and TTHR), organizers must identify sufficient numbers of personnel to support treatment facilities to direct patient flow, perform medical record keeping, fulfill logistics functions (resupply), and communicate patient needs (e.g., transport) [1, 13].

Healthcare providers must be credentialed in the provision of care, in accordance with event medical protocols. Prior to the mass gathering, the Event Medical Director must brief providers regarding medical oversight and command structures, the communications infrastructure, medical post locations and staffing, advanced medical care availability (e.g., location of on-site physicians or the nearest hospital for transport), EMS response times (with ingress and egress routes), mechanisms for public health surveillance, patient care documentation procedures, and logistics [1, 8]. All personnel should become familiar with event emergency response procedures, to include standard operating procedures to address mass casualty incidents and disasters. Physicians and EMS personnel must also understand their role in the Incident Command System [1, 8].

Emergency Medical Services

Emergency Medical Services providers are state and/or nationally certified at one of three levels: Emergency

Medical Responder, Emergency Medical Technician, and Paramedic. Progression through each of these levels comes with additional skills to include advanced life support at the paramedic level. When utilized at a mass gathering event, the providers need to be familiar with the event medical plan as well as governing protocols. Each level of certification has an approved scope of practice that they must adhere to and which is governed by and decided on by the National Association of State EMS Officials and the National Highway Traffic Safety Administration (NHTSA). EMS providers mostly work in the out-of-hospital environment, but may also be members of the care team within healthcare institutions. When employed at a particular event, they must be certified in the state in which the event is occurring [1]. Individuals should function within their scope of practice, delineated by state and local regulations, the Event Medical Director, and the jurisdictional EMS Medical Director [2, 3, 28].

Emergency Medical Responder

EMRs are an important link within the 911 and emergency medical services systems and function as part of a comprehensive EMS response, community, health, or public safety system with clinical protocols and medical oversight [29]. The EMR primary focus is to initiate immediate lifesaving care to patients while ensuring patient access to the EMS system. They possess the basic life support knowledge and skills necessary to provide lifesaving interventions while awaiting additional EMS response. They are often first responders and, as a result, await arrival of an EMS or public safety agency for higher-level medical care. They must quickly assess patient needs, initiate treatment, and request additional resources. EMRs often provide medical care in less populated areas and often have a low call volume. They may assist during the ambulance transport, but ideally should not be the highest-level person caring for a patient during transport.

Emergency Medical Technician

An EMT is a prehospital health professional whose primary focus is to respond to, assess, and triage emergent, urgent, and nonurgent requests for medical care, and apply basic knowledge and skills necessary to provide patient care and medical transportation to/from an emergency or health care facility [29].

EMTs are sometimes the highest level of care a patient will receive during an emergency and ambulance transport. With proper supervision, EMTs may serve as a patient care team member in a hospital or health care setting to the full extent of their credentialing. Since EMTs are often the first providers to arrive on scene; they are expected to quickly assess patient conditions, provide stabilizing measures, and request additional resources, as needed. As other prehospital providers, EMTs function as part of a comprehensive public safety system with defined clinical protocols and medical oversight.

Table 2.3 lists the various skills that can be performed by EMRs and EMTs.

Advanced Emergency Medical Technician (AEMT)

The AEMT has additional skills and education beyond EMT with the goal of improving patient care in common emergency conditions for which there are safe, targeted, and evidence-based interventions [29]. These more advanced and often invasive interventions within the AEMT scope of practice may carry more risk than interventions authorized for the EMR/EMT levels.

Paramedic

The paramedic has the highest level of certification and is trained to apply basic and advanced knowledge and skills necessary to treat the patient with a degree of autonomous decision-making [29]. This includes performing certain invasive procedures, advanced airway management, and administering a wide range of pharmacology. In addition, they are trained in advanced cardiac life support (ACLS) and interpretation of electrocardiograms. Advanced level medical interventions include endotracheal intubation, needle thoracostomy/decompression, cricothyroidotomy, and pericardiocentesis as per provider level of education and training, and event/local prehospital protocols. They are expected to utilize critical thinking skills to make complex judgments such as the need for transport from a field site, alternate destination decisions, the level of personnel appropriate for transporting a patient, and similar judgments. Paramedics facilitate medical decisions at an emergency scene and during transport and operate with collaborative medical oversight.

Table 2.3 Requirements for basic care at mass gathering events [28, 29]

Level of Care	Medical Care at Mass Gatherings			
	Requirements			
	Personnel	Equipment	Examples of Services Provided	Patient Disposition
Basic	Volunteer	First Aid Kit	Wound Care Hydration	EMS transport as needed
	EMR	BLS; With or without transport	CPR with AED Oral airway BVM Supplemental oxygen Extremity immobilization Hemorrhage control Eye irrigation C-spine stabilization	EMS transport as needed
	EMT-B	BLS; Transport	**EMR Plus:** Nasal airway Ventilation Spinal immobilization Patient extrication Extremity splinting Patient restraint Traction Splinting Mechanical CPR Assisted childbirth Administration of patient medications Tourniquet application Administration of OTC medications	Observation; release per treat-and-release protocols; transport as needed

(AED – Automated External Defibrillator; BVM – Bag-Valve-Mask Ventilation; CPR – Cardiopulmonary Resuscitation; OTC – Over-the-counter)

Calabro J, Kromer J, Rivera-Rivera E, Reich J, Balacombe J. Provision of emergency medical care for crowds. www.acep.org/globalassets/uploads/uploaded-files/acep/clinical-and-practice-management/ems-and-disaster-preparedness/ems-resources/emscrowd.pdf. Accessed November 6, 2021.

National Association of State EMS Officials. National EMS Scope of Practice Model 2019 (Report No. DOT HS 812–666). Washington, DC: National Highway Traffic Safety Administration.

Table 2.4 Requirements for advanced care at mass gathering events [28, 29]

Level of Care	Medical Care at Mass Gatherings			
	Requirements			
	Personnel	Equipment	Examples of Services Provided	Patient Disposition
Advanced	NRP, RN	ALS; Transport	EMT-B Plus: IV/IO access BiPAP/CPAP ACLS ATLS Needle chest decompression EKG interpretation Cardioversion Transthoracic Pacing	Observation; release per treat-and-release Protocols; transport as needed

(BiPAP – Bi-level Positive Airway Pressure; CPAP – Continuous Positive Airway Pressure; EKG – electrocardiogram; IO – intraosseous; IV – intravenous)

Advanced care (Table 2.4) at mass gatherings is provided by AEMTs, paramedics, and nurses.

Critical Care Nurses, Flight Nurses/ Prehospital Registered Nurses (PHRNs), and Registered Nurses

Critical Care Nurses, Flight Nurses (FNs)/PHRNs, and registered nurses should assist in evaluating and treating acutely ill and injured patients at mass gathering events. Similar to physician assistants (PAs) and nursing practitioners (NPs), nurses should be licensed in the state which the event is occurring, maintain current certification in ACLS and Pediatric Advanced Life Support (PALS), and be directly supervised by a licensed and qualified physician [1]. For individuals who possess prehospital credentials (FNs, PHRNs), the medical plan should address procedures for independent patient evaluation and treatment. The medical plan should also delineate specific roles for nursing personnel, which may include on-site medication dispensing and inventory [1].

Physician Assistants and Nurse Practitioners

In addition to, or as an alternative of physician employment, PAs and NPs may be utilized as members of the event healthcare team. In a prospective study of four mass-gathering events in the United Kingdom, attended by nearly 850,000 persons, the use of on-site nurse practitioners resulted in a statistically significant reduction in TTHR [26]. NPs were able to examine, diagnose, and prescribe medications for noncritical, ambulatory patients without the need for further healthcare referral [27]. PAs and NPs providing patient care must be licensed in the state in which the event is being held, certified in ACLS and PALS. Physician extenders and nurses must be directly supervised by a licensed and qualified physician, unless possessing appropriate prehospital credentials. In states such as Pennsylvania, Physician Assistants and Nurses can obtain certification as a prehospital physician extender (PHPE) or prehospital registered nurse (PHRN), respectively, and can function as independent EMS providers working under state regulated protocols. The medical plan should detail supervisory relationships and communication procedures. If providing medical coverage at events during which traumatic injuries are likely to occur, Prehospital Trauma Life Support (PHTLS) or International Trauma Life Support (ITLS) certification is advised [1].

Physicians

As previously stated, the presence of appropriately trained physicians at mass gathering events may significantly decrease the demand for local prehospital services. Physicians may perform advanced procedures such as splinting and suturing, allowing for on-site patient disposition. If trained and appropriately equipped, these providers may also deliver critical care interventions (e.g., cardioversion, rapid sequence intubation, central line insertion) to stabilize patients for transport. For mass gatherings events during which there is the high likelihood of traumatic injuries (auto racing, boxing, etc.), physicians experienced in emergency medicine, trauma resuscitation, and prehospital care are recommended [18].

Critical care (Table 2.5) is provided by physicians and medical providers trained at the critical care level, whether nurses or paramedics.

Legal Considerations

As previously discussed, medical providers should be credentialed by the Event Medical Director and/or applicable jurisdictional medical director, prior to providing patient care. If applicable, providers should be made aware of regulations regarding the storage and dispensing of controlled substances. Important considerations which should be addressed in the medical plan include liability and insurance coverage for medical providers. Expert legal advice should be solicited to ensure compliance with state and local regulations [19].

Equipment and Supplies

Basic, advanced, and critical care medicine may be performed at mass gatherings. The extent to which on-site medical care may be delivered is dependent upon provider resourcing. The medical plan must include a comprehensive list of on-site medical equipment, as well as an approved formulary. This information should be made available to all event healthcare providers and posted in on-site treatment facilities to facilitate inventory and resupply. Personnel responsible for event medical logistics

Table 2.5 Requirements for critical care at mass gathering events [28, 29]

Level of Care	Medical Care at Mass Gatherings			
	Requirements			
	Personnel	Equipment	Examples of Services Provided	Patient Disposition
Critical Care	CCP, CCN, FN	ALS; Transport	Advanced Care Plus: Ventilator Management Endotracheal Intubation Cricothyroidotomy	Observation; release per treat-and-release protocols; transport as needed
	Physician, PA, NP	Obstetric Packs Chest Tubes Thrombolytics Suggested: Ultrasound	Thoracostomy Emergent pericardiocentesis Thrombolytic administration Blood product administration Complicated child delivery	

(CCP–Critical Care Paramedic, CCN – Critical Care Nurse, FN–Flight Nurse, PA–Physician Assistant, NP–Nurse Practitioner)

should partner with event healthcare providers to modify daily resupply requests, such that the demand for healthcare resources is met. If on-site mobile response teams are not available, it is recommended that each treatment facility prepare a portable "go bag" to be carried in the event that staff members must depart to provide care [19, 31].

Patient Care Documentation

Documentation practices should be delineated by the Event Medical Director and published in the medical plan prior to the mass gathering event [2, 3]. It is recommended that demographics, chief complaint, assessment, treatment, and disposition information be documented for all patients seeking care [28]. Healthcare personnel and the Event Medical Director must ensure the security of patient health records from generation to storage [3]. Patients dispositioned on-site should receive a copy of their documented clinical encounter [8]. Transport units should utilize documentation procedures outlined by the EMS Medical Director responsible for the event jurisdiction.

Continuous Quality Improvement

Following a mass gathering event, the Event Medical Director and jurisdictional EMS Medical Directors should conduct a post-event debrief to discuss implementation of the medical care coverage – highlighting successes and identifying areas for improvement [30].

Each event medical provider should be given the opportunity to address concerns and offer recommendations regarding lessons learned to be published in the After-Actions Report (AAR). In addition to soliciting feedback from event healthcare staff, the Event Medical Director should obtain venue and jurisdictional EMS patient care reports, as well as local emergency department records to craft the event AAR.

The AAR should detail the event PPR, TTHR, and common patient illness and injury patterns [2, 3, 28]. A review of patient care documentation and patient safety concerns/patient complaints (reported to local emergency departments or EMS offices) should also be included. Utilizing this data, the Event Medical Director can inform local stakeholders regarding event resourcing and develop an improvement plan, proposing specific corrective actions for implementation during future events. In this manner the Event Medical Director plays a pivotal role in the continuous quality improvement process.

Summary

Consensus regarding medical staffing models for mass gathering events is lacking. As mass gatherings vary in terms of size, crowd demographics and behavior, type, and venue, a thorough risk assessment, created in partnership with local stakeholders, is essential to the development of a medical plan detailing medical resourcing requirements. Historical event data regarding PPR and TTHR should be utilized to inform staffing decisions.

Medical providers may deliver basic, advanced, and critical care at mass gathering events. The Event Medical Director must determine an appropriate level of care to be provided at the mass gathering event based upon the aforementioned risk assessment, and the availability of local healthcare providers and healthcare resources (medications, disposable medical supplies, and equipment). Physician staffing is recommended for events when there are limited transportation resources and prolonged transport times to higher levels of care.

Prior to the mass gathering, the Event Medical Director plays a vital role in guaranteeing the health and safety of event participants; ensuring that all providers are credentialed to provide care in accordance with local/event protocols. During the event, an on-site medical director is recommended to provide direct medical control. Following the mass gathering, the Event Medical Director ensures continuous quality improvement through the development of the AAR and improvement plan.

References

1. Yancey A., Milsten A., Luk J., Nafziger S. National Association of EMS Physicians. NAEMSP. https://naemsp.org/resources/store/. Published 2017. Accessed January 4, 2022.

2. Schwartz B., Nafziger S., Milsten A., Luk J., Yancey II, Arthur. Mass Gathering Medical Care: Resource Document for the National Association of EMS Physicians Position Statement. *Prehospital Emergency Care.* 2015;**19**(4):559–568. doi: 10.3109/10903127.2015.1051680

3. Margolis A. M., Leung A. K., Friedman M. S., McMullen S. P., Guyette F. X., Woltman N. Position Statement: Mass Gathering Medical Care. *Prehospital Emergency Care.* 2021:1–5. doi:10.1080/10903127.2021.1903632

4. Zeitz K. M., Zeitz C. J., Arbon P. Forecasting Medical Work at Mass-Gathering Events: Predictive Model Versus Retrospective Review. *Prehospital and Disaster Medicine.* 2005;**20**(3):164–168. doi:10.1017/s1049023x00002399

5. Arbon P. Mass-Gathering Medicine: A Review of the Evidence and Future Directions for Research. *Prehospital and Disaster Medicine.* 2007;**22**(2):131–135. doi:10.1017/s1049023x00004507

6. Koski A., Kouvonen A., Sumanen H. Preparedness for Mass Gatherings: Factors to Consider According to the Rescue Authorities. *International Journal of Environmental Research and Public Health.* 2020;**17**(4):1361. doi:10.3390/ijerph17041361

7. Arbon P., Bridgewater F. H. G., Smith C. Mass Gathering Medicine: A Predictive Model for Patient Presentation and Transport Rates. *Prehospital and Disaster Medicine.* 2001;**16**(3):150–158. doi:10.1017/s1049023x00025905

8. Public health for mass gatherings: Key considerations. World Health Organization. www.who.int/publications-detail-redirect/public-health-for-mass-gatherings-key-considerations. Accessed November 5, 2021.

9. Scholliers A., Gogaert S., Vande Veegaete A., Gillebeert J., Vandekerckhove P. The Most Prevalent Injuries at Different Types of Mass Gathering Events: An Analysis of More Than 150,000 Patient Encounters. *Prehospital and Disaster Medicine.* 2017;**32**(S1). doi:10.1017/s1049023x17003788

10. Goldberg S. A., Maggin J., Molloy M. S. et al. The Gillette Stadium Experience: A Retrospective Review of Mass Gathering Events from 2010 to 2015. *Disaster Medicine and Public Health Preparedness.* 2018;**12**(6):752–758. doi:10.1017/dmp.2018.7

11. Milsten A. M., Maguire B. J., Bissell R. A., Seaman K. G. Mass-Gathering Medical Care: A Review of the Literature. *Prehospital and Disaster Medicine.* 2002;**17**(3):151–162. doi:10.1017/s1049023x00000388

12. Mass Gatherings: Are You Prepared? Northwest Center for Public Health Preparedness. www.nwcphp.org/docs/mass_gatherings/mass_gathering_print_version.pdf. Accessed November 6, 2021.

13. Auerbach, P. S., Cushing, T. A., Harris, N. S., Townes, D., Waite, B. Wilderness and Endurance Events. In *Auerbach's Wilderness Medicine.* New York: Elsevier; 2017, pp. 2209–2218.

14. Federal Emergency Management Agency. (n.d.). Incident Command System Form 206: Medical Plan. Retrieved December 30, 2021, from https://emilms.fema.gov/IS201/assets/ICS%20Forms%20206.pdf

15. McQueen C., Davies C. Health Care in a Unique Setting: Applying Emergency Medicine at Music Festivals. *Open Access Emergency Medicine.* 2012:**69**. doi:10.2147/oaem.s25587

16. Smith S. P., Cosgrove J. F., Driscoll P. J. et al. A Practical Approach to Events Medicine Provision. *Emergency Medicine Journal.* 2016;**34**(8):538–542. doi:10.1136/emermed-2016-205805

17. Sanders A. B., Criss E., Steckl P., Meislin H. W., Raife J., Allen D. An Analysis of Medical Care at Mass Gatherings. *Annals of Emergency Medicine.* 1985;**14**(8):827. doi:10.1016/s0196-0644(85)80078-0

18. Grange J. T., Baumann G. W., Vaezazizi R. On-Site Physicians Reduce Ambulance Transports at Mass Gatherings. *Prehospital Emergency Care*. 2003;**7**(3):322–326. doi:10.1080/10903120390936518

19. Hiltunen T., Kuisma M., Määttä T. et al. Prehospital Emergency Care and Medical Preparedness for the 2005 World Championship Games in Athletics in Helsinki. *Prehospital and Disaster Medicine*. 2007;**22**(4):304–311. doi:10.1017/s1049023x0000491x

20. Parrillo S. J. Medical Care at Mass Gatherings: Considerations for Physician Involvement. *Prehospital and Disaster Medicine*. 1995;**10**(4):273–275. doi:10.1017/s1049023x00042163

21. Boyle M. F., De Lorenzo R. A., Garrison R. Physician Integration into Mass Gathering Medical Care: The United States Air Show. *Prehospital and Disaster Medicine*. 1993;**8**(2):165–168. doi:10.1017/s1049023x00040255

22. McDonald C. C., Koenigsberg M. D., Ward S. Medical Control of Mass Gatherings: Can Paramedics Perform Without Physicians On-Site? *Prehospital and Disaster Medicine*. 1993;**8**(4):327–331. doi:10.1017/s1049023x00040590

23. Feldman M. J., Lukins J. L., Verbeek P. R., Burgess R. J., Schwartz B. Use of Treat-and-Release Medical Directives for Paramedics at a Mass Gathering. *Prehospital Emergency Care*. 2005;**9**(2):213–217. doi:10.1080/10903120590924843

24. Hartman N., Williamson A., Sojka B. et al. Predicting Resource Use at Mass Gatherings Using a Simplified Stratification Scoring Model. *The American Journal of Emergency Medicine*. 2009;**27**(3):337–343. doi:10.1016/j.ajem.2008.03.042

25. Spaite, D. W., Criss, E. A., Valenzuela, T. D., Meislin, H. W., Smith, R., Nelson, A. A New Model for Providing Prehospital Medical Care in Large Stadiums. *Annals of Emergency Medicine*. 1998;**17**(8):825–828. doi:10.1016/s0196-0644(88)80563-8

26. Kemp, A. E. (2016). Mass-Gathering Events: The Role of Advanced Nurse Practitioners in Reducing Referrals to Local Health Care Agencies. *Prehospital and Disaster Medicine*. 2016;**31**(1):58–63. doi:10.1017/s1049023x15005543

27. Thompson J. M., Savoia G., Powell G., Challis E. B., Law P. Level of Medical Care Required for Mass Gatherings: The XV Winter Olympic Games in Calgary, Canada. *Annals of Emergency Medicine*. 1991;**20**(4):385–390. doi:10.1016/s0196-0644(05)81660-9

28. Calabro J., Kromer J., Rivera-Rivera E., Reich J., Balacombe J. Provision of Emergency Medical Care for Crowds. www.acep.org/globalassets/uploads/uploaded-files/acep/clinical-and-practice-management/ems-and-disaster-preparedness/ems-resources/emscrowd.pdf. Accessed November 6, 2021.

29. National Association of State EMS Officials. National EMS Scope of Practice Model 2019 (Report No. DOT HS 812–666). Washington, DC: National Highway Traffic Safety; 2019.

30. Cianca, J. Mass Participation Endurance Event Coverage. In *Clinical Care of the Runner*. New York: Elsevier Inc; 2020; 29–54.

31. Jaslow D., Yancy II A., Milsten M. Mass Gathering Medical Care. *Prehospital Emergency Care*. 2000;**4**(4):359–360, doi:10.1080/10903120090941119

32. http://ehspace.umbc.edu/ccemtp/. Accessed February 13, 2022.

33. www.ibscertifications.org/. Accessed February 13, 2022.

34. www.aacn.org/~/media/aacn-website/certification/getcertified/handbooks/ccrnexamhandbook.pdf. Accessed March 28, 2022.

35. Federal Emergency Management Agency (FEMA). Special Events Contingency Planning Job Aids Manual. March 2005 (Updated May 2010) 2501905270500

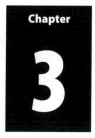

Chapter 3

Prediction of Medical Need and Event Risk Assessment at Mass Gathering Events

Thomas Hartka and Matthew A. Hewitt

Introduction

A key aspect of preparing to offer appropriate medical care during a mass gathering is anticipating the number and severity of patient contacts, as well as the number of patients who require transport to an outside hospital. Even though they are typically an assembly of well persons, mass gathering events have shown to produce a higher incidence of injury and illness than is apparent from the general population [1]. Planning for appropriate medical support is therefore not only critical to providing care to attendees of the event but also to minimize the strain on the surrounding region. The World Health Organization (WHO) defines a mass gathering as "an occasion, either organized or spontaneous, where the number of people attending is sufficient to strain the planning and response resources of the community, city, or nation hosting the manifestation" [2]. This definition illustrates the potential negative impact if insufficient medical resources are available at a mass gathering. While medical planning will optimally consider the impact on the local community and integrate with the existing resources [3], the focus of this chapter is the medical needs of attendees of a mass gathering event.

The problem of predicting medical needs at mass gatherings has been the subject of significant interest for the last several decades. Many groups who have experience providing medical support at these events have published data on the number and type of patient contacts [4–7]. The inherent variability between events and circumstances that are unknowable prior to the event makes estimations difficult [8, 9]. However, several prediction models have been developed to provide estimates for the number of medical resources that an event is likely to require [10–13]. The choice of model will depend on whether data is available from previous events, crowd characteristics, and environmental factors. It is important to also appreciate that there are additional features of a mass gathering that are known to lead to substantial underestimations of patient volumes.

This chapter first discusses the typical number of patient presentations, the required level of care, and hospital transports reported for mass gatherings. The next section provides an overview of the most important factors that influence patient volumes. This overview is followed by a review of several published models for predicting the medical resource needs. The next section covers the elements of an event that may lead to significant underestimation. Finally, the risk of critical illness occurring at mass gathering events is considered.

Definition of Terms

The medical needs for an event have been described using several different terms, which may vary slightly between authors. We will describe the most common terms and the definitions that we will use in this chapter. The patient presentation rate (PPR) is the portion of all attendees that seek any degree of care over the course of the entire event [10]. In contrast, the medical usage rate (MUR) often refers to the hourly patient presentations rate [9, 14], although some studies use MUR to describe the proportion of the entire event (the same as PPR) [14]. The Transport-to-Hospital Rate (TTHR) is the number of patients that require ambulance transportation to an outside medical facility. Since all of these terms refer to rates, the denominator must be specified. Most authors use incidence per 1,000 or 10,000, however, other values are occasionally used. In this chapter, we will primarily use the PPR and TTHR since these are the rates that are most commonly reported in the medical literature. Additionally, we will use rates per 1,000 attendees. This denominator was chosen because attendance is often reported in thousands and these rates facilitate easy calculation. For this chapter, we will assume that total patient presentations can be calculated by:

Total number = Rate per thousand * (Number of attendee/1,000) (Eqt 1)

The use of rates implies there is a linear relationship between the number of medical events and attendance. This relationship appears plausible since every additional person attending an event has the potential to require medical care, although it assumes that the probability that any one attendee requires care is independent of all the others at the same event. Given that medical emergencies are usually relatively rare, this assumption is reasonable. Indeed, several large studies confirm this linear relationship [6, 15]. Some authors advocate using total patient presentations (TPP) rather than PPR to avoid this issue [16, 17].

Typical Patient Presentation and Transport Rates

While every mass gathering is unique and has elements that are unpredictable, decades of experience with mass gatherings can provide typical ranges for patient volumes. There are many reports in the medical literature from events varying from the viewing of the Holy Shroud that had millions of attendees to wilderness races involving around a thousand people [18, 19]. There have been several systematic reviews that have examined the available evidence to identify the typical range for the number of patients, type of presentation, level of care, and age demographics. While the prediction models described later in this chapter can produce more specific estimates, these typical values can be used to provide quick approximations. The factors described in the next section will influence whether an event is likely to be closer to the upper or lower end of these ranges.

The United Kingdom (UK) has produced a guide for event organizers in order to improve health and safety at mass gathering events [13]. In addition to giving a more detailed algorithm to predict medical resource needs, the guide recommends the use of the heuristic that 1–2 percent of an audience will seek medical care. Of these patients, 10 percent will need further treatment on-site and 1 percent will require transport to the hospital. It is important to appreciate that the number of patient presentations often vary between different types of events [20, 21] and even similar events held at different times [5, 15, 22, 23].

However, these values represent reasonable estimates, especially when averaged over multiple events.

A useful general guide to predict patient-related medical need is as follows: rule-of-thumb: 1–2 percent of attendees will seek care. Of these patients, 10 percent will require full evaluation with ongoing care and 1 percent transport to the hospital.

Rate of Patient Presentations (PPR): There is a wide range in the number of patient presentations in the medical literature. PPRs have been reported to range from 0.01 to 198.9/1,000 attendees [20, 21]. When excluding multiday events and events where the medical staff also treated participants, a more reasonable range appears to be 0.5 to 2/1,000 [24]. In fact, a large study from Australia that included over 1.2 million people from 201 events reported an overall PPR of 1.0/1,000 [4] and a survey of 79 university events had an average PPR 0.8/1,000 [5]. These rates are typically more variable at small events, where one patient seeking care more directly impacts the overall rate [25]. It is worth noting that not all patients seeking care are spectators. Multiple studies have shown that event staff commonly present for care and may make up to 16 percent of all patients [5, 22].

Rate of Hospital Transports (TTHR)

Similar to the number of patient presentations, there is significant variation in the number of hospital transports between different studies. TTHRs have been reported to range from 0.003 to 10.2/1,000 attendees [20, 21]. The upper extreme of 10.2 was for a multiday camping event that had no on-site medical care [26]. Having on-site medical providers has been demonstrated to decrease the rate of ambulance transports [16, 20]. Excluding extreme events and those without medical services on-site, the range of TTHR was 0.003 – 0.27/1,000. The survey of Australian events found an overall TTHR of 0.027/1,000 [4]. Transports are typically necessary for between 1 percent and 9 percent of all patient contacts [5, 15, 16]. This rate of transport has been shown to be higher for intoxicated patients with or without additional medical or traumatic complaints [9].

Level of Care

The majority of patients present with only minor complaints, many of which may not require a full evaluation. The medical literature evaluating the level of care is complicated by the fact that level of care is presented in many ways which include Basic/ Intermediate life support [22], Green/Yellow/Red [14], Basic/Advanced [27], and Minor/Moderate/ Severe [5, 22]. Despite this heterogeneity of terminology, the ratios between different levels of care are remarkably stable across different events. Between 75 percent and 85 percent of patients will require the lowest level of care. Mid-range complexity patients represent 10–20 percent of all presentations. Most authors describe this mid-range as patients requiring a full evaluation. The highest level of care is required for 1–5 percent of all patients. The rate of patients with a life-threatening illness is discussed later in this chapter in the section Risk of Critical Illness.

Type of Complaints

Patient complaints can generally be classified as medical or trauma, and the ratio between these types of presentations may influence the staff and equipment that is needed. Different events have shown markedly disparate ratios between these categories, with traumatic complaints accounting for 6–84 percent of the total patient volume [20]. However, most studies show significantly less than 50 percent of presentations due to trauma [8, 16, 20, 28]. A university-based event medicine team found trauma accounted for 10 percent of patient presentations overall, but was 30 percent at sporting events [5]. Given this significant variability, it is important to prepare for a wide variety of both medical and traumatic patient presentations.

The most common medical complaints also show considerable variation between events, which is likely due to multiple demographic, environmental, and public health factors. Several analyses have found that the most frequent medical problem was headaches, often accounting for approximately half of all medical complaints [29–33]. In contrast, other studies have found few cases of headache, but are instead dominated by syncope, altered mental status, or other heat-related illnesses [5, 34, 35]. Weather conditions may be a significant contributor to these differences, which are discussed later in this chapter. Across most studies, there is a small but consistent fraction of patients presenting with asthma and other respiratory illnesses [4, 22, 36]. Despite the small percentage of patients with respiratory complaints, a relatively high proportion of these patients may require transport to a hospital [14]. Given this variability, resources to evaluate and treat headache,

heat-related illnesses, and respiratory illnesses are highly recommended in addition to general emergency care supplies.

Patients presenting with intoxication or acute psychiatric illness are typically classified as having medical complaints, but these disorders may also increase the possibilities of traumatic injuries [37]. The type of event significantly influences the number of patients who present for complications of alcohol intoxication, which may include altered mental status, vomiting, or traumatic injuries. The effect of alcohol specifically is discussed later in this chapter. Primary psychiatric presentations are relatively rare in all studies [8, 20, 23, 30, 32]. However, there is a paucity of data regarding the nature and severity of these psychiatric complaints. This is an area requiring further research to determine the psychiatric resources necessary to care for these patients.

Traumatic injuries are common at mass gathering events; fortunately, most are minor and can be treated and released [8, 20, 23, 32]. Abrasions, lacerations, and minor wounds are the majority of traumatic presentations. The next most common category of injuries is orthopedic (strains, sprains, fractures, and dislocations). Other types of injuries include closed head trauma, dental, blisters, insect bites, burns (sunburns and thermal), ocular injuries, and treatment for injuries sustained prior to the event [8, 20, 23, 32].

The management of traumatic injuries is largely driven by the resources available at the event. Patients presenting with traumatic complaints are less likely to require transport to a hospital than medical problems [23]. Minor wounds and abrasions can be rapidly cleaned and dressed. The decision about whether to close lacerations depends on the expertise of the medical personnel, the patient volume, and whether patients can be seen at an outside medical facility in a timely manner. At short events in populated areas, most lacerations can be dressed and referred to outside medical facilities as long as bleeding can be controlled. Fractures and dislocations can be splinted, then the necessity of ambulance transport is largely driven by the ability of the patient's level of pain and ability to ambulate.

Pediatric Presentations

Pediatrics patients will often make up a significant portion of all patient presentations for events that are not adult-only [18, 22, 38, 39]. The percentage of patients under the age of eighteen years depends upon the type of event, but usually ranges from 10 percent to 25 percent. Pediatric cases tend to have different characteristics than adults. They are more commonly minor and less likely to be related to alcohol and recreational drug use [38]. Injuries tend to be low in young children but begin rising after twelve years and peak in early adulthood (eighteen to twenty-five years). It is important to note that children usually require adult supervision, so adult presentations are common at events designed for younger audiences. For example, 50 percent of all patients were adults at a fair targeted for children [39].

Factors That Influence Patient Presentations

There are a number of factors that are known to influence the rate at which attendees will present for medical care; these factor include the following: crowd size, weather extremes (particularly high temperatures), attendee demographics, venue features, event type, and the presence of alcohol and recreational drugs. Determining the precise effect of these factors is difficult because there is significant heterogeneity in the elements collected by different researchers [10, 40] and because there is likely interaction between factors [10]. For instance, high ambient temperature and alcohol together can increase the number of patients presenting with dehydration more than would be expected by the individual effects of these factors. There are several conceptual frameworks that have been proposed, which typically divide factors into environmental, biomedical, and psychosocial [7, 10]. We will discuss the factors from each of these categories that are measurable and have been shown to have the most impact based on the available research.

Crowd Size and Density

The number of attendees to a mass gathering event is the principal determinant of the total number of patients that will seek treatment [13]. As discussed earlier, the concept using rates such as PPR and TTHR assumes a linear relationship between the number of attendees and the number of patients seeking care. A few studies have shown a nonlinear relationship at low attendance events, but this appears to be due primarily to small sample sizes [25, 41]. Some larger studies have shown that the number of patient presentations begins to plateau at very large events [16, 17]. However, most research has focused on calculating PPR and TTHR, therefore these rates will be used in our discussion. In planning for medical care, it should be noted that at low attendance predictions may be substantially wrong in terms of the percent error (e.g., if two patients present when one was expected, the prediction error is 100 percent). Whereas at high attendance, rate-based prediction algorithms may overestimate total patients.

It is likely that the density of crowds, the number of attendees per unit of space, also affect the PPR and TTHR [42, 43]. Denser crowds increase the possibility that patient presentations will not be independent. For example, an environmental hazard such as a falling piece of equipment will likely injure more people in a densely packed crowd. Additionally, dense crowds restrict mobility and may inhibit attendees from proactively taking measures to protect themselves from ailments such as dehydration [42]. While there have been attempts to model crowd behavior based on density, most observational studies do not report these values. It is therefore difficult to know the precise effect of crowd density of patient presentations. It also appears that crowd density has a minimal effect until a threshold is exceeded [42, 43]. Abiding by local fire and safety codes helps to avoid complications of excessive crowd density.

Weather

Weather conditions also show a very significant effect on the number of patient presentations [4, 8, 12, 14, 17, 44–46]. However, the research in this area is complicated by the fact that published analyses have captured different data elements about the weather and have studied events in very different climates. Despite this heterogeneity, there are some consistent findings regarding the effect of weather conditions on PPR. The importance of weather is illustrated by the fact that all of the predictive models that we will discuss later in this chapter use some derivation of expected temperature or season of the year.

Temperature is the most studied weather-related predictor of patient presentations. Extreme temperatures, either hot or cold, appear to increase PPR [6, 10, 12, 14, 44, 45]. Several analyses have shown that every degree Fahrenheit increase in temperature increases the number of PPR by approximately 0.3 PPR or 3–4 percent [44–46], however, these studies were chiefly focused on warm-weather events and the relationship between temperature and PPR is likely not linear across all possible temperatures. Another common approach has been to a threshold to analyze this effect, with temperatures above 74°F, 80°F, or 90°F all showing significant increases in patient presentations [9, 14, 17]. Cold weather also may increase the number of patients, with one study showing that PPR increases by 0.8 for every one degree Fahrenheit decrease in temperature below 40°F [23]. The UK model predicts more patients in summer and winter compared to the other seasons [13].

It appears that humidity combined with temperature is a better predictor than temperature alone [12, 45]. Early studies on the effect of weather examined temperature and humidity or dew point (the temperature needed for 100 percent relative humidity), with mixed results [15, 41]. These studies are confounded by the fact that there is a strong interaction between temperature and humidity and that relative humidity decreases as temperature increases. More recent studies have focused on the heat index, which combines temperature and relative humidity to determine the temperature that the human body perceives. Using the heat index has been shown to improve the accuracy of predictions of PPR [12, 45].

The relationship between precipitation and patient presentations is also complex. Every inch of precipitation was seen to decrease the total number of patient presentations, but it did not change the PPR [46]. An analysis of different types of events found that PPR increased at concerts when there was precipitation, but not at sporting events [14]. A study examining only concerts also found that precipitation above 0.5 inches increased the PPR. Overall, it appears that precipitation decreases total patient presentations due to decreased attendance, but may increase the PRR for those who chose to attend.

Venue Features

There are features of a venue that have a significant impact on healthcare needs at a mass gathering. The venue incorporates the location and infrastructure where an event is held, which are commonly sport stadiums, racetracks, open fields, exhibition halls, and concert arenas. The size, location, layout, and structural components can differ widely among event spaces. The extremes of venues are outdoor fields where patrons may roam freely to confined indoor spaces with limited points of ingress and egress. The venue space and its particular characteristics have

been found to influence the number of patients seeking care.

Venue spaces are often classified as bounded or unbounded. In bounded events there are clearly defined boundaries such as walls or fences, while unbounded events are open and attendees are free to move to and from the venue [4]. Examples of bounded events are sporting events in a stadium and ticketed concerts; in contrast, unbounded events include parades or marathons, which commonly span a large area. The data comparing PPRs among bounded and unbounded events are mixed. It has been shown that bounded venues lead to over a fourfold increase in PPR than those unbounded [4] and there are several theories for this finding. Bounded venues place patients in closer proximity to established medical services that may be more visible than those in unbounded venues. Also, potential patients are also thought to seek care at outside medical facilities in unbounded venues. Conversely, other studies have shown the higher PPR among unbounded events [28].

While the presence or absence of event boundaries can influence the degree of mobility of the crowd, perhaps a more fundamental determinate of crowd movement is whether the audience is seated or standing. It has been seen that a seated audience is generally associated with a lower PPR than mobile, unseated audiences. It is possible that mobile audiences are more prone to injury, or they are more likely to seek out or encounter medical services during their movement around the event space [4]. Related to seating and boundaries, outdoor events have statistically more medical presentations than indoor events [7]. Attendees at outdoor events may be more prone to illness stemming from injury, exertion, or exposure.

There are features of a venue that have been shown to reduce PPR, particularly the availability of free water. Dehydration is common at many mass gathering events due to exposure, exertion, and crowd density. Free water has been shown to decrease PPR [47]. The absence of free water was associated with a 71 percent increase in PPR in one study after adjusting for other cofactors [28]. When possible, it is recommended that water be provided free of cost or at least be inexpensive and easily accessible.

Crowd Demographics

Demographics of the attendees of a mass gathering may influence the medical resources needed during the event. While in general younger attendees have fewer baseline medical issues and comorbidities, they may be more prone to strenuous activity and injury, or may be more likely to experiment with alcohol and substance use [37, 48]. Several studies have tried to better characterize crowd demographics for use in predicting medical resource utilization.

The age of the expected attendees may affect patient volumes and severity of illness. In a retrospective analysis of past events at a single, large sports stadiums, the PPR increased with increasing decade of age until age sixty-five [23]. After age sixty-five, the PPR dropped. However, those over the age of sixty-five years had the highest rate of transport to the hospital. A review of multiple studies instead showed that PPR was highest among those less than thirty years of age, although these results may be driven by the overall demographics of the attendees [49].

The effect of gender is likewise difficult to determine. Some analyses have found that the gender distribution for those seeking care is equal [14], while others have found differences between genders [16, 23]. In a study that analyzed a patient set that was predominantly female, women were found to present more for physical and mental illness, while men were more likely to seek care for injury [32]. Conversely, another study found men preferentially presented for medical complaints, whereas most traumatic issues were found in women [23]. Given these results it is unclear if gender has a significant effect on medical utilization. However, certain events may be designed to target one gender, which appears to have an effect. Predominantly male events have higher PPRs than those with a more equal distribution [16]. A predominance of one gender over another may help determine what types of patient presentation to anticipate. Though small in proportion, obstetrical complaints made up about 1 percent of presentations at an analysis of multiple rock concerts [50].

Finally, one must consider special events that may attract a specific demographic of patrons who may be medically at-risk at baseline [49]. For example, cancer walks may attract a large number of older cancer patients or cancer survivors who may be more prone to exhaustion, dehydration, syncope, or other medical issues compared to other events. Concerts to benefit specific medical research programs may draw ill or immunocompromised attendees. The Concert for Life in Australia was known to have a large number of cardiac transplant patients, whereas the California AIDS Ride attracts a large number of cyclists with HIV or AIDS [49].

Event Characteristics

The characteristics of mass gathering events influence the number and type of patient complaints [1, 11, 16, 28, 51]. These event characteristics include the length of the event, the reason for the mass gathering (music, sporting, religious, festival), and subcategories of the event (genre of music, playoff or regular season sporting event). These factors appear to have a role in patient presentations beyond venue features and crowd demographics. To account for this dependency, most of the prediction models discussed in this chapter incorporate the type of event in some form.

The length of an event and time spent waiting to enter the venue influences the number of patients that present for care. Longer events tend to generate more medical needs, although the exact relationship is not clear [1, 6, 10, 49]. Care must be taken with planning the timing of medical staffing. Patient presentation and hospital transport rates may give the impression that patient presentations are uniformly distributed during an event, however, there are clear peaks and troughs in patient presentations [30, 34]. There is typically a ramp-up period at the beginning and end of events, as well as a decrease in the number of patients that present overnight in multiday events [30, 34, 52, 53].

The type mass gathering event has a significant impact on the patient volume [9, 14, 23, 28]. Concerts tend to have twice the rate of patient presentations compared to sporting events, although college football is an exception and had the highest patient volumes [23, 28]. In general, there are higher PPR and TTHR at football games compared to other sports [14, 23]. These rates were lowest for preseason games, then rose during the regular season and peaked in the postseason [23]. Among music genres, the highest PPR and TTHR were seen at rock and hip-hop concerts [9, 50]. The lowest rates were seen at classical and adult contemporary concerts, with country and pop having intermediate rates. Gospel and Christian music events were seen to have very high patient volumes in one study, but there were only a small number of concerts in this genre so it is unclear if this is a persistent trend [50]. Electronic dance music (EDM) concerts and music festivals have been shown to have the potential for very high patient volumes and discussed further in depth under the section Special Considerations.

Alcohol and Recreational Drugs

There is significant evidence that the presence of alcohol increases the number of patient presentations at mass gathering events, with higher PPRs observed at events where alcohol is readily available [4, 16, 32, 37]. A study of an indoor music event discovered that 79 percent of patients presenting for care were under the influence of alcohol and/or drugs [54]. Studies have shown that events with younger crowds with alcohol present had a higher PPR, as well as a greater proportion of alcohol-related complaints [37]. This was shown to be in contrast to older crowds that presented more frequently with musculoskeletal complaints and lacerations. More studies are certainly needed. The University of Virginia model described later in this chapter accounts for the degree of alcohol present at an event, reflecting prior research that had demonstrated greater patient volumes associated with alcohol use [12].

The relationship between patient volumes and the ingestion of alcohol and illicit substances is likely multifactorial. Alcohol and illicit substance use may predispose patrons to exacerbations of preexisting medical issues, as seen, for example, with the increased risk of cardiovascular events in the setting of sympathomimetic use [55]. Intoxicated patrons may have impaired balance or have lowered inhibitions, increasing the risk of inadvertent injury. There may also be an increase in violence among inebriated patrons, as lowered inhibitions combine with increased aggression often seen with alcohol use [56]. Alcohol and illicit substances may increase the frequency of headache, syncope, dehydration, palpitations, anxiety, or panic and increase the prevalence of relatively minor complaints [4].

Alcohol is often present at concerts, as well as professional and often collegiate sporting events. An event planner should consider the likelihood of tailgating, small gatherings before a sporting event that often involve consuming food and alcohol [57]. Attendees below the legal drinking age may imbibe alcohol prior to an event to circumvent age restrictions in place within the venue regarding the purchase of alcohol [58]. Westrol et al. reviewed medical resource utilization at a variety of concerts and found that, indeed, music genre could predict patients presenting with alcohol or drug intoxication. Intoxication was significantly more common in hip-hop, rock, electronic dance, pop, and country music as compared to classical, contemporary, or jazz music

[9]. Illicit substance use is common at outdoor concerts and especially music festivals. Studies have shown that illicit drug use is significantly more prevalent at these festivals as compared to the general population [58, 59]. Jam bands often draw attendees with heavier use of psychedelics such as LSD and psilocybin mushrooms, while electronic dance acts may see frequent users of stimulants such as MDMA and cocaine, or dissociative drugs such as ketamine [60].

It has been reported that young users of these drugs have little knowledge of the risk they are taking nor the potential long-term effects of repeated use [60]. Special consideration should be given to electronic dance music events, as they combine several of the highest risk elements for mass events, such as heat, active and mobile crowds, and frequent use of alcohol and illicit substances [61]. Furthermore, music festivals combine large crowds with relatively relaxed law enforcement. Many illicit substances are obtained on-site from other attendees, making many users unaware of the true strength or source of the drug ingested [62]. Special consideration must be given to the emergence of new synthetic designer drugs that may not fit into a classic toxidrome or may pose a danger to even experienced substance abusers.

A few studies have evaluated the medical care required *after* being transported from an event to local medical facilities. A study of music festivals with a young crowd with little to no past medical history and a high rate of self-reported alcohol and illicit drug use showed that patients transported presenting to the local emergency department did not require admission to inpatient units. Most patients required only intravenous fluids and supportive care, with 89 percent of patients discharged directly from the emergency department [63]. While further studies are needed, this data may imply that more patients might be successfully managed without transport to a hospital; a properly prepared medical staff may be able to care for patients on-site and reduce the need for transport. One study demonstrated that the on-site presence of a "higher level care" team of advanced care paramedics, nurses, psychiatric nurses, drug counselors, and/or physicians could significantly reduce the number of transfers to outside hospitals due to altered levels of consciousness [54]. However, it must be carefully considered that alcohol and/or illicit substance use is at times fatal, and the general health, comorbidities, and clinical presentation of each patient must be taken into account. A review of outdoor music festivals worldwide found that 13 percent of reported fatalities were due to drug overdose [64]. It is recommended that intravenous fluids, antiemetics, anxiolytics, and antipsychotics be supplied to providers for events with a high presence of alcohol and drug use [63].

It has been recommended that events provide on-site medical services to decrease risk and improve health outcomes at mass gathering events, especially to mitigate substance-related harms [48]. Interestingly, 50 percent of attendees surveyed about illicit substance use at an outdoor music festival stated that the presence of on-site medical services increased their likelihood of partaking in substance or alcohol use because they felt safer [48]. Forty-five percent of those same attendees said they would alter their planned use of substances if no medical services were present. While it has been hypothesized that easily accessible on-site medical services are perceived as safety nets that may increase the inclination of patrons to ingest alcohol and illicit substances, further research is needed to assess the overall harm reduction these services may provide.

Prediction Models

Accurate predictions of patients' needs at a mass gathering can significantly facilitate medical resource planning. The previous section discussed the event-level factors that are known to influence patient presentations. This section will describe the prediction models that utilize those factors to make specific predictions for mass gathering. Through these predictions, event coordinators can make decisions regarding medical personnel, supplies, and equipment.

Predicting medical needs for a mass gathering event is inherently a difficult problem. The same event held at different times with similar characteristics may have significant patient volumes [6, 8, 23]. Additionally, although certain factors may be known in advance, such as expected attendance and venue features, there are certain characteristics of the event that are challenging to anticipate in advance. The psychosocial factors including crowd mood and individual motivation impact may be difficult to know before the event. These types of unmeasured confounders will always add variability to the projections of patient volumes. However, while there are significant limitations to these predictions, they can provide a useful basis from which to formulate a plan for providing medical care.

There are several approaches to predicting medical needs at mass gatherings, we will review the most widely used and well-researched prediction algorithms. These models were designed to predict either the expected patient volume or the medical staffing that is likely needed for an event. The derivation of each model and variables that are needed to calculate each prediction are discussed, as well as the external validation if available. Each model has strengths and weaknesses which make it appropriate for different scenarios.

Australian (Arbon) Models

The Australian models, created by Paul Arbon and colleagues, are the most well-studied method for predicting medical needs at mass gatherings [4, 65–67]. These models were derived using data from 201 events in Australia, which varied from marathons to rock concerts. All the events used to develop this model had >25,000 attendees. The models were developed using linear regression, so a weight is given to each variable. Backward stepwise linear regression was used to identify which variables to include in the final models.

There are three distinct models that can be tailored to the information that is known about an event. The first model predicts total patient presentations (Table 3.1). The authors found that the PPR was lower for larger crowds, which is reflected in their model. While attendance does increase the predicted patient volume, there are a number of factors that are not dependent on the number of attendees. The second two models predict total hospital transports. One of the transport prediction models is used when the total number of presentations is known, while the other model uses the prediction from the total patient presentation model (Table 3.2). Since these models produce very similar results and the total number of patients is not known in advance of an event, only the model using predicted presentations is included.

Several analyses have compared the estimates from the Arbon model to actual patient presentations. A single week-long event in Australia held over several years found the Arbon model showed moderate predictive ability for each day. Overall, the model overestimated patient presentations by 20 percent and underestimated transports by 75 percent. Similarly, an analysis of motor races in the US found the model overestimated patient presentations by approximately 33 percent, but underestimated transport by a factor of 2.5 (prediction: 1.9, actual: 5.5) [68]. A study of electronic dance music (EDM)

Table 3.1 Arbon model for total patient presentations. Each variable in the left-hand column is multiplied by the weighing factor and the result is recorded in the right-hand column. Most variables are represented by one or zero, except for *Humidity* and *Attendance*. *Humidity* is represented by the percent (i.e., 50 is used for 50% humidity). *Attendance-humidity* is the number of attendees multiplied by the humidity. All of the values in the right-hand columns are then added together (including −78.18469) to determine the total predicted number of patient presentations.
*Both Indoor and Outdoor can be selected if there are components of both

Variable		Weighting Factor	
			−78.18469
Seats (1 if any portion seated, 0 if not)	*	−31.48856	=
Bounded (1 if bounded, 0 if unbound)	*	84.556898	=
Indoor (1 if indoor, 0 if no indoor component) *	*	42.370240	=
Outdoor (1 if outdoors, 0 if no outdoor component) *	*	81.31950	=
Sport (1 if sporting event, 0 if not)	*	−20.390940	=
Humidity (Expected % humidity)	*	−0.61613	=
Attendance (total number of expected attendees)	*	−0.000456	=
Attendance-Humidity (Product attendance and % humidity)	*	0.000016	=
Day-Night (1 is both day and night)	*	20.067439	=
			=
		Total predicted patient presentations (Sum of all rows above)	

Table 3.2 Arbon model to predicted number of total patient transportations. Each variable in the left-hand column is multiplied by the weighing factor and the result is recorded in the right-hand column. The predicted number of patient presentations is obtained from Table 3.1. *Seats* and *Bounded* are represented by one or zero. All of the values in the right-hand columns are then added together to determine the predicted number of patients requiring transportation to a hospital.

Variable		Weighting Factor	
			0.0
Predicted number of presentations	*	0.010980	=
Seats (1 if any portion seated, 0 if not)	*	−1.030687	=
Bounded (1 if bounded, 0 if not)	*	1.509155	=
			=
		Total predicted patient transports (Sum of all rows above)	

festivals, which had considerable variation, found that the Arbon model severely underestimated presentation by 35–96 percent (up to a factor of twenty underestimation); transports were likewise underestimated by 41–96 percent [65]. Another study of music festivals in Belgium, which included EDM, found the Arbon model was found to underpredict patient presentations [66]. As discussed later in this chapter, EDM festivals and concerts typically have higher patient volumes which likely contributed to these underestimates.

In general, the Arbon model appears to be reasonably accurate in predicting total patient presentations.

However, this model underpredicted transports in all external validation studies, often substantially. It is important to note that this model was developed using data from events with over 25,000 attendees and it is unclear from the validation studies how it performed in smaller events. Care should be taken if applying the Arbon model to events under 25,000 attendees.

University of Virginia Model

The University of Virginia model, published by Nicholas Hartman and colleagues, is the second most well-studied

29

Table 3.3 University of Virginia model for predicting patient presentations and transports. This scoring system is based on five event features. Points are assigned to each of the event features based on the predicted level (0, 1, or 2). The sum of all of these points and the individual scores are then used to determine the event category. Each event category has predicted numbers of total patient contacts, full medical evaluations, and patient transports to a hospital.

Weather (Heat Index)	Attendance	Alcohol	Crowd Age	Crowd Intention	Points
>90°F	≥15,000	Significant	Older	Animated	2
≤90°F	1,000–14,999	Limited	Mixed	Intermediate	1
Climate controlled	<1,000	None	Younger	Calm	0

Total Points	Event Category	Patient Contacts Mean [Range]	Full Evaluations Mean [Range]	Transports Mean [Range]
≥6 (or 2 points in two different categories)	Major	71 [24–127]	14.3 [4–57]	5.5 [1–17]
4–5 (2 points in one category)	Intermediate	6.3 [1–21]	0.9 [0–5]	0.4 [0–4]
≤3	Minor	2.3 [0–7]	0.2 [0–1]	0.1 [0–1]

method for predicting patient presentations and transports [12, 65, 66, 68]. This model uses a different approach compared to the Arbon model in that events are categorized into three levels based on various event features: "minor," "intermediate," or "major." A scoring system was developed using expert opinion based on event features. Hartman then used data from fifty-five events staffed by a university medical system to determine the average number of patient contacts, full medical evaluations, and hospital transports for each category of event.

The University of Virginia model is based on five different event features (Table 3.3). These features were determined based on a systematic review of the mass gathering literature at the time then a score was assigned to each based on expert opinion. The features include the heat index, attendance, alcohol use, crowd age, and crowd intention. Weather is classified based on whether the event is climate controlled or if heat index above 90°F non-climate-controlled events. Attendance is divided into three bins (<1,000, 1,000–14,999, and ≥15,000). Alcohol, crowd age, and crowd intention are similarly classified based on three levels, but the authors do not give explicit definitions for these levels. These selections are therefore largely up to the discretion of the event planners.

The points for each of the five event features are added together to determine the category of the event (Table 3.3). Additionally, having two points for one or more event features will increase the category level of an event. For each level, there is an estimate of the number of patient contacts, full evaluations, and

transports. The derivation paper also provides the range for each of these numbers, based on historical data.

There have been several attempts to externally validate this model. In a study at a US motor raceway, the University of Virginia model was found to overestimate patient presentations by a factor of two (prediction 200 percent of actual), however, the number of predicted transports were very accurate [68]. An analysis of electronic dance music festivals with high variation patient volumes found the University of Virginia model underpredicted patient encounters for some events and overpredicted others (–84 percent to +255 percent); however, it was significantly more accurate than the Arbon model for predicting patient transports [65]. A study of Belgium music festivals found that the University of Virginia model underpredicted at most events [69], although all the models examined in this study also underpredicted the majority events due to high average PPR.

Overall, the University of Virginia model seems to overestimate the patient encounters, but is reasonably accurate predicting hospital transports. The University of Virginia model has significant limitations due to subjectivity in assigning scores, but this subjectivity may allow for valuable judgment to be brought into the model if experienced medical planners are available. Some of the inaccuracy in predicting patient encounters is likely due to the coarseness of the classification system (i.e., "minor," "intermediate," and "major" events). It is useful to consider the ranges provided by the model in addition to the point estimates, since there will always be variation due to unmeasured factors.

United Kingdom and South African Models

The Health and Safety Executive in the United Kingdom first released *The event safety guide* in 1993 and then updated the guide in 1999 [13]. The guide provides a wealth of useful information on event planning and includes a section on medical management. While some of the information is specific to the UK laws and regulations, much of the information is applicable to other countries. This model differs from the University of Virginia and Arbon models in that it provides the recommended number of providers and ambulances, rather than predictions of patient encounters and transports. The derivation of the UK model is not explained, however, the distribution of points indicates a data-driven development process.

The model is based on twelve different categories, with points assigned to each based on event features. The categories are the nature of the event, venue, standing versus seated, audience profile, past history, attendance, waiting line times, season, proximity to emergency department, size of nearby emergency departments, additional hazards, and on-site resources. The sum of points for each of the categories determines the recommended medical resources. The tables are too large to reproduce in this chapter, but the guide is freely available through the UK's Health and Safety Executive's website (www.hse.gov.uk/event-safety/) or can be purchased through book retailers.

The South African model was deviated from the UK model for the purpose of planning medical resources for the 2010 World Cup [70]. This was motivated by the need to create a model that was appropriate for areas with more limited medical resources than the UK. Some categories were replicated without change, while others were altered based on expert opinion. For example, waiting line times were replaced with event duration. The most significant change was marked decrease in the number of recommended personnel and ambulances based on the overall score. The medical resources in the South African model tend to be half or less of those recommended by the UK model.

No external validations of the UK model could be found, but the South African model has been studied in both its country of origin and in the United Kingdom [51, 71]. The model was also compared to the actual medical needs for the 2010 World Cup [71].

It was found to overpredict the need for basic life support (BLS), immediate life support (ILS), and advanced life support (ALS) resources for larger events (>8,000 attendees), but underpredict ILS and ALS needs for smaller events (~2,000 attendees). However, this was based on the number of hours of medical personnel staffing compared to estimated care times based on fixed lengths of times to care for patients at each level (BLS: twenty minutes, ILS: thirty minutes, and ALS: thirty-five minutes). This approach does not take into account surge capacity of the staff and should be interpreted with caution since patient presentations are typically not uniformly distributed. The same validation methodology was applied to rugby matches in South Africa and the United Kingdom [51]. The South African model again tended to overpredict the need for medical staffing in both countries. There was underprediction for ILS for a minority of events, which tended to be smaller (<10,000 attendees). The need for ambulance transports was also underestimated for smaller events, but typically predictions were only underestimated by one transport.

In general, the UK and South African models appear to provide useful estimations for the number of medical personnel and ambulances needed at mass gathering events. The UK model estimates for medical resources are significantly higher than those of the South African model, and would appear to be preferred in resource-rich areas. It appears that it is safe to use the South African model where there are less resources available, since it still provides an adequate margin of error. Caution should be used when either model recommends that advanced providers are not needed because ILS and ALS care are sometimes needed at small events. Additional, further studies using actual provider time are needed for both models for definitive validation.

Baird (Heat Index-Adjusted Prior) Model

The Baird model is primarily based on prior patient presentation rates, with an adjustment of the change in predicted heat index from the previous event [11]. This model therefore can only be used when data from a prior similar event is known. The adjustment for heat index was based on a review of the available literature and assumes that there will be a 3 patient increase for every ten-degree increase in temperature (Figure 3.1). The UK and South African models also incorporate prior presentation rate, however, it is one

$$PPR = PPR_H + \frac{HI - HI_H}{100} \times 3$$

PPR = estimated patient presentation rate

PPR_H = average PPR from prior events

HI = predicted heat index

HI_H = average heat index at prior events

Figure 3.1 The Baird formula for patient presentation rate per 1,000 (PPR) based on historical data. The difference between the anticipated heat index and the average heat index from prior events is divided by one hundred and multiplied by three, then added to average PPR from previous events.

of many factors considered. Baird is unique in that it is only based on two factors (prior PPR and change in heat index).

It was previously shown that a regression model tailored to historical data for a recurring event performed better than a generalized model [67]. This is not surprising given that various factors will often have different effects at distinct types of events. For example, having seats for most attendees at a football game may have different effects than at a film festival. Baird extended this idea by using the previous PPR rate and assuming that factors besides heat index would stay the same between similar events.

The Baird model intuitively appears reasonable, but does not have published validation. This model is included in this chapter because it is most consistent with the National Association of Emergency Medical System Physicians (NAEMSP) position statement on Mass Gathering Medical Care [72]. This publication states that the "types of medical services and resources allocated to a mass gathering event should be determined by data from historically similar events." Additionally, the Baird model is used by the authors' event medicine group, which has prior data on the medical needs for many events.

In summary, the Baird model is used in practice but does not have rigorous validation. However, it is consistent with national recommendations regarding prediction of medical needs. It may be used when historical data from similar events is known. To ensure that an upcoming event is similar to prior, consider the elements discussed in the previous section on Factors That Influence Patient Presentations and the later section on Special Considerations. A significant limitation of this model is that it does not predict hospital transports and it is unclear if this methodology would be applicable.

Other Models

There are a number of other models described in the medical literature but are not yet recommended for use. Arbon and colleagues published a revised model using a decision tree [17]. This method may hold promise for the future models, but such approaches are prone to overfitting and will need significant external validation before it can be recommended. The Plan Risk Manifestation (PRIMA) was created in Belgium to predict in-event medical needs [69]. This model showed promise in a validation study comparing it to the Arbon and University of Virginia models [66], however, it is based on a spreadsheet with 160 questions that is not readily available. Zeitz et al. also created a prediction model based on historical data [67]. However, the method is specific to the individual events and may be prone to overfitting.

Recommendations for Model Selection

It is important to recognize that all mass gathering events are unique and there are unpredictable factors that will influence patient presentations. As such, all of the currently available prediction models have very significant limitations. However, it is necessary to have an estimate of the medical resource needs prior to an event. We recommend that a planner should consider a range of possible patient presentations and hospital transports. A reasonable range may be 25 percent lower and 25 percent higher than predicted (i.e., for a prediction of 100 patients, expect between 75–125 patients). There will be events where the actual numbers fall outside these extremes, but this approach will be appropriate for most events. Considering a possible range also helps because patient presentations are not uniformly distributed during an event and extra staff help to care for surges of patients.

The Arbon model is recommended for predicting the number of patient presentations when historical data is not available. If data from previous similar events is known, then we propose using the Baird model for predicting the number of patients. For predicting the number of transports, the University of Virginia model appears to be most accurate. The UK model is recommended for predicting the number of medical personnel and ambulances needed for an event. This model is especially useful because it can be used with or without historical data. It is also advantageous for groups that do not have experience determining the number of medical personnel needed to care for a certain number of patients. The South African model can be used where medical resources are sparser or if the UK model has been seen to over-predict needs based on experience with previous events.

Special Considerations

There are situations where the predicted number of patient presentations or transports substantially exceeds the number predicted by previously described models. Many of these circumstances are difficult to predict in advance, such as a natural disaster or a structural failure resulting in multiple injuries [64]. However, there are some event features that are known to pose an increased risk of very high medical needs. This section discusses these features and the reported increase in patient volumes. Medical care planners should consider whether an event is likely to have any of these features. Extra medical resources in terms of staffing, equipment, and ambulances are appropriate in those circumstances.

Caring for Event Participants

The patient and transport volumes may be much higher than predicted if the medical staff is respon-sible for caring for event participants. In many mass gatherings, especially sporting events, there is a med-ical team responsible for the attendees of an event and a separate team responsible for participants in the event. There are usually distinct medical needs for these groups of patients and this division helps to keep resources available to participants, who typically have a higher risk of injury. However, there are a number of events where a single medical team may be in charge of care of all patients. In some events there is not a clear distinction between observers and partici-pants, there are too many participants for specialized care, or the smaller size of the event may make spe-cialized teams impractical. These situations will often substantially increase both PPR and TTHR. The pre-diction models described previously only account for caring for non-participant attendees.

Most published accounts of events with very high patient volumes involved caring for participants [19, 34, 53, 73]. The 2009 World Police and Fire Games was an event in which there were more participants than attendees, sometimes referred to as a Category 3 mass gathering [53, 74]. These games had an average daily PPR of 10.9/1,000 and TTHR of 0.23/1,000 over a ten-day period [73], most of whom were partici-pants. This PPR is ten times higher than the rate typically seen at mass gathering, although the TTHR was only modestly increased since most presentations were for musculoskeletal complaints that did not require transport. Even higher rates were seen at two-day bicycle events held from 2010 to 2012, which had a daily average PPR of 80/1,000 and TTHR of 0.42/1,000 [73]. These rates are both well above what would be expected.

When caring for participants as well as attendees of an event, it appears common to see an order of magnitude increase patient presentations. There is also an increase in hospital transports, although not as large. The prediction models presented previously do not account for these increased needs. It is recom-mended that medical teams try to find published reports of medical needs at similar events when plan-ning for events in which they will care for participants.

Multiday Events

Multiday events are distinct in terms of both patient volumes and the type of patient complaints. The effect of a mass gathering event that extends for several days appears to vary depending on a number of factors. These factors include whether the same population is present for multiple days and if attendees will camp at the event site, in addition to the other factors dis-cussed earlier in this chapter. Chronic conditions are likely to become more common reasons for presenta-tion, such as asthma, diabetes, and psychiatric prob-lems [13].

Most multiday events appear to have higher daily patient volumes than single day events [52, 53, 75]. It is more appropriate to consider the daily PPR rather than the rate for the entire event for multiday events. There was an overall PPR of 42.9/1,000 at Burning Man; however, since this was a week-long event, the daily PPR was only 6.1/1,000 [52]. Similarly, the three-day US festival had a daily PPR of 6.9/1,000 [75] and a recurring five-day Austrian music festival had a daily PPR of 1.8–5.2/1,000 [8]. These were bounded events with overnight camping that had higher than average patient presentation volumes. In contrast, the Holy Shroud exhibition in Italy was an unbounded, forty-two-day event with a daily average PPR of 0.27, consistent with typical single day events. This type of event could be considered a series of forty-two single day events since new attendees were coming each day [18]. A nine-day agricultural and horticultural show held at a fairground with no overnight camping found an intermediate daily PPR of 1.6 [76]. In general, having the same population for multiple days appears to increase patient volumes, which is significantly higher if attendee camp at the event site.

There is typically a ramp up in the volume of patient presentations at the beginning of a multiday event and a ramp down at the end [52, 53]. The first and final days typically have the lowest patient volumes, with the highest seen in the middle of the event. This is similar to the pattern seen at single day events, but the ramp up and ramp down periods are measured in days rather than hours. Medical staffing should be maximal during the middle days of a multiday event.

It is not uncommon for patients to present before the start of a multiday event and continue after the end date [13, 52, 53]. There typically have significant build-in and load-out of infrastructure, so workers may present with injuries or other ailments outside of official event dates. Additionally, attendees may arrive early for a variety of reasons, especially those traveling long distances. Planners should consider having medical staffing during days immediately before and after a multiday event.

Electronic Dance Music Festivals

Electronic Dance Music (EDM) festivals have been shown to be at risk for significantly higher than expected patient volumes and potentially life-threatening presentations. In general, all music festivals have been shown to have patient volumes compared to other types of events [23] and this appears to be more significant at EDM festivals. While most of the reported patient volumes at EDM festivals are elevated above normal range, there are several published cases of dramatically high PPR and TTHR [8, 24, 65]. This is likely driven primarily by high rates of drug and alcohol use at these events [24].

Several large reviews of EDM festivals show persistently elevated rates of patient presentations. Analyses of patient presentations at EDM festivals in the Netherlands that spanned multiple years found PPRs in the range of 9–17/1,000 [8, 24, 77]. Data from the United States found PPRs in the range of 1.4–12/1,000 for most EDM events. However, there are several reports of markedly elevated patient volumes, with PPRs of 21–33/1,000. Patient transport rates are similarly elevated at EDM festivals [8, 30, 77]. At EDM events, most TTHR rates were 0.2–0.8/1,000, although rates as high as 1.1–2.0/1,000 were observed. This indicates more severe patient presentations. A review of a variety of music mass gathering events found that 75 percent of life-threatening presentations came from EDM festivals [66]. Overall, the medical needs at EDM festivals are significantly higher than other similar music mass gathering events and a number of these festivals showed extremely high patient presentation and transport volumes.

Drug and alcohol use appear to be significant causes of the increased medical needs at EDM events. The most commonly reported recreational drug patients reported at these events is 3,4-Methylenedioxymethamphetamine (MDMA, also known as "ecstacy" or "molly"), followed by marijuana, ketamine, lysergic acid diethylamide (LSD), stimulants, and benzodiazepines [61, 65]. Patients presenting with severe illness from EDM festivals were positive for drugs or alcohol in 95 percent of cases, with MDMA responsible for two deaths [78]. In a study of patients presenting with abnormal vital signs, 49 percent reported the use of MDMA [61]. Gamma-hydroxybutyrate (GHB) is also common at EDM festivals, but appears to be more common in Europe and Australia based on the published literature [24, 79, 80]. GHB is a sedative and is especially concerning because in overdose it produces somnolence, bradycardia, hypotension, and coma [80, 81]. These overdoses often occur in clusters and this can lead to multiple patients requiring critical care management and possible intubation.

When preparing to provide medical care for EDM festivals, planners should expect patient presentation rates significantly higher than other music festivals. This appears largely due to increased rates of alcohol and recreational drug use. There may also be higher severity of presentations and a greater proportion of patients requiring transport. Medical providers should be experienced with intubation and caring for patients with critical illnesses.

Mosh Pits

The presence of mosh pits at a music mass gathering event greatly increases the risk of injuries [82]. Moshing is "intense and violent physical activity; slamming into other audience members and throwing mock punches and kicks" [83]. This is a violent type of dancing most commonly seen in rock and punk music concerts, although it may also be seen at

EDM events. Moshing typically concentrates in informally designated areas known as mosh pits. These mosh pits tend to spontaneously emerge and dissipate based on crowd activity, and are usually not planned or approved by event organizers. Events that will likely, or have previously, included mosh pits should raise the concern for increased patient presentations for injuries, some of which may be very severe.

Given their violent nature, it is not surprising that events with mosh pits have higher patient volumes, transports, and injury severity than other similar music events. A retrospective study of six such music festivals found PPR of 5.6–13.0/1,000 and TTHR of 0.7–2.0/1,000, with an average of one quarter of patients injured in a mosh pit [82]. Another study of a four-day event found a mean daily PPR of 2.1/1,000 and TTHR of 0.05/1,000, which is similar to typical rates; however, 37 percent of all presentations and 74 percent of transports were due to mosh pit-related injuries [84]. Even more concerning, there were seventy reported deaths from injuries sustained in mosh pits between 1994 and 2006 [82].

Medical staffing should be increased when there is a significant probability that there will be mosh pits at a music event. While no model directly includes moshing and mosh pits, several indirectly incorporate this type of violent activity. The University of Virginia model includes a variable to assess for "Crowd intention," which can be classified as "Animated." The Baird model uses previous presentation rates, so this model may capture the increased risk if mosh pits were present in past similar events. However, event planners should have increased caution even when using these models, since mosh pit-related injuries are often unpredictable.

Remote and Austere Environments

Remote and austere environments both pose unique challenges in terms of patient volumes, variety of patient conditions, and the need for specialized care. These locations lack the flexibility to utilize nearby community resources, so the staff and equipment are limited to that which is brought to the site. There are often unique environmental risks that are not common to most mass gathering events, which may include rock falls, animal attacks, and altitude sickness [19]. Because of limited resources, medical providers are often responsible for all attendees, staff, and participants at such events. Additionally, participants may be engaging in activities that are strenuous and have a high risk for injury, as in adventure or wilderness races. Careful planning is necessary for events held in these environments.

There are a number of published accounts about the experience providing medical care in remote or austere environments. In addition to common ailments, the medical staff at the Burning Man festival had to treat injuries due to sun and sand exposure. There was also an ailment unique to this location in the Black Rock desert, known as "playa foot" caused by the low pH of the sand [52]. The medical providers at this event found that including physicians was necessary because much of the care provided was beyond the scope of paramedics. A review of multiple wilderness mass gathering events found most events require medical care for 10–40 percent of participants, which would be equivalent to PPR of 100–400/1,000 [19]. Additionally, mortality rates appear to be elevated at 0.1–0.3/100,000 for wilderness events, but may be as high as 1–3/100,000 for adventure races and kayaking.

The medical resources required to provide care in remote and austere locations will vary substantially based on unique characteristics of the environment [85]. Organizers should expect to care for a significant proportion of people at the event and should account for caring for observers, participants, and staff. There should be equipment to care for critically ill patients until they can be safely extracted, which may be hours or even days. It is recommended that a physician typically be part of medical staff, even if the number of participants is relatively small because of the potential for critical illnesses. Plans should be in place to care for the unique risk of these remote and austere environments.

Risk of Critical Illness

Mass gathering events demonstrate a greater incidence of medical and traumatic complaints than the general population. Fortunately, the large majority of these complaints are minor, as demonstrated by low transport rates to external medical facilities. However, catastrophic illness does occur, though fortunately at a very low rate [33]. Planners should be aware of these risks and have the resources necessary to treat these conditions if they occur.

Cardiac Arrest

In an analysis of nearly 12,000 patient presentations, 0.05 percent suffered cardiac arrest and less than 1.5 percent of patients suffered cardiac issues (non-arrest) [4]. There were over 12 million attendees at these events, resulting in a rate of cardiac arrest of 0.5 for every million spectators. A meta-analysis, which reviewed 35 previous studies with an average PPR of 3.2/1,000, found the rate of cardiac arrest was 0.7 per one million spectators [6]. Weaver et al. observed the 1986 World's exposition, where 4 out of every 1,000 patrons sought medical care; the rate of cardiac arrest was 0.3 per million visitors [86].

The rate of cardiac arrest appears to be related to the type of event. A review of multiple sporting and non-sporting events examined the difference in the incidence of cardiac arrest [6]. The incidence was found to be higher than average at sporting events, with 1.7 arrests per one million spectators. The highest incidence, however, occurred at papal masses, with 3.1 arrests per one million spectators; although this might have been due to the high average age of the attendees. At the 1995 papal visit to New York City, 64 percent of attendees were over the age of fifty years; elderly populations may be at higher risk of cardiac arrest due to the greater prevalence of preexisting medical conditions [49].

A study of multiple events at the Melbourne Cricket Ground found there was an incidence of cardiac arrest of 2 cases per 1,000,000 patrons [87]. Eighty-six percent of the patients experiencing cardiac arrest left the venue alive (return of spontaneous circulation had been achieved) and 71 percent were discharged from the hospital. All cases of cardiac arrest were patients initially found to be in ventricular defibrillation and 93 percent were defibrillated within five minutes from documented time of collapse. This highlights the importance of early intervention in cardiac arrest. Rapid intervention with early CPR and defibrillation has been shown to positively affect patient outcomes [88]. Although cardiac arrests are a very small percentage of medical occurrences at mass gathering events, lack of preparation by event planners can be devastating. Most events should have automated external defibrillators present and medical staff should be trained in delivering high quality CPR. In a review of thirteen cardiac arrests at a football stadium, early defibrillation and CPR led to return of spontaneous circulation in 77 percent of cases, with 80 percent of those cases surviving to discharge without a neurologic deficit [89].

While cardiac arrest is relatively rare among case presentations, very large gatherings are likely to have a higher absolute incidence. Studies of the annual Hajj pilgrimage, which drew nearly 3.2 million visitors in 2012, have provided better insight into the demographics of cardiac arrest. A prospective analysis over multiple years of 426 patients diagnosed with cardiac arrest found that two-thirds were male and one-third female [90]. Seventy-three percent were over the age of fifty years, and over one-third had documented preexisting cardiovascular disease.

Other Critical Illnesses

Studies have shown that death is infrequent at mass gathering events, however, some events may have a higher risk. A literature review of music festivals occurring between 1999 and 2014 highlighted 722 deaths [64]. Eighty-two percent of these documented deaths were traumatic, most of which were caused by trampling (81 percent of traumatic deaths). Other traumatic fatalities of note were related to motor vehicles (6.5 percent of traumatic deaths), structural collapse (4.7 percent of traumatic deaths), acts of terror (4.3 percent of traumatic deaths), with drowning, assaults, and falls at less than 4 percent of traumatic deaths each. Most nontraumatic deaths in this review were due to overdose, which accounted for 13 percent of all deaths.

Other studies have evaluated the risk of head injuries at concerts, with a higher incidence found at rock concerts versus other music genres. One such study found that 17.6 percent of presentations at rock concerts were head injuries versus 5.8 percent at non-rock concerts [50]. The higher incidence of head injury at rock concerts is thought to be due to the frequent presence of mosh pits, crowd surfing, and the higher risk of being hit by thrown projectiles. Another study found that head injury accounted for 11.6 percent of patient presentations at rock concerts, with half of these injuries the result of being hit by thrown objects [91]. Fortunately, the majority of these head injuries were minor and without loss of consciousness.

The data on respiratory arrest are very limited [32]. It is possible that cases of respiratory arrest are not identified until cardiac arrest has occurred, and the patients are classified as experiencing the latter. Respiratory arrest may result as a consequence of prolonged traumatic asphyxiation. There is a higher incidence of traumatic asphyxiation events in which stampedes occur [92]. Stampedes can be highly fatal;

in a 27-year span, 215 reported stampedes resulted in the death of 7,000 and injury of 14,000 [93].

References

1. Arbon P. Mass-Gathering Medicine: A Review of the Evidence and Future Directions for Research. *Prehospital and Disaster Medicine.* 2007;**22**(2):131–135.

2. *Preparedness Team. Public health for mass gatherings: key considerations [Internet].* World Health Organization; 2015 [cited September 20, 2021]. www.who.int/publications-detail-redirect/public-health-for-mass-gatherings-key-considerations

3. Turris S. A., Lund A., Hutton A., Bowles R., Ellerson E., Steenkamp M., et al. Mass-Gathering Health Research Foundational Theory: Part 2 – Event Modeling for Mass Gatherings. *Prehospital and Disaster Medicine.* 2014;**29**(6):655–663.

4. Arbon P., Bridgewater F. H., Smith C. Mass Gathering Medicine: A Predictive Model for Patient Presentation and Transport Rates. *Prehospital and Disaster Medicine.* 2001;**16**(3):150–158.

5. Locoh-Donou S., Guofen Y., Welcher M., Berry T., O'Connor R. E., Brady W. J. Mass-Gathering Medicine: A Descriptive Analysis of a Range of Mass-Gathering Event Types. *American Journal of Emergency Medicine.* 2013;**31**(5):843–846.

6. Michael J. A., Barbera J. A. Mass Gathering Medical Care: A Twenty-Five Year Review. *Prehospital and Disaster Medicine.* 1997;**12**(4):72–79.

7. Van Remoortel H., Scheers H., De Buck E., Haenen W., Vandekerckhove P. Prediction Modelling Studies for Medical Usage Rates in Mass Gatherings: A Systematic Review. *PLoS ONE* [Internet]. June 23, 2020 [cited June 11, 2021];**15**(6). www.ncbi.nlm.nih.gov/pmc/articles/PMC7310685/

8. Maleczek M., Rubi S., Fohringer C., Scheriau G., Meyer E., Uray T., et al. Medical Care at a Mass Gathering Music Festival: Retrospective Study over 7 Years (2011–2017). *Wien Klin Wochenschr* [Internet]. April 26, 2021 [cited June 11, 2021]. https://link.springer.com/10.1007/s00508-021-01856-5

9. Westrol M. S., Koneru S., McIntyre N., Caruso A. T., Arshad F. H., Merlin M. A. Music Genre as a Predictor of Resource Utilization at Outdoor Music Concerts. *Prehospital and Disaster Medicine.* 2017;**32**(3):289–296.

10. Arbon P. The Development of Conceptual Models for Mass-Gathering Health. *Prehospital and Disaster Medicine.* 2004;**19**(3):208–212.

11. Baird M. B., O'Connor R. E., Williamson A. L., Sojka B., Alibertis K., Brady W. J. The Impact of Warm Weather on Mass Event Medical Need: A Review of the Literature. *American Journal of Emergency Medicine.* 2010;**28**(2):224–229.

12. Hartman N., Williamson A., Sojka B., Alibertis K., Sidebottom M., Berry T., et al. Predicting Resource Use at Mass Gatherings Using a Simplified Stratification Scoring Model. *American Journal of Emergency Medicine.* 2009;**27**(3):337–343.

13. The Event Safety Guide: A Guide to Health, Safety and Welfare at Music and Similar Events. 2nd ed. Norwich: HSE Books; 1999. 218 p.

14. Milsten A. M., Seaman K. G., Liu P., Bissell R. A., Maguire B. J. Variables Influencing Medical Usage Rates, Injury Patterns, and Levels of Care for Mass Gatherings. *Prehospital and Disaster Medicine.* 2003;**18**(4):334–346.

15. Zeitz K. M., Schneider D. P. A., Jarrett D., Zeitz C. J. Mass Gathering Events: Retrospective Analysis of Patient Presentations over Seven Years. *Prehospital and Disaster Medicine.* 2002;**17**(3):147–150.

16. Anikeeva O., Arbon P., Zeitz K., Bottema M., Lund A., Turris S., et al. Patient Presentation Trends at 15 Mass-Gathering Events in South Australia. *Prehospital and Disaster Medicine.* 2018;**33**(4):368–374.

17. Arbon P., Bottema M., Zeitz K., Lund A., Turris S., Anikeeva O., et al. Nonlinear Modelling for Predicting Patient Presentation Rates for Mass Gatherings. *Prehospital and Disaster Medicine.* 2018;**33**(4):362–367.

18. Bortolin M., Ulla M., Bono A., Ferreri E., Tomatis M., Sgambetterra S. Holy Shroud Exhibition 2010: Health Services During a 40-Day Mass-Gathering Event. *Prehospital and Disaster Medicine.* 2013;**28**(3):239–244.

19. Burdick T. E. Wilderness Event Medicine: Planning for Mass Gatherings in Remote Areas. *Travel Medicine and Infectious Disease.* 2005;**3**(4):249–258.

20. Alquthami A. H., Pines J. M. A Systematic Review of Noncommunicable Health Issues in Mass Gatherings. *Prehospital and Disaster Medicine.* 2014;**29**(2):167–175.

21. Ranse J., Hutton A., Keene T., Lenson S., Luther M., Bost N., et al. Health Service Impact from Mass Gatherings: A Systematic Literature Review. *Prehospital and Disaster Medicine.* 2017;**32**(1):71–77.

22. Burton J. O., Corry S. J., Lewis G., Priestman W. S. Differences in Medical Care Usage Between Two Mass-Gathering Sporting Events. *Prehospital and Disaster Medicine.* 2012;**27**(5):458–462.

23. Goldberg S. A., Maggin J., Molloy M. S., Baker O., Sarin R., Kelleher M., et al. The Gillette Stadium Experience: A Retrospective Review of Mass Gathering Events from 2010 to 2015. *Disaster Medicine and Public Health Preparedness.* 2018;**12**(6):752–758.

24. Krul J., Sanou B., Swart E. L., Girbes A. R. J. Medical Care at Mass Gatherings: Emergency Medical Services at Large-Scale Rave Events. *Prehospital and Disaster Medicine.* 2012;**27**(1):71–74.

25. Woodall J., Watt K., Walker D., Tippett V., Enraght-Moony E., Bertolo C., et al. Planning Volunteer Responses to Low-Volume Mass Gatherings: Do Event Characteristics Predict Patient Workload? *Prehospital and Disaster Medicine.* 2010;**25**(5):442–448.

26. Bossarte R. M., Sullivent III E. E., Sinclair J., Bixler D., Simon T. R., Swahn M. H., et al. Injury, Violence, and Risk Among Participants in a Mass Gathering of the Rainbow Family of Living Light. *Journal of Health Care for the Poor and Underserved.* 2008;**19**(2):588–595.

27. Sanders A. B., Criss E., Steckl P., Meislin H. W., Raife J., Allen D. An Analysis of Medical Care at Mass Gatherings. *Annals of Emergency Medicine.* 1986;**15**(5):515–519.

28. Locoh-Donou S., Yan G., Berry T., O'Connor R., Sochor M., Charlton N., et al. Mass Gathering Medicine: Event Factors Predicting Patient Presentation Rates. *Internal and Emergency Medicine.* 2016;**11**(5):745–752.

29. Dutch M. J., Senini L. M., Taylor D. J. Mass Gathering Medicine: The Melbourne 2006 Commonwealth Games Experience. *Emergency Medicine Australasia.* 2008;**20**(3):228–233.

30. Feldman M. J., Lukins J. L., Verbeek R. P., MacDonald R. D., Burgess R. J., Schwartz B. Half-a-Million Strong: The Emergency Medical Services Response to a Single-Day, Mass-Gathering Event. *Prehospital and Disaster Medicine.* 2004;**19**(4):287–296.

31. Grange J. T., Baumann G. W., Vaezazizi R. On-Site Physicians Reduce Ambulance Transports at Mass Gatherings. *Prehospital Emerg Care Off J Natl Assoc EMS Physicians Natl Assoc State EMS Dir.* 2003;**7**(3):322–326.

32. Hutton A., Ranse J., Verdonk N., Ullah S., Arbon P. Understanding the Characteristics of Patient Presentations of Young People at Outdoor Music Festivals. *Prehospital and Disaster Medicine.* 2014;**29**(2):160–666.

33. Varon J., Fromm R. E., Chanin K., Filbin M., Vutpakdi K. Critical Illness at Mass Gatherings Is Uncommon. *Journal of Emergency Medicine.* 2003;**25**(4):409–413.

34. Chang W.-H., Chang K.-S., Huang C.-S., Huang M.-Y., Chien D., Tsai C.-H. Mass Gathering Emergency Medicine: A Review of the Taiwan Experience of Long-Distance Swimming Across Sun-Moon Lake. *International Journal of Gerontology.* 2010; **4**(2):53–68. https://doi.org/10.1016/S1873-9598(10)70025-9.

35. Morimura N., Katsumi A., Koido Y., Sugimoto K., Fuse A., Asai Y., et al. Analysis of Patient Load Data from the 2002 FIFA World Cup Korea/Japan. *Prehospital and Disaster Medicine.* 2004;**19**(3):278–284.

36. Steffen R., Bouchama A., Johansson A., Dvorak J., Isla N., Smallwood C., et al. Non-Communicable Health Risks During Mass Gatherings. *Lancet Infectious Diseases.* 2012;**12**(2):142–149.

37. Bullock M., Ranse J., Hutton A. Impact of Patients Presenting with Alcohol and/or Drug Intoxication on In-Event Health Care Services at Mass-Gathering Events: An Integrative Literature Review. *Prehospital and Disaster Medicine.* 2018;**33**(5):539–542.

38. McQueen C. P. Care of Children at a Large Outdoor Music Festival in the United Kingdom. *Prehospital and Disaster Medicine.* 2010;**25**(3):223–226.

39. Thierbach A. R., Wolcke B. B., Piepho T., Maybauer M., Huth R. Medical Support for Children's Mass Gatherings. *Prehospital and Disaster Medicine.* 2003;**18**(1):14–19.

40. Hutton A., Ranse J., Zimmerman P.-A. Rethinking Mass-Gathering Domains for Understanding Patient Presentations: A Discussion Paper. *Prehospital and Disaster Medicine.* 2021;**36**(1):121–124.

41. Bowdish G. E., Cordell W. H., Bock H. C., Vukov L. F. Using Regression Analysis to Predict Emergency Patient Volume at the Indianapolis 500 Mile Race. *Annals of Emergency Medicine.* 1992;**21**(10):1200–1203.

42. Johansson A., Helbing D., Al-Abideen H. Z., Al-Bosta S. From Crowd Dynamics to Crowd Safety: A Video-Based Analysis. *Advances in Complex Systems.* 2008;**11**(04):497–527.

43. Khademipour G., Nakhaee N., Anari S. M. S., Sadeghi M., Ebrahimnejad H., Sheikhbardsiri H. Crowd Simulations and Determining the Critical Density Point of Emergency Situations. *Disaster Medicine and Public Health Preparedness.* 2017;**11**(6):674–680.

44. Kman N. E., Russell G. B., Bozeman W. P., Ehrman K., Winslow J. Derivation of a Formula to Predict Patient Volume Based on Temperature at College Football Games. *Prehospital Emergency Care.* 2007;**11**(4):453–457.

45. Perron A. D., Brady W. J., Custalow C. B., Johnson D. M. Association of Heat Index and Patient Volume at a Mass Gathering Event. *Prehospital Emerg Care Off J Natl Assoc EMS Physicians Natl Assoc State EMS Dir.* 2005;**9**(1):49–52.

46. Selig B., Hastings M., Cannon C., Allin D., Klaus S., Diaz F. J. Effect of Weather on Medical Patient Volume at Kansas Speedway Mass Gatherings. *Journal of Emergency Nursing.* 2013;**39**(4):e39–44.

47. Van Remoortel H., Scheers H., De Buck E., Haenen W., Vandekerckhove P. Prediction Modelling Studies for Medical Usage Rates in Mass Gatherings: A Systematic Review. *PLoS ONE* [Internet]. June 23, 2020 [cited June 11, 2021];**15**(6). www.ncbi.nlm.nih.gov/pmc/articles/PMC7310685/

48. Hutton A., Munn M. B., White S., Kara P., Ranse J. Does the Presence of On-Site Medical Services at Outdoor Music Festivals Affect Attendees' Planned Alcohol and Recreational Drug Use? *Prehospital and Disaster Medicine.* 202;**36**(4):403–407.

49. Milsten A. M., Maguire B. J., Bissell R. A., Seaman K. G. Mass-Gathering Medical Care: A Review of the Literature. *Prehospital and Disaster Medicine.* 2002;**17**(3):151–162.

50. Grange J. T., Green S. M., Downs W. Concert Medicine: Spectrum of Medical Problems Encountered at 405 Major Concerts. *Academic Emergency Medicine.* 1999;**6**(3):202–207.

51. Smith W. P., Tuffin H., Stratton S. J., Wallis L. A. Validation of a Modified Medical Resource Model for Mass Gatherings. *Prehospital and Disaster Medicine.* 2013;**28**(1):16–22.

52. Bledsoe B., Songer P., Buchanan K., Westin J., Hodnick R., Gorosh L. Burning Man 2011: Mass Gathering Medical Care in an Austere Environment. *Prehospital Emerg Care Off J Natl Assoc EMS Physicians Natl Assoc State EMS Dir.* 2012;**16**(4):469–476.

53. Gutman S. J., Lund A., Turris S. A. Medical Support for the 2009 World Police and Fire Games: A Descriptive Analysis of a Large-Scale Participation Event and Its Impact. *Prehospital and Disaster Medicine.* 2011;**26**(1):33–39.

54. Lund A., Turris S. A. Mass-gathering Medicine: Risks and Patient Presentations at a 2-Day Electronic Dance Music Event. *Prehospital and Disaster Medicine.* 2015;**30**(3):271–278.

55. Lange R. A., Hillis L. D. Cardiovascular Complications of Cocaine Use [Internet]. http://dx.doi.org/10.1056/NEJM200108023450507. Massachusetts Medical Society; 2009 [cited December 8, 2021]. www.nejm.org/doi/10.1056/NEJM200108023450507

56. Evans C. Alcohol, Violence and Aggression. *Br J Alcohol Alcohol.* 1980;**15**:104–117.

57. Anthenien A. M., Fredrickson G., Riggs N. R., Conner B. T., Jurica J., Neighbors C. Tailgating Protective Behavioral Strategies Mediate the Effects of Positive Alcohol Outcome Expectancies on Game Day Drinking. *Journal of Primary Prevention.* 2019;**40**(3):357–365.

58. Puryer J., Wignall R. Tobacco, Alcohol and Drug Use among Dental Undergraduates at One UK University in 2015. *Dentistry Journal.* 2016;**4**(1):2.

59. Lim M. S. C., Hellard M. E., Hocking J. S., Spelman T. D., Aitken C. K. Surveillance of Drug Use Among Young People Attending a Music Festival in Australia, 2005–2008. *Drug and Alcohol Review.* 2010;**29**(2):150–156.

60. Bahora M., Sterk C. E., Elifson K. W. Understanding Recreational Ecstasy Use in the United States: A Qualitative Inquiry. *International Journal of Drug Policy.* 2009;**20**(1):62–69.

61. Friedman M. S., Plocki A., Likourezos A., Pushkar I., Bazos A. N., Fromm C., et al. A Prospective Analysis of Patients Presenting for Medical Attention at a Large Electronic Dance Music Festival. *Prehospital and Disaster Medicine.* 2017;**32**(1):78–82.

62. Lu T. S., Flaherty G. T. Tuning into the Travel Health Risks of Music Tourism. *Journal of Travel Medicine* [Internet]. January 1, 2018 [cited November 4, 2021];**25**(1). Available from: https://academic.oup.com/jtm/article/doi/10.1093/jtm/tay106/5139594

63. DeMott J. M., Hebert C. L., Novak M., Mahmood S., Peksa G. D. Characteristics and Resource Utilization of Patients Presenting to the ED from Mass Gathering Events. *American Journal of Emergency Medicine.* 2018;**36**(6):983–987.

64. Turris S. A., Lund A. Mortality at Music Festivals: Academic and Grey Literature for Case Finding. *Prehospital and Disaster Medicine.* 2017;**32**(1):58–63.

65. FitzGibbon K. M., Nable J. V., Ayd B., Lawner B. J., Comer A. C., Lichenstein R., et al. Mass-Gathering Medical Care in Electronic Dance Music Festivals. *Prehospital and Disaster Medicine.* 2017;**32**(5):563–567.

66. Spaepen K., Haenen W. A., Kaufman L., Beens K., Vandekerckhove P., Hubloue I. Validation of a Belgian Prediction Model for Patient Encounters at Music Mass Gatherings. *Prehospital and Disaster Medicine.* 2020;**35**(5):561–566.

67. Zeitz K. M., Zeitz C. J., Arbon P. Forecasting Medical Work at Mass-Gathering Events: Predictive Model Versus Retrospective Review. *Prehospital and Disaster Medicine.* 2005;**20**(3):164–168.

68. Nable J. V., Margolis A. M., Lawner B. J., Hirshon J. M., Perricone A. J., Galvagno S. M., et al. Comparison of Prediction Models for Use of Medical Resources at Urban Auto-racing Events. *Prehospital and Disaster Medicine.* 2014;**29**(6):608–613.

69. Spaepen K., Haenen W. A., Hubloue I. The Development of PRIMA – A Belgian Prediction Model for Patient Encounters at Mass Gatherings.

Prehospital and Disaster Medicine.
2020;**35**(5):554–560.

70. Smith W. P., Wessels V., Naicker D., Leuenberger E., Fuhri P., Wallis L. A. Development of a Mass-Gathering Medical Resource Matrix for a Developing World Scenario. *Prehospital and Disaster Medicine.* 2010;**25**(6):547–552.

71. Allgaier R. L., Shaafi-Kabiri N., Romney C. A., Wallis L. A., Burke J. J., Bhangu J., et al. Use of Predictive Modeling to Plan for Special Event Medical Care During Mass Gathering Events. *Disaster Medicine and Public Health Preparedness.* 2019;**13**(5–6):874–879.

72. NAEMSP. Mass Gathering Medical Care. *Prehospital Emergency Care.* 2015;**19**(4):558–568.

73. Lund A., Turris S. A., Wang P., Mui J., Lewis K., Gutman S. J. An Analysis of Patient Presentations at a 2-Day Mass-Participation Cycling Event: The Ride to Conquer Cancer Case Series, 2010–2012. *Prehospital and Disaster Medicine.* 2014;**29**(4):429–436.

74. Hodgetts T. J., Cooke M. W. The Largest Mass Gathering: Medical Cover for Millennium Celebrations Needs Careful Planning. *BMJ.* 1999;**318**(7189):957–958.

75. Ounanian L. L., Salinas C., Shear C. L., Rodney W. M. Medical Care at the 1982 US Festival. *Annals of Emergency Medicine.* 1986;**15**(5):520–527.

76. Zeitz K., Zeitz C., Kadow-Griffin C. Injury Occurrences at a Mass Gathering Event. *Australasian Journal of Paramedicine* [Internet]. 2005 [cited December 3, 2021];**3**(1). https://ajp.paramedics.org/index.php/ajp/article/view/307

77. Krul J., Girbes A. R. J. Experience of Health-Related Problems During House Parties in the Netherlands: Nine Years of Experience and Three Million Visitors. *Prehospital and Disaster Medicine.* 2009;**24**(2):133–139.

78. Ridpath A., Driver C. R., Nolan M. L., Karpati A., Kass D., Paone D., et al. Illnesses and Deaths Among Persons Attending an Electronic Dance-Music Festival – New York City, 2013. *MMWR (Morbidity and Mortality Weekly Report).* 2014;**63**(50):1195–1198.

79. Dijkstra B. A. G., Beurmanjer H., Goudriaan A. E., Schellekens A. F. A., Joosten E. A. G. Unity in Diversity: A Systematic Review on the GHB Using Population. *International Journal of Drug Policy.* 2021;**94**:103230.

80. Dutch M. J., Austin K. B. Hospital in the Field: Prehospital Management of GHB Intoxication by Medical Assistance Teams. *Prehospital and Disaster Medicine.* 2012;**27**(5):463–467.

81. Caldicott D. G. E., Chow F. Y., Burns B. J., Felgate P. D., Byard R. W. Fatalities Associated with the Use of Gamma-Hydroxybutyrate and Its Analogues in Australasia. *Medical Journal of Australia.* 2004;**181**(6):310–313.

82. Milsten A. M., Tennyson J., Weisberg S. Retrospective Analysis of Mosh-Pit-Related Injuries. *Prehospital and Disaster Medicine.* 2017;**32**(6):636–641.

83. Kahn-Harris K. *Extreme Metal: Music and Culture on the Edge.* Oxford: Berg; 2006. 204 p.

84. Janchar T., Samaddar C., Milzman D. The Mosh Pit Experience: Emergency Medical Care for Concert Injuries. *American Journal of Emergency Medicine.* 2000;**18**(1):62–63.

85. Laskowski-Jones L., Caudell M. J., Hawkins S. C., Jones L. J., Dymond C. A., Cushing T., et al. Extreme Event Medicine: Considerations for the Organisation of Out-of-Hospital Care During Obstacle, Adventure and Endurance Competitions. *Emergency Medical Journal.* 2017;**34**(10):680–685.

86. Weaver W. D., Sutherland K., Wirkus M. J., Bachman R. Emergency Medical Care Requirements for Large Public Assemblies and a New Strategy for Managing Cardiac Arrest in This Setting. *Annals of Emergency Medicine.* 1989;**18**(2):155–160.

87. Wassertheil J., Keane G., Fisher N., Leditschke J. F. Cardiac Arrest Outcomes at the Melbourne Cricket Ground and Shrine of Remembrance Using a Tiered Response Strategy: A Forerunner to Public Access Defibrillation. *Resuscitation.* 2000;**44**(2):97–104.

88. Weisfeldt M. L., Becker L. B. Resuscitation After Cardiac Arrest: A 3-Phase Time-Sensitive Model. *JAMA.* 2002;**288**(23):3035–3038.

89. Luiz T., Kumpch M., Metzger M., Madler C. Management of Cardiac Arrest in a German Soccer Stadium. *Anaesthesist.* 2005;**54**(9):914–922.

90. Shirah B. H., Al Nozha F. A., Zafar S. H., Kalumian H. M. Mass Gathering Medicine (Hajj Pilgrimage in Saudi Arabia): The Outcome of Cardiopulmonary Resuscitation during Hajj. *Journal of Epidemiology and Global Health.* 2019;**9**(1):71–75.

91. Hewitt S., Jarrett L., Winter B. Emergency Medicine at a Large Rock Festival. *Emergency Medicine Journal.* 1996;**13**(1):26–27.

92. Madzimbamuto F. D., Madamombe T. Traumatic Asphyxia During Stadium Stampede. 2004 [cited December 9, 2021]; https://opendocs.ids.ac.uk/opendocs/handle/20.500.12413/6305

93. Hsieh Y.-H., Ngai K. M., Burkle F. M., Hsu E. B. Epidemiological Characteristics of Human Stampedes. *Disaster Medicine and Public Health Preparedness.* 2009;**3**(4):217–223.

Medical Logistics and Operational Planning for Patient Care at Mass Gathering Events

Scott A. Goldberg, L. Scott Nichols, Michael S. Molloy, and Gerald W. (Jerry) Meltzer II

Introduction

Patient recognition, retrieval, tracking, evacuation, and transport decisions are key components of operational planning for mass gathering events. Optimal medical care during mass gatherings relies upon rapid identification and retrieval of those persons who need to be assessed and treated, as well as rapid access and egress from the venue for ambulances needing to transport patients. Planning and advanced designation of appropriate receiving facilities for the illness or injury encountered is a key element of a high-quality response plan. At the same time, even when hospital transportation is not indicated, or possibly deferrable pending on-site evaluation, therapy, and periods of observation, patient encounters, either on-scene or at on-site medical aid facilities, can still be quite difficult and dynamic across a myriad of circumstances.

Beyond climate, the nature of the event and other risk factors, it is intuitive that the larger the event, the greater the challenge, not only in terms of locating the patient but also with respect to the sheer volumes of attendees and on-site workers that can often approach 100,000 persons or more for a single daytime or evening event.

Beyond the noise of the event itself and the compacted crowds of thousands, traditional radio and mobile phone communications become extremely limited and the ability of bystanders to call for help when someone near them feels unwell or has a syncopal episode, can be very difficult. As a result, alerts to responders regarding persons needing help can be unfortunately delayed. The inherent obstacles to medical response in mass gatherings not only apply to those reaching out for help, but also in terms of rescuers who, understandably, have received limited information and are often unable to pinpoint the patient's location in an unfamiliar, crowded setting.

These challenges of alerting rescuers, finding the patient's location, and facilitating retrieval under mass gathering conditions can be observed in a variety of circumstances. These variations on the same theme can range from a noisy, concentrated crowd of viewers spread along a lengthy parade or marathon route to the packed center of a general admission (GA) audience site on a stadium pitch or meadow during a loud rock concert (Figure 4.1). Medical response may be needed in an undetermined location somewhere in a sprawling dark and rain-slickened parking lot or some ambiguous location for a water rescue. Whether within a fixed venue or along a lengthy race route, retrieving ill or injured patients can be difficult, particularly in higher stadium seats (Figure 4.2) or trying to find someone within a teeming crowd pressing together. Such situations are not only frustrating for the prudent medical responder, but they can also compromise optimal medical care.

Beyond the logistics of patient identification and retrieval, information gathering regarding the patients and their conditions is also an integral consideration. Efficient record-keeping and subsequent information conveyance are pivotal for those who become ill or injured during mass gatherings. Considering that transporting ambulance teams often are not the on-site first-in responders who had direct, first-hand knowledge about the on-scene events and findings, record-keeping should therefore be as informative as possible and yet be accomplished as efficiently as possible.

Beyond the care and tracking of individual patients, these medical records are also critical for future event planning as well as important considerations for event risk management teams and their typical "after-action" reviews of the event. Collation of medically related information assists promoters, security teams, and

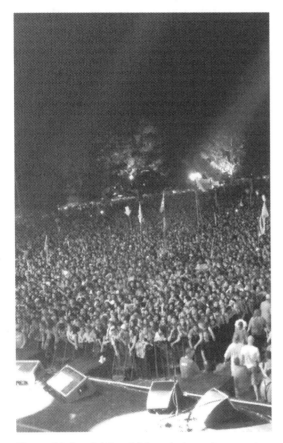

Figure 4.1 Poor lighting, tightly packed crowds, rampant inebriation, and the accompanying loud noise from the event can all create special risks and threats as well as pervasive obstacles to providing rapid medical response, patient retrieval and eventual proper treatment of those becoming ill and injured at mass gathering events.

Photograph (October, 2012) taken and provided with the permission of Dr. Paul Pepe

event planners in their preparations to properly manage future events, be it those involving the home teams' next game or match or those involving upcoming performances in some other city hosting a popular entertainment artist's tour. Accordingly, contingency planning and coordination with promoters, organizers, security teams, and public safety agencies need to involve knowledgeable, experienced medical leaders who are all involved well ahead of time to help optimize outcomes and to better ensure that any prospective patient will be more readily identified, located, and logistically easier to retrieve.

There is, however, no singular roadmap for such considerations. Depending on the type of event, its geographic spread, its anticipated patient volumes, and historical rates of transport, the logistics and staging of medical teams may vary greatly, even for the same type of event. With this understanding, the following chapter will attempt to highlight some of the key components of patient identification, retrieval, dispositions, and transportation planning, but again with the understanding that such planning will need to be adapted and modified depending on the specifics of any given event, the venue, and the timing of the event.

Patient Identification

While patient identification is the first step in providing medical care, finding, assessing, and differentiating very ill or seriously injured patients among all other attendees can be challenging during a mass gathering event. In addition, many attendees manifesting a potential illness or injury may be extremely reticent to even leave their coveted spot in the audience, let alone miss any of the event. In many cases, the attendee may have paid significant amounts of money for premium passes or tickets, traveled from afar to be there, and, in many cases, they may have waited for many months, or even years, to attend the specific event at hand. This understandable and yet concerning refusal to leave the location can lead to awkward and difficult decision-making for responders, especially when dealing with somewhat intoxicated persons or those avoiding the disclosure of any serious underlying medical conditions in that public forum. The psychological and emotional aspects of crowd demographics and dynamics has become a science in itself.

Even beyond the mass gathering situation, on a daily basis, most human beings will also feel embarrassed about needing medical attention especially when friends or family call for help in public places. Be it stoicism, modesty, or simply not wanting to be seen in a vulnerable light among others, the most common and predictable iteration will inevitably be affirmations from that person that he or she is "just fine." Moreover, for similar reasons, they will also most adamantly avoid the embarrassment (in their mind) of being transported by ambulance crews in full view of others. In essence, the psychological aspects of receiving medical attention in public places is a common challenge, particularly when it occurs during a long-awaited, "one-time-only" cherished event for the loyal fan/attendee. Not only should it be well-understood and recognized, but appropriate tactics to manage

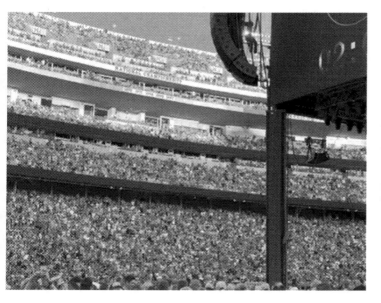

Figure 4.2 Beyond immensely crowded and less controlled floor dynamics, steep stairwells and multifloored buildings can also create significant challenges to medical professionals in terms of rapid response, carrying medical equipment and transport devices to rapidly retrieve and evacuate patients out of the stands. Heat and direct sunlight at these higher levels can also cause additional stressors for at-risk persons attending the mass gathering as well as the rescuers. Among the excitement and common inebriation of celebrating crowds or fans, these elevated perches can also pose additional risks from falls, inter-personal skirmishes, and even falling objects.

Photograph (August 14, 2021) taken and provided with the permission of Dr. Paul Pepe

these psychosocial challenges should be prospectively entertained and include sensitive strategies to enhance privacy, minimize the embarrassment, and yet gain trust using a compassionate demeanor and tone.

While the would-be patient may ultimately decline help altogether and has the capacity to do so, medical responders may still invoke other strategies to ensure the safety of those attendees. At all times, there should be compassionate caring and negotiation and not angry confrontation, not only with such patients, but also with the surrounding bystanders who will be witnessing and often video-recording the encounter. It should be clear that every attempt was made to offer care for the patient and convince him or her to leave with the rescuers for better assessment and management. In some cases, it may involve a discretely negotiated movement to an observation area that may even have better views of the event. Coordination of these situations with security leads is therefore recommended, especially as these interactions under noisy conditions can also be disruptive to other attendees, and particularly if they become prolonged. Alternatively, if the persons still decline to leave their position in the audience, medical and security teams may assign a person to post nearby and continue observation of the person in question.

As previously discussed, even among cooperative persons or those without capacity, there are challenges to persons receiving help. For the patients and bystanders assisting them, not only are there profound obstacles in terms of alerting anyone for assistance within the compacted crowds surrounding them, but also because of the exceptional levels of noise emanating from shouting and cheering crowds and the ambient entertainment for which they came to enjoy.

These factors raise the evolving concept of those requesting help being able to send texts to predesignated emergency numbers, utilize special social media sites or even consider the use of special geospatial locator applications (apps). When crowds are large or if event sites are in more austere locations, standard mobile phones texts or internet use may be slow or inoperative altogether. Also, the request for assistance may require more information to try to describe the exact location from which they are texting. More recently, specialized apps for geospatial locators have been introduced in some locales. Utilization of these mobile apps such as "What3words" may hold great promise in terms of better assisting rescuers in terms of localizing potential patients across widely dispersed sites. However, they are not yet widely used and, in some respects, may have some of the potential limitations that standard texting encounters when there are large audiences or austere conditions. Nonetheless, when these apps have been used, to date they have been shown to be capable of geolocating individuals within a three-meter square zone and do so almost anywhere on the globe using only three words. Using this simple platform, the victim or bystander can quickly relay the three words to a dispatcher enabling them to deploy a more appropriate and targeted resource to a now better defined location.

At the same time, even if eventually alerted to the need for assistance, incoming responders still need to find those persons and reach them under the same obstacles of packed crowds, loud noise, and/or distances from medical aid centers. At other times, the hurdles for rescuers could be a steep stairwell in a stadium and or arena, or they could be incidents occurring at upper levels of a large venue or at some poorly defined location along a longitudinal raceway, parade, or beachside festival.

For the purposes of crowd medicine intelligence gathering and subsequent reporting and planning, it is also important to define what constitutes a reportable patient. Most would define a patient as any person who receives medical care, medical advice, or related supplies from a medical professional [1]. In many situations, patients may just ask for hydration (even just water bottles) for some dizziness or over-the-counter (OTC) medications for headache (e.g., acetaminophen). When otherwise very busy with truly ill and injured persons, these requests may not need to engender a full medical assessment and report. However, medical providers rendering support and advice should still tabulate or annotate such requests to help inform future stocking needs, relevant logistics and planning, and even risk management for future events. Naturally, advice about where to get food or find a toilet does not fall within the specific realm of medical advice, but these frequent interactions should still be anticipated and managed with a knowledgeable, courteous, public service orientation as part of the overall positive experience being provided to attendees.

As previously stated, quickly identifying patients and matching them with an appropriate level of medical response that ensures the most appropriate care and disposition can be challenging under the circumstances of crowd medicine. While this may include providing care on-site in close quarters, extrication of the patient to an aid station, or rapid evacuation from the event premises, logistics planning should always address all of these considerations and be considered integral parts of mass gathering medicine as well as the reporting of logistical difficulties, including how many patients were difficult to reach/retrieve due to barricades, high floor rescue or how often patients decline to leave their cherished spot in the audience.

Despite all of the aforementioned patient-locating and retrieval challenges, at most events, patients will self-identify themselves or, more often, accompanying friends and families will bring them directly to medical aid stations or direct them to event personnel. To facilitate patients being able to readily locate medical resources, medical aid stations should be well-marked with additional signage well above crowd height. Aid stations should be easily accessible, often with accessible pathways and they should be established in sufficient quantities to support anticipated patient presentations. Many of these strategic implementation plans will be based on event history if available, but should also consider potential differences for presumed identical events based on time of year, climate/weather, air quality, and other modifiers. Medical stations should preferably provide room and stools or folding chairs for designated companions as these persons can be invaluable in terms of reporting what happened, relaying any symptoms or signs observed, conveying any known past history, medical or otherwise. They may even have knowledge of current medications or allergies and they can also provide some key emergency contacts especially when the patient is incoherent, significantly intoxicated or otherwise noncommunicative or noncooperative. Being able to interact with these companions and observe them directly, medical practitioners can better judge that they would likely be competent persons who can reliably accompany and observe the patient if they were to be treated and released on-site. This can diminish the need for more extended observation and thus help with turnover and free up beds at the on-site medical stations. Many times they serve well as additional patient "monitors" sitting and communicating with their loved ones/companions.

In large stadiums and arenas, medical care sites may be staged on numerous levels, or they may be supplemented with makeshift temporary locations when very large crowds are anticipated, or if the geography of the event is expansive. Again, while on any given day there can be variation from one similar event to another, patient presentations and transport patterns from previous or similar events should still be taken into account to help address predictable staffing patterns, particularly for these more challenging events [2]. As noted in other chapters of this text, patient presentation and transport rates will most often be determined by on-site attendance, attendee density, event geography, weather and climate factors, distance traveled to the event, and the type of mass gathering populations including the demographics and historical behaviors of audiences usually attracted to the specific event in question.

As previously stated, most patients will self-identify or be identified by accompanying friends and families [3]. Many others will be identified by bystanders or event staff. Designated event staff groups, or specific individuals, should be leveraged for this role, including ushers, vendors, and, very often, security staff. The addition of dedicated spotters can be particularly helpful during certain events, particularly those activities allowing on-site camping or events known to have high patient presentation rates such as endurance sports or those very crowded events involving exceptional levels of alcohol consumption and events transpiring during days of high heat and humidity.

Such dedicated spotters are usually nonmedical personnel who can assist with medical reconnaissance, but also can be trained to provide basic first aid training. Spotters ideally will have basic first aid training and even know how to provide immediate lifesaving interventions, including hemorrhage control and CPR.

Simple protocols can be put in place that will better enable these individuals to support the medical staff when they identify potential patients, pinpoint their precise location, and begin basic first aid. They would also be knowledgeable about the location of the closest automated external defibrillator (AED), opioid reversal medications or bleeding control kits.

In some circumstances, spotters may even fall under the auspices of embedded law enforcement or tactical teams that are already scanning and observing the crowd for suspicious behaviors or other possible criminal activities. Again, basic first aid should already be part of those persons' basic training as well.

Whoever they are, spotters would also have a working knowledge of seating set-ups or predefined location markers. They should be familiar with "stage left" or "stage right" or "front of house console" terminology or be familiar with mile-marker or light post numbering systems and the like. Ability to communicate with medical and security personnel, effectively and accurately, is also a critical related function. Texting abilities and well-delineated directions and meeting points are key components of training and preparation.

Spotters should be strategically positioned to have a wide view of attendees, while also being close enough to see the potential patients. Elevated positions are usually best for visualizing large crowds and the spotters may be placed higher up in a post that does not obstruct views of the event, and ideally positioned on the periphery of the audience or in a watch tower, such as a police tower seen at some fairgrounds or racing venues. Binoculars should be a routine consideration depending on the venue size. Spotters can also be embedded within the crowd depending on audience density and event type. In all circumstances, spotters should be protected from the elements, including protection from precipitation, and provided with appropriate heating or cooling strategies.

Once identified by such spotters, or other event staff, the patient's location must be effectively, efficiently, and accurately communicated to responsible event medical personnel and/or public safety incident commanders. Communications protocols and back-up mechanisms must be established in advance and should include a "care escalation" pathway. Surrounding noise, dense crowds, dark conditions, and extended, unmarked geography may make communicating a patient location exceptionally challenging or make a medical cart retrieval unfeasible.

Beyond the crowd, gaining access to patients over a barricade fence poses physical challenges to rescuers. At the same time, in situations in which the patient care needs to be provided on the ground, finding the patient is even more difficult as incoming responders may not have a direct line of sight. Clearly marked and well-defined event locations can help guide the medical response. Asking rescuers or a bystander to alert incoming rescuers with light signals or specialized flagging can help when there is a deep crowd and dark conditions. In contrast, in widely dispersed events, such as ultra-marathons, electronic trackers can be used to provide precise global positioning satellite (GPS) locations such as those seen with ride-share applications. Mile markers or utility poles marked with large numbers or different colors can be used in road races or longitudinal events such as beachside festivals or inner city parades. Likewise, stadiums, large arenas, and all other venues should use consistent naming conventions for venue landmarks. Temporary event sites, including Black Rock City, have effectively used named street addresses, and, as mentioned before, flagging or specialized alerting light systems to help medical personnel identify patient locations in crowds [4]. Other organizers will use numbering systems that can be seen at great distances or will encourage event attendee use of apps such as the What3Words app.

For rescuers, one area of grave concern and compromised access is when sudden stampeding or crowd crush innately blocks access to injured patients. This challenge was highlighted following a crowd crush incident in Houston, Texas (USA) in November 2021 that resulted in eight deaths and many more injuries. In that sense, logistical planning and security protocols should take such potential events into account to set up mechanisms for responder access and rapid crowd decompression and egress as well as *immediate* interruption of the event itself if not already halted.

Consideration must also be given to patients located outside of the immediate event area or venue. Systems must be in place to monitor for and identify patients in parking lots or in event entrance queues. Some long-awaited events will engender lengthy outdoor queues extending for several days in a variety of challenging climates and limited access to food and water. Therefore, event staff, spotters, or even medical personnel should also be positioned external to the event venue in areas where attendees are expected to congregate over many hours, if not days, in advance.

In certain unbounded events, the areas of concern may encompass substantial geography. Accordingly, mutual aid agreements between local jurisdictions and event personnel should be established beforehand. Substantial local resources may be used for a major multiday music festival such as the Electric Daisy Carnival ("EDC"), a Formula One event or a National Football League championship. The additional populations coming in to attend or work at the event, and those driving home inebriated after the event, or simply those enjoying a typical weekend away evening in the affected community, can tax local EMS response capabilities. This is compounded by any additional associated traffic obstacles or event-driven detours, purposeful diversions, and additional pedestrian traffic.

The logistics and patient identification concerns for multiday mass gatherings can also benefit from partnerships with public health organizations performing syndromic surveillance for early identification of potential disease outbreaks or climate, environmental and air quality concerns [2, 5, 7]. Of particular concern are those mass gathering events that involve communal living, such as camping festivals or large-scale havens quickly formed for evacuees sheltering together after leaving a major disaster or military conflict zone. Local disease outbreaks can occur rapidly and should be monitored closely such as the local measles outbreak that occurred just prior to the 2010 Fédération Internationale de Football Association (FIFA) World Cup in South Africa. Similarly, following the landfall of Hurricane Katrina in the US gulf coast in 2005 and prior to instituting strict hygiene and sanitizer interventions at the shelter, gastrointestinal viral outbreaks were routinely seen after several days of harboring tens of thousands of displaced evacuees in various respective convention center shelters throughout Texas and elsewhere [7]. Public health interventions have now become an important consideration in the mass gathering events, particularly in the wake of the COVID-19 pandemic in 2020 and 2021.

Surveillance systems monitoring local healthcare centers are now routinely used for mass gatherings [5, 8] and this surveillance capability is easier when such systems are already in place [9]. Surveillance may include data from agencies supporting the event, as well as other area healthcare facilities or pharmacies. For example, a sudden uptick in the purchase of over-the-counter (OTC) antidiarrheal medications can be a signal. Likewise, an uptick in patients presenting with pulmonary problems may identify the actual severity of air quality problems despite the reported level of the local air quality index (AQI). Knowing the endemic presence or increased presence of snakes, ticks, or other pests, often instigated by the event itself, is also helpful. In many circumstances, communications with local EMS and other public health or emergency facilities can also help to identify local toxicology concerns including the latest profile of recreational and illicit drugs or tainted legal substances. All these considerations impact planning, anticipated logistical demands, and the resources that will be needed to assist in more rapid identification of persons or groups of persons who may need attention.

Documentation and Patient Tracking

Every mass gathering event should have an internal documentation system and every relevant patient encounter should be documented. All applicable local, state, county, and federal regulations for documenting patient care must be followed as if it were occurring in any other routine medical facility. Event attendees will often visit aid stations for medically related supplies without any expectation of evaluation or treatment, such as requests for sunscreen, hearing protection or small bandages. As stated previously, in those cases for which no medical assessment or care was rendered or required, a preestablished protocol should still be established to account for and tabulate all of these visits and any supplies used or distributed. As these individuals do not meet the appropriate definition of a patient [1], the detail and need to document these cases will vary particularly in events where the medical providers are overwhelmed by unanticipated challenges such as a sudden outbreak of overdoses, heat exhaustion, or injuries. Otherwise, any patient for whom medical care was rendered, including distribution of OTC medications, should be documented as a patient, even if in a separate, expedited, simpler record or tracking system to help predict future stocking needs.

For smaller events, the electronic medical record of the EMS agency or local healthcare system staffing the event may be used, or that of any other participating emergency care entity. For larger events, custom-built medical records may be preferred to help expedite efficiency and optimal content by tailoring it to likely issues that arise, be it intoxication-related, injury/laceration-related, heat-related, or other common conditions in mass gatherings including cardiac arrest, coronary artery syndromes, stroke, hypoglycemia, or respiratory problems. Of course, in case of digital failure, back-up charting mechanisms should be part of the stocking portfolio.

Whatever system is used, it should facilitate conveyance of key information that receiving facilities will need to know considering that the on-site treating responders will usually be transferring care and information to secondary responders who must relay secondhand information. At the same, there may be little time to create comprehensive medical records if on-site teams are overwhelmed with cases. Some first aid tents and on-site clinics will thus assign knowledgeable medical care practitioners such as an experienced nurse or medical resident or registrar to act as a scribe. They can create the bulk of reports while others are providing direct medical care, a configuration frequently used in hospital resuscitation rooms.

Once patients are identified and care is initiated, it is important that all patient care and movements are tracked for situational awareness and accountability. Patient tracking will help to ensure appropriate allocation of healthcare resources and patient distribution across receiving healthcare settings, particularly during multiday events. Furthermore, it will facilitate family or companion reunification and also accountability in

the event of a missing person. Finally, patient tracking is important for reporting, financial information and data collation that will help in planning for future events.

The patient tracking system should be established prior to the event whenever possible and it should utilize resources already available in the community and at corresponding receiving centers. When developing tools for patient tracking, all agencies and organizations involved in patient care and transportation should be collaborating ahead of time to establish and have knowledge of the working protocols for tracking. Those collaborating stakeholders should include event organizers, on-site healthcare providers, public safety personnel, and particularly EMS agencies and receiving facilities, including both hospitals and relevant clinics.

Despite best efforts to track all patients, as seen in the Route 91 Harvest Festival sniper shootings (October 1, 2017) near the Las Vegas Boulevard in Clark County, Nevada (USA), many persons will be taken from the scene by rideshare vehicles, police or other private vehicles and hospitals may be overwhelmed with untracked patients. While having tracking, demographic, and clinical information integrated into a comprehensive electronic medical record is an idealistic concept, it may not always be practical for most events. In such circumstances, designated public safety personnel in the command center can be assigned to constantly survey receiving facilities in real-time for their latest sense of relative capacities. Depending on the number of unanticipated arrivals at a given hospitals, this capacity capability may change rapidly and proceed up and down in a dynamic manner.

As previously indicated, in certain events, particularly some endurance sporting events involving mass gatherings such as marathons or ironman triathlons, electronic participant tracking tools, including GPS trackers and microchip imbedded bibs, lend themselves well to improved patient tracking. Accordingly, these electronic patient tracking tools have significant advantages over traditional tracking methods, including real-time assessments of resource allocation [10]. Radiofrequency identification (RFID) tracking systems are another option, as are bar-coded identification and tracking systems.

The US city of Chicago recently implemented a patient tracking system using bar-coded wristbands during mass gathering events [11]. Patients can be evaluated on-site and have a wristband placed by EMS which, in turn, can be scanned by the attending EMS agency (or other transporting entities) and then rescanned at the receiving hospital. This allows for real-time patient tracking via a web-based platform. Such regionwide tracking systems are not only useful to know when, where and how many patients are moved from the scene to receiving centers, but it can also help with resource allocation and hospital load-leveling, especially during the much larger events or a multicasualty incident (MCI). In addition to incorporating a standardized patient tracking format, standardized nomenclature for patient identification and triage is also useful, particularly when anticipating a potential MCI. During the 2013 Boston, Massachusetts (USA) marathon-related bombings, one lesson learned to avoid was the confusion created when unstandardized, random identifiers were used to identify unknown patients [12].

In general, the technological concept of incorporating an electronic tracking system into every attendee's credentials, as part of their ticket purchase or event registration, could conceivably become part and parcel to the evolving future of mass gathering medicine and its effectiveness. Beyond identification and accounting for attendees following an evacuation for MCIs or the identification and location of a child who is lost or abducted, the concept of incorporating a GPS component to help track attendees' whereabouts could be invaluable in many respects. In fact, it could also be applied to all staff working at the event, including the medical staff who could even receive a medical response assignment based on their proximity and other logistics.

Akin to the marathoner runner's bib microchip previously discussed, this concept could be extended to help locate on-scene victims, dead or alive, after an MCI or help to find departed attendees after being transported by means other than ambulance to an area hospital. It may help to better pinpoint the location of an ill or injured persons within a crowd, but, better yet, such a microchip may also be capable of providing very basic but important demographics and information (age, emergency contacts, and even an optional component for prospectively providing important medical information). This would be helpful if the person being attended is found unconscious or unable to communicate. If used for that purpose, special microchip reader devices would be used and only provided in confidential manner to certain senior on-site medical professionals who maintain professional confidentiality.

In some countries or cultures, such a tracking concept may seem unacceptable and portrayed as an Orwellian technique or unnecessary invasion of privacy. However, during the early stages of the COVID-19 pandemic, several technologies did arise that linked a negative COVID-19 test to the ticket purchase or registration to the event which, in ensuing months, also was applied to electronic tracking of vaccinations or negative COVID-19 testing as a criterion for admission. While some patrons may have objected, organizers of such events generally received positive feedback as participants believed that they felt safer with such policies and mechanisms in place.

Surveys have shown that, in the post-9-11 era, when airport security was heightened, most travelers eventually agreed with the much stricter policies as it provided a better sense of safety and security and eventually was accepted as the norm. Today, when presenting one's "real-IDs" or passports at the time of moving through security checkpoints, those identification data are already linked in many cases to the airline data bases. The linked data provide the passport holder's individual flight number and destinations in real-time to the airport security official checking the passenger at the time of departure, or the customs and immigration agents checking at the time of arrival. In essence, forms of tracking are now better accepted for the purposes of safety. It is also well-known in today's society that mobile phones can be readily tracked and video cameras abound. In that respect, in the case of tracking event attendees with the event credential, such tracking would be limited to the event only and inactivated soon after the end of the event (assuming no MCI has occurred) and disposed of by the attendee. In essence, while such concepts would seem conceptually threatening at first glance, their eventual implementation and routine use in one form or another during mass gatherings is neither inconceivable nor unfeasible. This is particularly acceptable when considering the public's overriding expectation to have organizers do whatever they can to better ensure the safety and security of all attendees so that the event itself can be consistently enjoyed.

In the meantime, in terms of record-keeping and patient tracking, third-party solutions and web-based applications do exist and have been used successfully in some scenarios [13, 14]. In the end, the best attempts to account for each and every patient should be made, especially for the sake of family and loved ones needing to reunite or identify their injured (or ill) mass gathering event attendee.

As a final note, paper tracking tools are readily available and straightforward to use. Importantly, with power system failures, malevolent hacking, or some type of device malfunction, the paper tools are required as a back-up system in case of any digital system collapse. Nonetheless, they also are subject to loss, human error, and are often illegible. In many cases, they have limitations in terms of the amount of patient information that they can capture. In addition, paper tracking tools, including triage tags in particular, are subject to weather and environmental exposure and may be easily torn, lost, or become unreadable or stained in wet conditions. Plans should account and prepare for such circumstances.

Patient Transportation

During a mass gathering event, intra-venue patient transportation may occur within the event site, or patients may be transported off-site to a receiving medical center. Transportation within the event site will depend on multiple factors, including the terrain, barricades, geographic spread of the event, vertical challenges, and crowd density. For example, transportation within a sports venue on a paved concourse will vary significantly from the transportation required within a music festival covering a large area on open terrain and particularly on a sandy beachside or on a soggy grass field or muddy desert after a heavy rain. Extricating patients out of stands or seats (Figure 4.2) can be challenging depending on the steepness and configuration of seating and stairwells. In this case, patient movement may require transport via a stair chair or even folding military cots. Alternatively, patients may even need to be carried a short distance. Once out of the seats or stands and on traditional stretchers, patients will need to be moved to a definitive care area via elevators or ramps, either directly on a stretcher or by a cart vehicle. Dedicated elevators or access to situationally cleared elevators are important parts of the plan but also anticipation of power failure should be considered.

In certain situations, medical personnel should expect to be accompanied by security personnel and event staff during many phases of access and egress. Those support personnel would help to facilitate

crowd penetration, adequate space for patient assessment, and rapid patient extrication. Crowd control is essential to facilitate patient movement, and security therefore should be there for assistance, especially in dense crowds where access to the patient may be limited or obstructed. Likewise, the crowds themselves, often intoxicated, may pose a potential threat to the safety of responding personnel [15]. As such, ingress and egress plans for mass gatherings should be carefully planned far in advance of the event and should account for crowd size. Lack of sufficient access points not only provides a significant risk to attendees but makes transportation of patients challenging [16]. Again, the November 2021 stampede and crush injury event at a musical festival in Houston, Texas (USA) highlights that medical care and extrication can be affected by such issues. Dedicated transportation routes and emergency access lanes for emergency personnel and vehicles are often used and can be exceptionally useful for both medical and security purposes. In essence, security and medical teams should be well-integrated and actions choreographed long before the event. As discussed in another chapter (Chapter 24), some leading event medicine physicians are assigned often as part of the security team to help facilitate that choreography.

Once extricated from the crowd or stands, the retrieved patient must be brought rapidly to an area that is appropriate for evaluation and intervention. A resuscitation area may not always be a first aid center, but rather right on-site or a reasonably feasible location proximal to the incident site when time-sensitive interventions such as CPR need to be initiated immediately, even if it disrupts the event. In March of 2014, a professional hockey player in Dallas, TX (USA) experienced a cardiac arrest during the game and was immediately resuscitated next to the team's rink-side bench, facilitating a good patient outcome. Of note, for a remarkable few minutes, this incident rapidly quieted the entire crowd of 20,000 onlookers while rescuers provided immediate CPR and resuscitated this surviving athlete with a well-placed AED and well-drilled medical choreography. The player regained consciousness within minutes and, as a result of this rapid intervention, eventually returned to normal health and function. A similar cardiac arrest event occurred in Cincinnati, Ohio, on January 2, 2023, during a live professional American football television broadcast with millions of observers. The incident halted the game and care began at the site mid-field. With well-placed equipment and a pre-planned, well-choreographed pit crew approach, the player was revived and was soon back to work because of the rapid mid-field actions that continued on-site until the patient was resuscitated.

During rapid extrication, thorough evaluation and monitoring may not be feasible. However, a brief assessment including a quick look at the mucous membranes of the conjunctiva bilaterally to see if they are pink in an impaired or unconscious person may be helpful. Evaluating with a portable (battery-operated) finger pulse oximeter can also provide useful information, including heart rate, its regularity and peripheral tissue oxygen saturation, which may also help to guide decision-making regarding immediate extrication to a medical aid station or even more emergent intervention is required immediately on-site.

Within a venue, multiple means of patient transport may be necessary. Nonambulatory patients may require lifting or being carried for a short distance out of seats or spectator stands or they may need to be hoisted over a barricade. In either situation, they should be transitioned quickly to a stretcher or other transport device/vehicle. For sports arenas or other venues with hard or paved surfaces, wheeled chairs or transport stretchers and electric carts can be used. For transport over longer distances or over softer ground (sand, soggy grassland, mud) all-terrain vehicles (Figure 4.3) can be employed with the understanding that their heavier weight can also be a compromising factor. In turn, routes should be tested ahead of time and retested throughout the event if, as often happens, the environment changes.

Likewise, when responsible for larger areas, transportation by ambulance or utility vehicle may be considered, depending on terrain. While the use of motorized vehicles can be helpful, event planners should also consider risks to other event attendees as these vehicles may need to move in densely populated, crowded, and highly trafficked areas. Dense crowds may prohibit patient access, and vehicles should be prestaged whenever possible to reduce response times and to increase reliable and timely egress within the event site.

When moving a patient within an event venue, additional consideration should be given to sociological and environmental factors. For example, efforts should be made to maintain patient privacy during public areas of transport. As mentioned, the patient should be shielded from attempts at bystander

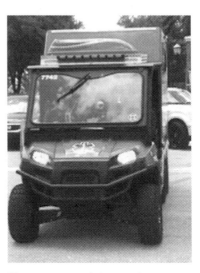

Figure 4.3 Particularly at outdoor events, smaller all-terrain vehicles and similar electric carts can be very useful in mass gatherings, particularly those vehicles capable of holding a patient stretcher and capable of maneuvering more facilely through dense crowds, often in amply allotted lanes. It is preferred if these transport unit can also shield patients from direct sunlight and other weather-related or sociological elements including shielding the patients from opportunistic photography and other behavioral challenges from the passing crowds.

Photograph (March 24, 2018) taken and provided with the permission of Dr. Paul Pepe

videography or any type of encounter from other attendees. This protective spirit should also include a professional and congenial countenance despite attempted confrontations by difficult and often intoxicated persons. Again, the coordination with security teams is important.

At the same time, one should anticipate that, during the movement process, the patient could vomit, seize, or otherwise rise up suddenly. Tactics that anticipate those occurrences should be entertained proactively. In addition, the patient should be further protected from the environment whenever possible during assessment and transport, especially when outdoors. In direct sunlight or on a hot day, someone should be positioned to block direct sunlight on the patient and even provide some fanning. Transport through a concourse or other covered area is ideal if possible. In contrast, with cold weather, blankets should be provided, and the patient should be protected from rain or snow, both for comfort and to maintain body temperature. Eye protection may be necessary depending on the weather and terrain, and efforts should be made to protect the patient from exposure to insects, fumes, or other noxious conditions.

Regarding videoing and photographing of the patient, rescuers should also keep in mind that their own behavior and performance and on-scene discussions will be recorded for posterity and left to public scrutiny. Confrontation with surrounding audience members or others witnessing the incident should be avoided even if these behaviors are combative or inappropriately confrontational. All efforts to exude confidence and control under such challenging circumstances are critical to a good outcome for both patients and rescuers alike and it improves the respect and acceptance of event medicine practice.

After temporizing care is provided on-scene, the patient may require transport to a receiving hospital for definitive care. This type of disposition will often require a priori partnerships with local or regional public transporting EMS agencies or designated private ambulance services in some cases. Depending on anticipated patient transport rates, it may be beneficial to have transporting ambulances and their crews staged within the event venue to facilitate a smooth handover and timely transport. In certain cases, it may be in the patient's best interest to be transported immediately, bypassing on-site facilities. For example, a patient with major trauma or one with acute-onset hemiparesis and normal glucose levels might be extricated from the stands and moved directly to an ambulance for transport to a designated trauma center or comprehensive stroke center as indicated. Accordingly, the actual process and designated locations for the handover of patient care from event medical staff to transporting EMS providers should be established well ahead of time.

Outside of the venue site itself, many organizers purposely create several wide-laned roadways, often newly formed by barricades that maintain bidirectional lanes for rapid evacuation. These rapid evacuation lanes would be used for motorcaded principals, but also for outbound emergency vehicles transporting to hospitals as well as responding (inbound) or returning ambulances and law enforcement vehicles. Anticipating and preparing for the reality of a potential MCI or other security-based circumstance is a critical component of the overall transportation planning component and several of these protected lanes and entry points should be created in case one is compromised by a sudden structural collapse, explosion, active shooter incident, or other forms of obstruction.

Usual access routes to a mass gathering location, especially during a mass evacuation, may be compromised due to crowds, road closures, or traffic. Again, mass gathering event organizers (and medical staff) must plan for dedicated public safety lanes, preferably multiple, at the event site and on local roads to facilitate unobstructed ambulance access to the event as well as unimpeded departure as needed. The inability to rapidly transport patients in previous mass gatherings has resulted in avoidable morbidity [15].

In some circumstances, ground transportation may be impractical, heavily delayed, or severely compromised. Also, the venue may be very distant to optimal receiving facilities for the particular condition. In turn, air medical evacuation may be necessary. Landing zones for air ambulances, and possibly in the future, "reclining passenger" single operator drone units, may be utilized with safe landing zones that are well-identified and well-marked. Again, the event terrain itself must also be considered. For example, dust clouds caused by helicopter rotor wash at Burning Man festivals have created helicopter transportation challenges. Manned drones or fixed-wing transport may eventually become necessary alternatives or ground to air transportation intercepts at a location some distance away from the primary site [4]. For MCIs challenged by rapid extrication or structural collapse, drones might even be used in the future to deliver large numbers of blood products as indicated.

During planning, it should be appreciated that patient transport rates from mass gathering events have varied quite widely from 0.5 percent to 12 percent of patient presentations [3]. Ironically, beyond bombings and active shooter events, some of the events generating very high rates of transport have been among young, relatively healthy persons who are attending festivals with intra-site to site movement, lengthy hours of festivity and consumption of indeterminate types of drugs that have proven to be quite toxic. The number of resources needed to meet the expected patient transport rate should be carefully considered far ahead of time with back-up plans in anticipation of a potential MCI including large numbers of intoxications and drug overdoses. Efforts should be made to minimize ambulance turnaround time at hospitals and thus improve ambulance availability under these circumstances. Transporting multiple patients in the same transport vehicle can increase efficiency and especially if they are from the same family. This option also assumes that there is sufficient staff for safe patient care and that the vehicle is appropriately licensed for multipatient transport.

Finally, consideration should be given to others requesting to be transported with the patient. This may include friends or family members, athletic trainers, or VIP/dignitary protective details. As noted in the earlier discussion, their involvement may be critical to identifying appropriate patient assessment and management. Whenever possible, accompanying personnel should be allowed to ride along, but the ultimate decision will rest with the transporting agency, dependent on available space, regulatory prohibitions, patient acuity and exposure of that accompanying person to a potential psychologically traumatic experience or even physical harm.

Evacuation

Evacuating a mass gathering event is a challenge and not always free of several downsides and complications. While mass evacuation is a relatively infrequent endeavor, it still needs to be anticipated and mitigated. For example, mass evacuations can lead to severe falls, tripping, and even crush injuries among other complications. It also creates a spectrum of emotions ranging from apprehension and being frightened to frank anger for having to leave and miss the purchased entertainment, match or rally of which the guest is now being deprived. In turn, it requires the careful coordination of event staff and public safety personnel. Common reasons for sudden evacuation may be accidental fire or smoke in an arena, a concerning bomb threat or an open stadium about to experience a sudden severe weather event or lightning strikes.

Plans for mass evacuation should be made far in advance of any event and egress routes tested. There should be multiple well-marked egress routes positioned to eliminate bottlenecks and ensure smooth outbound flow, which ideally should be unidirectional [15, 16]. Plans should consider the movement and transport of multiple nonambulatory patients by litter, stair chair, or stretcher especially with many attending persons with disabilities (see Chapter 18). Depending on the reason for the needed evacuation, elevator service may be unreliable or unavailable and alternate routes must be established, especially for the disabled and other vulnerable populations who are at higher risk of injury. Finally, the location of a designated casualty clearing station (or two) should

be identified prior to the event [17]. For reasons stated, plans should be in place for mobilizing regional MCI resources, including multipatient transport vehicles and mutual aid.

Stampedes and crowd crush are a concern in any evacuation of a mass gathering site [18]. They are often triggered by an incident that causes mass panic and a rush to exit the venue such as an explosion or perceived gunshots being fired. Again, these events can result in trampling, body crush, and even death from asphyxiation or traumatic injury. Therefore, attendees should be escorted and guided through the venue in a calm and orderly fashion. A clear incident command structure will help to provide order and effective guidance. The decision to evacuate should be made by the incident commander or designated decision makers, such as production and security staff in conjunction with venue leadership. Those roles must be designated ahead of time and drills to help orchestrate a flow of attendees guided by security personnel must be part of training before the event. Such a process enabled the successful evacuation of 70,000 attendees at Spain's Santiago Bernabeu stadium in just 8 minutes without incident in 2014 following a bomb threat [19].

Communication

A communications plan is essential for any mass gathering and the medical practitioners working within that context. Communications plans must consider not only internal communications but communications with external partners as well. Prior to the event, a medical communication plan should be established, including direct contact information or dedicated phone lines or alert systems for receiving facilities, local public safety agencies, transporting EMS agencies, and the on-site command staff as well. Such communications may involve the use of runners with written messages in case mobile systems failures.

Best practices for the incident command structure should be identified ahead of time and followed, including a dedicated medical communication channel and the establishment of a medical sector command post, whether or not it is embedded within the main command post [2]. Nonmedical personnel should be familiar with the medical communications plan and know how to hail medical personnel in the event of an emergency. Some event venues will have readily available communication systems, including phone lines, public address systems, and even repeaters for radio communications. For other events, communication equipment and systems will need to be installed on-site prior to the event. Whatever mechanisms are used, redundancies and back-up systems are critical including texting capabilities, voice phones, and specialized radio systems with noise buffering as indicated.

As very loud noise pollution is indeed an anticipated and significant challenge in dense crowds and especially at particularly loud events and concerts, redundant methods of communication among staff are truly essential. As noted, text or SMS messaging is one option to help contend with noise pollution [20]. However, direct, in-person communication via runners may also be useful to facilitate communication or to fill requests for supplies or equipment. Specialized flagging or flashing light systems are other options for communicating important information that cannot rely on radio systems.

Mass gathering event considerations include not only communications between event personnel and venue staff, but also communication between event staff and attendees. Clear signage should alert attendees and participants to the location of medical resources, including aid stations, hydration and cooling facilities, and locations of AEDs and bleeding control kits. Oftentimes, prospective communications by news outlets or social media can help to alert persons as to how to remain safe, stay hydrated, use a buddy system, or provide information on how to find event staff, medical care, or a public safety official in a crowded circumstance. For example, for a major professional championship celebration parade held on a hot, humid day with over 100,000 persons packed along several miles of a major city's streets and the spectators having positioned themselves many hours before to gain an optimal viewing, prospective public communication could be invaluable. Beyond media recommendations for wearing the "3 L's of light-colored, loose-fitting, light-weight clothing" and staying well-hydrated, the prospective recommendations could also give instructions to companions to look out for each other using a "buddy system" with each one knowing how to identify nearby public safety personnel such as police, fire, or EMS.

Egress and evacuation routes should also be easily identifiable and communicated in advance as is done on an airplane flight or during an elementary school fire drill. Signage should be clear and information

should be provided in multiple languages. Additional notifications, including weather alerts, can be amplified through pre-event announcements, public address systems, mass text messages, stadium "mega" videoboards, or event "apps." Social media is a growing mechanism for the real-time communication of important information to event attendees.

If an on-site PSAP has been established, protocols for routing calls to this on-site, event-specific PSAP should be established. A centralized dispatcher is helpful to coordinate communication between medical personnel, including responding and transporting personnel [4]. It is likely, however, that event attendees may call the local public safety answering point (PSAP) if encountering a medical emergency (e.g., 999 in the United Kingdom, 911 in North America, 112 in Europe, 0-0-0 in Australia). Prospective communication and provision of the relevant local numbers to attendees is vital, especially if international audiences are expected to be large and those guests will need the applicable country code and a relevant multidigit number [3].

At the same time, with all of the excessive noise from the stadium, parade or race site, PSAP operators may not understand what the mobile caller is saying, especially with windy or other noise-generating conditions. In that respect, some PSAPs have considered having a dedicated texting app that allows them to text back to the caller (using their caller identification number) and thus exchange information through that format.

Event-dedicated medical staff should be able to communicate via a dedicated radio channel established specifically for medical communications. Unified command should be established to ensure effective communication between medical staff, security staff, and other essential intra-venue personnel. Ideally, this central command area will have a good view of the event area, supported by closed circuit cameras. Likewise, communication with external partners is also essential for a successful medical response to a mass gathering event. Receiving facilities should be notified prior to any patient transports, and event command staff should maintain situational awareness as to the fluctuating capacity at receiving facilities [21]. Particularly in an MCI or other events generating many hospital transports, a dedicated medical staff person (or persons) should be assigned who can establish and maintain a bidirectional communication with all receiving facilities that will help to better ensure patient load-leveling at all appropriate facilities and thus reduce the likelihood that any facility will become over-extended with event-related patients. Effective communication between event staff, public safety, and receiving hospitals was integral to the effective and efficient medical response observed during and following the April 15, 2013, Boston marathon bombing [22]. Beyond the risk for MCIs, receiving hospitals should be alerted and informed of the event size, its duration, and anticipated patient transport volumes far in advance of the event to ensure adequate resources and staffing.

As previously indicated, prospective and real-time communication with local or regional public health and law enforcement authorities is also important. Effective communication will maintain awareness of local medical threats and mitigate event impacts [23]. For larger events or gatherings spanning a larger geographic region, not only are mutual aid agreements with additional public safety agencies important, but a clear process for communicating and activating this mutual aid response and how the concomitant incident command systems can be contacted and the applicable communications protocols will be rolled out.

Special Circumstances

Specialized plans should be established to address the medical care of high-profile event attendees, including dignitaries, celebrities, public figures, or other high-profile personnel, especially those requiring special security details or insulation from media and other privacy-compromising sources. Most mass gatherings occur because of such persons including rock stars providing the music on-stage, professional athletes competing on the pitch or raceway, religious leaders such as the Pope visiting the faithful, or a political figure running for office. In addition, fellow celebrities or political figures may be in attendance as friends or guests of the principals and family members may also be in attendance as well.

While the medical care provided to all event attendees, including these celebrated personalities, should be of the highest quality, such individuals still pose certain challenges that bear advanced planning and preparation as previously alluded (Chapter 14). Among considerations will be establishment of an alternative care space, safe places and evacuation points that allow for added safety and security, maintenance of privacy, and avoidance of crowd interference with treatment. Plans for tracking such individuals and identification of appropriate destination facilities should be made ahead of time, including how these persons should be identified and to whom inquiries from the media should be directed. Such protocols are often preemptively established by agencies such as the US Secret Service (USSS) and its counterpart agencies or military for other nations. To maintain security, access to information regarding the location and movement of these individuals should be limited and directed by the assigned security teams.

Protocols for media inquiries should be established, with all media inquiries ideally routed to a prospectively designated public information officer (PIO) or media relations personnel. As noted, many high-profile individuals travel with additional security and medical personnel. Event medical staff should therefore understand the nuances of those existing relationships and work closely with those counterparts to ensure that any concerns are being addressed while also ensuring that all local protocols are followed.

As previously mentioned about the psychological and emotional aspects of dealing with the medical response to fans and attendees, declination of transport is also common among those serving the dignitary whether it is the personal assistant to a prime minister or celebrity entertainer who are assigned to what are considered essential tasks that only they can perform. Their sense of loyalty and concerns over abandonment can be quite passionate and they will often defy concerns over their own potential life-threatening conditions as a result. Creative accommodations may need to be considered when faced with their informed declination of evaluation and transport. One might consider assigning a designated and qualified medical care professional to provide individualized stand-by monitoring and observation of that person. In turn, when such dedicated members of the entourage perceive that they are relatively freed from their urgent duties, hopefully, they will then be ready and willing to receive proper evaluation and treatment. If feasible, developing trust during the stand-by period is also a key strategy. Such situations can occur frequently and they can be unsettling and angering to a prudent medical professional. However, the most successful patient advocates in these situations exhibit a demeanor of cheerful patience, compassion, and understanding for those who have full capacity but still possess an intense and overriding loyalty to the greater cause and willing to risk themselves accordingly.

Depending on the possible medical threat, security threat, and cleared background checks, a dedicated medical detail may be necessary for the principals and their entourage. Nonetheless, such special assignments should be adopted as long as they are planned as such and will not adversely affect the medical care provided to other event attendees. Detailed approaches and contingencies for these added complexities are addressed in Chapter 14 of this textbook.

Other special circumstances that are of additional concern are those that involve at-risk populations such as the elderly, the very young and the displaced. Be it a papal visit bringing out the elderly faithful onto a sun-drenched Sunday afternoon park site or an encampment receiving several convoys of refugees arriving from war-torn countries like Afghanistan, Syria, the Gaza or Ukraine, these are special populations that require a much broader span of attention and resources. Accordingly, a detailed discussion regarding this additional level of complexity affecting medical logistics is addressed in Chapter 18 of this textbook.

Summary

Mass gatherings create special challenges for medical responders, both logistically and medically. However, well-organized systems of care, excellent record keeping, and novel patient tracking techniques can help to hopefully mitigate these obstacles and improve planning and patient outcomes. Prospective coordination and real-time communications with local public health authorities, law enforcement teams and receiving facilities are key elements to help identify patient management resource needs and well-implemented retrieval and evacuation plans as are specialized logistical coordination with on-site security teams.

References

1. Yancey A., Luk J., Milsten A., Nafziger A. *Mass Gathering Medical Care Planning: The Medical Sector Checklist*. National Association of EMS Physicians; 2017.

2. Margolis A. M., Leung A. K., Friedman M. S., McMullen S. P., Guyette F. X., Woltman N. Position Statement: Mass Gathering Medical Care. *Prehospital Emergency Care*. 2021;**25**(4):593–595.

3. Locoh-Donou S. M. S., Guofen Y. P., Welcher M. E. M. T., Berry T. M. P. H., O'Connor R. E. M. D. M. P. H., Brady W. J. M. D. Mass-Gathering Medicine: A Descriptive Analysis of a Range of Mass-Gathering Event Types. *The American Journal of Emergency Medicine*. 2013;**31**(5):843–846.

4. Bledsoe B., Songer P., Buchanan K., Westin J., Hodnick R., Gorosh L. Burning Man 2011: Mass Gathering Medical Care in an Austere Environment. *Prehospital Emergency Care*. 2012;**16**(4):469–476.

5. Centers for Disease C, Prevention. Surveillance for Early Detection of Disease Outbreaks at an Outdoor Mass Gathering–Virginia, 2005. *MMWR Morbidity and Mortality Weekly Report*. 2006;**55**(3):71–74.

6. Khan K., Freifeld C. C., Wang J., et al. Preparing for Infectious Disease Threats at Mass Gatherings: The Case of the Vancouver 2010 Olympic Winter Games. *CMAJ*. 2010;**182**(6):579–583.

7. Abubakar I. P., Gautret P. M. D., Brunette G. W. M. D., et al. Global Perspectives for Prevention of Infectious Diseases Associated with Mass Gatherings. *The Lancet Infectious Diseases*. 2012;**12**(1):66–74.

8. Centers for Disease C, Prevention. Public Health Aspects of the Rainbow Family of Living Light Annual Gathering–Allegheny National Forest, Pennsylvania, 1999. *MMWR Morbidity and Mortality Weekly Report*. 2000;**49**(15):324–326.

9. Lombardo J. S., Sniegoski C. A., Loschen W. A., et al. Public Health Surveillance for Mass Gatherings. *Johns Hopkins APL Technical Digest*. 2008;**27**(4):347–355.

10. Ross C., Basdere M., Chan J. L., Mehrotra S., Smilowitz K., Chiampas G. Data Value in Patient Tracking Systems at Racing Events. *Medicine and Science in Sports and Exercise*. 2015;**47**(10):2014–2023.

11. Farcas A. M., Zaidi H. Q., Wleklinski N. P., Tataris K. L. Implementing a Patient Tracking System in a Large EMS System. *Prehospital and Emergency Care*. 2021:1–9.

12. Landman A., Teich J. M., Pruitt P., et al. The Boston Marathon Bombings Mass Casualty Incident: One Emergency Department's Information Systems Challenges and Opportunities. *Annals of Emergency Medicine*. 2015;**66**(1):51–59.

13. Juvare. EMTrack. 2021; https://emtrack.juvare.com/. Accessed October 27, 2021.

14. Hospital Association of Southern California. ReddiNet. 2021; www.reddinet.com/. Accessed October 27, 2021.

15. Johansson A. D., Batty M. P., Hayashi K. M. D., Al Bar O. P., Marcozzi D. M. D., Memish Z. A. P. Crowd and Environmental Management during Mass Gatherings. *The Lancet Infectious Diseases*. 2012;**12**(2):150–156.

16. Soomaroo L., Murray V. Disasters at Mass Gatherings: Lessons from History. *PLoS Curr.* 2012;**4**: RRN1301.

17. Hardcastle T. C., Samlal S., Naidoo R., et al. A Redundant Resource: A Pre-Planned Casualty Clearing Station for a FIFA 2010 Stadium in Durban. *Prehospital and Disaster Medicine.* 2012;**27**(5):409–415.

18. Memish Z. A. P., Stephens G. M. M. D., Steffen R. P., Ahmed Q. A. M. D. Emergence of Medicine for Mass Gatherings: Lessons from the Hajj. *The Lancet Infectious Diseases.* 2012;**12**(1):56–65.

19. Sid Lowe G. T. Eta Bomb Scare Clears Madrid Stadium as Real Play Basques. *The Guardian.* December 12, 2004.

20. Lund A., Wong D., Lewis K., Turris S. A., Vaisler S., Gutman S. Text Messaging as a Strategy to Address the Limits of Audio-Based Communication During Mass-Gathering Events with High Ambient Noise. *Prehospital and Disaster Medicine.* 2013;**28**(1):2–7.

21. Madzimbamuto F. D. A Hospital Response to a Soccer Stadium Stampede in Zimbabwe. *Emergency Medicine Journal.* 2003;**20**(6):556–559.

22. Fielding R., Bashista R., Ahern S. A., et al. After Action Report for the Response to the 2013 Boston Marathon Bombings. Multi-Agency Report. 2014:1–130.

23. Basdere M., Ross C., Chan J. L., Mehrotra S., Smilowitz K., Chiampas G. Acute Incident Rapid Response at a Mass-Gathering Event Through Comprehensive Planning Systems: A Case Report from the 2013 Shamrock Shuffle. *Prehospital and Disaster Medicine.* 2014;**29**(3):320–325.

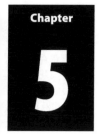

Medical and Medical Support Staffing at Mass Gathering Events

Lucian A. Mirra

Introduction

In medicine, having adequate staffing and fostering an environment of teamwork and mutual trust are correlated with improved patient outcomes [1]. This is especially true in the emergency department [2] and prehospital settings [3]. With medical care during a mass gathering event predominantly occurring in the prehospital setting on an emergent or urgent basis, it is reasonable to consider the right type and amount of staffing for such an event as the most imperative consideration toward its success. While the most obvious planning consideration is the total number of medical providers needed, additional considerations include the type of staff, and the need for support staff. Additional key considerations include provider training, provider mindset, models of staff deployment, and how characteristics of specific events may alter the number and type of staff necessary.

Ideally, medical care services provided at events would be comprehensive and plentiful. Treatment rooms in this ideal world operate like a small, well-staffed emergency department, with a fleet of vehicles and personnel to bring the ill and injured to the treatment area. In reality, venues and event organizers are confined by space and financial resources. An in-venue clinic takes up valuable space that could potentially make the venue profit such as seating or vendor stalls. Additionally, the budget necessary to equip and staff these resources are costs that directly impact the cost of the event. As a result, planners are asked to do more with potentially less space, equipment, and resources. The venue and event organizers are focused on delivering an experience to event patrons, while at the same time mitigating risk posed by the event [4]. In essence, planners are asked to deliver high quality, but cost-effective care while also providing a positive customer service experience.

Event medicine operates in a hybrid world of prehospital as well as in a hospital-like environment in some cases. Medical care teams are tasked with not only providing high quality patient care, but also the movement and transportation of patients, medical equipment logistics, and even incident command roles – all within the confines of a specific medical budget. A team of all one discipline (such as all physicians or all paramedics) may be able to accomplish one or more of the tasks but may not be proficient at all tasks. For example, an emergency medical technician (EMT) is trained to proficiency in patient movement using devices such as stretchers, stair chairs, and backboards. An EMT cannot, however, administer advanced cardiac life support (ACLS) drugs. Conversely, a physician who may be skilled in ACLS is likely not trained in patient movement in the prehospital environment.

This chapter will first discuss general considerations for event medical staffing and break down different capabilities of various medical provider types. It will also address medical support roles such as logistics and incident command positions. The next sections will address provider training and mindset during an event. This chapter will also review staffing best practices and examples of staffing models and positions. Lastly, special considerations of specific event types will be addressed.

General Staffing Considerations

Mass gathering events, by definition, has enough attendees that a potential emergency could overwhelm the local emergency response system [5]. In other words, a mass gathering event is by definition a potential multiple casualty incident (MCI) due to this characteristic to potentially overwhelm a local emergency response system [6]. When considering the staffing needed for the event, planners must consider two groups of individuals: medical care personnel who provide direct clinical care, and medical support personnel who fill logistics and supervisory roles. Medical care providers must be of sufficient numbers and capabilities to address the expected number of patients. They must be positioned to allow for quick access to the patient. Support personnel must be of sufficient number to provide necessary logistical and administrative support to the medical care team.

While no single standard exists for "response time" (time of being alerted to the need of medical services to patient contact), consider the scenario of a cardiac arrest within the venue. The American Heart Association suggests that brain death begins to occur within four to six minutes after cardiac arrest, and that a victim's chance of survival decreases by approximately 10 percent with every minute without defibrillation for patients with ventricular fibrillation (VF) or pulseless ventricular tachycardia (VT) [7]. Assuming all responding teams (walking team, bike team, etc.) are equipped with an AED, staffing should be deployed such that initial responders with an AED can access the patient prior to this four to six minute window expiring.

The ideal staffing plan combines the right medical care providers with the necessary support staff. It ensures that those providers are assigned proper roles and properly deployed and supervised, and also allows for meal and rest breaks. Starting from the different types of personnel necessary, this section will explore how the medical and medical support teams come together.

Medical Support Personnel

Incident Command Staff

As described in Chapter 7, the Incident Command System (ICS) is part of the National Incident Management System (NIMS) promulgated by the Federal Emergency Management Agency (FEMA). ICS, among other functions, provides a clear organizational structure for the management of incidents. This structure allows for a limited span of control and ensures that all personnel at the event have a clear line of reporting and information flow. The other advantage of the ICS is that it is scalable and modular – as it is intended to provide a limit on the span of control of

any one individual, the number of levels utilized varies based on the size of the event.

As described in Chapter 7, positions specific to the medical management of mass gathering events include the Medical Branch Director, Group or Division Supervisors, and Unit Leaders. Refer to Figure 5.1 for a depiction of a collegiate athletic organizational chart.

Medical Branch Director

The Medical Branch Director is typically the highest appointed position that is directly dealing with medical operations. This position generally reports to the Operations Section Chief or may report directly to the Incident Commander in smaller events. In many instances, this position sits equal to the Law Enforcement Branch Director and Fire Branch Director, with each individual controlling their specific resources at an event, under the Operations Section Chief or Incident Commander's overall direction. At larger events, the Medical Branch Director is generally located in the command post or emergency operations center (EOC) and as best practice, should not be involved in the tasks of providing medical care. This individual should be well-versed in not only the overall goals of medical care, but also in the incident command system and their role within that structure. It should be noted that while this position is operationally in charge of medical operations at an event, it does not mean that they are the highest medical authority. Medical direction can and in most cases should be separate from operational oversight of medical providers.

Group and Division Supervisors

In the Incident Command System, a Group and a Division are the same hierarchal level with a Group being a supervisory level of a specific function, while a Division is a supervisory level of a specific geographical area. Operating under the Medical Branch Director, these supervisors are intended to provide forward operational oversight with a direct link back to the Medical Branch Director in the command post or EOC. The idea of this level is to provide frontline supervision to teams operating in the event environment. An example of the utilization of Group Supervisors is using groupings of Extraction Group, Treatment Group, and Transport Group. In this case, the Supervisor is overseeing teams with similar tasks. This is typically seen in smaller venues where there does not need to be divisions based on geography.

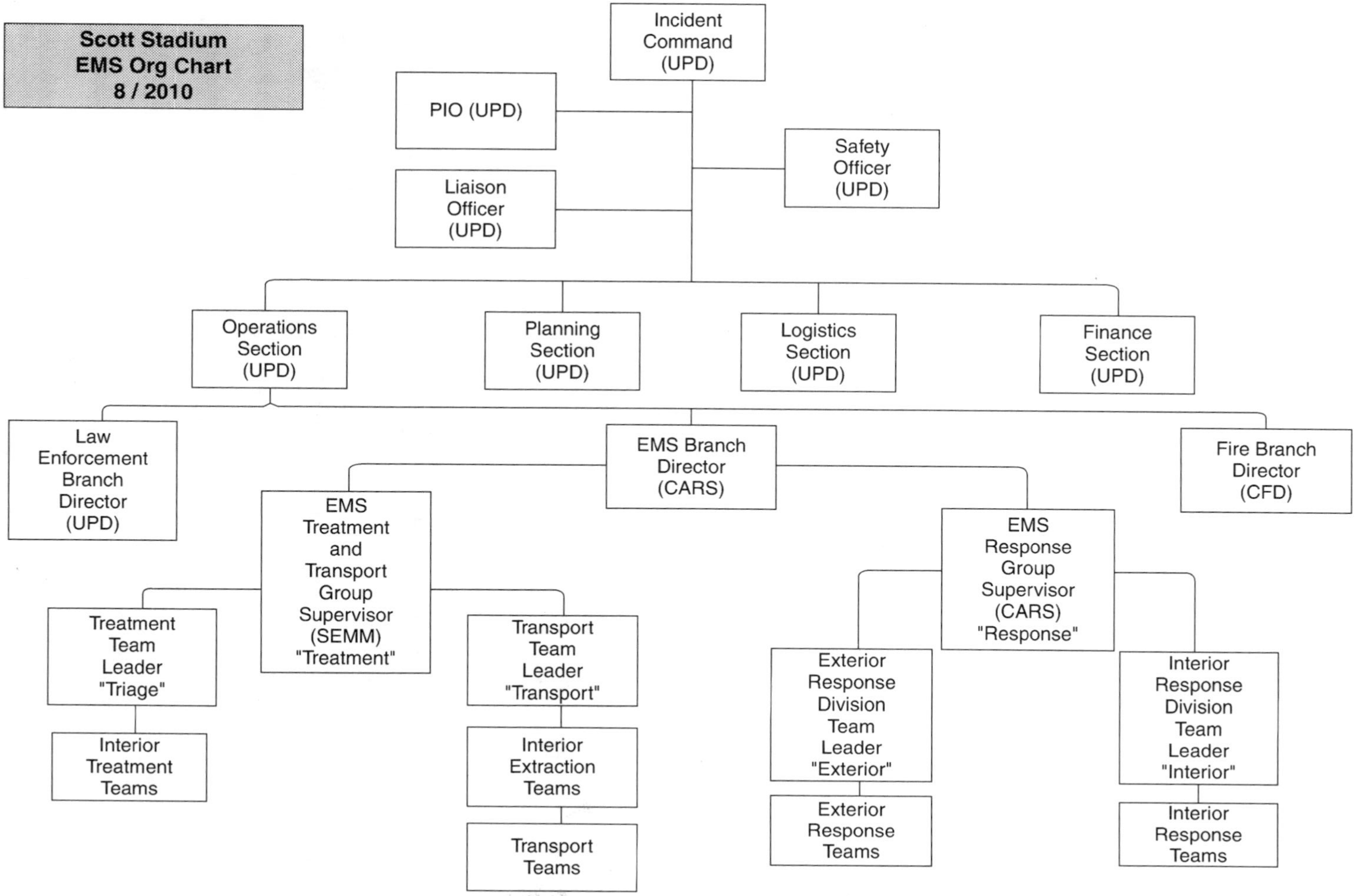

Figure 5.1 Incident command structure for a collegiate football game, University of Virginia Special Event Medical Management.

Divisions, on the other hand, would be a geographical supervisor such as Interior Division, Exterior Division, West Division, and so on. In this case, Supervisors are overseeing teams who may have different tasks but are within a specific area.

Groups and Divisions may be used on the same incident as well – for example at an NCAA Division 1 football game, there may be an interior and exterior division (referring to the interior and exterior of the stadium) and a Transport Group. In either case, the Supervisor needs to be knowledgeable as a clinician, of the incident command structure, and the plan of operations as they would be delegating tasks directly from the Medical Branch Director.

Unit and Team Leaders

Under Supervisors are Teams and Units, though typically these are given more practical designations based on the event. There are two FEMA defined teams – the Strike Team and the Task Force. These are described in more detail in Chapter 7. Units represent individual teams, partners, or single resources that are within the medical operation. This may be a walking team, a bike team, a medical cart team, ambulance, or treatment area. The expectation is that the unit function as one resource – for instance, a common staffing model at both indoor and outdoor events is a two-person walking team. This walking team is its own "unit" and should have a designated leader. This may be assigned as the more experienced or higher credentialled provider and may be tasked with communicating directly with Supervisors and other resources as well as ensuring the safety of the team.

Logistics Personnel

To ensure that the event runs smoothly from a supply perspective, there needs to be consideration given to staffing a logistics position. In larger incidents this may be a function under the event's Logistics Section Chief, but events of any duration will need direct support. Personnel are needed before the event to ensure that adequate supplies are checked and in place in the venue if treatment areas are being used. Additionally, any equipment carried by walking teams must be checked to ensure they are fully stocked and ready to be used. In smaller events, it may be possible for medical teams to work together to accomplish logistical tasks such as restocking supplies and

ensuring there is food and hydration for medical teams. In larger events, a person or persons may need to be specifically dedicated to logistical tasks including running errands. If multiple trips off-site may be needed for things like restocking supplies or procuring refreshments and food during the event, it may not be prudent to pull a medical provider away from an assignment to accomplish the task and have someone dedicated to filling this role.

Dispatch and Documentation

The manner by which medical personnel are alerted to the need for medical services varies widely based on the event and the venue. It may be as simple as medical providers staffing a static first aid area and receiving walk-up patients, or as comprehensive as being dispatched by radios. In many geographically or demographically large events, it makes most sense to utilize two-way radio communications, especially if a link can be established with the local 911 or 112 emergency dispatch center. In larger events it is likely that patrons with a medical issue may use cell phones to call for help, and a link with the center receiving those calls will allow for more efficient response of personnel assigned to the venue. In this case, staffing for a dispatch position may be required. This person may be sitting in the local emergency dispatch center, emergency operations center, or event command post and is responsible for handling radio and telephone traffic. They should have sufficient training in the use of the equipment as well as dispatching procedures if necessary.

In larger events, it may also be necessary to have a position assigned to documentation. This may fall under an overall Documentation Unit Leader under the Planning Section Chief, but if not and there are multiple patient contacts, a documentation position may be required. Typically, this position would work in conjunction with, and depending on volume may be one in the same with the dispatch position. This would allow for accurate tracking of resources assigned to the event, as well as ensuring accurate documentation of patient records and counts.

Personnel Training

Medical providers at an event must have basic training and credentialing to properly provide care to the event participants and to protect the medical provider. Whether the medical staff for an event are full-time employees of a venue or department, part-time

Table 5.1 Suggested minimum training for event medical staffers

All Staff (Clinical and Support)
• CPR/AED certification
• FEMA IS–100, 200, 700
Basic Life Support Providers
• Valid EMT certification
• Emergency vehicle operator certification (if vehicles being utilized)
Advanced Life Support Providers (RN, MD/DO, Paramedic)
• Valid provider certification or license
• ACLS certification
• PALS certification (if event involves children)
• Emergency vehicle operator certification (if vehicles being utilized)

or contract staff, or even volunteers, it is important to ensure that they meet the minimum requirements for practice for their respective clinical level. Specific requirements for practice are typically defined by state departments of health or other similar bodies. For example, many states require that all emergency medical services (EMS) providers are certified in cardiopulmonary resuscitation (CPR) and the use of an automated external defibrillator (AED). Providers with advanced life support abilities (such as paramedics, nurses, and physicians) should hold current certifications in Advanced Cardiac Life Support (ACLS), and depending on the population served at the event, Pediatric Advanced Life Support (PALS). A listing of suggested minimum certifications by level can be found in Table 5.1.

It is imperative that event organizers ensure that all medical providers have the proper certifications and licenses needed to practice. If the medical providers are employed by an agency that provides medical event staffing, it is likely that the agency is responsible for ensuring all certifications are on file and up to date. Organizers must check with local, state, and national bodies to understand what requirements are necessary. For example, some states may have a requirement that a paramedic have an advanced cardiac life support (ACLS) certification to be allowed to practice. While it may be easy to ignore or take a person for their word, it is critical to ensure proper credentialing prior to a negative outcome occurring. Once all personnel are cleared to practice, they should be credentialed with identification. This credential may be issued by or a requirement for the venue, but some form of visible identification and their level of practice of all providers should be a requirement.

Because of the unique setting of some mass gathering events, emergency medicine planners must also ensure a clear understanding of treatment protocols. Emergency medical services (EMS) providers generally operate under the auspices of a physician medical director and have standing orders or protocols to treat patients. These orders may be specific to a company or department, or to a region or state. If planners are soliciting EMS personnel outside of their own agency, there must be a clear understanding of patient care guidelines to go along with the credentialing of providers. Because scopes of practice are defined at the state or local level in the United States, the level of care that a particular EMT or paramedic can provide could differ based on their training and region or state of practice [12]. If recruiting providers across state lines, be sure to check with the office of emergency medical services in the state of the event to ensure that providers from out-of-state have the proper credential to practice in that state and to the full extent of their licensure.

Medical Care Personnel

The core of the medical team serving a mass gathering event is focused on providing high quality medical care. Because of the atypical environment, however, both prehospital providers, such as emergency medical technicians (EMTs) and paramedics, as well as hospital providers such as nurses and physicians may mix to form a multidisciplinary team. The amount and type of medical care personnel should be directly reflective of the overall objectives of mass gathering medical care, which include (1) stabilize injury and illness in participants, staff, and patrons, (2) reduce the demand on local medical systems, and (3) be poised to respond to a catastrophic event [8]. This section better defines the capabilities and skill set of each group in order to facilitate recruiting the right type and number of providers.

Prehospital Providers

In the United States, the levels of emergency medical services (EMS) personnel who provide care in the prehospital setting vary by state. While the delivery of EMS is left up to the states, the National Highway Traffic Safety Administration (NHTSA) is the federal coordinating body for emergency medical services. This body maintains the National EMS Scope of Practice Model, which defines four levels of EMS provider, divided between basic life support (BLS) and advanced life support (ALS). The specific names of levels of providers and their specific skill sets vary across states and countries, however generally there is a delineation between basic and advanced life support providers [9].

The National EMS Scope of Practice model defines the basic life support levels as emergency medical responder (EMR) and emergency medical technicians (EMT). These providers may also be known as emergency care assistants or ambulance technicians in other countries. Generally, BLS providers have the training and certification to perform CPR, use an AED, assess and stabilize life-threatening injuries, and provide trauma and wound care, administer a limited number of medications such as epinephrine or naloxone auto-injectors and assist with emergency childbirth. In the United States, the EMR level differs from the EMT level in regard to training on patient movement and transportation. The EMR is meant for first responders such as police officers, park rangers, or firefighters who may have to stabilize an ill or injured patient. The EMT level is generally seen as the entry into the emergency medical services field.

An EMT is trained to assess and stabilize medical, trauma, obstetric, and psychiatric patients, and safely move them to a higher level of care. This means that the skill set of an EMT is ideal for being the initial level of patient contact at many mass gatherings. They are able to rapidly assess an ill or injured patient and make a quick decision on how and where to transport the patient. They are trained in and proficient at both routine and emergent moves and are familiar with movement devices such as stretchers, stair chairs, and other devices outlined in Chapter 3.

The National EMS Scope of Practice Model defines advanced life support levels as Advanced EMT (AEMT) and Paramedic. Both the AEMT and Paramedic levels have the same basic training as an EMT, and between 200 hours (AEMT) and over 1,000 hours (Paramedic) of additional advanced training. Both AEMTs and Paramedics have additional training on anatomy, physiology, and pathophysiology, as well as pharmacology and have an expanded scope of practice that includes venous access, advanced airway procedures, and medication administration.

The Advanced EMT level in the United States is somewhat analogous to the Primary Care Paramedic (Canada) and may take on other names in various states such as EMT-Intermediate. These providers undergo approximately 200–300 hours of instruction beyond the EMT level which allows these providers to perform certain advanced skills. AEMTs generally are able to initiate vascular access using intravenous or intraosseous cannulation, place supraglottic airway devices, and deliver a limited number of medications such as bronchodilators, epinephrine, naloxone, corticosteroids, and intravenous fluids [9].

Paramedics represent the highest level of care in the prehospital setting. In the United States, paramedics must have graduated from a paramedic program accredited though the Commission on Accreditation of Allied Health Education Programs (CAAHEP) [10]. These programs are generally well over 1,000 hours of classroom, lab, and clinical education which in many areas is equivalent to 40–50 college credits. The paramedic level in the United States is equivalent to the Advanced Care Paramedic in Canada and can generally administer a wide variety of medications including antidotes, advanced cardiac life support (ACLS) drugs, and narcotic analgesics. Some providers in certain jurisdictions may also be credentialed to perform more advanced skills such as rapid sequence induction (RSI) procedures. Paramedics are trained in ACLS and have the ability to work a cardiac arrest as the team leader, as well as care for patients with complex medical and traumatic pathologies.

Hospital-Based Providers

Hospital-based providers, such as nurses and physicians, can provide a high level of medical care at mass gathering events. The presence of hospital-based providers may actually increase the number of patients referring to medical care when properly advertised in order to seek care for medical issues such as chest pain and dizziness as patrons may feel as it is an opportunity to speak with a physician [11]. Both nurses and physicians have training in advanced life support and work in conjunction with one another in hospital settings, allowing an easy transition to an event treatment area.

Medical oversight at larger events is typically provided by an on-site physician. While smaller events can be managed by a combination of EMTs, paramedics, and nurses, having an on-site physician is advantageous as it provides more clinical decision-making ability. Physician staffing on site may also reduce the percentage of patients requiring transport to the emergency department [11]. When utilized, physicians are most valuable in a fixed treatment area that patients can either self-refer to or be brought to by EMS providers. Depending on the amount and type of equipment, this treatment area can be as simple as a first aid station or as advanced as a field hospital. The physician should have sufficient training in emergency medicine to be able to make clinical decisions regarding patient disposition. They also may be called upon to provide medical oversight to EMS providers functioning at the event [12].

Students of Various Medical Training Programs

The mass event setting offers a unique opportunity for students in a variety of medical education programs to gain valuable experience in assessing and treating patients. Under proper supervision of an approved preceptor, as well as approval from the students' educational program, students enrolled in emergency medical services (i.e., EMT, paramedic) programs, nursing programs, or even medical school can gain valuable experience treating patients. For example, students in paramedic programs must achieve a minimum number of IV initiations, patient assessments, and other skills which can take place in a variety of field or clinical settings [13].

The nature of mass gathering medicine being an interface between the clinical and prehospital environment also make it ideal to provide interdisciplinary training. Allowing students across the EMS, nursing, and medical professions to partake in this interdisciplinary clinical setting may lead to improved learning outcomes [14]. Specifically, it allows prehospital providers such as EMTs and paramedics the opportunity to work in a more hospital-like environment while maintaining elements of the prehospital environment. Similarly, it allows traditionally clinical-based providers such as nurses and physicians a view into prehospital care. This builds a sense of camaraderie among the team [14, 15] and may persist past the end of the specific event when team members work together in their normal work environments.

The mass gathering event also offers a unique opportunity for graduate medical education (GME) physicians during residency or fellowships. As previously mentioned, the mass gathering event blends the hospital-based clinical environment with the prehospital environment. This offers unique opportunities for emergency medicine residents to hone their skills in a more austere environment than the hospital emergency department, while still maintaining a high level

of control and safety. It may be coupled with prehospital experiences on ambulance shifts for GME physicians to gain exposure to the prehospital environment.

Event Medical Training

Event Specific Training

Mass gathering events can be anything from a high school graduation in an auditorium, to a professional sporting event, a multiday music festival, or a protest rally marching through a city. While in a certain sense the medicine is the same, the type of event is a critical variable to predict the type of patients likely to be seen, and injury patterns presenting. As discussed further in Chapter 8, factors such as weather, event characteristics, and the availability of alcohol and/or drugs had an effect on the number and type of patients presenting for medical care.

While it is unlikely that training will prevent patients from appearing, ensuring that staff is trained properly for the event will likely allow them to provide higher quality medical care. This training can be formalized such as in a continuing education session or meeting or can be part of the briefing done before the event. Examples of training could include how to package football players in pads, how to treat heat stroke, or the types of drugs likely to be seen. This training could be delivered in person, virtually, or even as a "just-in-time" model during the event briefing, as covered later in this chapter.

Event-specific training should also include other medical staff on site such as sports medicine providers at athletic events or medical teams assigned to VIPs. While these providers typically only are focused on their assigned populations (the athletes or VIP, respectively), they provide a valuable resource for both treating and interacting with those populations as well as potentially providing additional support in a mass casualty setting. For medical teams providing regular support for athletic events, the team athletic trainers provide a valuable resource. Athletic trainers have specialization in working with injured players, and at top levels of competition, often have specific high-level experience with the specific sport they work in. With the large number of athletic events that are in themselves mass gathering events, the medical team may be called to also treat an athlete depending on the agreement between the provider of medical care and the team and venue. Building the relationship with the athletic training staff, including of the opposing team when possible, allows the teams to understand roles and expectations. These relationships can also lead to additional specific training sessions such as how to properly move a player in football equipment.

Venue Specific Training

All staff members need to have venue specific training. This consists of multiple facets. Most importantly, staff members should know the general layout of the facility, and the location of all emergency equipment including emergency exits. In many cases, staff members are alerted to the need to respond to a patron with an emergency via a communications device such as radio, cell phone, or word-of-mouth. In order to access the patient, staff members must be familiar with the access and egress points of the facility. Each staff member should be afforded time to do a walkthrough of the facility or venue and any walking or other response teams should have a map of the venue on hand with their equipment. A walkthrough of the facility or venue also affords providers the opportunity to preplan routes and identify areas that could be used as casualty collection points (CCP) if not pre-identified.

Personnel working in the venue should be aware of where emergency equipment is stored or located. Depending on the venue, items such as automated external defibrillators (AEDs) may be mounted, or items such as stretchers or wheelchairs stored in a specific forward location. Part of this training should also include how to use equipment being used at the venue. For example, there are multiple different cardiac monitors/defibrillators used in the clinical setting and depending on the staffing of the event, an advanced level provider may be using a cardiac monitor that they are not familiar with. Ensuring providers are comfortable with using the venue-specific medical equipment is a critical pre-event task.

Incident Command Training

The Incident Command System (ICS), covered in detail in Chapter 7, provides a specific structure for managing emergency incidents including many mass gathering events. The ICS is a modular, scalable organizational structure that provides resource management, communications and information management, and command and coordination [16]. Because many events utilize ICS as an organizational structure, it is imperative that all medical team members have a basic understanding of

the system. Providers in leadership roles such as Incident Commanders, Medical Branch Directors, Group/Division Supervisors, and Unit Leaders should have additional training in the National Incident Management System (NIMS) as well as ICS. This training is provided free online from the Federal Emergency Management Agency (FEMA). A list of suggested training can be found in Table 7.1.

Triage and Multiple Casualty Incident Training

Due to their inherent nature, mass gathering events are a multiple casualty incident (MCI) waiting to happen. As has been evidenced in recent history, active threats, weather, or even the crowd itself can be catalysts for the mass gathering even to turn into a multiple casualty event [17]. Because of this potential, all providers should have an understanding of managing an MCI as well as be proficient in the triage system used by the local response system. Medical teams should also be briefed on what actions to take for a potential MCI at the venue, including the location of casualty collection points (CCPs).

Providing Care at Mass Gathering Events

For many providers, the provision of medical care at a mass gathering event is not a regularly scheduled aspect of their job. This requires the provider to be mentally prepared for staffing such an event. These events may involve large crowds of people, loud noise, extreme weather, and physical exertion. Providers should also be prepared for the worst-case scenario. A mass gathering event always has the possibility of turning into a multiple casualty incident. Providers should mentally review contingency plans and triage systems prior to arriving. Even a quick mental overview beforehand may be beneficial in an actual event.

Preparing for an Event

In addition to the mental preparation of providing care at a mass gathering event, providers should also be physically prepared for the event. This involves both individual providers as well as the medical care team collectively to take steps to ensure they have all equipment needed for an event. It also requires the provider to be physically prepared for the event. If the provider is working an outdoor event during the summer, they should begin hydrating days in advance. Similarly, if the provider is working an extreme outdoor sports event, they should ensure that they are physically capable of working in the environment required.

Weather Considerations

Perhaps the most important practical consideration for a medical staff member is the environment. In addition to being one of the most important variables in predicting patient numbers, the weather can pose a particular challenge for medical teams. While outdoor venues are more affected by weather, medical care teams at indoor venues must consider access and egress from the venue, particularly if the teams are providing transport to the hospital. Especially rainy or snowy conditions may impact travel times or make conditions dangerous as teams and patrons are entering the venue which could be a source of injury. Teams operating in outdoor venues should be cognizant of the weather, including potential changes in the event. Providers should dress appropriately for the weather – preferably dressing in layers with protective items such as hats and gloves as necessary.

Personal Equipment

Providers working in forward posts such as walking, bike, or cart teams should be particularly prepared for providing care in an austere environment. In addition to ensuring they have appropriate weather equipment; providers should ensure that they have any additional items with them that they may need. This includes any tools, personal protective items, comfort/personal items, and anything else that may be needed during the event. A list of suggested items for walking, bike, or cart teams to carry with them is found in Table 5.2.

Team Provisions

When events last more than just a few hours, it is critical to ensure that the medical team members themselves have basic needs met. This includes ensuring access to restroom facilities, break areas, water, and food. Medical organizers should work with the venue and event organizers to understand how these items will be provided. If food and water must be provided by the medical teams themselves this often must be ordered or arranged in advance. Additionally, staffing

Table 5.2 Suggested equipment for medical teams

Walking and Bike Teams (teams of 2)
- 2-way radio for each team member with backup such as personal cell phone
- Automated external defibrillator (AED)
- Basic life support equipment including:
  - Assessment equipment (blood pressure cuff, stethoscope, etc.)
  - Minor wound care supplies
  - CPR pocket mask or bag-mask device
  - Major hemorrhage control supplies (tourniquets, hemostatic gauze, etc.)
- Triage supplies
- Personal protective equipment including:
  - Medical gloves
  - Surgical and/or N95 mask
  - Eye protection
  - High-visibility clothing if operating in or adjacent to vehicle traffic

Cart (UTV) and Ambulance Teams
- All equipment listed above
- Patient transportation device (stretcher)
- Advanced life support equipment (if service provided)

of long duration events should account for the need for providers to take rest and meal breaks. This may include building in an additional position(s) as a relief to rotate teams to rest and meal areas. This need increases in outdoor events in weather extremes where teams should be rotated more frequently.

Pre-event Briefing

The pre-event briefing is one of the most important aspects of providing care at any mass gathering event. It should occur with sufficient time allowed before the event for a full briefing and questions prior to providers needing to be on post. The briefing may occur at a central site prior to arriving at the event (such as at a station or hospital prior to being transported to the event) or may occur upon arrival at the venue. In either case, it is also important to conduct the briefing when all providers can be present. Additionally, if the event is a multiple day event (such as a music festival or athletics tournament), a briefing should be conducted prior to each operational period or shift.

The briefing can be formal or more informal as the event dictates. In larger-scale events, these will likely be done in a formal fashion by the Medical Branch Director or other similar position. Even if there is a general briefing for all workers at an event, there should be a medical specific briefing with medical personnel. In smaller events, it may be a more informal team huddle, similar to what is done often times at the beginning of a shift in the hospital or prehospital setting.

A copy of the Event or Incident Action Plan should be distributed at least to Supervisors and Leaders prior to or during the briefing. This plan outlines much of the information to be covered during the briefing and should also include such items as a venue map, communications list, and staffing assignments. Major topics to be covered in the briefing include any pertinent event or venue specific items, weather forecast (if applicable), staffing, communications plan, and emergency action plans and the safety message.

During the Event

Whether or not the medical providers work directly for the venue or event, in the eyes of patrons, all staff members represent the venue and the event. Medical staff should always conduct themselves professionally, especially when in public. Event plans dictate the position of any pre-stationed providers or areas for walking, bike, or cart teams to cover. Venue and event rules also govern whether staff can use seating, be in public view, or watch the event when not engaged in patient care. Whatever the local guidelines, staff members should be ready and alert to respond to any calls for assistance before, during, or after the event. As soon as uniformed medical services providers are on site, they are visible to others and while they may still be setting up, if they are there, they are subject to be called upon. Staff should monitor proper communications channels during the event and follow proper procedure to acknowledge the request for service and relay any important information.

To provide optimal patient care, providers must understand the objectives and philosophy of the event plan. The staffing model discussed later in this chapter are centered around the philosophy of moving the patient quickly to a defined treatment area unless it is a very minor encounter. Depending on the type, venue, and staffing of the event, this philosophy may be different. Knowing the expectations of the event management staff is imperative to a successful operation. In this model, providers must be able to perform an assessment in under a minute to decide disposition and call for the proper resource. This requires the provider to have solid medical assessment skills and decision-making ability but does not require advanced medical knowledge. In other cases, more treatment may be done at the patient's side which may require less patient movement skills but more medical knowledge. Understanding the medical objectives and philosophy will help ensure the proper providers are in the proper roles.

In addition to filling their primary role as a medical or support provider, teams are an extension of the venue and event. Patrons will often ask medical team members about venue or event information. When possible and practical, medical teams should serve as good customer service agents. Teams assigned to walking, bikes, or carts, should have a venue map and be able to answer questions such as "where is the rest room?" Additionally, having a program or schedule of the event tends to be an important tool from a customer service perspective. With this in mind, medical care should come first. Also, if the provider does not know the answer, they should try to seek out a staff member who does.

After the Event

The conclusion of the event for the medical team may be the end of the event, or shift change with an oncoming group of providers. In longer duration events, providers should handle shift change as directed by their incident command structure and typically on a one-for-one basis. Teams should not leave their posts until properly relieved either by their oncoming relief or by their supervisor. Upon arrival of the oncoming team, providers leaving should provide an overview of the objectives, a brief review of the role or area of responsibility, and any significant events of note. Equipment should be checked and handed off if required. If handing off care of a patient in a treatment area, providers should use generally accepted patient hand-off rules.

At the end of the event, providers should ideally gather for a post-event or post-shift briefing. This allows for a "hotwash" or a quick review of positives as well as any areas for improvement. Importantly this is not a full after-action review, but especially in events covering multiple operational periods or multiple days, it can be an opportunity to provide valuable feedback to improve care or operations. It also is a time to ensure all equipment is checked back in and all reports are completed or have a plan for completion. Lastly, it is important to provide thanks to the team, especially when they are volunteering their time and to remind the team to report any injuries or other issues prior to leaving the event site for documentation.

Staffing Models

Patient presentation rates at mass gathering events vary widely [18], with numerous mitigating factors such as weather, the type and duration of event, crowd demographics, and venue characteristics [19]. Specific models for predicting patient presentation rates (PPR) and transport to hospital rates (TTHR) are discussed in Chapter 3, giving planners a resource as they consider the number of staff members needed. The remainder of this chapter will take a broad lens to discuss various staffing models and considerations based on various special circumstances.

The most important consideration before any model or deciding on a specific number and type of provider is ensuring that those providers remain safe at all times. Some events such as an indoor graduation, or classical music concert may not come with much inherent risk to the providers. On the other hand, a heated sporting rivalry on a summer day, a politically volatile public speaker, or a remote music festival may pose certain risks to medical providers, especially when operating outside of the medical care area or treatment room. Two important safety strategies should always be implemented: providers should work in teams and should always have a communications link.

While often a supervisor may operate as a sole resource, medical teams should always operate as a team. Specific considerations of this team composition are described later in this chapter, but from a safety perspective having two team members ensures a safer environment than a solo provider. This allows one provider to be able to focus on the surroundings while the partner assesses and treats the patient. Each team must also be equipped with a way to communicate with other team members if operating away from a fixed location. Importantly, this communications device (usually a two-way radio to alleviate potential cellular service disruption) is a method of calling for assistance if required.

Philosophy of Planning

A major consideration of the staffing model is based on the philosophy of the event organizers regarding what is to be provided. For example, do event organizers want the event medical team to provide transport services, or will that rely on the local emergency medical services (EMS) system? Is the expectation that both minor and moderate illnesses and injuries be treated on-site and attempt to divert potential patients away from the local emergency department when possible? It is important to also remember that event organizers are likely trying to provide a service for the most reasonable cost and there is a very real tendency to underestimate the amount of medical services needed at an event or the ability of the local EMS system to handle the potential patients from the event.

Planners with knowledge of the best practices of event medical management, the incident command system, as well as local knowledge of available EMS and hospital services are critical to the process. In some instances, this may mean involving multiple subject matter experts. For large events and events with a high probability of a higher PPR or TTHR based on the type of event, meetings with local public safety entities (police, fire, EMS) and hospital representatives should take place early. This allows event planners to understand what the local public safety system is able and willing to provide, as well as the capabilities of the local hospital systems. In some instances, involvement of local government authorities such as city, town, or county governing bodies, is required for certain types of events. Additionally, some localities may have ordinances requiring their public safety entities to be used to provide medical standby services. In any case, whether required or not, event planners should involve local public safety and hospitals from the beginning of the planning process. While the majority of patrons seeking care are for minor complaints [11, 12], a heuristic from the United Kingdom estimates that 10 percent of the patients presenting to care will require treatment beyond very basic care, and that 1 percent of those patients needing medical care will require transport to the emergency department [20]. Understanding whether the event medical team will provide medical transportation to the hospital and what the expectation is on the event to mitigate the burden to local hospitals are major philosophical considerations that directly affect staffing.

The second major overall consideration regarding staffing is how patients will present to medical services, or how they will seek medical care. Many requests for event medical services starts with a request to staff a first aid area (such as a room, booth, tent). Event organizers

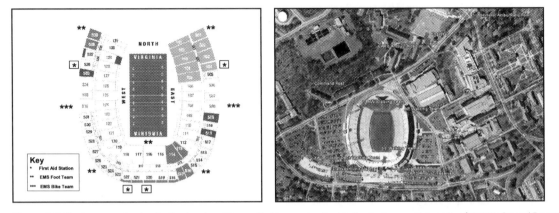

Figure 5.2 Deployment planning for fixed and mobile medical teams at collegiate football game, University of Virginia Special Event Medical Management.

may be under the impression that people seeking medical care will self-report to this area, likely seeking minor care. While many patrons do self-report to a designated area, in events over a larger area, or when patrons have a more serious medical issue, they may call the local emergency number, flag down an usher or other event staff member, or even have someone come to the first aid area on their behalf. In this case, the medical care team must retrieve the patient and decide a disposition – to return to the first aid area, or to have the patient transported to the emergency department. As part of the planning process, representatives from the medical team should ensure that event organizers are aware of the challenges of moving patients and the resources needed. From a staffing perspective, it means ensuring that there are enough team members trained in moving patients, and in some cases, trained to operate bicycles and powered carts to safely move patients.

Staffing Models

The number and type of providers needed to staff an event should be aligned to providing sufficient resources to handle the predicted patient presentation rate (PPR) and transport to hospital rate (TTHR). The manner in which these providers are deployed are dependent on numerous factors in addition to simply the number of projected patients and transports. Major factors for the deployment of providers at an event include the size and scope of the venue and the type of event. Larger indoor venues or stadiums likely have designated first aid or treatment rooms, but at the NCAA Division 1 and

professional levels, these may require additional responders who are mobile. The types of teams used are described in more detail below. Refer to Figure 5.2 for a depiction of staffing model for a collegiate football game at the University of Virginia.

Walking Teams

For events with defined boundaries such as arenas, stadiums, amphitheaters, or other similar venues, the "walking team" is perhaps the most common staffing model. Walking teams are typically stationed strategically throughout the venue so that they can quickly respond to injured or ill patrons on foot. In the model used by the University of Virginia (UVA), the goal of the walking team is to establish patient contact, perform a rapid assessment of any life threats and the chief complaint, form a disposition and communicate needs. In most cases this disposition is either to (1) treat a very minor injury on site, or (2) to transport the patient back to a treatment area for further treatment and evaluation. Walking teams are typically a two-person team and can be either basic or advanced life support providers, or a combination of both. Teams carry a small aid bag with limited equipment for a quick assessment, minor wound care, and immediate lifesaving care (such as tourniquets, nasal airways, and a pocket mask). The teams also typically carry an automated external defibrillator (AED). They should also have at least one two-way radio or other communication device assigned to them. In larger venues, several walking teams are spread out within the venue and assigned a specific geographic section, such as shown in Figure 5.2.

Extraction Teams

In this model, extraction teams (Figure 5.3) are centrally based or spread out in a venue and specialize in moving patients from where they present to the treatment area. While it may be natural to assume that the walking teams can transport their patients to a treatment area, it is often impractical for each team to have all the devices necessary to transport the patient (such as a stretcher and a wheelchair). The walking team does a quick assessment of the patient and communicates the needs back to the extraction team. If the walking team is going to treat and release, or if the patient is ambulatory, the extraction team stands down. If the walking team decides to transport the patient to the treatment area, they relay the device necessary. The extraction team is also able to provide additional lifting and moving assistance if the patron is in a seat and non-ambulatory. While extraction teams do not usually provide medical care, they may continue care started by the walking team, or may themselves be flagged down for assistance. A team of two emergency medical technicians (EMT) work well as an extraction team. This also allows this team to serve as a backup medical walking team or in the treatment area if the need arises.

Bike and Cart Teams

In outdoor venues, or venues where event medical teams have responsibilities for parking lots or tailgate areas, increased mobility beyond foot speed may be required. Depending on the venue, equipment available, and training of providers, this may consist of either bicycles or utility carts such as 4x4 or 4x6 wheel utility terrain vehicles (UTVs; Figures 5.4 and 5.5). With properly trained and equipped riders, bicycles offer a way to carry a limited amount of equipment, such as what is carried by a walking team, but with increased speed and maneuverability. In this sense, the bike team functions as a walking team especially in the outdoor setting such as tailgate areas, outdoor concerts, or festivals. Upon arrival at the patient, the bike team assumes the role of a walking team and performs a rapid assessment, initiates any lifesaving treatment, and communicates a disposition to an extraction team. While riding a bicycle may sound like an easy skill, many amateur bicyclists have little experience navigating through a crowd, over terrain and even stairs. For this reason, it is imperative that providers serving on a bike team are properly trained and certified.

Utility carts or UTVs offer the advantage of increased speed over walking in outdoor settings, and often come with the added ability of transporting a patient and limited equipment. These carts vary from a simple modified stock 4x6 UTV to specially designed ambulance carts. These teams can typically serve as both a walking team and an extraction team for incidents occurring outdoors. They may be part of a roving medical presence or stationed at a central location during an event. Like bicycles, while carts add an added measure of maneuverability and capability, they come with an increased risk of injury to the operators and other patrons. Those operating medical carts should be properly trained, and certified if required by local statute.

Treatment Teams

Many events have a fixed location for providing medical services. These areas may provide basic (BLS) or advanced life support (ALS) and may be rooms, tents, tables, booths, or even the back doors of an on-site ambulance. Capabilities of these areas may range from an area that has some basic first aid supplies to a nearly full-scale emergency department suite. Using the rule of thumb that approximately 10 percent of patients encountered at a mass gathering event will require some level of advanced assessment or treatment, it may be prudent for a treatment area to provide some level of advanced care. While equipment is covered further in Chapter 3, having advanced level providers such as physicians capable of making informed medical decisions regarding whether a patient needs to be transported may lead

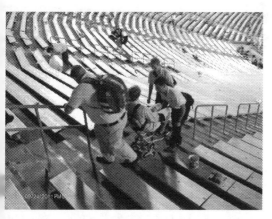

Figure 5.3 Extraction team, removing a nonambulatory patient from the stadium seating area

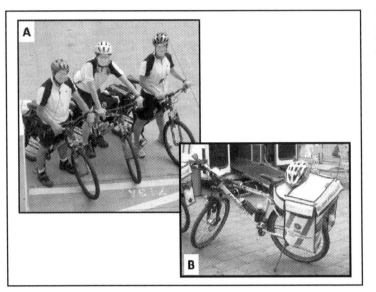

Figure 5.4 Bike teams allow for coverage of a larger area with rapid response times (A) with appropriate emergency equipment (B), including an automatic external defibrillator

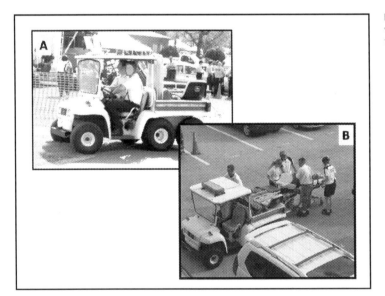

Figure 5.5 Gators, or all-terrain vehicles, allow for wider coverage areas with enhanced response times (A) as well as patient transport (B)

to a lower rate of transports to hospital emergency departments [11].

Treatment areas should be staffed with providers appropriate for the level of care to be provided. Minor first aid areas (first aid rooms, tents, etc.) can be staffed with BLS providers such as an EMT. More advanced treatment areas with cardiac monitoring, medications, and airway supplies should be staffed with providers capable of providing advanced care.

If physicians and registered nurses are used as part of staffing, the treatment area is the natural location for them to operate from. It allows a similar handoff of care from a patient encounter to hospital arrival as is seen in the typical prehospital setting – the ambulance crew, or in this case the walking and extraction teams, assess and transport the patient, and may begin treatment while en route. The patient is then handed off to the nurse and physician at the bedside in the treatment area similar to how it occurs in the hospital emergency department. The treatment area is also typically the best area for students as well. Because anything beyond a simple bandage will be transported, it allows students to be in the more controlled setting of the event, while also seeing all moderate to severe illnesses or injures at the event.

Transport Teams

A major part of the event planning from a medical perspective is how patients requiring treatment at an emergency department will be transported. If this transportation will be done by the local EMS system, ensure there is a proper route of communication to facilitate this. In some instances, however, the event medical team will be responsible for providing transportation. If the event medical team will be transporting patients to the hospital, ensure there is adequate staffing for the transport ambulance(s). At minimum, two people are required to transport a patient to the hospital, one who is certified to drive the ambulance, and one who is certified to provide care during transport. Laws vary by state and country on ambulance staffing and their requirements. Using models to predict transports to hospitals, along with understanding hospital transport and turnaround times will help planners provide an adequate number of ambulances and staffing for them.

Supervisors

Supervisors serve many roles. Perhaps most importantly, they are responsible for the safety of the teams reporting to them and provide support to those teams as required. Supervisors should be mobile and able to respond to provide assistance, whether operational or customer service based, to all teams under their control. They should also coordinate the rotation of their assigned teams on longer duration events to allow time for meal and comfort breaks. Supervisors also function to disseminate information to ensure that all teams have the information necessary to successfully complete the objectives of the event and ensure that each team has a place within the incident command structure and has adequate resources.

While some events can be managed with one supervisor, larger events will need to consider the span of control of any one supervisor. The ideal "span of control" defined by the Federal Emergency Management Agency (FEMA) ranges from three to seven, with an optimal number of five [21]. This means that no single individual should be supervising more than seven teams at a time. The specific number varies by the complexity of the event or teams supervised and the skill of those in supervisory roles, however, adequate staffing should allow for a proper span of control. As detailed in Chapter 7, teams or units typically report to a Division (geographic) or Group (function) Supervisor. How these are used depends on the event and the venue. Larger events may need to be divided geographically, or it may make more sense for the functions to be supervised by task such as treatment and transport. It is acceptable to use both Divisions and Groups during the same event – for example a typical large college football game may have an Interior Division, Exterior Division, and a Treatment/Transport Group. This results in three supervisors each with less than seven teams reporting to them and those three supervisors reporting to the Medical Branch Director.

Support Teams

In events with a long duration, large area, or other challenges, additional personnel are needed beyond those required to directly provide medical care. As previously discussed, logistics personnel may be required to ensure that supplies are restocked and personnel have basic needs met such as food, water, and rest facilities. Based on the staffing level, having an extra person or persons to serve in this logistics role, almost as a "runner," may be beneficial. Like the extraction team, while this person would not likely be providing direct patient care, they should at least have basic first aid knowledge in case they are flagged down for assistance. Additionally, depending on the organization of the event and the management structure, personnel for dispatching and documentation may also be required. Lastly, consider the use of relief teams for events that are long duration or in extreme climates. This team can rotate into any position to provide each team with a break, especially for meals and during hot weather.

Special Considerations

Weather Issues

Any outdoor event is subject to changes in and extremes of weather. Extremes in weather, particularly high temperatures, can increase the number of patients seen by medical teams. When planning for an outdoor event, organizers should pay careful attention to the weather and temperature forecast and use accepted standards such as the wet bulb globe temperature (WBGT) risk chart, commonly known for its use by the military and for the most extreme conditions being considered "black flag" [22]. During times of extreme temperatures, planners should ensure an adequate amount of hydration supplies for staff, and supervisors should help ensure staff stay hydrated and have time for breaks. Staff should be alert to patrons or event participants who may be exhibiting early signs of heat injury and take appropriate cooling actions. Outdoor events also carry the possibility of severe weather events. In many areas, hot days correspond with the risk of severe storms. Staff should be briefed on sheltering procedures and their role during a lighting event and should be familiar with the treatment of lightning injury.

Large Area and Mobile Events

While venues with defined walls such as concert halls, sports arenas, stadiums, and amphitheaters can present challenges to event medical teams, venues with much larger and less defined boarders pose an even greater challenge. As an example, the Bonnaroo Music and Arts Festival, held annually in Tennessee hosts 75,000–100,000 attendees, and takes place at a 650-acre (1.02 square mile) farm [23, 24]. Events such as street festivals may take up multiple city blocks, and some protest rallies may not even have defined boarders. Additionally, some events such as adventure races, marathons, or some auto races may be mobile events. In either case, planners should understand the general boundaries of the event and have staffing based geographically. This also may necessitate the use of motor vehicles for response to incidents or movement of personnel.

EDM Festivals

Electronic dance music, or EDM, festivals are a popular source of entertainment for certain demographics. With names like Electric Daisy, Electric Zoo, and Beyond Wonderland, these festivals combine the pumping beats of electronic dance music, with light shows, and dense, dancing crowds in a warm environment, often with the easy availability of alcohol and drugs such as MDMA (or "Molly"). Due in part to these factors, these festivals have patient presentation rates that surpass generally accepted models for other types of events [25]. Medical staff working events such as these should be prepared for proportionally more patients, and patients with a higher likelihood of toxicological involvement.

Wilderness Events

Outdoor adventure events, such as triathlons, adventure races, and others, continue to be an exciting way for some to seek both fitness and being outdoors. These events often combine extreme athletics performance, over hours to even days, often in a wilderness, rural, or backcountry setting. Because of the extreme nature of these events, patient presentation rates can be high [26]. Providing medical care to these types of events can pose several unique challenges. Besides dealing with issues previously mentioned such as weather and being across a large area, adventure races and other activities often take place in backcountry settings. Should an injury or illness occur along the route of one of these events, teams may need special knowledge, physical ability, and equipment beyond that used in a more static large area event such as a music festival to extract the patient. Due to the characteristics of the event, patients who are participants in the event may have more severe orthopedic or soft tissue injuries, or even complex medical issues in endurance events [27].

Conclusion

Providing high quality medical care at a mass gathering event starts with the people providing care. Organizers must ensure that they plan for the proper types of medical staff, as well as adequate support staff to ensure a successful operation. Training must go beyond the clinical ability to provide care and include specifics on how to provide care during the event, on the venue itself, and on triage and incident management theories. Providers must ensure that they are prepared mentally and physically for their assignments and organizers should ensure that teams have the proper equipment and provisions to provide care at the event. The key to a successful event comes down to this careful planning and preparation, as well as regular sharing of information and effective communication among all staff members.

References

1. Manser T., Teamwork and Patient Safety in Dynamic Domains of Healthcare: A Review of the Literature. *Acta Anaesthesiol Scand.* 2009;**53**:143–151.

2. Ajeigbe D. O., McNeese-Smith D., Searle Leach L., et al. Nurse-Physician Teamwork in the Emergency Department. *Journal of Nursing Administration.* 2013;**43**:142–148.

3. Herzberg S., Hansen M., Schoonover A., et al. Association Between Measured Teamwork and Medical Errors: An Observational Study of Prehospital Care in the USA. *BMJ Open*. 2019;**9**:e025314.

4. van der Wagen L. and White L. *Events Management: For Tourism, Cultural, Business and Sporting Events*. Richmond: Pearson; 2010.

5. Preparedness Team. Public health for mass gatherings: Key considerations [Internet]. World Health Organization; 2015. www.who.int/publica tions-detail-redirect/public-health-for-mass-gather ings-key-considerations

6. Office of the Assistant Secretary for Preparedness and Response. Mass casualty and mass effect incidents: Implications for healthcare organizations [Internet]. US Department of Health and Human Services; 2012. www.phe.gov/Preparedness/planning/mscc/health carecoalition/chapter1/Pages/implications.aspx

7. Link M. S., Atkins D. L., Passman R. S., et al. Part 6: Electrical Therapies: Automated External Defibrillators, Defibrillation, Cardioversion, and Pacing: 2010 American Heart Association Guidelines for Cardiopulmonary Resuscitation and Emergency Cardiovascular Care. *Circulation*. 2010;**18**:706–719.

8. National Association of EMS Physicians. Position Statement: Mass Gathering Medical Care. *Prehospital Emergency Care*. 2015;**19**:558.

9. National Highway Traffic Safety Administration. National EMS scope of practice model [Internet]. US Department of Transportation; 2007. www.ems.gov/pd f/education/EMS-Education-for-the-Future-A-System s-Approach/National_EMS_Scope_Practice_Model.pdf

10. National Registry of EMTs. Paramedic program accreditation policy [Internet]. www.nremt.org/ Policies/Certification-Policies/Paramedic-Program-Acc reditation-Policy

11. Martin-Gill C., Brady W. J., Barlotta K., et al. Hospital-Based Healthcare Provider (Nurse and Physician) Integration into an Emergency Medical Services-Managed Mass-Gathering Event. *American Journal of Emergency Medicine*. 2007;**25**:15–22.

12. Schwartz B., Nafziger S., Milsten A., et al. Mass Gathering Medical Care: Resource Document for the National Association of EMS Physicians Position Statement. *Prehospital Emergency Care*. 2015;**19**:559–568.

13. Commission on Accreditation of Allied Health Education Programs. Standards and Guidelines for the Accreditation of Educational Programs in the Emergency Medical Services Professions 2015. https://coaemsp.org/resource-library.

14. Lockeman K. S., Appelbaum N. P., Dow A. W., et al. The Effect of an Interprofessional Simulation-Based Education Program on Perceptions and Stereotypes of Nursing and Medical Students: A Quasi-Experimental Study. *Nurse Education Today*. 2017;**58**:32–37.

15. Croen L. G., Hamerman D., Goetzel R. Z. Interdisciplinary Training for Medical and Nursing Students: Learning to Collaborate in the Care of Geriatric Patients. *Journal of the American Geriatrics Society*. 1984;**32**:56–61.

16. Federal Emergency Management Agency. ICS-100 Student Manual 2018. https://training.fema.gov/emi web/is/is100c/student%20manual/is0100c_sm.pdf

17. Soomaroo L. and Murray V. Disasters at Mass Gatherings: Lessons from History. *PLoS Curr*. 2012;4: RRN1301.

18. Milsten A. M., Maguire B. J., Bissell R. A., et al. Mass-Gathering Medical Care: A Review of the Literature. *Prehospital and Disaster Medicine*. 2002;**17**:151–162.

19. Moore R., Williamson K., Sochor M., et al. Large-Event Medicine: Event Characteristics Impacting Medical Need. *American Journal of Emergency Medicine*. 2011;**29**:1217–1221.

20. Health and Safety Executive. *The Event Safety Guide* 2nd ed. 1999. [Internet]. www.gov.gg/CHttpHandler .ashx?id=107111&p=0

21. Emergency Management Institute. IS-200: ICS for Single Resources and Initial Action Incidents. Federal Emergency Management Agency 2020. https://train ing.fema.gov/is/coursematerials.aspx?code=IS-200.c

22. Casa D. J., DeMartini J. K., Bergeron M. F., et al. National Athletic Trainers' Association Position Statement: Exertional Heat Illness. *Journal of Athletic Training*. 2015;**50**:986–1000.

23. Rau N. and Paulson D. After Big Attendance Drop, Bonnaroo 2019 Sells Out in Dramatic Turnaround. *Tennessean* 2019. www.tennessean.com/story/enter tainment/music/bonnaroo/2019/06/10/bonnaroo-20 19-sells-out-dramatic-turnaround/1370144001/

24. Great Stage Park. Property info, 2008. www.greatsta gepark.com/greatstagepark.pdf

25. KitzGibbon K. M., Nable J. V., Ayd B., et al. Mass-Gathering Medical Care in Electronic Dance Festivals. *Prehospital and Disaster Medicine*. 2017;**32**:563–567.

26. Burdick T. E. Wilderness Event Medicine: Planning for Mass Gatherings in Remote Areas. *Travel Medicine and Infectious Disease*. 2005;3:249–258.

27. Mort A. and Godden D. Injuries to Individuals Participating in Mountain and Wilderness Sports. *Clinical Journal of Sport Medicine*. 2011;**21**:530–536.

Mass Gathering Medicine: Equipment and Planning Considerations

Robert Alexander, Tatum Lemly, Melanie Welcher, and Kostas Alibertis

Introduction

"Amateurs talk strategy. Professionals talk logistics."

Providing emergency services to event gatherings of any size goes far and beyond simply having medical providers present. Small events may not need a large cache of supplies or equipment, or even a medical tent to stage out of; however, as events grow, the resources required to provide effective care grows exponentially to the number of staff required. Ambulances, medical supplies, and even self-contained medical shelters are often essential to ensure a comprehensive and capable provision of services to manage any on-site emergencies. Large events necessitate extensive preplanning and support logistics in order to become self-reliant and sustainable. Establishing an effective IMT (Incident Management Team) with multiagency inclusion early in the planning process allows the designation of roles, responsibilities, scope, and associated logistics. As events expand, being able to provide care requires the incorporation of complex algorithms of operations and careful pre-event acquisition of everything from Band-Aids and OTC (over the counter) medications to ACLS standard medications and critical care equipment to compliment capability. Setting up a "base of operations" will allow coordination of a hospital-like treatment area, a command tent/trailer, stretchers, equipment, personnel, and supplies to support the extended events. An equally important, and often overlooked component of a successful event also includes the infrastructure necessary to provide care. Generators, Heating, Ventilation, and Air Conditioning (HVAC) units, support trailers, and lodging campers for staff are key components of large scale, multiday events. In addition, providing meals, snacks, respite, and rehabilitation areas are essential for maintaining the mental and physical health of the support staff. Staffing of nonmedical personnel for logistics and maintenance needs prevents gaps in service delivery and helps preserve medical personnel for health-care needs. Without careful planning and the presence of a strong support system, any event's success can be functionally and medically compromised.

Event Assessment

The first step to providing quality care for any event begins well before the actual event date. A careful assessment of the event is required to determine what equipment and personnel will be necessary to provide on the day or days of the event. Knowledge of everything from the median age of attendees, demographics, type of venue, and weather can influence the number and types of patient contacts that a provider can expect to experience. See Figure 6.1. These variables will ultimately determine staffing and what equipment should be available. In addition, other important variables to consider are time to definitive care, duration of the event, and even what budget a venue is willing to provide.

Size of the Event

One of the most important determining factors of expected patient contacts is the size of the event in question. Naturally, one would expect to need more personnel and equipment on hand to appropriately staff a multiday heavy metal band concert over a large area, than the local high school football game, although each presents its own unique challenges. See Figure 6.2. While the number of personnel required scales fairly linearly, the amount of equipment needed increases exponentially as an event moves from the levels 1, 2, and 3 to the levels 4 and 5.

Weather (heat index)	Attendance	Ethanol	Crowd age	Crowd intention	Point value
>90°F (heat index)	>15,000	Significant	Older	Animated	2
<90°F (heat index) climate not controlled	1,000–15,000	Limited	Mixed	Intermediate	1
Climate controlled	<1,000	None	Younger	Calm	0

Major events: total score greater than 5, or scores of 2 in 2 different categories.

Intermediate events: total score greater than 3 but less than 5, or a score of 2 in any 1 category.

Minor Events: total score less than 3.

Figure 6.1 Predicting resource use at mass gatherings using a simplified stratification scoring model. (Hartman N, Williamson A, Sojka B, Alibertis K, Sidebottom M, Hamm J, O'Connor RE, Brady WJ. Predicting Resource Utilization at Mass Gatherings Using a Simplified Stratification Scoring Model. *American Journal of Emergency Medicine*. 2009;27:337–343.)

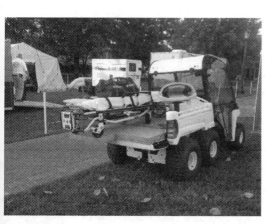

Figure 6.2 Gators effectively used for patient access and transport during large events where vehicular travel is prohibitive

Venue

The type of venue in which an event will be hosted can cause huge variations in the number and type of patient presentations a provider team must be able to anticipate. Significant infrastructure variations (indoor versus outdoor, daytime versus nighttime) alters the amount of logistics and specialty equipment. This goes beyond simply understanding that outdoor events in the peak of summer will see more cases of heat exhaustion, bites and stings, and even sunburns than an indoor event. Medical calls for service are not only limited to patrons but also event staff who often make up a significant number of patient contacts. Providers must prepare for a number of different logistical complications that may arise with outdoor venues and night operations in addition to the medical complaints that accompany them.

One of the first questions providers need to answer may be whether they will need to provide a covered area for both the staff as well as the patrons that are being treated. While a two-hour outdoor sporting event may not necessitate a covered workstation, a longer event or an event in places without natural shade may benefit from a roof to shelter from the elements. See Figure 6.3.

Providers may also need to vary their approach based on the size of the venue itself. Larger venues may require multiple aid stations to be staffed across the event and/or a means of transporting patients to and from the aid station. Walking teams, bike teams, and medical gators/carts are all essential to provide comprehensive responses to the venue, parking areas, and walking routes. In addition, it is not uncommon to also provide primary 911 service to neighborhoods and local residents whose access to timely jurisdictional

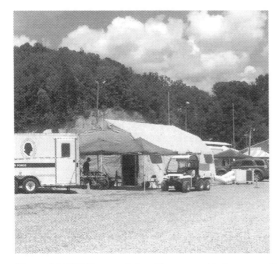

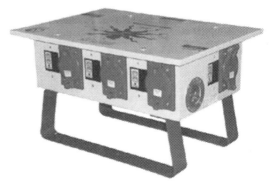

Figure 6.4 Power distribution box like the one pictured can allow for more efficient utilization of power

Figure 6.3 EMS Treatment site with command trailer, covered tent for triage and patient drop off and mobile hospital facility

emergency medical services (EMS) is delayed or restricted by traffic congestion and/or established event perimeters. Providers will also need a reliable means of communication to help direct resources where they are needed. In terms of communication, cell phones may not be useful as cell towers are easily overwhelmed with the added numbers of users and the bandwidth consumption from live transmissions. At times mobile cell towers can be a part of logistics to ensure wireless communications but those come at a high price. Typically radios (VHF, UHF, or 800 MHz) are the most common (and reliable) means of communication on existing municipal radio systems with the utilization of special assigned event or special operations channels. Areas outside of reliable network reception can rely on the utilization of direct communications (talk around frequencies or nonrepeated channels). This may necessitate access to a cache of radios either through a local Emergency Communication Center or a state Emergency Operation Center. Modern technology with group texts can include the whole team and keep people informed of what is happening in each venue as a secondary or concurrent system. Notably text messages require much less bandwidth. Communication decorum is expected at all times and "just in time" training may be required for some staff. An added resource in this setting would be a dedicated dispatcher (one point of contact) that not only assigns

staff to calls for service, but also aids in prioritizing responses and ensuring adequate resources are responding to treat and transport as needed. The tracking of incidents and their dispositions and monitoring for accountability and safety of staff is just as critical. Lastly, this system is used for logistics of supplies that need to be replenished at aid stations or staff that need to be rotated or relieved from their shifts, this means of communication allows for not only the provision of care but also the ability to integrate multiple agencies or partners. Despite the advances of technology, there are still plenty of areas in the country where cell phone service is not readily available and/or reliable even for back-up communications, therefore, radios are always preferred. This allows for large broadcasts to the whole team and can be used in almost every situation.

While access to electricity is an assumption in most cases, *adequate* electricity can be a challenge. Even at the most modern stadiums having access to an adequate electrical supply to power a stand-alone HVAC unit for a cooling tent or medical treatment tent is not always available. Remote venues almost always need the inclusion of generators for primary services. These vary from small 5kw units for basic lighting and fans to more robust 40kw units that can power whole medical compounds with support operations equipment. Having a power distribution box like the one pictured above allows for better utilization of the available electricity. See Figure 6.4. Electricity is critical to so many aspects from climate control to recharging radios and equipment to maintaining readiness by ongoing charging of stand-by ambulances. Lighting is another often taken for granted need. Even day-long events often require setup and takedown in the dark not to mention tent lighting. Water is also an essential need for all operations, both potable water and nonpotable should be available in quantity for long-term events. Dehydration is a primary concern during summer events both in participants and staff as well as the need to be able to wash and decontaminate equipment.

Duration

Another key consideration when planning for an event is to consider the time of the day the event will be held and how long the event is expected to run. The longer the event, the higher volume of patient's that can be expected to be treated and the more infrastructure needed to provide extended services for patrons and staff.

For events lasting up to a half-day there will not be the need for multiple shifts or relief teams for the providers and while certainly appreciated, meals and snacks are likely not a necessity, however having water available should always be a priority. As the events stretch to full day or multiday affairs, it is important to plan how and when snacks, meals, and hydration will be provided. Always encourage staff to bring a snack or hydration to any event to meet what might be a personal requirement. Some events may dictate that meals will need to be catered as there have been examples of venue food not always meeting the need or even being reliably safe. All of these should be factored into the budget process. With these longer events, careful consideration must be put into how and when teams are going to be scheduled to work. Staggering shifts to ensure redundant coverage during peak hours helps alleviate the individual provider workload but may not always be feasible depending on the particular event. Also, there are often specific requirements for the needs of "talent" or athletes in addition to those for the participants. Surge capacity is important for multiple reasons and should be included in any contractual negotiations. This becomes especially challenging for multiday events in places away from larger urban centers. Will shelter/housing need to be provided for staff overnight? Will providers be shuttling back and forth? Is there the need to have a fresh set of staff for each day? Given longer ambulance transport times it may be advisable

to add additional units, also preplanning (LZ locations) and arranging for air evacuations if needed. All of these are important questions that need to be answered before the event begins.

While longer events take a toll on staff, it also affects attendees as well. Longer events that include drugs/alcohol also increases the complexity of care that needs to be provided. Attendees may have preexisting medical conditions that would require them to seek assistance and care. After all, a goal for any mass gathering is to keep patrons at the event which helps minimize the impact on local EMS and community healthcare resources. For instance, with microbreweries becoming more popular throughout the country, there are more outdoor related brew crawls that are being held. These usually happen in the summer which couples sun/heat/humidity with ample amounts of alcohol. This combination always poses risks to the patrons that include heat emergencies, dehydration, and alcohol-related emergencies.

Weather

Expected weather conditions are important to account for when planning an event. During cold weather months it may be important to provide an enclosed shelter to house the triage and treatment teams. Portable heaters can be rented and run off of generators or propane and these can quickly and efficiently warm a staging area and provide a refuge for staff and patients while providing care in a more controlled environment. During the summer months the heat index can take a toll on attendees and one can expect to see more people suffering from heat exhaustion and dehydration, especially during day long or multiday events. While smaller events may only need some form of shade to escape the sun. For larger events, acquisition of an HVAC system is beneficial and allows the venue to create a cool sheltered environment from which to operate and provide medical care. Misting fans, cooling tents, and hydration stations can help lessen the impact of weather/heat-related complaints. When considering the use of generators and HVAC systems, the team has to keep in mind that there will need to be at least one person with adequate knowledge of the systems to be able to serve as a mechanic to troubleshoot any complication that may arise with the systems being used. Adequate food and supplies need to be considered as well when staffing large/long events especially when considering the elements. Water supply must always be present during these events for the staff and patrons needing care.

Event Profile

Profiling events is an important component of event medical services. Knowing the population of people expected to attend an event can also drastically alter the types of patient encounters a provider will experience. The presence of alcohol at an event will dramatically increase the number of medical encounters that are expected and the number of intoxicated attendees will most likely increase as the event goes on. Concerts and festivals also tend to coincide with increased recreational drug use which increases the likelihood of adverse events or injury requiring medical intervention. Predicting current needs from previous experiences is very helpful. Reaching out to venues that have hosted similar events or talent (concerts) as a preview of what to prepare for and what services will be needed is always a wise choice.

Other events such as high school sporting events or graduations have a significantly different attendee profile and while the attendees themselves are usually relatively young and healthy, they usually bring an older patient population with more chronic medical conditions. While generally tamer and with less medical encounters, we see a higher incidence of transport to definitive healthcare sites for presentations such as chest pain or shortness of breath. Lastly, all large event gatherings should have a very robust MCI plan with mutual aid agreements in place as well as a command and control agreement.

Definitive Healthcare

The reality remains that while event medical staff are hired to provide medical care, there is always a limit to what can be provided in a remote setting. Inevitably, they will have to transport patients to a definitive healthcare setting for additional workup and treatment. However, depending on location and settings this can occupy a team of medical providers and an ambulance for at least an hour and up to several hours. This time only increases the further out from a healthcare setting medical providers are located and it is not always feasible to rely on local EMS systems for

transport especially in the remote setting. The more remote, the fewer local resources that are available as a rule. For these remote events, it may be necessary to have three or four teams to ensure they always have one ambulance and a provider team onsite and ready in case of emergency and in this case having dedicated transport teams that do not factor into the primary care team staffing.

For events located within city limits or with definitive healthcare readily available this often takes a huge burden off of the event staffing as transport times are short and they can often utilize local EMS systems in the case of overflow or surge to provide transport should it become necessary. However, particular traffic flow and access, for security reasons, do not allow nonvetted entry (security clearance), thus rendezvous and transfer of care options may be necessary.

Infrastructure and Logistics Summary

When planning what equipment is necessary to properly staff the event, one of the important things to ask is what infrastructure is already in place that can be utilized. Being able to secure an indoor area with access to heating and cooling as well as electricity can obviate the need for enclosed tents, HVAC or heating and generators and significantly reduce the cost required to provide an adequate working area from which to stage a medical response. However, the absence of these niceties necessitates event management procuring and providing essential supplies, infrastructure, and equipment, in addition to the medical and nonmedical staff needed to support an operation.

Service Level

When approached by venues it is beneficial to probe their expectations of the medical service provider. Often medical providers are hired as a legal necessity and when laying out the budget to provide the medical care of the venue there is usually a degree of reluctance. While it is important to be flexible with some of the less medically necessary equipment, as the expert in mass gathering medicine event medical providers will be responsible both ethically and *legally* for managing any emergencies that may arise. It is important to clearly define equipment and resource expectations that are required to operate safely and make sure that medical provision needs are well known to the event organizers and recorded in writing. At the end of the day if there is a poor outcome at an event one can easily become a victim of an organizer that claims, "they didn't tell me I needed that."

There will almost always be discrepancies between the equipment which is felt to be necessary and what the venue is willing to provide. One must also consider what level of care is expected by the attendees. With longer and higher profile events, attendees may expect to be able to access physician providers who can suture, treat asthma exacerbations, and offer rehydration along with OTC medications that are not readily available. Intervening to treat and release or treat and delay allows patrons to continue to enjoy the event.

Equipment by Event Category

Category 1

Overview: Category 1 events are considered to consist of an expected small number of attendees (usually a few hundred or less). In addition, these are typically low risk based on demographics and event profile and duration. Few patient contacts are anticipated. Other factors (alcohol and/or weather extremes) independent of the expected total number to attend the event can raise the risk profile of the event to higher categories that would require additional staffing and supplies.

Staffing: A single EMS provider is usually adequate to provide service at these smaller events where there is not expected to be a large burden on the health care providers. One must also consider the training of the staff according to event size as well as risk profile of the crowd. An individual with EMT training is usually acceptable staffing for these events. Occasionally, these events may be events within larger events. This would allow other crews with higher training, such as paramedics, to be centrally located and respond as needed.

Equipment: For these category one events, very minimal equipment is needed outside of the EMTs standard equipment (oxygen, medical bag, and Automated External Defibrillator [AED]). Granted, one has to consider the comfort and safety of the crew during these events. If the crew is expected to be outside during the event, something as basic as a place of shade to protect from the sun and a chair/seat will serve the crew well and

allow them to continue to concentrate on providing medical care. Communication with the individual is key in terms of preparing them not only for medical events that may take place at the event but also what kind of supplies they will need to keep them comfortable and safe.

Equipment list: AED, fanny pack with bandaging and splinting supplies, blood pressure cuff, stethoscope, pulse oximeter. Basic meds to include ASA, MDI (inhaler), epi pen, oral glucose.

Logistics: The EMT providers will be expected to provide on-scene medical care and utilize the local 911 service for transport to hospitals. This actually simplifies the logistical aspect of making sure enough staff will be on scene while the patient is being transferred to the hospital due to the providers not being responsible for both medical care and the actual transport.

Category 2

Overview: Category 2 events usually consist of less than 2,500 patrons. These usually consist of small entertainment events such as a small outdoor concert or sporting event such as a local high school football game.

Staffing: These events usually require two EMS providers with or without an ambulance but not transport capable. These providers will need to be trained at recognizing and treating life threatening emergencies as well as other more basic medical care such as addressing small wounds. At these category 2 events, there may be niche training involved in order to best serve the patients at these events. For example, if an EMS crew is working a high school football game they will need to know the proper way to stabilize the cervical spine for athletes given current standards of care and other orthopedic injuries that they will be expected to treat.

Equipment: Both EMT providers will have their standard medical equipment. Ambulance can be used as a base of operations and a cache of medical supplies but not utilized as a primary transport. As with any scenario, keeping the integrity of the crew is paramount. Having communication equipment and protocols in place, along with options for food, shelter, and water is key.

Logistics: The EMT providers will be expected to provide on-scene medical care and utilize the local 911 service for transport to hospitals. This actually simplifies the logistical aspect of making sure enough staff will be on scene while the patient is being transferred to the hospital due to the providers not being responsible for both medical care and the actual transport.

Category 3

Overview: Category 3 events are usually less than 3,500 patrons. In addition, this may be an event with fewer patrons that has a higher risk profile due to crowd demographics, event profile, duration, or other factors that may add to the anticipated number of patient contacts.

Staffing: Recommend three to four EMS providers with onsite transport available. This team may be expected to work in multiple configurations. As a group in a three to four person team, a base team of one to two members and one to two functioning as a walking/roving team, or two two-person teams positioned strategically for the event. This event should have a team supervisor that can be one of the care providers. It should also be anticipated to be ready to downsize to a two-person team if a patient needs to be transported via onsite ambulance. Utilization of local EMS for surge assistance.

Equipment: Standard medical equipment along with backup equipment should the ambulance be needed for transport. Shelter and chairs for outdoor events and provisions for water and meals for longer events. Portable radios for communication.

Logistics: The logistically challenging part of only three to four providers and an ambulance is that they can only transport one patient to the hospital at a time. This mitigates the challenge if multiple people need medical attention and/or transport. If one of the available teams is transferring a patient to the hospital, then the secondary team will be left to treat the other patients. When this happens in largely populated metropolitan areas with adequate resources, this usually does not pose a large risk due to other units most likely being immediately available nearby. This tends to pose higher risk when these events occur in more rural areas with longer transport time to hospitals as well as larger distance between various EMS crews and location of the event. Therefore, having more than one EMS crew available on scene at these events, has multiple benefits. It provides for surge capability, the ability to provide transportation for patrons, multiple points

of contact for the provision of medical care and for teams to rehab during longer events.

Category 4

Overview: These are larger sporting events such as a college basketball game or low risk concert or entertainment event where an expected 3,500–10,000 will be attending the game/event.

Staffing: Minimum of eight EMS providers with two to three on-site ambulances to transport. Dedicated field supervisor(s) is necessary and potentially a dedicated supervisor to staff a command post for interagency coordination. This would be comprised of representatives from medical, law enforcement, event staff, and possibly a facilities representative.

Equipment: At this point equipment needs begin to rapidly expand as it may not be optimal to use the ambulances as an equipment cache. Additional medical bags and AEDs for walking teams, either a designated room or tent(s) setup as a base of operations to provide evaluation and treatment. This area should have its own dedicated equipment and staffing. It should have Advanced Life Support (ALS) (paramedic) capability, medications, cardiac monitors, and a treatment area with cots. Extraction equipment should be available like a Reeves stretcher, stair chair, med sleds, and ambulance cots for moving patients from point of contact to the care area. Radios are necessary to coordinate responses and a dispatcher may be needed to monitor activity and responses. Depending on the venue a bike team or medical cart may be utilized. Once again, the duration, demographic, risk profile, weather, and other factors of the event will also dictate what type of equipment is needed to keep the medical staff that is working the event safe and ready to respond to emergencies.

Logistics: Coordination between teams is always key when it comes to delivering patient care, therefore roles must be assigned and an accountability system in place. In addition, there needs to be a robust means of receiving and dispatching calls. At these events requests for service are often by direct contact and in rare instances a patron may call 911. Every crew member must know who is on site and what operations are ongoing, that is, teams available, responding or transporting at any given time, and if there are multiple crews transporting patients at the same time. The teams must know that more

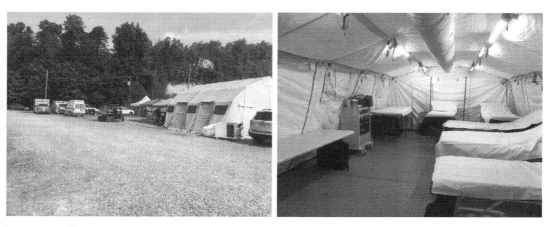

Figure 6.5 Left: Category 5 base of operations. Right: Base-X Model 305 (18'x25') Climate controlled with flooring

responsibility will fall on their shoulders in terms of continuing patient care at these events and backfilling empty assignments or expanding areas of responsibility. Arguably, single resource assignments in a safe controlled atmosphere where other event staff are also present provide more points of contact for patrons and a faster response time due to proximity. This is in contrast to standard EMS models that often deploy in two to three-person teams. This determination is contingent on a low risk profile that has large crowds like a university graduation. Also note that most of these events also have nonmedical staff that can assist so medical responders are rarely alone.

Category 5

Overview: Category 5 events are considered the most complex and involve 10,000+ people at an event that may be extended in duration or even multiday. Some of these necessitate twenty-four-hour service coverage and are often influenced by multiple other factors (type of event, camping/overnight facilities, and patient characteristics to name a few)that enhance the risk profile and effect the number and type of patient contacts and the need to provide physician level services, critical care, and even resuscitations. These events take months to prepare for and several days to set up and take down. College football, equine events, car races, outdoor concerts, and large music festivals are examples.

Staffing: Minimum of fifteen EMS providers and scalable based on event. A dedicated multiagency command post and IMT, along with multiple supervisors assigned to sectors or divisions not involved in direct patient care. Staff dedicated to logistics, event dispatchers, bike teams, medical carts/gators, and multiple transport ambulances on site with dedicated crews. Physicians typically staff the medical care areas.

Equipment: the equipment list is extensive from basic EMS supplies to multiple STIP (Stabilize Treat In Place) tents that function as mobile hospitals. See Figure 6.5. Given the expected large crowd with potential high volume of patients, a large amount of planning is needed in order to ensure adequate health care delivery. Stand-alone HVAC systems, generators to provide electricity, portable bathrooms and showers, decontamination supplies patient monitoring systems, a pharmacy cache and ventilators. Trailers and tents setup for storage of supplies and backup equipment. Areas for staff to take breaks and get meals.

Logistics: The logistics behind these events are large and complex. One must consider every aspect from both the medical team perspective as well as the expected patients. The longer the event, the more complex this will become. How long are the shifts? What type of overlap will there be between providers? In these situations, there has to be at least one and often multiple staff whose job is to solely be handling the logistical side of the event. This person should have a list of all supplies needed and how much there is of said supplies readily. See Figure 6.6. Philosophically it means

Category 5 Event Checklist:

Equipment:

Bags

- MCI
- Medication
- Airway
- Trauma
- Immobilization
- Fanny pack

Ambulances

Quick response vehicles

Gators

Bikes

AEDs

Extra multifunction defib/pacers

Medical carts

Cots

Radio cache and bank chargers

Linens

Structures:

E-Z UP® tents

Enclosed trailers with climate control

STIP (SeT up In Place) tents with flooring

Miscellaneous supplies:

Chairs

HVAC/Environmental Control Units (ECU) units

Generators

Power distribution boxes(ex Ericson Oscar box, spider boxes)

Privacy partitions

Water key

Tools and power equipment

Lighting indoor and outdoor

Jump box

Ambulance charging cords

Misting fans

Fire extinguishers

Coolers

Coffee pot

Medications

EMS drug box

Rapid Sequence Intubation (RSI) medications

Oxygen fixed and portable

IV fluids

Event specific medications

OTC medications (aspirin, acetaminophen, ibuprofen, Benadryl, tums, antacid Imodium, Zofran)

Figure 6.6 Supply list for Category 5 event

establishing a structure and a service delivery model that is independent and self-sufficient from hot coffee to critical care medicine.

Setting up these tents requires expertise and at least four to six individuals led by a well-trained seasoned supervisor and ideally all should have basic training on set-up and repair. There are countless examples of costly damage to equipment due to lack of proper training and experience. There should be another individual that is well-versed in handling the mechanical questions, repairs, and is responsible for the equipment such as the generators. If the event is outside and no means of power is readily available, then generators are required for the powering. Even if there is power available, access and utilization is often difficult because of design constraints.

Summary

Preparing for an event from simple to complex involves preplanning and robust communication between the involved agencies and the sponsor. Failure to adequately plan, prepare, and have the necessary equipment invites failure. A complex medical mission is often a lot more logistics and equipment than actual care.

Events that are small and simple require little more than basic thought and supplies. Large events that are complex require preplanning, complex implementation, and can have event-specific medical protocols and terms not standard to the industry of healthcare. One example is when asking for a cot to be brought to evacuate a patient the term "light cot" means just the cot and a provider, while "heavy cot" may mean suction, cardiac monitor, airway bag, and medications. The ability to be dynamic and flexible working outside the norms both with equipment and mindset is a necessity in mass gathering medicine, and mass gathering medicine is not just about providing care but providing customer service!

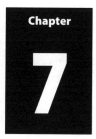

Incident Command System at Mass Gathering Events

Lucian A. Mirra

Introduction

A Case for the Incident Command System

A rush of patrons onto a field after a hard-fought victory in a rivalry game. The surge of a crowd to the front of a concert venue. A sudden summer microburst at an outdoor festival. An active threat, fire, or any other catastrophe that could affect a mass gathering event and cause a multiple casualty incident. An event, so sudden, chaotic, and often unexpected, that it causes pandemonium and chaos among event attendees, and often, among event staff as well. As a medical provider assigned to the event, we must consider how we would manage the incident beyond just the treatment of patients. Who commands, controls, and coordinates the response? What is the proper reporting chain, who is in charge of what, and what tasks need to be accomplished? The answers to these questions lie in the Incident Command System (ICS).

History of the Incident Command System

Like many concepts adopted in medicine and emergency services, the roots of the ICS can be dated to the military. When veterans returned from World War II, they brought with them a more modern idea of a command-and-control structure. In this structure, each person had a specific reporting line in a chain of command, and battlefields were managed by completing specific objectives. This direct line of order, along with focusing on accomplishing specific mission objectives, was successful and has been taught as strategy in military training programs for decades.

With the end of World War II, numerous highly trained professionals returned to the United States with extensive training on this command-and-control strategy. Many veterans continued public service by joining the ranks of the fire department. Coinciding with a large wildland-urban population growth in Southern California, there were numerous new jobs in the fire service. These firefighters faced not only traditional building fires similar to their colleagues in fire departments on the east coast, but also large wildfires that threatened development. These veterans, who by the 1960s and 1970s were often in superior ranks, applied the strategies which were learned on the battlefield to these large incidents. The first application of a formal command-and-control structure was the Large Fire Organization (LFO), which was an incident management structure built to coordinate wildfire management in Southern California. The LFO primarily organized the effort to fight a fire locally but lacked centralized coordination, particularly between multiple jurisdictions or agencies.

The Incident Command System that exists today was a result of a particularly devastating wildfire season in 1970. In addition to a large volume of fires, the effort to combat them lacked coordination which resulted in critically low resource levels due to inefficiencies. During a thirteen-day period, sixteen people were killed, over a half-million acres burned, causing over $200 million dollars in damage. In reaction to this, Congress allocated funding to the United States Forest Service (USFS) with the goal of establishing a centralized command-and-control system that provided for both multiagency and multijurisdictional coordination. The USFS partnered with the California Department of Forestry (CDF), the California Office of Emergency Services (OES) and several local jurisdictional fire departments in Southern California, including the City and County of Los Angeles. The resulting organization, FIRESCOPE (Firefighting Resources of Southern California Organized for Potential Emergencies), developed the Multiagency Coordination System (MACS), and the Incident Command System (ICS) that exists today [1].

Early Incident Command System Development

The Incident Command System that was developed by FIRESCOPE had the primary objective of command, control, and coordination. Understanding that large wildfires can often cross multiple jurisdictions, and involve services besides the fire department, a more advanced structure was needed to ensure that like on the battlefields, crews were fighting with a united front. The developers of ICS also realized that numerous ancillary services were necessary as well. Wildfire incidents often last several days, and even several weeks. Crews would need to have rest areas, food, and a plan for medical treatment. Additionally, with the passage of the Disaster Relief Act of 1974, a plan was in place to reimburse states and local governments for disasters, necessitating expenditures be tracked. The Incident Command System accounted for not only the operational needs but the ancillary needs of these large incidents as well.

Nationwide Adoption

Throughout the 1970s and 1980s, the use of the Incident Command System was largely concentrated in the management of wildfires. In addition to wildfires, the City and County of Los Angeles began using ICS for other incidents such as structure fires and

technical rescues. Despite this, the use of ICS was still limited. One of the first uses outside of the Southern California and wildfire management communities was by the United States Coast Guard. After the *Exxon Valdez* spill in 1989, the Coast Guard recognized the need for a more coordinated way to respond to large incidents and ICS became a standard practice in all Coast Guard responses through the 1990s [1, 2].

The terrorist attacks of September 11, 2001, also marked a key milestone in the propagation of ICS as a nationwide standard. In response to these incidents, President George W. Bush issued Homeland Security Presidential Directive 5 (HSPD-5), which called for the selection and development of a nationwide incident command and management system [3]. In 2004, this resulted in the launching of the National Incident Management System (NIMS), which includes MACS and the Incident Command System. Since 2004, the Department of Homeland Security (DHS), specifically through the Federal Emergency Management Agency (FEMA) has administered the NIMS, including offering both asynchronous online courses as well as in-person courses as well as tying the completion of specific courses to federal grant funding. Suggested courses for medical personnel staffing mass gathering events can be found in Table 7.1.

The Incident Command System

Overview of the Incident Command System

NIMS is a "systematic, proactive approach to guide all levels of government, nongovernmental organizations (NGOs), and the private sector to work together to prevent, protect against, mitigate, respond to, and recover from the effects of incidents" [4]. NIMS has three major components: resource management, communications and information management, and command and coordination. The Incident Command System is a component of NIMS, and is the pillar of the command and coordination component.

The ICS, still largely unchanged from its original version published by FIRESCOPE, is a scalable solution to managing any incident. While it was originally designed to handle wildfires, the flexibility, scalability, and portability of the ICS mean that it may be used for any incident of any size and duration. It is used daily by fire departments across the United States on incidents as simple as a minor motor vehicle crash or a fire alarm sounding, in which the response may consist of one or two apparatus and may only be active

---

Table 7.1 Suggested courses

Courses Recommended for All Responders

FEMA Independent Study Courses: http://training.fema.gov/is

- FEMA IS–100.c – Introduction to the Incident Command System
- FEMA IS–200.c – Basic Incident Command System for Initial Response
- FEMA IS–700.b – An Introduction to the National Incident Management System

Advanced Courses (In Person)

- FEMA ICS–300 – Intermediate ICS for Expanding Incidents
- FEMA ICS–400 – Advanced ICS
- TEEX AWR–167 – Sport and Special Event Risk Management
- TEEX MGT–404 – Sports and Special Events Incident Management

for several minutes. In this example, many of the ICS functions go unfilled, and the ICS may consist just of an Incident Commander. Conversely, the ICS has also been used at large-scale and/or long-term events.

Key Concepts of the Incident Command System

The ICS draws on fourteen characteristics from the NIMS. These concepts are the foundation on which the ICS is built and functions on and include: unity of command, span of control, modular organization, management by objective, common terminology, incident action planning, incident facilities and locations, comprehensive resource management, integrated communications, establishment and transfer of command, unified command, accountability, dispatch/deployment, and information and intelligence management.

Unity of Command

The fundamental concept on which the ICS is built is an established chain of command. Within the ICS, each individual has one, and only one, supervisor. This means that each individual knows who they should report to, and with rare exception such as a safety issue, only report to their designated supervisor. This is meant to ensure accountability, coordinate the flow of information, and cut down on "freelancing," or individuals acting without direction.

Span of Control

In order for the concept of unity of command to be effective, each supervisor within the Incident Command System must be able to effectively coordinate their subordinates. Even in the most effective leader, at a certain point the number of inputs exceed what the individual is capable of processing and the leader becomes too focused on the tasks of their subordinates and loses the "big picture" of an incident. ICS therefore limits the number of individuals who should report to a supervisor to a maximum of seven, with an ideal number of five. The ICS achieves this by its modular structure that can be expanded as the incident and number of resources expands.

Modular Organization

As previously stated, the ICS is used on incidents which may only involve a small number of resources for a short amount of time, or an incident that involves a large number of resources over a long period of time. The ICS allows for the structure to be scaled based on the size, complexity, and type of event. A fire department responding with two fire apparatus to a fire alarm sounding may only need an Incident Commander and perhaps an Investigation Group Supervisor, and the structure may only exist for a few minutes while the cause of the alarm is investigated. On the other hand, a three-day music festival with thousands of attendees will require multiple different agency types from medical, to law enforcement, to public works, and thus will need many more positions of the ICS filled. In unplanned events such as a major fire, crash, active threat or otherwise, the positions are filled in as the incident unfolds.

Management by Objective

Much like in medicine, the ICS has a system of triage for managing parts of the incident. Incidents are managed using objectives, which are ranked by priority. For instance, objectives dealing with preserving the lives of others are ranked ahead of objectives dealing with preserving property. These objectives give a building block for specific tactical decisions as they provide a common operating picture.

Common Terminology

The ICS, through NIMS, establishes common terminology so that everyone operating on an incident understands what is meant. This is especially important when multiple agencies of differing missions or multiple jurisdictions are involved. Specifically, NIMS addresses the common terminology of organizational functions (as described later in this chapter), resources, and facilities. This makes requesting the specific, correct resource and understanding the flow of command and coordination easier by using the same language. An anecdotal example from the wildfire origins of ICS illustrates the importance of common terminology. In some jurisdictions, a "tanker" is a large fire apparatus capable of carrying large amounts of water, normally between 1,000 and 3,000 gallons. In other jurisdictions, this is called a "tender," and a "tanker" is an aircraft capable of dropping water. Imagine the confusion that would ensue if a "tanker" was requested, and instead of a large truck with water, an airplane showed up.

Incident Action Planning

An Incident Action Plan (IAP) is a standardized planning tool that captures and communicates the incident objectives and priorities. It also addresses specific tactics and assignments, as well as support activities such as resource and communication management. An IAP can take many forms, and in smaller, short-term incidents may even be verbal. The IAP addresses a specific time period, known as an operational period, which may be for the duration of a planned event (in the case of a sporting event or concert) or broken up into increments such as in longer-term events. The IAP should answer four basic questions:

1. What are the incident objectives and priorities?
2. Who is responsible for completing each objective?
3. How is communication accomplished?
4. What are the procedures in the case of a safety hazard or injury?

Incident Facilities and Locations

Depending on the extent, type, and duration of the incident, several specific incident facilities and locations may be established. When established, these positions should be communicated through the Incident Action Plan. Specific incident locations which are likely to be designated in mass gathering events are listed in Box 7.1.

Comprehensive Resource Management

Large-scale incidents, whether planned or unplanned, require many different types of resources to be successful. These resources include not only things needed to complete the actual objectives, but also logistical items to support the operation. For example, at a multiday music festival, not only are medical resources required, but the ICS must also address things like food, water, and rest facilities for staff. Comprehensive resource management addresses and implements systems to

> **Box 7.1** Incident locations for mass gathering events
>
> - Incident Command Post
> - Staging Area
> - Triage Area
> - Casualty Collection Point
> - Emergency Shelters

identify an incidents needs, assets acquired, mobilization and tracking of personnel and assets, and demobilization of these personnel and resources.

Integrated Communications

With the basis of the ICS being coordination and sharing information, a common communications plan must be established. Often included as part of an IAP, the communications plans should address connectivity of systems and how information will be shared. Communications plans may include radio, cellular phones, internet, face-to-face, and other methods and designate specific ways of leveraging these technologies such as incident channels and phone numbers.

Establishment and Transfer of Command

As is described in the next section, each incident that uses the ICS has at minimum an Incident Commander. Depending on how the event unfolds, the initial Incident Commander may or may not serve in that capacity for the duration of the event. The establishment of command should be done as early as possible in the incident in order to establish a command and control structure. When the responsibility of Incident Command is transferred it should occur with a briefing to ensure the incoming Incident Commander is ready to step into the role.

Unified Command

In some incidents, due either to size, complexity, or the number of different agencies or jurisdictions involved, it is not feasible to have a single incident commander. This is common in mass gathering events, as typically there is a need to have a law enforcement/security, medical, and event management components of Incident Command. In these instances, a Unified Command may be established. Unified Command allows multiple inputs into a command function and is ideal when the event has multiple facets to the management. See Box 7.2.

Accountability

With the number of resources involved in the management of any large-scale event, it is important to maintain accountability. This accountability applies to both personnel resources as well as logistical resources. This is both for ensuring the safety and well-being of personnel, but also to ensure that a common operating picture is maintained and resources can be properly allocated.

Box 7.2 Single incident commander versus unified command incident examples

Single incident commander: At a structure fire, the objectives center around saving lives and extinguishing the fire. Support activities, such as the police department providing traffic control, is still centered around this primary objective. In this case, a fire department officer is likely to be a single incident commander during this incident.

Unified command: At a major music festival, the police department is responsible for traffic flow, security screening, and general order inside the venue. The emergency medical services agency is responsible for the treatment and stabilization of patients. In this case, while the entities are operating at the same incident, it would not be prudent to have a police officer over the medical care, and vice versa. In this case, a unified command structure may be implemented.

Dispatch and Deployment

In addition to accountability, resources must be dispatched and deployed when needed. Importantly, this also means that resources should not self-dispatch to an incident until called. The temptation to go to where a major incident is occurring is natural to most first responders and medical professionals, however, this may come at the cost of missing a key safety concern or another key aspect in the overall operating picture.

Information and Intelligence Management

Part of the planning process within the ICS is gathering intelligence and information. Even information such as weather can play a pivotal role in incident planning. A football game taking place in August with predicted temperatures in the 90s with a chance of severe thunderstorms has a completely different hazard profile than one in December with temperatures in the 30s with a chance of snow. In order to ensure a common operating picture, information and intelligence must be continually reassessed and shared.

Incident Command System Organization and Positions

One of the key characteristics of the ICS is that it is modular and scalable to the event to which it is being applied. In a smaller incident, the Incident Command position may be the only formal role filled and the IAP existing as a preplanned response template or in verbal form. In a large-scale or long-term incident, additional functional areas may be phased in as required and dictated by the incident objectives. There are five functional areas of the Incident Command System: Command, Operations, Planning, Logistics, and Finance & Administration. Each of these functional areas have specific positions within them, and collectively all of the staff

assigned to the Command area are known as the "Command Staff" and all of the staff assigned to Operations, Planning, Logistics, and Finance & Administration are known as the "General Staff." It is important to note that many agencies use a paramilitary type of command structure (such as sergeants, lieutenants, and captains in police and fire organizations). The Incident Command System is unique in that it operates outside of any single entities organizational structure. When setting up the Incident Command System, personnel should be placed into positions based on their area of expertise, not necessarily by rank.

Command Functional Area and Positions

The Incident Command System is successful in part due to the idea of unity of command. In reality, ICS is a rank structure that is scalable to an incident and exists outside of traditional rank structures. In order for this to be successful, there must be an individual, or in some cases, a small group of individuals, with the responsibility of being in charge. In the ICS, this is known as the command function. While ICS is modular and scalable, the Incident Command position is always required. Broadly, this command position has the responsibilities of establishing incident objectives and priorities in order to facilitate management by objectives. The command function is also responsible for ensuring appropriate safety precautions are in place, determine and approve resources, establishing a command structure and incident command post, and authorize and implement the IAP.

Incident Command

The Incident Commander (IC) is the person ultimately responsible for a given incident. The IC is responsible for the overall development of incident objectives, resource management, and the incident operations including safety, in conjunction with the Safety Officer when staffed. While on larger incidents, these responsibilities are delegated to respective General Staff positions, the incident commander maintains the overall responsibility and oversight, and often gives the final approval for any important decision. This position is uniquely the only position that is always staffed when the Incident Command System is operationalized.

Ideally, ICs should have significant expertise, experience, and training. Because the IC is the only position which must be filled in the Incident Command System, the initial IC in some incidents may not be the most appropriate selection for a larger event. In unplanned events such as a natural disaster or active threat in everyday life, the initial IC is the first arriving responder – which could be an entry-level police officer, firefighter, or emergency medical technician (EMT). Planned events, like those found in mass gathering medicine, allow for careful selection of the right person for the role of IC.

The IC must be able to ensure the safety of all personnel and establish objectives, and in many cases, tactics. The IC must have the technical knowledge to understand the tasks at hand and have the right people in the right positions to assist with technical decisions where necessary. In a mass gathering event where medical services are being provided, ideally the IC would have some medical background or knowledge or expand the ICS to ensure that there is a technically knowledgeable medical leadership position filled. The ideal IC should also be knowledgeable about incident management, strategic planning, and the ICS. This allows the IC to be comfortable in the environment in which they are operating. Lastly, ICs must have the "soft skill" of diplomacy, decisiveness, and the management of personnel. In a high-stress environment as found when responding to an emergent incident, the IC must be able to give orders directly and succinctly, make and articulate decisions, and be able to put the right person in the right place to be successful at their objective.

In many incidents, the position of Incident Command may need to be transferred. Transfers of command may take place when a more qualified IC arrives, the jurisdiction or primary mission of the incident changes, or at the end of an operational period. Ideally a transfer of command occurs face-to-face, but no matter the medium, an overview of the incident, review of objectives and priorities, and the status of resources must be shared. Additionally, notification should be made to personnel when the transfer of command occurs. When a subordinate position is established, that person assumes the title of Deputy Incident Commander. The Deputy IC may be delegated any or all tasks of the IC as required. The Deputy IC position may also be used to mentor new ICs. Uniquely, because mass gathering events are generally planned events, they offer a vital training opportunity for new ICs who may serve in a deputy or shadow capacity to an experienced IC.

Unified Command

In some instances, having one single individual in the Incident Command position is not feasible. This may occur on large incidents, or in certain mass gathering events where several disciplines are required to execute the event. This usually involves multiple agencies and/or jurisdictions participating in an incident or event with several different categories of objectives. In a Unified Command (UC) system, the responsibility normally held by an individual IC is spread among two or more individuals called the Unified Command Group. This is typically implemented when the objectives of the incident are distinct to several different agencies or jurisdictions. This Unified Command Group acts as a single entity in decision-making and is often comprised of senior representatives from the participating agencies or jurisdictions.

Mass gathering events are often run as Unified Command incidents. From a public safety standpoint, mass gathering events have security objectives, medical objectives, and event management objectives. Because the IC should have some technical knowledge of the objectives, it would be difficult for a police commander or medical commander to make tactical decisions for one another. Thus, in many mass gathering events, a Unified Command may be implemented and involve senior leaders from police and security services as well as from medical services, and potentially event management services. Typically, one representative will act as the group's spokesperson, but this does not imply any difference in rank or priority within the group.

Area Command

When an incident has multiple separate geographic locations, an Area Command may be established.

An Area Command is often implemented when a similar event affects multiple different specific incidents. In this instance, each geographic incident has its own Incident Commander who then reports up to an Area Command (which may be an individual or a Unified Command structure). The Area Command is set up in a separate location, such as an Emergency Operations Center (EOC) (discussed later in this chapter) and exists primarily to provide logistical support to each incident under its purview. This is especially helpful when managing a local disaster or a mass gathering event with multiple separate sites across a jurisdiction. This allows these separate incidents to share the Logistics, Planning, and Finance & Administration Sections. Typically, Area Commands do not have an Operations Section, as they exist at the individual incidents.

Command Staff

The Command Staff consists of the IC, Unified Command (UC), or Area Command as well as personnel who support the command function. In most incidents these staff include a Safety Officer, a Public Information Officer, and a Liaison Officer. If subordinates to these positions need to be appointed, such as additional Safety Officers on incidents covering a large geographic area, these would be known as an Assistant (i.e., Assistant Safety Officer). The Command Staff representatives fill specific functions that directly support the IC and typically report directly to the IC.

Safety Officer

The Safety Officer reports directly to the Incident Commander and is part of the Command Staff. When this position is staffed, the Safety Officer is responsible for monitoring operations for any safety issues that may arise. Specifically, the Safety Officer is concerned with the health and safety of all incident personnel, and in many cases, carries the delegated authority of the Incident Commander to stop, suspend, or alter operations for safety reasons. If an additional Safety Officer needs to be appointed, such as due to the size or scope of an incident, they hold the title of Assistant Safety Officer, and report to the Safety Officer.

Public Information Officer

The Public Information Officer (PIO) is the member of the Command Staff delegated with interfacing with the media and the general public. The PIO may be responsible for drafting press releases, speaking to news media,

monitoring and updating social media, and fielding questions from the public. The PIO often works directly with the Incident Commander or their designee to compile what information will be disseminated at what time. Additional PIOs may be necessary and would carry the title of Assistant Public Information Officer.

Liaison Officer

The Liaison Officer is the Command Staff position with the responsibility of being the point of contact with outside agencies. Often this role is seen as somewhat of a "Chief of Staff" position. An additional Liaison Officer would carry the title of Assistant Liaison Officer.

Additional Command Staff Positions

In addition to the established Command Staff positions, additional positions may be appointed by the IC based on the incident. Most often, the additional positions appointed by the IC are technical specialists. In a mass gathering event with a high potential of the need of medical services, a physician, nurse, or paramedic may serve as a technical specialist to the Command Staff to serve as a medical advisor.

General Staff Functional Areas and Positions

The General Staff are responsible for the four noncommand functional areas of the Incident Command System: Operations, Logistics, Planning, and Finance & Administration. Each of these functional areas are called "Sections" (i.e., Operations Section) and are led by a Chief (i.e., Operations Section Chief).

Operations Section

The Operations Section is typically the first expansion of the ICS beyond the Command functional area. The Operations Section, headed by the Operations Section Chief, is primarily responsible for developing and executing the specific tactics needed to achieve the objectives of the incident. In many events, the Operations Section is the largest area in terms of personnel assigned and is where those providing medical care would typically be categorized.

Because the Operations Section can often exceed the seven individuals allowed by span of control, it is often subdivided further. The first division of the Operations Section is by functional area of the assets or resource type and mission, called a Branch, led by a Branch Director. Examples of Branches would be a Medical Branch or Law Enforcement Branch. Within Branches, incidents may be further divided by geographic area or functional task. When divided by geographic area, each area is known as a Division (i.e., East Division), and when divided by functional task, each area is known by a Group (i.e., Triage Group). Both Divisions and Groups are led by a Supervisor. These divisions carry consistent terminology to both ensure unity of command and span of control is maintained and to provide for a common operating picture to all individuals regardless of jurisdiction or agency.

Planning Section

The Planning Section is responsible for coordinating the dissemination of information for the incident. Led by the Planning Section Chief, the Planning Section is responsible for ensuring all information and intelligence is current and disseminated. The Planning Section is also responsible for the preparation of the Incident Action Plan in using the priorities outlined by the Incident Commander/Unified Command. On larger incidents, the Planning Section is also responsible for tracking incident resources along with the Logistics and Finance and Administration Sections.

Logistics Section

The Logistics Section has the responsibility of providing resources for the management of the incident. These resources can range from personnel, to vehicles, to supplies, to food and water for staff, and external services. The Logistics Section, led by the Logistics Section Chief, is who the IC turns to in order to ensure there are sufficient resources to mitigate the incident. The Logistics Section is also responsible for ensuring communications abilities.

Finance and Administration Section

Nearly any incident, no matter the size and scope, has a cost associated with it. The Finance & Administration Section led by the Finance/ Admin Section Chief is responsible for keeping a tally on all financial resources utilized during the incident. This includes not only resources purchased and procured, but also often includes serving as the timekeepers for personnel. The Finance/ Admin Section works closely with the Logistics

Section to ensure that resources are provided and are paid for.

Medical Services Specific Positions

In a mass gathering event, there is likely to be a Medical Branch within the Operations Section. Functions of delivering medical care to event attendees will typically fall under the direction of the Medical Branch Director. The Medical Branch Director, who reports to the Operations Section Chief, leads the Medical Branch, and may be assisted by a Deputy Branch Director. This functional level, seen in larger-scale incidents, allows for reporting directly to a supervisor who is knowledgeable both about the common operational picture, Incident Command Structure, and about medicine. This supervisor role is typically staffed with someone who has experience in both incident management and medicine. When a Medical Branch is established, any Divisions and Groups would report to the Medical Branch Director in order to assure unity of command and a proper span of control.

Groups and Divisions

As previously described, Groups and Divisions are on an equal level to one another and fall between a Branch and a Unit. Groups are an organizational unit established based on a functional task. In some instances, there may be a Medical Group in lieu of a Medical Branch if the Branch positions are unfilled. More commonly at a mass gathering event, there may be a Treatment Group and/or Transport Group. A Division, on the other hand, is an organizational unit operating within a specific geographic area. At a sporting event, for instance, there may be an Interior Division and an Exterior Division. Divisions may have similar tasks or may be mixed in tasks. Both Groups and Divisions are led by Supervisors. The decision to use Groups versus Divisions is based on the type and scope of the incident. In some cases, both Groups and Divisions may be used. See Figure 7.1 for an example of this division for a large outdoor sporting event.

Units

Depending on the size and scope of an incident, a further functional unit below Groups and Divisions, called Units, may be established. Units are led by a Unit Leader and have a specific task within a General Staff function. Units are unique because they exist also in the Logistics, Planning, and Finance/Admin

Sections – because those sections typically have smaller staffs, additional organizational units above the Unit are not usually required. For medical services at mass gathering events, units may include a Triage Unit or Treatment Unit. Because Groups and Units both organize based on functional tasks, Units tend to be used in conjunction with geographic-based Divisions.

Strike Teams, Task Forces, and Individual Resources

To execute specific missions, a Strike Team, Task Force, or an Individual Resource is utilized by the Operations Section. These groups are the task-based operators on an incident and include things like an ambulance crew or engine company. Specifically, a Task Force is a group of individual resources of different types, with the mission of carrying out a specific task. For example, a medical Task Force may consist of ambulances, supervisors, and fire engines. Conversely, a Strike Team is a group of the same type of resources designated to carry out a specific task.

Incident Command System Locations

In order to maintain common terminology, the ICS designates several specific locations. Each of these locations carry out a specific function and may or may not all be co-located with the incident itself. Applicable to mass gathering events are Incident Command Posts, Emergency Operations Centers, Staging Areas, Casualty Collection Points, Helibase and Helispots, and Joint Information Centers.

Incident Command Post

The Incident Command Post (ICP) is normally established very early in an incident and is the designated location for the Command Staff to carry out their functions. There is only one ICP for an event, and it typically is located close to the incident or event, ideally within sight of the incident or event. Critically, the ICP should not be within the direct hazard area. It may be as simple as a supervisor's vehicle, a mobile command post vehicle, or in a more permanent location such as a nearby building. In mass gathering events at a venue, there is likely a predesignated ICP location that is activated for events.

Emergency Operations Center

An Emergency Operations Center (EOC) is a coordination facility responsible for emergency management at the strategic level. EOCs may be open and staffed at all times in larger jurisdictions or may just be opened for large incidents or events at smaller jurisdictions. The goal of the EOC is to provide for strategic oversight. It also often serves as a central resource coordination center and may be co-located with an Area Command overseeing multiple individual related incidents. An EOC in most jurisdiction is in a predefined location and is often not at the scene of the incident or event.

Staging Area

The staging area is a location near an incident or event scene that allows resources that are not currently being utilized to wait prior to a specific assignment. The idea of a staging area is to reduce congestion in and around the actual incident or event, protect equipment from damage, as well as a method of ensuring accountability of resources. For example, should a multiple casualty incident (MCI) occur at a mass gathering event, additional ambulances would initially be dispatched to a staging area, run by a staging officer. As the Transport Unit Leader or Transport Group Supervisor calls for additional resources, ambulances are released from the staging area to respond directly to the incident or event in an orderly fashion. Depending on the location and type of incident, as well as potential access issues, multiple staging areas may be utilized and should be named geographically. Staging areas should be carefully selected to ensure adequate ingress and egress for responding resources.

Casualty Collection Points

Casualty collection points (CCP) are designated areas in a triage system that victims are evacuated to emergently. CCPs are most often designated during active threat type events and are where patients are quickly moved to while the threat is ongoing. Situations such as the loss of the playing field (i.e., a "field rush" as seen at the end of an exciting sporting event) also warrant the designation of a CCP. Extraction teams (described later) can evacuate patients to this point to be further triaged and moved to appropriate treatment areas.

Emergency Shelters

Emergency shelters are designated locations that provide refuge from weather events. In the mass gathering event setting these are most commonly found for outdoor events. Shelter locations should be predesignated and shared with event attendees so that they can quickly move to shelter if need be. A consideration for the mass gathering event is the potential to have to move treatment teams to these shelter locations to provide medical response during an event that causes an evacuation.

Helibase and Helispot

Depending on the type and location of an event, planning for aeromedical evacuation may be required. Using ICS terminology, helicopters operate from a helibase. These locations are usually permanent in nature and offer fueling and storage of the aircraft when not in use. In the case of many air medical resources, this is an airport or other base location for the helicopter. Helibases are designated by their geographic or political name. A helispot, on the other hand, is a more temporary location that allows a safe location for a helicopter to land and take off. In events that take place in areas where air medical resources may be used, the predesignation of multiple helispots is ideal. Helispots are typically identified by phonetic alphabet letter (i.e., Helispot Alpha, Helispot Bravo, etc.).

Joint Information Center

On large scale incidents, a Joint Information Center (JIC) may be established to coordinate and manage the media. A JIC is used as a media staging area and is often where press conferences may occur. A JIC also has the technological capability of supporting the needs of the media, such as adequate internet, power, and telephone lines.

Implementation and Application of the Incident Command System

Utilizing the Incident Command System (ICS) has numerous benefits. ICS allows for a standard organizational structure that can be applied to all incidents, from a small-scale local incident, to a wide-reaching disaster, such as one that may affect a mass gathering event. ICS implements a coordinated command and control structure that focuses on safely responding to objectives based on priorities established. Because of the established modular command and control structure, all individuals responding to an incident know their role, and have a single supervisor based on the incident.

Effective Command Procedures

In order for an ICS to be effective, all agencies must have established procedures relating to ICS. Command procedures should detail how and when command structures will be established. One major pitfall of an improperly implemented ICS is an agency or group of individuals who surreptitiously undermine the existing command structure whether maliciously or not. To combat this, procedures should be established codifying the use of the ICS. Additionally, upon implementation of a command structure, whether before an event or once an event has started, all parties need to be notified. The command role must be clearly designated, and the person or persons filling the Incident Command role must be able to establish an effective incident management organization. The designation of the IC should be verbal (such as using the call sign of "Command" on a radio) as well as visual through the use of labeled vests or the use of an Incident Command Post.

Because one of the core characteristics of the ICS is management by objective, both the IC as well as all subordinates must be willing to work toward specific tasks and goals. This may also mean subordinate staff must take orders from someone other than their normal day-to-day supervisor. Medical providers may not be routinely in positions to take task-based orders from others and may normally make independent decisions. With the implementation of the ICS, each individual has a direct supervisor and decisions are task-based, working toward incident objectives. Individual providers must understand that during events where the ICS is implemented, that tasks will be assigned and must be completed as directed. These incidents are generally larger than a specific task and drives the organization toward the goals established in the IAP.

Incident Command Responsibilities at a Mass Gathering Event

The individual designated as the IC for a mass gathering event may or may not be a medical professional. No matter who is filling the role, the primary objective in any incident should be preservation and protection

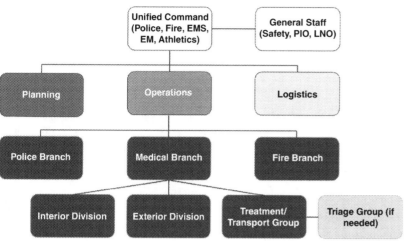

Figure 7.1 Example of establishment of medical specific branches under Operations Section of Incident Command System

of life (life safety). Specifically for medical operations, the IC has the ultimate responsibility to ensure that all victims are rescued, extricated, treated, and transported to appropriate medical care. Additionally, the IC should work to stabilize the incident ensure the safety and accountability of all responders.

Implementation of the Incident Command System for a Mass Gathering Event

By definition, mass gathering events are scheduled events, which allow time to plan thoughtfully for the potential for response. In a spontaneous incident such as a fire in a building or active threat in a school where there was no preexisting event plan, the first individual or unit to arrive on scene must establish command. In a preplanned mass gathering event, however, the Incident Commander, as well as other key incident personnel, are able to be selected and appointed prior to the event, and are often directly involved in event planning and the drafting of the IAP. Before a specific Incident Action Plan is developed, the event specific hazards should be understood and addressed. In addition to an IC, an Incident Command Post must also be established on all incidents where the Incident Command System Structure is established.

When planning for the implementation of the ICS, planners should consider the proper span of control. The idea of the ICS is to ensure that each individual or resource has a direct supervisor, and that supervisor's responsibility is no more than seven individuals or resources. When planners find that supervisors have more than seven direct reports, it is an indication to expand the module structure of the system. In nearly all large scale, planned events, there is an IC and an Operations Section Chief. If the Operations Section Chief is supervising more than just medical services, then a Medical Branch or Medical Group should be established with organizational units consisting of geographic-based Divisions, and task-based Groups or Units.

Medical Branch Specific Positions within the Incident Command System

When the ICS is utilized at a mass gathering event, it is likely that several medical-specific positions will be utilized in the Operations Section. In many cases this involves the opening of a Medical Branch, led by a Medical Branch Director. Below this position, or in lieu of this position depending on the incident size, are Groups and Divisions led by their respective Group or Division Supervisors. Additionally, Units, such as a Triage Unit may also be designated. Many of these positions have predefined roles that are established within the existing Incident Command System. An example of how a Medical Branch or Medical Group would be established within the ICS is seen in Figure 7.1.

Medical Branch Director or Medical Group Supervisor

Depending on the size and scope of the event, a Medical Branch may be established within the

Operations Section, or may report directly to the Incident Commander. Alternatively, a Medical Group may be established if no Branches are established, which also may report to an Operations Section Chief, or in the absence of an Operations Section, the Incident Commander. A Branch would be established in instances where it is expected that Divisions may be created or there will be the need for an additional layer of supervision at the Group level. Whether a Medical Branch or Medical Group, the Director or Supervisor respectively has similar responsibilities. This individual is responsible for implementing all assigned objectives, which usually involve providing assessment or triage, extrication, transport, and transportation. The person filling this role also participates in Branch or Operations Section planning activities and, critically, determines the types and the amounts of resources needed. The Medical Branch Director or Medical Group Supervisor also typically serves as the lead medical officer of the event and is also likely the liaison to other healthcare agencies. For example, it is likely this position that coordinates with local hospitals and emergency medical services units. Lastly but perhaps most importantly, the Medical Branch Director or Medical Group Supervisor is ultimately responsible for the safety and accountability of their assigned staff.

Medical Branch Groups

The standard configuration of the ICS accounts for a Treatment Group (referred in the original ICS model as the Medical Group) and a Patient Transportation Group (sometimes referred to just as the Transport Group). These Group Supervisors report either to a Medical Branch Director, or to the Operations Section Chief if a Medical Branch is not in use. The Medical Group Supervisor typically oversees both Triage and Treatment Units, discussed later. The Patient Transportation Group is primarily responsible for providing transportation to receiving facilities. In many mass gathering events, there are several ambulances on site that would report to the Patient Transportation Group Supervisor. Additionally, this position would also coordinate outside ambulances that respond into the event if there is a need for additional transport units such as in a multiple casualty incident. The Patient Transportation Group Supervisor tracks patient flow once they leave treatment areas, and

also coordinates with the Medical Branch Director or Operations Section Chief as applicable to request additional ground or air ambulance resources, as well as coordinating staging areas.

Divisions

Depending on the size and scope of the event, there may be a need to divide the event site geographically. This is typically seen in outdoor events such as large sporting events, festivals, or other events that span a large footprint. This may allow for better accountability of personnel and resources as the supervisor is only managing resources within their specific geographic areas. Divisions can be used in conjunction with or in lieu of Groups within the ICS. For example, at a large sporting event held at an outdoor stadium, there may be an Interior and Exterior Division created. When Divisions are created, the supervisors will generally take on responsibilities that would normally be split between different Groups. In the Interior and Exterior Division example, these Supervisors may take on the role of the Medical (or Treatment) Group Supervisor and Patient Transportation Group Supervisor for their respective Divisions. More commonly, the Divisions take the place of the Medical (or Treatment) Groups, and the Patient Transportation Group is left unchanged and serves multiple Divisions.

Triage Unit

In mass gathering events, the goal is to prevent an MCI, but in cases that an MCI does occur, patients must be rapidly triaged in order to progress to the treatment area and progress to definitive care. Appointing a Triage Unit and a Triage Unit Leader in the planning stages will prevent confusion if and when an incident during the mass gathering event causes multiple casualties. The Triage Unit members may have other tasks during the event, such as being assigned to mobile treatment teams or support duties but would be activated into the Triage Unit in the event an MCI occurs. Triage Unit members should be trained in a common triage system (such as SALT or START triage) and should have the ability to rapidly move from patient to patient. Triage Unit members should also either be equipped with or have direct access to triage equipment such as tape and tags, as well as emergency treatment equipment such as tourniquets.

The Triage Unit Leader would be the supervisor of this group. The Triage Unit Leader's role is to coordinate triage activities, including providing their supervisors (usually the Medical Branch Director or Medical Group Supervisor) with updates on patient counts. The Triage Unit Leader would also ensure that proper triage supplies such as triage tags and tape are available for team members. Additionally, the Triage Unit Leader may be asked to preplan triage areas and casualty collection points, as well as provide oversight and ensure the overall efficiency of the triage operation. As the supervisor, they would also be responsible for the safety and accountability of team members assigned to them.

Treatment Unit

The Treatment Unit is responsible for the delivery of patient care during the event. In a more traditional application of the ICS the Treatment Unit is typically set up in the moment as an area to transport patients to after triage but before transport. In an MCI, the treatment area is often very temporary and may be denoted by different color tarps or flags based on the triage color of patients. In mass gathering events, treatment areas are often predesignated and often already staffed. In permanent venues such as stadiums and arenas, treatment areas may be areas such as first aid rooms. In other venues, especially outdoor events, these may be a treatment tent that is set up in advance. Depending on the geographic size and scope of the event, multiple treatment areas may be established.

Unique to mass gathering events, members of the Treatment Unit may be assigned to a treatment area or may be assigned as mobile treatment teams. Mobile treatment teams are usually pairs of individuals equipped with basic supplies to assess and provide initial treatment to patients. These teams may be static or roving teams. Treatment teams may employ many methods to respond to emergencies. In many indoor venues, and even smaller outdoor venues, treatment teams may simply respond to calls for assistance on foot. In larger or more spread out venues, teams may use other means of transportation such as bicycles, all-terrain vehicles or utility vehicles, or even ambulances.

The Treatment Unit Leader is often responsible both for treatment teams as well as treatment areas. They also coordinate closely with the Triage Unit and Extraction Unit, as well as the Patient Transportation Group. The Treatment Unit Leader should also keep their supervisor informed, specifically providing regular updates regarding numbers and conditions of patients. They also must ensure that the treatment areas and teams have the resources they need. Additionally, because members of the Treatment Unit may be out in the elements, the Treatment Unit Leader must ensure that these team members are provided adequate rest and nutrition. As with all supervisors, the Treatment Unit Leaders are responsible for the safety and accountability of those resources assigned to them.

Extraction Unit

Depending on the event venue, an Extraction Unit may be necessary, and is not a predesignated role in the traditional Incident Command Structure. The goal of the Extraction Unit would be to move patients from the point of encounter to a Treatment Area. Because of challenging geography, architecture, crowd sizes, and other issues, moving the patient from the point of first healthcare encounter to the point of more definitive treatment is often more complex than wheeling them back from the waiting room or placing them on an ambulance stretcher. The Extraction Unit and the Extraction Unit Supervisor specialize in the movement of patients and have the proper resources to accomplish patient movement. Depending on the event venue, this may mean special stretchers, stair chairs, sleds, or even all-terrain vehicles.

The Extraction Unit Supervisor monitors the resources assigned to their unit, and communicates needs to their supervisor. Unique to mass gathering events, the Extraction Unit Leader is also tasked with preplanning patient flow and movement. For instance, the Extraction Unit Leader must consider how crowds, and thus potential patients, are moving during event ingress and egress, as well as during a possible evacuation or shelter-in-place order. This may mean prepositioning teams within the unit to designated locations during key times to be able to maintain access to, and egress with potential patients.

Application and Flexibility of the ICS for Mass Gathering Events

The nature, location, and duration of the mass gathering event will dictate what level of the ICS must be used. The advantage to the ICS is that it is modular and scalable. There is no requirement for any position except for an Incident Commander. A high school football game may have simply an ambulance crew standing by, with one member serving as the de facto

IC. Smaller events likely do not have a specific written IAP, but rather operate based on standard procedures and protocols. Despite the small scale of this event, should an emergency happen, an influx of responders would be best managed by implementing the ICS as personnel arrive. In the case of a high school football game with an MCI, a Triage Unit Leader would likely be chosen from the first arriving emergency medical services (EMS) crew, and depending on the number of patients, a treatment area, under the direction of a Treatment Unit Leader may also be established. Another officer would assume the role of Patient Transport Supervisor to managing the Staging Area and ensure the safe and efficient flow of patients to higher levels of care.

As incidents scale up in size, attendance, and risk, the Incident Command System Structure is likewise expanded. A large college or professional sporting event will likely utilize a Unified Command model involving police, emergency medical services, and event operations superiors. From a medical perspective, at a larger event, it is likely to have either a Medical Branch or a Medical Group established which reports to the Operations Section Chief. In these larger incidents, many of the positions described are already filled, and if additional resources are required, they will likely fill task-level positions. In larger events, such as an outdoor music festival, Divisions may also be filled to mitigate the large geographic area of the event.

In any of the examples, from a high school football game to a large, multi-day outdoor music festival, the ICS provides a constant command and coordination structure for responders to operate within. In each of these events, it is critical to adhere to the characteristics of the ICS for it to be effective. Ensuring that there are designated, prioritized objectives, a linear and unified chain of command, and using common terminology allows all responders to maintain a common operating picture no matter their role in the event.

Conclusion

The ICS is a proven command, coordination, and control system that streamlines the operations of many different incident types. Because mass gathering events are planned, it allows for time for the ICS to be implemented ahead of time and built out to the needs of the specific event. While ICS may put individuals in positions they are not used to being in, it ensures a standardized chain of command and that the incident is mitigated according to the outlined priorities and objectives. Whether it is a small incident with only an Incident Commander and individual responding units, or a large scall incident with all positions filled, or anywhere in between, the ICS is an ideal way to measure that all responders keep the common operating picture in mind.

References

1. California Office of Emergency Services. History of ICS. https://firescope.caloes.ca.gov/SiteCollectionDocuments/ICS%20History%20and%20Progression.pdf

2. Sylves R. T. How the Exxon Valdez Disaster Changed America's Oil Spill Emergency Management. *International Journal of Mass Emergencies and Disasters*. 1998;**16**:13–43.

3. U.S. Department of Homeland Security. Homeland Security Presidential Directive-5. 2003. www.dhs.gov/sites/default/files/publications/Homeland%20Security%20Presidential%20Directive%205.pdf

4. Federal Emergency Management Agency. ICS-100 Student Manual. 2018. https://training.fema.gov/emiweb/is/is100c/student%20manual/is0100c_sm.pdf

Chapter 8

Security and Other Nonmedical Logistical Support Issues at Mass Gathering Events

Mark Shank, Colleen Shank, Emily Wheeler, Amy Lowther, and Courtney Kirkland

Introduction

Event Medicine is a new subspecialty of Emergency Medicine that deals with the management of event services during events of all sizes and locations. While the scope of practice varies depending on event size, the allocation of the various support services represents a unique challenge to organizers, medical support staff, and law enforcement. These requirements may vary depending on event-specific characteristics, however it is imperative that medical directors have a clearly defined framework from which to predict medical needs as to provide necessary interventions or services should the need arise. Careful attention should be paid to general logistical concerns such as communication, crowd size, venue characteristics, available emergency medical personnel resources, and the ability of staff to recognize and report any adverse events in real time. A multidisciplinary approach to meeting medical needs ensures the safety and health of both staff and attendees.

One of the most challenging aspects of Event Medicine includes the designation of law enforcement at various levels. Most events will be staffed either by contracted security personnel or local police/sheriff departments. However, recent terrorist attacks such as the Boston Marathon bombing in 2013 demonstrate how medical directors should also be familiar with protocols set in place by the Federal Emergency Management Agency as it pertains to SWAT teams, bomb threats, illegal substances, and hazardous materials. Additionally, medical support staff such as firefighters, EMTs, and practitioners must be properly briefed on available resources to treat patients on site as well as transport them via ground transport or helicopter to nearby hospitals.

Event medical directors must have proficiency in the coordination of nonmedical support staff as well. Recognizing various hurdles in healthcare access from crowd flow such as trams, shuttles, or simply parking lots can prevent unnecessary patient harm. Protocols for entrance to a given event, as well as evacuation in case of an emergency, should be carefully planned well in advance. Additionally, event staff should be briefed on disaster protocols in the case of extreme weather, an active shooter scenarios, sexual assault, and missing persons. Ultimately, excellent communication among agencies, providers, event staff, and event participants will be instrumental in making events safe and successful. In this chapter, we outline the various security and other nonmedical logistical support issues involved in mass gathering events.

Communications

Communication is the most critical area of planning for a large event. Not only do event planners focus on the technological means of communication, but they must also learn how to communicate and whom to communicate with in a large event setting. Commonly, events will have an integration of civilians and professional first responders who must have direct lines of communication with each other, higher level planners, and incident commanders as needed. Event leaders should also be able to contact external agencies as well as the authorities should the need arise. Communication must be able to occur even if first line technologies were broken by disasters, weather, or technology failure.

Common communication standards are vitally important when it comes to organizing a large-scale event and these standards must be planned well in advance to ensure a seamless integration. Centralized communication areas are locations where all vital information is available to event coordinators and commanders during any large-scale event (SECP job aids manual).

Planning Stage

The three communication planning stage tenets include: education, integration, and practice. All first responders and event staff should be educated on their communication systems, radio etiquette, and what to do if the primary means of communication is cut off. Incident command systems can be modified or adjusted to better suit specific event needs and sizes. These incident command systems can be easily taught to civilian and private security staff, so they understand who to report to in the chain of command during an emergency. Each member of the event team should have an opportunity to practice using the specific type of communication technology they will be operating or any back-up technology that could be used during an event. We suggest planning a training day to review pertinent topics with all participants and providing a reference card-type booklet that describes the incident command system in place for the specific event with instructions on how to reach others at the event. These instructions may help stressed workers remember radio frequencies and phone numbers during emergencies.

It is important to reiterate that event contingency plans must be in place. Typical "first-line" communication technologies (radios, cellular phones) are easy to use, familiar, and commonly available. However, "first-line" communication technologies are prone to failure and require back-up systems in place to ensure consistent communication among the authorities and staff during the event.

Communication Within the Event

Radio communication is the most used modality for communication among staff at large-scale events. While longer-distance radios are dependent on towers and limited by terrain, two-way radios (i.e., handheld transceivers or walkie-talkies) have remarkable range allowing for communication without having to rely on radio towers. Radios can talk on semiprivate channels with a variety of people by switching among frequencies. Digital and satellite radios have gained popularity by marketing the resilient communication capabilities toward first responders and public safety organizations around the world. The most popular of these is P25, a digital radio technology made specifically for public safety agencies. RAVE mobile safety is a mobile and internet-based platform that integrates critical event data, emergency response coordination,

and mass notification of users under one umbrella to facilitate rapid and fluid responses to critical events. Every year, a new host of technologies, apps, and internet-based communications sources are created.

Thus far, we have primarily discussed the communication between staff, security, and event leaders. However, it is also vitally important that event information and emergency alerts be conveyed to event participants. In the last few years, we have seen an increase in the number of phone applications that can be used to communicate essential information to all event participants in real time. However, these applications are dependent on cellular or Wi-Fi service and are only useful in situations where a large majority of the participants are using smart devices. Common back-up systems include intercoms, PA systems, closed circuit television, or bullhorns can also be employed to deliver real-time vital information. Another consideration is if the announcement should be made in many different languages, so all the participants understand and receive the information [10].

There are several federally supported and private mass notification systems that can be used to convey alerts to large groups of mobile phone users at or near mass gatherings. Each of these modalities must be planned with the appropriate applications and rights to post through state and local government agencies must be obtained. The Integrated Public Alert Warning System (IPAWS) is FEMA's national system that allows emergency alerts to be sent to the public. It uses the Wireless Emergency Alerts (WEA) system to send alerts to mobile phones, the Emergency Alert System (EAS) to alert through radio and television, and the National Oceanic and Atmospheric Administration's weather radio system. The CodeRED mobile alert system can be integrated with the IPAWS WEA system to send emergency alerts ONLY to those mobile phone users in the path of the emergency. FEMA has a large network of free information on emergency alerts and how to use them on their IPAWS Program Planning Toolkit site.

Although cellular phones' familiarity makes them the easiest form of communication, event planners should anticipate that cellular phone service may be limited and hinder communication outside the event, with high volumes of people using a cellular network, their speed and reliability will decline sharply. However, several cellular carriers do provide "first responder" packages that provide preferential service to police and emergency medical providers that may enhance their cellular phone usability in these types of circumstances.

Guest Services/Customer Service

At large-scale events, consider setting up a small guest services tent within the VIP section or in an established hospitality area. The purpose of guest services is to direct guests to critical areas of the venue including restrooms, ATM, or coat check. Guest services are available to attendees to provide additional assistance whenever necessary. Position guest services away from access routes and in less densely occupied areas. Consider locations that would not obstruct pathways. Crowd pressure at the entrance can be reduced by keeping activities, including guest services, well clear of entry points.

National Weather Service

The National Weather Service is a federal program through the US Department of Commerce that tracks global weather patterns via satellite monitoring. Along with this, surface measurements such as barometry can predict shifts in weather with high accuracy. NOAA also utilizes a special radio system called the NOAA Weather Radio All Hazards, to provide uninterrupted weather reports and warnings, with coverage over 95 percent of the United States. Additional information can be found at the National Weather Service's website (weather.gov), which includes meteorologic data and tracking, active storm watches, and satellite imaging.

Event Local Air Traffic Control

Air monitoring is another helpful tool that can be utilized to improve public safety during large-scale gatherings.

Event Security

Identification of all involved agencies and establishing a hazard analysis are the initial steps when planning event security for a mass gathering. The responsibilities and roles of security personnel should be clearly defined before any event. A pre-event briefing for security personnel is recommended and should include clear directions for managing unacceptable behavior, medical aid post locations, and any pertinent spectator information.

Pre-event Planning

Pre-event planning for any mass gathering is the major portion of security efforts should begin at least twelve to eighteen months in advance. Hosting a large-scale event is an intense and exhaustive process. Planners should begin as soon as possible and should not wait for federal guidance. Pre-event security planning should include developing a strategic vision, identifying a lead planner for the department, determining authorities of participating agencies, and establishing a local core planning team. Next, any event risk should be assessed, security roles should be clearly defined, and a plan for the worst outcome should be established [1].

Internal Risks

Hot weather can place attendees at risk for becoming victims of heat-related illnesses. This scenario can cause a mass casualty incident if shade and a water supply is not readily available. Events with high rates of alcohol or illegal drugs may lead to more disruptive behavior and the requirement of emergency medical services due to serious side effects of these substances. Recognize that fights, stabbings, and shootings frequently arise at protest rallies or meetings of politically inflammatory groups if not mitigated early [3].

External Risks

External risks may include the attendance of a national or international politician or dignitary. These events may attract terrorists who use the opportunity to make statements through assassinations, explosions, or release of a variety of toxic substances. Two aspects that may not be found in "ordinary" mass gatherings are emergency medical services (EMS) dedicated to the dignitary(s) and EMS readiness for a mass-casualty incident. To properly prepare EMS, they must be provided an intense framework of security and readiness to conform to requirements unfamiliar to their routine practice [3].

Uniformed Police Officers

Private uniformed security guards are best suited for nonconfrontational roles, such as taking tickets and parking cars. Recruiting from reputable sources will ensure competent and suitably trained personnel. Private uniformed security personnel can have a deceiving authoritative appearance but provide neither the power of police nor the rapport achieved by peer security [1]. As evidenced by the recent 2021 Travis Scott Astroworld Music Festival, excessive crowd surge can lead to catastrophic consequences. Failure to meticulously plan for crowd control resulted in a massive and uncontrolled crowd surge at this event leading to ten casualties and leaving hundreds injured. Crowd control is an integral aspect of event security, and the appropriate personnel should be utilized based on both their training and abilities. In addition to their skill set, it is also essential to recognize that the attitude of event security personnel also plays a significant role in crowd control by helping spectators feel more welcome [1].

The role of local law enforcement should include security control at all entrances and exits, crowd management, control of vehicle traffic, and marshaling of the event. Crowds that are composed of mostly families typically require a less aggressive approach and therefore one officer for every one thousand spectators should suffice. This number increases to two officers per one thousand spectators for more active participants (e.g., sporting events with alcohol consumption) [1].

High-Risk Mass Gatherings: Threat Assessments

Attendance of national or international politicians or dignitaries are known as high-risk mass gatherings and place attendees at higher risks for physical harm. In 1998 the President issued Presidential Decision Directive 62, which gave the planning role to federal agencies once events were designated a National Security event by the Department of Homeland Security. After consultation with the Homeland Security Council, the US Secret Service assumes the role as the lead agency for the design and implementation of the operational security plan, the FBI is the lead agency for crisis management, and FEMA is the lead agency for consequence management [4]. In the event of a terrorist act, the role of the Secret Service or DSS is to remove their protected individual, allowing the FBI to take over the crime scene. The FBI is the lead federal agency for intelligence during any federally managed major events. The FBI has an operations system developed for managing the entire intelligence cycle during unique events including establishment of requirements,

collection, analysis, production, and dissemination. Local FBI field offices will send representatives from their interagency Field Intelligence Group (FIG) to help with the planning and operations for major events. If state and local officers are participating in special event security with federal agencies, they may need security clearances to receive intelligence information [4].

Three security zones or perimeters are typically established when a protected individual of the Secret Service of DSS attends an event. The "cold zone" (outer perimeter) is under surveillance for any threat but is open to the public. The "warm zone" may be accessed by ID or people may be accompanied by security personnel. The "hot zone" (inner zone), typically staffed by Secret Service or DSS, requires a special ID badge for admittance and typically has the highest level of protection. Fire and EMS personnel will need access to all three zones [3].

SWAT

Depending on the nature of the event and the perceived threat level, event planners may need to involve specialized tactical units, like the SWAT (special weapons and tactics) teams to work the event or be on standby. Some examples of SWAT tactical capabilities include hostage negotiation, counter assault, counter sniper, and counter surveillance.

HAZMAT

Event organizers should seek advice regarding potential hazards at the proposed venue. HAZMAT is an abbreviation for "hazardous materials" and includes such substances as toxic chemicals, fuels, and biological, chemical, and radiological agents. An appropriate risk management and emergency plan should be developed to manage any potential hazardous material that pose a risk to health, property, or the environment [2]. The FBI planning for HAZMAT incidents includes availability of subject matter experts for rapid assessment, procedure for venue protection, development of assessment teams, and response for law enforcement in the event of a HAZMAT incident.

Event Transportation

Strategic planning should be done to ensure transportation during an event is both safe and enjoyable for the attendees. Transportation as a topic involves initial ticketing, routes/detours, parking, and availability of public transit. From a nonemergent standpoint, having well thought out and implemented instructions will create a positive impression on all affected. If an emergency of any magnitude were to occur, special attention should be placed on the diverse types of transportation available for emergency medical purposes. Planning should focus on the size, number, and location of these vehicles. Establishing separate routes and staging plans for emergency medical personnel would allow for better access and treatment of those involved.

When planning nonemergent transportation, the venue size, number of expected attendees, routes attendees may take to arrive (flying, walking, driving), the community layout, and pathways the attendees would ingress or egress need to be addressed as a part of planning. The amount of traffic created by the event will have a significant effect on the community. The timing of the event may determine how much of the community is impacted [10].

Simply notifying the community of an upcoming event and posting signs/detours in advance can limit most of the impending traffic concerns. Establishing a traffic management group can also help to prevent anticipated issues that may occur during the event. A traffic management group could entail all or some of the following: professional traffic planners, local public safety, traffic service providers, local law enforcement, department of transportation, local media, and public transportation authorities [10].

Parking is a major element in transportation that needs to be well planned out long before the event is to take place. There are a variety of essential elements involved in nonemergent transportation planning. Parking layouts should address overflow parking, road conditions, parking attendants, and clearly marked parking signs. One vehicle for every three people attending the event is typical. However, this may vary depending on the community and ease of public transportation. Therefore, public transportation is another essential element when it comes to non-emergency event transportation. Public transportation can help transport attendees to and from the event, help minimize overall traffic, and decrease parking demands.

Major events will require the involvement of multiple other nonemergent vehicles. These vehicles could include tow trucks, law enforcement vehicles, garbage trucks, water tankers, public works, and a variety of utility vehicles [10]. Consider establishing a safety screening for these vehicles prior to entering the event. Also, planning their strategic locations and routes of transportation should be considered. An example of strategic location planning could involve placing tow trucks in prohibited parking areas to deter attendees from illegally parking [10].

Emergent Transportation Planning

Goals for planning emergency transportation during an event include minimizing response times, establishing safe patient loading areas that are easily accessible, and clearing safe pathways to treatment facilities [9]. Predicting the utilization of emergency needs during an event is the next step to meeting these goals. This could be accomplished by reviewing the event during previous years or comparing similar events elsewhere [9]. However, if this is a new or different event, focus should be placed on evaluating the venue for safety risks and attendee characteristics, such as age and socioeconomic status. Another important detail to evaluate when attempting to prepare emergency transportation is the length and type of event, such as multiday events with camping onsite. There must be established treatment plans for anticipated illnesses including alcohol, carbon monoxide toxicity, dehydration, heat exhaustion, exacerbations of chronic diseases, and sexual assaults.

The plan must also anticipate injuries from falls, cuts, vehicle accidents, or bicycle accidents. Recognize that these injuries/illnesses can affect one or multiple people, therefore the ability to increase resources on demand is a necessity [9].

Types of Emergency Vehicles

Emergency vehicles only make up a small portion of total vehicles that may be utilized during an event. All acting or assisting emergency vehicles should be clearly marked and highly visible. All vehicles should also meet state regulations and licensure standards. For any nonmedical vehicles, there should be at least one medically trained (EMT-B level) aboard [9]. Strategies for staging emergency vehicles are of utmost importance when attempting to minimize vehicle transit time. The key is to geographically select an area that has proximity to the crowd and an easily accessible egress route. Distinct types of emergency vehicles may be essential depending on the venue site, environment, number, and location of attendees. Options can vary from simple foot patrols or "roaming crews" on all-terrain vehicles (ATVs) and bicycles to accessing aeromedical helicopters. All vehicle types can play a significant role in emergency treatment and transportation.

Foot patrol or "roaming crews" allow emergency personnel to survey the crowd for attendees with emergent signs/symptoms indicating dehydration or drug/alcohol intoxication [11]. Once identified, roaming crews can quickly gain access to the patients and direct them to "Casualty Collection Points (CCP)" or emergency vehicles [11].

Bike crews can also roam areas of events unable to be accessed by larger vehicles. This crew is often an advanced life support (ALS) first responder team, which allows for rapid initial triaging and treatment of those in need. Bike crews often quickly coordinate with alternative modes of transportation. This crew will carry "paniers" on their bikes, which are bags with ALS emergency equipment and supplies [11]. Riders should wear approved gear making them recognizable as emergency crew and have approved riding gear/supplies.

Utility vehicles (UTV) can have similar equipment and supplies as an ambulance while allowing for access to rougher, smaller terrain. Other transportation vehicles that can be transitioned or utilized as emergency vehicles include boats and golf carts. All vehicles need to have their equipment checked and updated on a regular basis. Operators should have a good understanding of the terrain they are approved to drive upon as well as the vehicle's capabilities [11].

Finally, rotary and fixed wing transportation is a consideration depending on the type of venue and its location. The main purposes of aeromedical transport include transporting the acutely ill or injured off-site and delivering additional personnel or equipment to disaster incident sites [9].

To do this, they must have an established and secure landing zone coupled with a standard operating system with security for fire suppression [9]. However, depending on the venue, many of these standards may not be accessible. The weather can affect take-off and landing conditions, thus also limiting their usefulness [11].

There are many topics that encompass both nonemergent and emergent event transportation. Every transportation detail is integral when it comes to running a smooth event and quickly adjusting to any unforeseen emergencies. From parking to foot traffic, the transportation of all event attendees is a critical aspect that needs to be well planned and all contingencies must be covered to prevent unforeseen issues.

Resources Section

Missing Persons Protocol

During and after events, there may be reports of a missing person that had attended. Reports could involve an attendee temporarily separated from their group, someone who left the premises without notifying others, or even someone taken against their will. As discussed earlier, we must recognize that cell phone service can be scarce during major events due to high data traffic volumes. All missing persons notified to staff members should be reported through an incident command system (ICS). A missing person's protocol has a few objectives; primarily to locate the missing person, to document information for follow-up of the missing person and possible court proceedings, and to prevent reoccurrence.

There are two levels of responses composing the missing person's protocol: Level 1 being the higher of the two. Level 1 may include a multiagency response that uses a significant amount of comprehensive labor and equipment. This type of response should be activated when the missing person is twelve years old or younger or if the person has diminished capacity. This response should also be initiated if there is compelling evidence, like a witness or ransom note, that the missing person was abducted, and the abduction is not custodial related. Lastly, thisresponse should be used if there is a strong reason to believe that the person is in danger of bodily harm or death. All other reports of missing persons should be considered Level 2 responses.

Disaster Planning

Emergency planning should be considered an integral aspect of the event planning process and the importance increases exponentially with the size of the event. Start the planning process by assessing the venue prior to the event and take note of any potential hazards. Staff should be familiar with preexisting emergency and disaster plans to facilitate planning. Prior incidents that have occurred within the event or venue should also be taken into consideration.

Instructions should be prepared to brief medical staff on their specific role during an emergency response. Finally, there should be a plan for evacuation of EMS and then a reestablishment of EMS at a secondary location if there is a catastrophic emergency.

It is especially important to be familiar with all evacuation routes in the event of a fire. It is imperative to discuss the evacuation plan with staff before the event. It may even be helpful to run fire drills prior to the event. Safety is the most important priority in a fire, with the goal of evacuation coming first. Employees may be useful in extinguishing small fires if they are professionally trained to use a fire extinguisher. The local fire department should be kept up to date on event plans so they can be readily available in case of a fire. A sufficient number of exits should be available to event attendees and staff. If the event is contained in a building, make sure there are at least two exits on every floor. Prior to the event, a walk-through is recommended to ensure that every exit has adequate lighting and marked with an exit sign. Remove any objects that are blocking exits.

In the event of an active shooter, the most important thing to remember is to protect your own life. Event staff should be familiar with the exits and have an evacuation plan ready. Event attendees are most likely to follow the lead of employees and staff members. If there is an active shooter, the main priority should be escaping the situation. This may include leaving your belongings behind and evacuating the area despite those around you. While evacuating, everyone must remember to follow the instructions of police officers that arrive on the scene and keep your hands visible. Those who reach safety should call 911 to let them know you are safe. If evacuation is not an option, then the next best option is to hide. Ideally, choose a hiding place out of the active shooter's view that provides protection, like a closed room with a locked door. Keep the door locked or consider blocking the door with heavy furniture to keep the shooter out.

Staff members should also be familiar with the policies regarding sexual assault. If a sexual assault is reported during the event, EMS and local law enforcement should be contacted. The victim should be taken to a safe location and examined by medical professionals.

Bombings and explosions remain one of the most common deliberate causes of disasters and instruments of terrorism that involve many casualties.

Attacks are almost always made against unsuspecting and untrained civilians. Most bomb threats are reported via telephone. There are a few important steps to be taken if staff members receive a call reporting a bomb threat. First, the staff members should take the caller seriously and take notes during the conversation on everything including voice characteristics, background noise, etc. The next step is to keep the caller on the line for as long as possible. Attempt to call the police either immediately after the caller hangs up or discreetly from another phone during the conversation. Someone should also immediately notify the event supervisor. The entire event should be evacuated using the previously determined evacuation strategy. Security staff should conduct thorough inspections of the area for explosives before and during the event. Any suspicious appearing packages should be reported immediately. Also, a triage plan should be in place for staff members and first responders if a bombing does take place.

Weather events such as storms, flooding, earthquakes, and fires are another crucial factor to consider when planning for a large-scale event. As climate change has emerged the frequency of catastrophic storms, extreme shifts in weather patterns, and severe flooding occurrences have increased. For example, many musical festivals take place in tropical or arid climates predisposing attendees to heat exhaustion and dehydration. Tropical climates also have a risk of extreme storms, such as hurricanes or flash flooding. To plan for weather events, a designated staff member should oversee following local weather alerts. The staff member should have a clear system for distributing any alerts such as a PA system, text message, or handheld device. Preferred monitoring from the National Weather Service or National Oceanic and Atmospheric Service is recommended.

North American Free Trade Agreement Regulations/Recommendations

The North American Free Trade Agreement (NAFTA) is an integral part of commercial trading between the United States, Mexico, and Canada. This agreement was enacted in 1994 and created a free trade zone, and in 2007, all tariffs and quotas were eliminated on US exports to Mexico and Canada. NAFTA provides coverage to services apart from maritime, aviation transport, and basic telecommunications. This agreement also provides protection of intellectual property rights.

References

1. SECP – Special Events Contingency Planning Job Aids Manual, IS-15. March 2005, FEMA, www.training.fema.gov

2. GMP – Guidelines for the Management of Public Health & Safety at Public Events. Government of South Australia Department of Health. October 2006. www.sahealth.sa.gov.au

3. Leonard R., Winslow J., Bozeman W. Planning Medical Care for High-Risk Mass Gatherings. *The Internet Journal of Rescue and Disaster Medicine.* 2006;**6**(1); www.ispub.com

4. Conners E. (2007, March). Planning And Managing Security for Major Special Events: Guidelines for Law Enforcement. Publications https://cops.usdoj.gov/RIC/Publications/

5. Endericks T., et al. Public Health for Mass Gatherings: Key Considerations, World Health Organization. (2015).

6. Topic Collection: Mass Gatherings/ Special Events. ASPR TRACIE. (n.d). https://asprtracie.hhs.gov/technical-resources/85/Mass-Gatherings-Special-Events/0

7. Bertram C. D. *Preparing for Planned Events: National Security Special Events. In the Role of Law Enforcement in Emergency Management and Homeland Security.* Bingley: Emerald Publishing Limited; 2021.

8. Emergency Response Plan. Emergency Response Plan | Ready.gov.(n.d.). www.ready.gov/business/implementation/emergency

9. Jaslow D., et al. Mass Gathering Medical Care. National Association of EMS Physicians Standards and Clinical Practice Committee. *Prehospital Emergency Care.* 2000;**4**(4): 359–360.

10. Special Events Contingency Planning: Job Aids Manual March 2005 (updated 2010). FEMA Training. https://training.fema.gov [PDF]

11. Fitzpatrick C., ACEP: Event Transportation, www.crowdrx.org

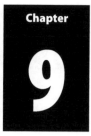

Chapter

9

Understanding Local, State, and Federal Public Safety, Health Care, and Support Agencies

William Fales and William Selde

Introduction

Nearly every special event or mass gathering of sufficient size to warrant dedicated medical services will likely have opportunities to interface with other agencies and organizations providing support services. In general, the larger or more complex the event, the more agencies will be involved. Law enforcement, most often local, is almost always involved in the planning and operations of a special event. Other public safety agencies such as local or mutual aid emergency medical services (EMS), the fire service, and emergency management are also commonly involved. It is important that event medical planners and leaders also interface with local and regional hospitals, including those providing specialty services for important time-critical problems (e.g., trauma, cardiac, stroke). When event venues are in rural areas, more distant from hospitals, including the area helicopter EMS provider(s) in planning is important, and often neglected. There are a number of other local, state, federal, and private organizations that may be involved in event planning and operations. This chapter is intended to provide an overview of many of these important partners that help to assure the event has sufficient resources to provide safety and security to all.

National Incident Management System and Interagency Planning and Coordination

In response to the terrorist attacks of 9/11, Homeland Security Presidential Directive 5 (HSPD-5) created the National Incident Management System (NIMS) to improve the way that all levels of government and the private sector can effectively collaborate with one another to prevent, prepare for, respond to, and recover from terrorist attacks, major disasters, and other emergencies [1]. NIMS includes the Incident Command System (ICS), Emergency Operations Center (EOC) structures, and Multiagency Coordination Groups (MAC Groups) providing guidance and a framework of how personnel work together during incidents. While NIMS applies to incidents of all sizes, it also includes planned events [2] (see Table 9.1). The Emergency Management Institute offers a variety of NIMS-related training courses, including many free, online courses that are highly recommended for those providing medical planning and leadership to events and mass gatherings [3]. These include the items shown in Table 9.1.

- IS-100.b (ICS 100) Introduction to Incident Command System
- IS-200.b (ICS 200) ICS for Single Resources and Initial Action Incidents
- IS-700.a National Incident Management System (NIMS), An Introduction
- IS-800.b National Response Framework, An Introduction

Interagency Planning

While the expectation of HSPD-5 is that incidents, including events and mass gatherings, be managed in a NIMS-compliant manner, the reality is that this remains highly variable throughout the nation. For an experienced event medical planner, it should usually be quickly apparent if the event organizers and other support partners are following NIMS principles. Even if the broader event organizer is not following NIMS, the medical plan should still be developed in accordance with NIMS. This includes establishing objectives for medical services, developing a medical operational plan, and establishing an incident command system (ICS) for managing medical resources, ideally fully integrated with other public safety elements.

Table 9.1 Overview of NIMS [2]

NIMS It	NIMS Is Not
• A comprehensive, nationwide, systematic approach to incident management, including the command and coordination of incidents, resource management, and information management	Only the ICS Only applicable to certain emergency/incident response personnel A static system
• A set of concepts and principles for all threats, hazards, and events across all mission areas (Prevention. Protection. Mitigation. Response. Recovery)	• A response plan
• Scalable, flexible, and adaptable, used for all incidents, from day-to-day to large-scale	• Used only during large-scale incidents
• Standard resource management procedures that enable coordination among different jurisdictions or organizations	• A resource-ordering system
• Essential principles for communications and information management	• A communications plan

Using NIMS for all size of events is highly recommended and leads to a more efficient and safe operation. However, the value of NIMS becomes even more important as events grow in size and complexity. Event organizers often fail to or are delayed in convening an interdisciplinary planning meeting that brings together the key public safety and support partners. Developing an interdisciplinary, NIMS-compliant public safety event operational plan is a best practice. When the event organizer is a private entity with little experience with NIMS, an individual or agency should be identified to take on this important planning function.

Unified Command

Managing the event through ICS is a fundamental and essential component of NIMS. Smaller events and those with a single jurisdiction/discipline expected to dominate the operational activities (e.g., law enforcement/security) may be effectively managed by a single incident commander. However, when more than one agency has event jurisdiction (e.g., law enforcement and medical), or when events cross political jurisdictions (e.g., a marathon), the use of Unified Command is called for. This enables multiple organizations to collaboratively perform various Incident Commander functions. Each Unified Command agency maintains its own authority, responsibility, and accountability for its resources while jointly managing and directing event activities through the establishment of common event objectives and strategies, resulting in a single Incident Action Plan (IAP). With a Unified Command, there is not a sole "commander" but rather the event is managed through jointly approved objectives. Unified Command allows the primary event organizations to work collaboratively while putting aside issues like competing authority, jurisdictional boundaries, and resource control and ownership. Instead, they establish clear event priorities and objectives producing unity of effort and allowing resource allocation regardless of ownership.

Local and State Emergency Operations Centers

Depending on the size, complexity, and associated risks and threats associated with an event or mass gathering, a local emergency operations center (EOC) may be activated. Under NIMS, the EOC is part of the Multiagency Coordination (MAC) System. The local EOC physically (or increasingly virtually) brings together a variety of both governmental and nongovernmental representatives to effectively support the on-scene incident command system. These might include public safety agencies, hospitals, public works, utilities, elected or appointed government officials, and other stakeholders. Rarely will there be a need to activate a state EOC for an event or mass gathering. A common practice by EOCs is to partially activate for an event, bringing in only the agencies that are felt to be needed to support the event.

Fusion Centers

Each US state, territory, and the District of Columbia, in collaboration with the US Departments of Homeland Security and Justice have established fusion centers. These state-owned and operated centers primarily support law enforcement by providing intelligence regarding criminal activities and terrorism. They serve as focal points for the receipt, analysis, gathering, and sharing of threat-related information between local, state, federal, private sector, and other partners [4]. While Fusion Centers are primarily law enforcement related, they may produce actionable intelligence that can impact medical plans. For example, they could identify a new supply of high-potency opioids that have recently entered the area of the event that might result in increased numbers of overdoses.

Overview of Interdisciplinary Functions

Law Enforcement

Almost any event worthy of on-site medical operations will have some degree of involvement by one or more law enforcement agencies. This may range from a small number of police officers from a single agency to hundreds of officers from multiple agencies. In most cases primary law enforcement operations will be handled by local and/or state law enforcement. Private security services often contracted by the event organizer do not typically obviate the need for at least some sworn law enforcement personnel to be on-site for the event. In addition to enforcement of the law, crowd and traffic control are areas in which law enforcement is often partially or completely responsible. Other specialized roles may include intelligence gathering, tactical operations (e.g., SWAT), bomb detection and disposal, dignitary protection, and counter-terrorism. In addition to their primary policing responsibilities, law enforcement officers assigned to an event may be a valuable resource to support medical operations, although not typically their primary responsibility.

Fire and Hazardous Materials

Most events do not have significant involvement of (non-EMS) fire service or hazardous materials (HAZMAT) response teams. When the event includes special fire or hazardous materials risks (e.g., fireworks), appropriate personnel should be involved in the event planning and resources should be on-site during the event, as circumstances warrant. Additionally,

firefighters typically have training at least at the emergency medical responder level and can potentially be used to augment event medical staffing during routine operations or in the event of a multicasualty incident.

Emergency Medical Services

The involvement of local EMS in a special event or mass gathering will vary from minimal involvement to local EMS providing all event medical services. If event medical services are not being provided by local EMS, the event medical leadership should fully integrate local EMS into the event medical plan to the extent warranted by the nature and scope of the event. Helicopter EMS may be an important consideration, especially for events in rural areas and/or where EMS vehicle ingress and egress to the venue will be limited. Event medical leadership should also be in contact with EMS agency/system medical director(s) and be familiar with applicable local and state regulations that might impact the event medical plan.

Hospitals

Local hospitals and regional specialty facilities should be included in the event medical planning. A special event can potentially have significant impact on hospitals, especially when the event medical plan fails to provide sufficient resources to effectively manage lower acuity medical problems on-site. It is important that event medical plans recognize the hospital capabilities for routine and specialty care (e.g., trauma, cardiac, stroke, pediatric) and are fully familiar with any established regional systems of care protocols that might exist.

Emergency Management

Medium to large events and those with special hazards or risks may warrant the services of the local emergency management agency. Emergency management does not typically provide direct services but rather they help other emergency and public safety agencies obtain and coordinate the additional resources needed to accomplish the mission. For large events, emergency management may elect to partially or fully activate their emergency operations center (EOC), an off-site multiagency coordination center. For some events emergency management may deploy a mobile command post or other specialized resources.

Law Enforcement and Security

Law Enforcement Overview

Almost any event worthy of on-site medical operations will have some degree of involvement by one or more law enforcement agency. This may range from a small number of police officers from a single agency to hundreds of officers from multiple agencies. In most cases primary law enforcement operations will be handled by local and/or state law enforcement agencies. Private security services often contracted by the event organizer do not typically obviate the need for at least some law enforcement at the event. Regardless of the degree of law enforcement involvement, there should be a primary point of contact from law enforcement leadership that can serve as a liaison with medical planning and operations.

While the primary purpose of law enforcement in an event is providing security, protecting attendees, and enforcing the law, they can also be an important resource in support of medical operations. Most law enforcement officers are trained in cardiopulmonary resuscitation (CPR), automated external defibrillator (AED) operations, bleeding control, and naloxone administration with many trained at the emergency medical responder level or higher. Law enforcement officers are often the ones to identify a medical emergency, summon medical services, and coordinate medical responders to the patient. Law enforcement officers should be briefed on the event medical plan and have interoperable communications with medical personnel.

Mounted police may be used in some events and, given the high vantage point of the officer, can often identify medical emergencies in dense crowds. Teams of mounted officers can be valuable in helping to escort medical responders through a crowd by forming a V-shaped pattern with EMS vehicles or personnel protected in the center of the "V" (see Figure 9.1).

Local Law Enforcement

Most large events involve local law enforcement agencies. Depending on the venue this may involve city, county, or other regional/municipal police departments and/or county sheriff's offices. Larger municipalities may have sufficient personnel to provide law enforcement services through their agency alone. Events occurring in smaller jurisdictions and larger events occurring in more populated communities may require additional support from other local and state police agencies. Events that span multiple jurisdictions (e.g., a marathon) might require various law enforcement agencies for their specific jurisdiction, with or without mutual aid support. When multiple agencies are involved in providing law enforcement services, it is essential that they operate under a unified command system with central command and control and with interoperable communications that include integration with other public safety and emergency services (e.g., EMS and medical).

Local law enforcement agencies often utilize reserve or auxiliary officers to augment their personnel. These individuals may have no, limited, or full police powers. While many reserve and auxiliary officers are well-trained, their training is usually

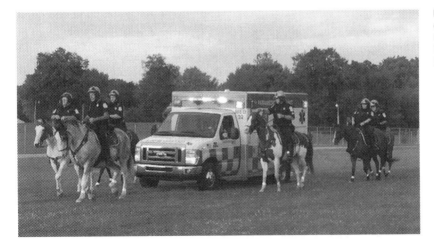

Figure 9.1 Mounted Police demonstrating ambulance escort for use large event, depicting the Kalamazoo County Sheriff's Mounted Division

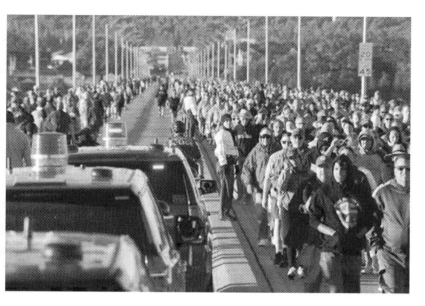

Figure 9.2 Michigan State Police provide law enforcement services during annual Mackinac Bridge Walk, depicting State of Michigan resources at work

considerably less than full-time officers. However, some may have health care backgrounds that could be beneficial to medical operations.

State Law Enforcement

Law enforcement at the state level varies across the United States from large, resource-rich state police departments to considerably smaller and more focused highway patrol agencies. In general, those states with highway patrol as their primary state law enforcement agency will often have relatively larger sheriff's offices, especially to cover rural and unincorporated areas. Events occurring in more rural areas may have state police as their primary law enforcement agency. State police and highway patrol are also often used to augment law enforcement coverage of larger events where additional personnel are needed (see Figure 9.2).

Federal Law Enforcement

It is very rare for a federal law enforcement agency to be the primary provider of law enforcement services for a major event. Involvement of federal law enforcement agencies is typically limited to intelligence gathering, information sharing, and providing general or specialty support. Federal law enforcement agencies that may interact with medical planning or operations include the FBI and the US Secret Service. Certain major events of significant importance may receive special designation through the US Department of Homeland Security.

- *Federal Bureau of Investigation (FBI):* The FBI rarely will serve as the event's primary law enforcement agency. In an era that includes the potential for terrorism, the FBI is increasingly involved in intelligence gathering and dissemination and field support for large or otherwise high-risk events. Involvement of the FBI in planning or event operations does not indicate a higher risk of a terrorist incident or the presence of a credible threat. Limited FBI involvement has become commonplace in special events ranging from highly politically charged rallies to large sporting events. The FBI often serves as the liaison between local and state law enforcement and the federal law enforcement community. The FBI also has specialty teams including tactical, explosive, and hazardous materials, that may be used to augment local and state resources.

- *United State Secret Service (USSS):* Most known for assuring the safety and security of the President of the United States, the Vice-President, and visiting heads of state, the USSS will always be involved in events that involve these individuals. In such events, the USSS, supported by other local, state, and federal law enforcement agencies, will be primarily responsible for event security. However, their focus is primarily on dignitary protection with other law enforcement activities typically being managed by local and/or state law enforcement. During political rallies and other events involving qualifying Presidential and

Vice-Presidential candidates, the USSS provides a security detail for the candidate which involves considerably less personnel than with an event involving the incumbent President or Vice-President. It should also be understood that the White House Medical Unit is primarily responsible for medical care to the President and Vice-President. This is not typically a responsibility of the event medical providers. Additionally, an advanced life support ambulance is routinely incorporated in the motorcade but should be viewed by event medical planners as having a very focused mission in support of the dignitaries and others directly associated with the motorcade.

- *Other Federal Law Enforcement Agencies:* Depending on the nature and location of the event, a number of other federal law enforcement agencies may be involved, typically in a support role. These may include:

  - *Homeland Security Investigations (HSI):* For events that may require special intelligence or involve areas in which HSI has ongoing investigations (e.g., human trafficking).
  - Bureau of Alcohol, Tobacco, Firearms and Explosives (ATF): For events at higher risk for an explosive incident.
  - *National Park Service and/or US Park Police:* For events occurring on or near US National Parks.
  - *United States Coast Guard:* For events involving large waterways or with a maritime component.
  - *US Border Patrol:* For events occurring near a US border or where border security is identified as a concern.

- *Special Event Assessment Rating (SEAR) Events:* These events are submitted by the primary law enforcement agency to the US Department of Homeland Security (DHS) on a voluntary basis for special events with high security concerns. Past SEAR events have included Super Bowls, the Indianapolis 500, and the Kentucky Derby. DHS applies a risk-based process to submitted events resulting in the assignment of a SEAR rating which considers the threat, vulnerability, and consequences for each event. The event may receive a rating from 1 to 5 designating the degree of international, national, or state significance (see Table 9.2) [5].

Table 9.2 Special Event Assessment Rating (SEAR) Categories [6]

Level	Description
1	Significant events with national and/or international importance that require extensive federal interagency support.
2	Significant events with national and/or international importance that may require some level of federal interagency support.
4	Events with limited national importance that are managed at the state and local levels.
5	Events that may be nationally recognized but generally have local or state importance.

The federal government may provide additional resources to SEAR events assisting state and local officials in filling gaps in capabilities. Historically, this support included:

- Explosive detection canine teams.
- Cyber risk assessments.
- Venue screening and field intelligence teams,
- Air security and tactical operations support

- *National Special Security Events (NSSE):* Nationally significant federal government or public events may be designated by the President – or his representative, the Secretary of DHS – as National Special Security Events (NSSE). In such events the USSS is the lead federal agency responsible for coordinating, planning, exercising, and implementing security. Factors that may lead to an NSSE designation include the anticipated attendance by senior US officials and foreign dignitaries; size of the event; and significance of the event. Some events categorized as NSSEs include the following:

  - presidential inaugurations
  - major international summits held in the United States
  - major sporting events, and
  - presidential nominating conventions.

NSSE operational plans include the use of security fencing, barricades, special access secure badges, K-9 teams, and other security technologies. To ensure consequence management, DHS pre-positions federal specialty teams such as the Domestic Emergency Support Teams, Urban Search and Rescue Teams,

National Emergency Response Teams, Nuclear Incident Response Teams, and assets from the Strategic National Stockpile [6].

Private Security

Most special events will include the use of private security personnel. These individuals usually lack or have very limited police powers. They may or may not be armed. Training requirements for private security personnel are highly variable, and usually related to requirements to be armed. Their training is usually far less than a sworn law enforcement officer, if they have any training at all. That said, occasionally off-duty police officers may work for private security companies. Occasionally, private security personnel may have current or past training as an EMS provider, or, at least in basic life support, providing a potential for assisting medical operations

Law Enforcement/Security Support of Medical Operations

Law enforcement and security personnel can be a valuable and often underappreciated resource for supporting medical operations. While, patient care is not typically their primary purpose, increasingly law enforcement agencies encourage (if not expect) their officers to provide basic lifesaving care until the arrival of EMS. Often the effectiveness of law enforcement support of medical operations directly correlates to the degree of joint planning, unified incident command, and interoperable communications.

Examples of medically related activities event law enforcement and security may provide include:

- Early recognition of medical emergencies (e.g., heat-related illnesses, altered mental status, cardiac/respiratory arrest)
- Administering direct lifesaving patient care before arrival of medical personnel (e.g., CPR, AED use, bleeding control, naloxone administration)
- Locating patients in crowded areas and directing medical personnel to them
- Escalating or de-escalating the medical response based on their initial assessment
- Escorting medical personnel to patients located in secure or restricted areas
- Providing crowd and traffic control to facilitate medical/EMS ingress and egress
- Establishing a landing zone for air evacuation

- Placing behavioral health crisis patients at risk of harming themselves or others into protective custody in accordance with authority under a state's mental health code
- Assisting in patient handling and movement
- Helping to protect patient privacy
- Securing any weapons or illegal substances found with patient

Fire Departments

Most events do not have significant involvement of (non-EMS) fire service. Especially when the event includes special fire or hazardous materials risks (e.g., fireworks), appropriate personnel should be involved in the event planning and resources should be on-site during the event, as circumstances warrant. Additionally, firefighters typically have training at least at the emergency medical responder level and can potentially be used to augment event medical staffing during routine operations or in a multicasualty incident.

Fire service is typically provided by a city, county, or other municipal fire department or through a multijurisdictional fire district. In urban and suburban communities, the fire department is often staffed by full-time career firefighters, while in more rural areas volunteer or paid-on call firefighters are common. Some fire departments are staffed by a combination of career and volunteer/paid-on call personnel. Many, but not all, fire apparatus carry basic and (occasionally) advanced life support equipment with their personnel trained accordingly.

While the fire service is a primary provider of EMS throughout much of the nation, many events will use private, non-fire-based EMS as the primary EMS resource for the event. Conversely, the fire department may be the sole EMS agency supporting the event. In other cases, fire department personnel may assist in medical operations by deploying roving basic life support-capable first response teams, while paramedic and transport services are provided by a different agency. When the fire department is not the lead EMS agency for an event, it is important to have clearly established incident management/command roles and responsibilities, understanding that these may change in the event of a mass casualty or other catastrophic incident, with the fire department taking a more active role in the incident command structure.

Depending on the nature, size, hazards, and location of the event, the nonmedical role of the fire department may vary considerably. Especially for events involving indoor activities, the fire department may be present in a fire prevention and code enforcement role. In most communities the fire department is empowered to cancel or prematurely end an event if they identify fire code violations are present, particularly those that have life-safety implications (e.g., more event attendees than the occupancy of the building is permitted).

The proximity of the event to community fire stations will often determine the need to preposition fire suppression vehicles at or near the event site. Similarly, events with increased risk for fires may warrant fire-suppression equipment and personnel to be on-site. In general, the larger and more complex the event the more likely it will be to have fire suppression resources on-site. Racetracks may have their own fire–rescue resources.

Emergency Medical Services

The use of EMS agencies and personnel in event medical operations may vary considerably based on numerous factors including the event size, location, activities, and risks, as well as the availability and willingness of local and area EMS agencies to participate. In some events a single local EMS agency will manage the entire event medical operation with no additional support. Conversely, in other events, local EMS may have little involvement, outside of unanticipated emergencies that may result in their response. Regardless of the involvement of the local 911 EMS agency, most events must consider and have plans for BLS and ALS care, including nontransporting EMS response and transporting ambulances. Particularly in events in rural areas with long transport times to hospitals capable of providing definitive care (e.g., trauma centers), event medical plans should have provisions for using helicopter EMS. Event medical leadership should also be aware of local or state regulations that may impact staffing for special events. In some cases, the jurisdiction(s) in which the event is held may have a jurisdictional EMS medical director and/or EMS regulatory agency that may have some authority over the EMS resources used to support the event.

Local (911 Responding) EMS Agencies

Unlike law enforcement and the fire service where delivery local models are usually limited to agencies of city, county, or other municipal governmental jurisdictions, local EMS in the United States is delivered by a myriad of methods. As mentioned above, the fire service is one of the most common providers of both transport and nontransport BLS and ALS services. However, in many communities the fire service limits their role to providing BLS or ALS nontransporting services or, especially in rural areas, may provide no EMS at all. There are many alternatives to the fire service for transporting EMS including municipal "third service" EMS agencies, private for-profit and not-for-profit services, hospital-based services, and volunteer services. While the fire service is the primary provider of nontransporting medical first response services, in some communities these services are provided by law enforcement agencies, independent rescue squad/quick responder teams, or other organizations.

In smaller and lower-risk events, it may be appropriate to simply have plans to use the local 911 EMS resources to respond to a serious medical incident while event medical staff provide BLS and (potentially) ALS care. In larger or higher-risk events, multiple BLS and ALS units from one or more EMS agencies may be needed on-site to meet anticipated medical demands. Regardless, it is important that the event medical leadership reach out to the local EMS community to assure mutual appropriate integration of local EMS resources into the event medical operations.

The ability of local EMS agencies to provide dedicated on-site resources is often dependent upon the event organizers to provide financial support sufficient to cover all (or at least most) of the direct costs incurred by the agency, primarily personnel and usually involving overtime pay. Event organizers routinely provide reimbursement to law enforcement agencies to cover their personnel costs. Unfortunately, in contrast, event organizers often reportedly believe EMS agencies should provide their services at no cost. In some cases, private EMS agencies may be willing to absorb the cost of dedicating resources to an event in exchange for free event sponsorship and with the expectation that revenue generated from some transports may at least partially cover their staffing costs.

EMS operations at a special event may take on several forms. A common model is for dedicated EMS units or personnel to provide the initial stabilizing care and then hand the patient off to a nondedicated ambulance for hospital transport.

In other cases, on-site ambulances may be used to transport patients understanding that this could potentially deplete the available resources needed to respond to further medical incidents. When robust medical services (e.g., physician staffed) are available at the event, a staged operation works well in which nonemergent patients are transported to an event medical facility for evaluation and treatment, potentially preventing the need for transport of lower acuity patients to the hospital. In smaller events or when local EMS resources are limited, a nondedicated EMS standby may be proposed in which the EMS agency offers to position an EMS unit(s) on-site with the understanding that they may be pulled to respond to 911 and other nonevent requests for service. Nondedicated EMS standbys are generally the least desirable option for using local EMS and planners should base their plans on EMS units not being able to remain on standby for the event.

Even if the involvement of local EMS in an event is minimal, it is important that EMS still be involved in the planning process. Local EMS can provide extensive information on the community and regional healthcare system, potentially assist in identifying sources to augment staffing, and provide insight into any unique regulatory requirements that might be applicable. If nothing else, EMS should develop joint plans in the event of a mass casualty incident (MCI) that incorporate both event medical and local EMS personnel.

Air Medical and Helicopter EMS

Events occurring in rural areas and those in locations in which traffic congestion or other factors may delay ground ambulance transport to definitive care hospitals should consider including plans for using air medical services, specifically helicopter EMS (HEMS). Additionally, if after consultation with local EMS leadership, the joint MCI plan includes the potential for using one or more EMS aircraft as part of an MCI response, then a section on HEMS should definitely be a part of that plan.

HEMS agencies are typically hospital-owned or affiliated organizations or private for-profit or not-for-profit agencies. In a few states (e.g., Maryland and Delaware), the primary HEMS provider is the state police. A few large city or county fire departments may also use other potential but much less common HEMS providers including the US Coast Guard, the National Guard, or other active duty or reserve air medical units. These units often have minimal medical capabilities making them less desirable for use in most plans, except in extreme circumstances.

Planning for the use of HEMS at a special event should be done in collaboration with the event organizer, the venue management, local EMS, and other public support safety agencies. Identification and emergency contact information for the nearest HEMS agencies should be obtained. Clinical conditions (e.g., major trauma, acute myocardial infarction) should be predetermined and agreed upon by appropriate stakeholders.

An important HEMS planning consideration is where to safely establish a landing zone (LZ), assuming the venue does not have an existing helipad. Pre-identifying an LZ prior to the emergency will help to assure a safe and efficient integration of HEMS into the event medical operation. Similarly, it should be predetermined which personnel will be responsible for securing the LZ if needed. The local HEMS agency is often willing to help identify the best site for the LZ, increasingly using, open-source web-based mapping applications to remotely assess the proposed site(s). The MCI plan should also consider pre-identifying multiple LZs in the event multiple aircraft are simultaneously needed.

Safety Considerations for EMS Helicopter Landing Zones [7]

- Minimum of 100 x 100-foot area free of overhead obstructions (e.g., wires, trees, poles).
  - Any overhead obstructions unable to be cleared should be communicated to pilot.
- The LZ should be a flat surface that is firm, and free of debris.
- Consider the wind direction. Helicopters land and take off into the wind.
- The LZ perimeter should be walked and checked for hazards.
- 45 Degree Angle Test: Stand in the middle of the LZ with one arm extended at a 45-degree angle. Any objects at or above the line projected from the outstretched arm are potential obstacles that need to be reported to the incoming aircraft. Sweep 360 degrees.

- Do not use landing zones that contain loose material such as gravel. The rotor wash will cause stones or gravel to become airborne, striking personnel and damaging vehicles.
- Do not use flares or cones to mark the landing zone, as they will become airborne during the landing. However, weighted cones/lights designed for LZ operations are acceptable.

EMS Medical Direction and Physician Oversight

Physician direction of EMS varies considerably throughout the United States. Most EMS agencies are required to have an agency medical director. In other systems there may be a system (e.g., county or region) medical director that has authority over all licensed EMS agencies in the jurisdiction. Regardless of the way physician oversight is provided it is an essential component of an effective EMS system with the EMS medical director having numerous responsibilities, often statutorily defined [8]. Event medical leaders should understand that EMS medical directors may be unwilling to credential EMS personnel who are not from agencies they oversee. Such credentialling may be required for outside EMS personnel to legally function at an event.

Event medical planners and leaders are encouraged to contact local EMS medical directors for large or complex events, events in which local EMS agencies or personnel are likely to be involved, or for additional information on the local EMS and healthcare system. Commonly, local agency/system medical directors welcome the opportunity to assist in the event planning and operations. Medical directors are also often well aware of local and state regulations and laws that may be applicable and could impact the event medical plan. Additionally, medical directors can often connect event medical staff with other key stakeholders within the EMS and healthcare system.

EMS Regulatory Considerations

Event medical planners should understand that there may often be local and/or state regulations and laws that might impact the ability to use certain EMS resources. For example, a local jurisdiction may have an exclusive contract with a particular ambulance service in which that agency is the only agency authorized to provide EMS transport service in that jurisdiction. A commonly reported misunderstanding is that events occurring on private property are somehow exempt from complying with local and state regulations and laws. Event medical planners and leaders should be fully familiar with applicable regulations and laws governing EMS (including personnel licensing and credentialling) that might impact the medical event plan.

Public Safety Specialty Teams

Large or complex special events may involve various specialty teams such as hazardous materials, tactical (SWAT), and bomb response team. Event medical leadership should be aware that these and other specialty teams may be prepositioned for an event or may be requested for various real or potential threats that warrant the specialized capabilities of these teams.

Hazardous Materials Response (HAZMAT) Teams

FEMA defines a HAZMAT Team as "A Hazardous Materials Response Team is an organized group of hazardous materials (HAZMAT) technicians who respond to HAZMAT incidents, including those involving Weapons of Mass Destruction (WMD)" [9]. HAZMAT teams typically have specialized equipment and training to identify unknown potentially harmful chemicals, to mitigate dangers to people, and to protect the environment. While these teams almost always have the ability to decontaminate their own personnel and equipment, they may or may not be capable of providing large scale decontamination to multiple patients. These teams may also have limited antidote capabilities.

- *Local/Regional HAZMAT Teams*: Local and regional HAZMAT Teams are usually provided through the fire service. Less commonly the teams will be provided by law enforcement or EMS agencies or through multidisciplinary teams. A HAZMAT team may be provided by a single larger department or through multiple departments forming a multijurisdictional or regional team. It is not common for a HAZMAT team to regularly standby at a special event unless the event involves hazardous chemicals or there is a credible threat that hazardous materials might intentionally be used as a weapon.
- *Weapons of Mass Destruction (WMD) Civil Support Team (CST)*: Each state, US territory, and

the District of Columbia have at least one WMD CST team made up of twenty-two full-time members of the National Guard and Air National Guard. These teams are on-call and available to rapidly respond to incidents involving chemical, biological, radiological, nuclear, and explosive (CBRNE) agents as part of the nation's preparedness for terrorism incidents. WMD CST teams may be assigned to large or complex special events and to events associated with a heightened threat for terrorist activity. Team members receive over 650 hours of specialized training that usually far exceeds that of most local/regional HAZMAT teams. These teams usually have a small medical component including a physician or advanced practice provider that may be an excellent source of medical and toxicologic information but are otherwise limited in their abilities to provide large-scale patient care [10].

Tactical (SWAT) Team

More commonly known as SWAT teams, in an era of terrorist incidents, law enforcement tactical teams are increasingly standing by at large special events, particularly those that have political, religious, or particularly controversial themes. Tactical teams are usually made up of officers from local or state law enforcement, or less commonly from federal agencies such as the FBI or USSS. Increasingly more tactical teams have an embedded medical element capable of providing BLS and/or ALS in high threat zone areas, including care under fire. If event medical leadership is made aware of the presence of a tactical team, they should attempt to determine their internal medical capabilities. Often, for security reasons, the presence of staged tactical teams will be kept confidential and information on the teams will be shared on a need-to-know basis.

Bomb Response Team

Often referred to as a "bomb squad," bomb response teams are specialized units with equipment and training to investigate, render safe, and dispose of suspected hazardous devices, explosives, pyrotechnics, and ammunition [11]. Most bomb response teams are usually affiliated with local or state law enforcement agencies. Like tactical teams, bomb response teams may be requested to standby on-site for large events and those with heightened risks for terrorist activity or when a credible threat is received. Bomb response teams do not usually have their own medical support.

Interfacing with Hospitals and the Healthcare System

Hospitals and healthcare systems may be particularly impacted by special events and mass gatherings. Indeed, the effectiveness of the event medical plan may very well determine the degree that nearby hospitals are impacted. Events that have poor medical planning and/or are under resourced can overwhelm area hospitals and adversely affect the quality of care afforded to both event and nonevent patients. Conversely, events that are well planned and properly resourced may mitigate unnecessary emergency department (ED) visits and their consequences. Event medical planners and leaders should work collaboratively with the closest hospitals as well as area or regional specialty hospitals to help assure the right patient is delivered to the right hospital in the appropriate amount of time. In some events, local hospitals may be a source of supplemental personnel or even be the primary provider of event medical services.

Closest Community Hospital(s)

In most cases, the closest community hospital(s) to the event is most vulnerable to the medical consequences associated with the event. An effective event medical operation will reduce the number of patients that present to the local hospital ED. Event medical planners are encouraged to make early contact with area hospitals to discuss the potential impact the event might have on ED and hospital operations. In many cases, hospitals may wish to add additional staff to better handle anticipated increases in event-related patient visits. Hospitals may be willing to help supplement the event medical operation to help reduce the potential ED burden. It is important that the event medical and ED leadership have a means to communicate with one another during the event, especially when relatively large patient volumes are occurring. When the closest hospital ED is experiencing high patient loads (event or nonevent), event-related medical patients may be better served by being transferred to more distant EDs that have greater capacity.

Regional Specialty Hospitals

While the closest community hospital(s) is the most common recipient of event-related patients, it is important to recognize that certain time-critical problems are best treated by bypassing community hospitals and transporting the patient directly to specialty care facilities. These types of time critical conditions include major trauma, pediatrics, acute myocardial infarction, stroke, and cardiac arrest (after return of spontaneous circulation). Since the 2010 report from the Institute of Medicine's report on Regionalization of Emergency Care, increasing efforts have been made to develop regional systems of care that are designed to assure patients have rapid access to definitive care. Ideally, the location of the event will be in an area where such systems are well-established and fully integrated into the local EMS system. However, this may not always be the case necessitating event planners to develop various contingencies in the event of time-critical medical emergencies.

Local, regional, and state protocols will often be in place that designate certain types of specialty hospitals. Trauma centers became the first widespread hospitals to become designated to deal with a specific time sensitive condition. Since then, specialty centers dealing with acute ST-segment elevation myocardial infarction (STEMI), acute stroke, sepsis, pediatric emergencies have developed. Various national organizations have established processes for evaluating and verifying or accrediting these types of facilities. However, it is ultimately up to local, regional, and/or state regulatory agencies to formally designate these facilities as part of a comprehensive regional system of care.

An important aspect of effective regional systems of care is the establishment of evidenced based criteria that identify the types of patients that should preferentially be transferred to these specialty facilities. Like facility verification, various national organizations have established criteria for their respective conditions. However, it is again up to local, regional, or state regulatory agencies to promulgate protocols to operationalize the criteria which may or may not be fully or partially aligned with the criteria established by national organizations.

Regional Health Care Coalitions

Following the attacks of 9/11, the US Department of Health and Human Services (HHS) have worked to better prepare the nation's hospitals and healthcare organizations to better prepare, respond, and recover from disasters and other catastrophic incidents. HHS's Administration for Strategic Preparedness and Response (formerly, the Office of the Assistant Secretary for Preparedness and Response, ASPR) has established the national Hospital Preparedness Program (HPP). Among the many HPP initiatives is the promotion of regional health care coalitions, a collaboration of hospitals, EMS, emergency management, public health and other healthcare organizations within a defined geographic area. HCCs are intended to better prepare hospitals and health care systems to respond to emergencies and disasters. HCCs vary considerably between different states, with some states having highly developed and effective coalitions while other states have no HCCs.

Event medical planners should determine if the event is served by an HCC and determine what resources the HCC might be able to make available to support the event. In some cases, especially for large or complex incidents, HCCs may be able to provide technical support and guidance to event planners. Some HCCs have procured specialized equipment that might be valuable or have developed volunteer teams of medical providers that might be able to augment the event medical staffing (see Figures 9.3 and 9.4). Some HCCs have developed regional medical coordination centers to coordinate healthcare resources in an emergency.

Potential Support from Health Care Coalitions

- Planning assistance and information on regional healthcare resources
- Provide medical equipment and supplies
- Preposition mass casualty supplies
- Provide temporary shelters (e.g., inflatable tents)
- Coordinate communications between the event, EMS, and hospitals
- Solicit volunteer medical providers to augment staffing
- Provide a single point of contact for information sharing
- Coordinate the distribution of patients to area hospitals
- Request additional specialty resources from the state

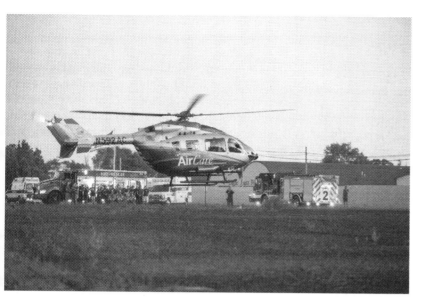

Figure 9.3 EMS helicopter from West Michigan Air Care takes off from landing zone at a large event

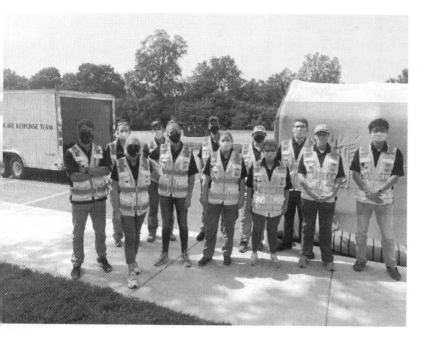

Figure 9.4 Regional HCC from the Michigan 5th District Medical Response Coalition provides inflatable tent and assists with staffing for college football game

Special Health Care Teams and Programs

Medical Reserve Corps

The Medical Reserve Corps (MRC) Program is administered through ASPR and consists of a network of more than 200,000 volunteers in approximately 800 local or regional units located throughout the United States. MRC volunteers come from throughout the community and are willing to contribute their time to support the healthcare and public health systems during disasters and other emergencies. MRC volunteers represent a diverse group of medical and public health professionals as well as well as individuals with little or no health care background. MRC units and members are often willing to provide support during special events and mass gatherings [12].

Emergency System for Advance Registration of Volunteer Health Professionals

The Emergency System for Advance Registration of Volunteer Health Professionals (ESAR-VHP) is a federal initiative of ASPR administered at the state level. ESAR-VHP establishes standardized volunteer registration programs for disasters and public health and medical emergencies. The program verifies health professionals' identification and credentials so that they can respond more rapidly to emergencies. Essentially, a statewide registry of health care professionals as well as individuals with no health care background who are willing (but not obligated) to volunteer during emergencies. Like MRC members, ESAR-VHP registrants are often willing to volunteer for special events and can be an important means to augment staffing.

Event planners can receive additional information on using ESAR-VHP volunteers by contacting their state health department's preparedness program and or through regional healthcare coalitions [13].

Disaster Medical Assistance Teams

Disaster Medical Assistance Teams (DMAT) are part of the National Disaster Medical System. Comprised of physicians, nurses, advanced practice providers, respiratory therapists, paramedics, and pharmacists, these teams are located throughout the United States. While primarily intended to provide medical care when public health and medical emergencies overwhelm state and local, resources, these teams are also used to provide medical support at national special security events such as the presidential inauguration. DMAT is a resource that is reserved for extremely large, national events. As such, it is unlikely for them to be a resource for most special events [14].

Summary

This chapter provides a brief overview of some of the many types of governmental and nongovernmental agencies and organizations that event medical planners and leaders may interact with. In some cases these interactions will be brief and minimally significant while in others they may be quite extensive. In general the larger or more complex the event, the more agencies will likely be involved. While some agencies may complicate your event medical operation, in most cases, expressing a willingness to understand and respect the agencies' roles and responsibilities will result in cooperation and collaboration. Indeed, in many cases these agencies and organizations can contribute very positively to event medical operations. Event medicine is most definitely a "team sport." It is hoped that this chapter contributes to an appreciation for just how big the expanded team can be.

References

1. Office of the President of the United States. (2003, February 28). *Homeland Security Presidential Directive 5*. Publication Library. Retrieved March 6, 2022, from www.dhs.gov/sites/default/files/publications/Homeland%20Security%20Presidential%20Directive%205.pdf

2. Federal Emergency Management Agency. (2017, October). *National Incident Management System, 3rd Edition*. Retrieved March 6, 2022, from www.fema.gov/sites/default/files/2020-09/pda-report_fema-1977-dr_ia.pdf

3. Federal Emergency Management Agency. (2021, June 30). *NIMS Implementation and Training*. FEMA National Incident Management System. Retrieved March 6, 2022, from www.fema.gov/emergency-managers/nims/implementation-training#training

4. US Department of Homeland Security. (2019, September 19). *Fusion Centers*. Fusion Centers | Homeland Security. Retrieved March 7, 2022, from www.dhs.gov/fusion-centers

5. US Department of Homeland Security Office of Operations Coordination. (2019, September 5). *Special event assessment rating (SEAR) events fact sheet – DHS*. Retrieved August 28, 2022, from www.dhs.gov/sites/default/files/publications/19_0905_ops_sear-fact-sheet.pdf

6. Congressional Research Service. (2021, January 11). *National Special Security Events: Fact Sheet*. Retrieved August 28, 2022, from https://sgp.fas.org/crs/homesec/R43522.pdf

7. Maryland State Police. (n.d.). *Optimal Landing Zone Set-up*. Maryland State Police. Retrieved September 5, 2022, from https://mdsp.maryland.gov/Organization/Pages/SupportServicesBureau/AviationCommand/OptimalLandingZoneSetup.aspx

8. Physician Oversight of Emergency Medical Services. *Prehospital Emergency Care*. 2017;**21**(2):281–282, doi:10.1080/10903127.2016.1229827

9. Federal Emergency Management Agency. (2020, March 26). *Resource Typing Definition – Hazardous Material Response Team*. View Resource Typing Definition. Retrieved September 6, 2022, from https://rtlt.preptoolkit.fema.gov/Public/Resource/View/4-508-1248?p=11

10. National Guard Bureau. (2017, December). *Weapons of Mass Destruction (WMD) Civil Support Team (CST)*. National Guard. Retrieved September 6, 2022, from www.nationalguard.mil/Portals/31/Resources/Fact%20Sheets/CBRNE%20Fact%20Sheet%20(Dec.%202017).pdf

11. Federal Emergency Management Agency. (2019, November 15). *Resource Typing Definition – Bomb Response Team*. View Resource Typing Definition. Retrieved September 6, 2022, from https://rtlt.preptoolkit.fema.gov/Public/Resource/View/6-508-1176?q=bomb

12. US Department of Health and Human Services Administration for Strategic Planning and Response. (n.d.). *About the Medical Reserve Corps.*

ASPR –=Administration for Strategic Preparedness and Response. Retrieved September 6, 2022, from https://aspr.hhs.gov/MRC/Pages/About-the-MRC.aspx

13. US Department of Health and Human Services Administration for Strategic Preparedness and Response. (n.d.). *The emergency system for advance registration of volunteer health professionals*. ASPR-Public Health Emergencies. Retrieved September 6, 2022, from www.phe.gov/esarvhp/pages/about.aspx

14. US Department of Health and Human Services. (2021, May 21). *Disaster Medical Assistance Teams*. Administration for Strategic Preparedness and Response. Retrieved September 6, 2022, from www.phe.gov/Preparedness/responders/ndms/ndms-teams/Pages/dmat.aspx

Common Themes and General Considerations across Mass Gathering Event Types

Erica Simon, Jonathan D. Trager, and Bryan Wilson

Common Themes and General Considerations Across All Event Types

A mass gathering is often a preplanned event, like a concert or sporting event, held at a specific location for a defined duration that strains planning and response resources. However, a mass gathering can also be spontaneous, such as the gathering of mourners associated with the death of a celebrity or a protest. Over the last few years, we have seen an increase in the number of protests, some events that are preplanned and organized but others that are not and that can quickly become out-of-control and end in tragedy. The Federal Emergency Management Agency (FEMA) uses the term "special events," to describe a nonroutine event that strains the resources of the hosting community and requires special permitting or additional planning, preparation, and mitigation. Rather than focusing on the number of people, the emphasis is placed on how the event will affect the hosting community's ability to respond. Consideration must be given for the potential of a delayed response to emergencies because of limited access to patients or other features of the environment and location. Planning and preparation are paramount to mitigating the hazards inherent in a mass gathering and ensuring timely access to appropriate medical care is available [79, 85]. The bottom line is that despite the many years of dealing with and researching mass gatherings, there remains a lack of in-depth understanding of the mass gathering and, despite often being attended by reasonably healthy or well people, the gatherings seem to be more hazardous than expected [6].

Planning and preparing for potential risks and hazards with the goal of preventing incidents is paramount to the success of the event and critical to public safety. Planning will be challenging and depending on the size of the gathering, will often involve the cooperation of multiple agencies and jurisdictions. A multidisciplinary planning team may include representatives from Emergency Management, Law Enforcement, Fire and Rescue, Public Works/Utilities, Public Health, and Transportation Authority as well as the promoter or sponsor. Essentially any person, organization and agency that holds a functional stake in the event should be part of the planning team – all stakeholders [45, 79, 85].

It is crucial that the lead agency be identified early in the process and that all involved agencies are present from the outset of the planning process. Remember that each community's resources are different and what may be classified as a special event in one community may not in another. Planning for a mass gathering should thus begin well in advance of the event and should be a team approach. At the initial meeting, the planning team should assess and consider the promoter's or sponsoring organization's purpose and experience, event risks (including crowds, staffing, food and shelter, parking, transportation, medical facilities), previous event concerns, relevant local concerns, weather, and community impact. Three main objectives should be achieved by the planning team: (1) Develop a mission statement, (2) develop event objectives, and (3) determine the necessary components of the public safety plan. This team must thus plan, prepare, execute, coordinate, and effectively communicate among themselves to ensure a good outcome [79].

Preparing for a special event can be daunting. First and foremost, the team must develop a mission statement. Some questions that should be answered include: (1) What is the purpose of the special event? (2) What is being done to address the purpose? (3) What benefits or values will result from the event? (4) How will public health and safety be protected? Next the team is tasked with developing event objectives which should be "SMART": Specific, Measurable, Achievable, Realistic, and Time Based. Additional common special issues that must be considered include the permit-approval process, legal issues, liability issues, political issues, economic issues, and attendee issues [79]. The National Association of Emergency Medical Services Physicians (NAEMSP) 2021 Position Statement: Mass Gathering Medical Care [53] recommends the following when planning for a Mass Casualty Incident (MCI):

(1) Event planners should utilize the Incident Command System for command and control of resources responding to an MCI.

(2) The ability to quickly, and efficiently, expand the scope of response to an incident should be considered in the development of all mass gathering plans.

(3) Triage algorithm(s) and casualty collection point(s) should be identified.

(4) The plan should be practiced via tabletop exercise or live drills involving all stakeholders to ensure it meets the needs for the event and possible threats.

(5) The plan should be regularly reviewed and updated.

There are numerous advantages to working collaboratively with other teams. Planning together will hopefully instill a sense of ownership and make it more likely that the plan will be adhered to. Furthermore, cooperative efforts enhanced by good communication foster the creation of enduring relationships. The more players involved, the more resources, knowledge and expertise that can be brought to bear on the planning efforts enhancing the plan and ultimately the operation. As an example, a novel approach to assist in the planning process involves domain ontology, the study of the interrelationships of the properties of a set of concepts and categories of a particular subject area. Specifically, the domain would represent, in a standard format, knowledge of the main concepts and characteristics of mass gatherings and the relationships between concepts. The process of creating the domain requires the specification and classification of the components, such as individuals (instances of objects), determining the attributes of each and relations between each and understanding the restrictions, rules, and axioms. The goal is to create a formal unifying, shareable and reusable model of mass gatherings that can be applied to all events to support decision making. Essentially, it is

creating an emergency management decision support system by using the Intelligence-Design-Choice-Implementation decision support model. This would require collaboration with personnel skilled in computer science and information technology [14, 41].

To prepare and plan successfully, it is helpful to address the common themes and general considerations noted across the spectrum of mass gatherings Some of the factors or common themes that must be considered and that can influence patient presentations and contribute to successful planning and outcomes include: (1) Location and geography of the venue and the associated weather patterns (especially temperature and humidity), (2) type and scope of event, (3) the People (crowd demographics and population modeling), (4) security and safety challenges posed, (5) public health concerns, (6) resources required and production elements, and (7) regulatory issues and the logistics of the gathering [44, 55, 62].

The following flow charts (Figures 10.1 and 10.2), constructed from the perspective of rescue authorities addressing factors that must be considered when preparing for mass gatherings, can serve as an organized guide for the planning process [44].

Location

As the expression goes, location is everything … or is it? It is certainly a factor that must be considered when planning for a mass gathering. Celebrations and mass gatherings occur all over the world and during all seasons, and it behooves event planners to consider the environment and weather patterns that may be expected [6, 55, 56].

Environmental factors frequently contribute to the need for medical resources at large events [8, 55, 56, 62]. Inclement weather can complicate a well-designed event plan and can have a significant impact on a mass gathering event as it simultaneously affects all in attendance and can result in illness and injury. Drastic changes in the weather, especially if severe, like a tornado, can interfere with the response of medical personnel [15, 40].

When planning a mass gathering event, the factors of season, temperature, and humidity must be considered [46, 55, 70]. Heat-related illnesses are defined as an elevation of core body temperature and due to exposure to high environmental temperatures and/or strenuous physical activities and can result in fatality. The heat index (Figures 10.3 and 10.4), defined as the

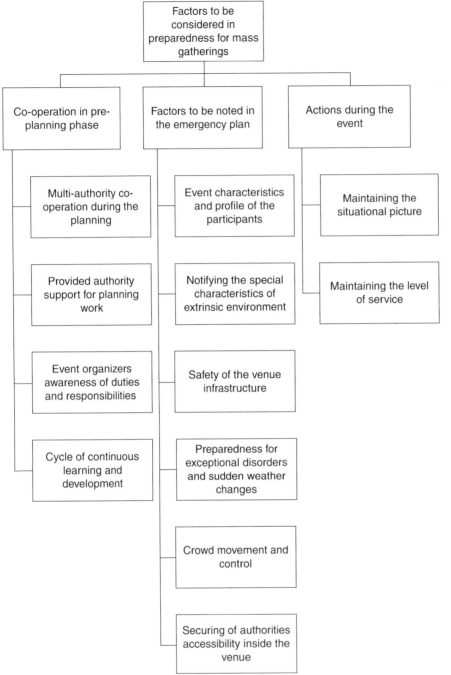

Figure 10.1 Main categories and generic categories

Koski A., Kouvonen A., Sumanen H. Preparedness for Mass Gatherings: Factors to Consider According to the Rescue Authorities. *International Journal of Environmental Research and Public Health.* 2020;17(4):1361. doi:10.3390/ijerph17041361

temperature felt by the human body when relative humidity is combined with the air temperature, can amplify the effects of heat and lead to increased illness. This effect can be enhanced by the consumption of anticholinergics, sympathomimetics, and neuroleptic agents [55, 59, 62]. One study showed a linear effect of heat index resulting in increased patient presentations, 3 per 10,000 patrons for every 10-degree increase in the heat index [58]. There is a concern that there may be more issues due to heat-related illnesses with climate change [63] toward hotter temperatures and this is a point that must be considered

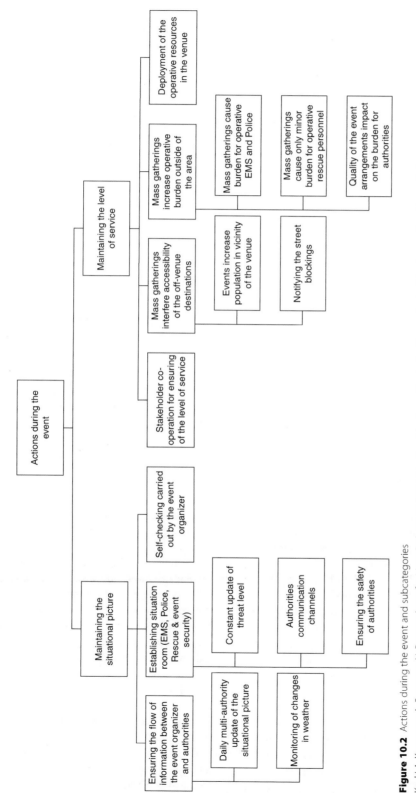

Figure 10.2 Actions during the event and subcategories

Koski A, Kouvonen A, Sumanen H. Preparedness for Mass Gatherings: Factors to Consider According to the Rescue Authorities. *International Journal of Environmental Research and Public Health.* 2020;17(4):1361. doi:10.3390/ijerph17041361

NWS Heat Index — Temperature (°F)

Relative Humidity (%)	80	82	84	86	88	90	92	94	96	98	100	102	104	106	108	110
40	80	81	83	85	88	91	94	97	101	105	109	114	119	124	130	136
45	80	82	84	87	89	93	96	100	104	109	114	119	124	130	137	
50	81	83	85	88	91	95	99	103	108	113	118	124	131	137		
55	81	84	86	89	93	97	101	106	112	117	124	130	137			
60	82	84	88	91	95	100	105	110	116	123	129	137				
65	82	85	89	93	98	103	108	114	121	128	136					
70	83	86	90	95	100	105	112	119	126	134						
75	84	88	92	97	103	109	116	124	132							
80	84	89	94	100	106	113	121	129								
85	85	90	96	102	110	117	126	135								
90	86	91	98	105	113	122	131									
95	86	93	100	108	117	127										
100	87	95	103	112	121	132										

Likelihood of Heat Disorders with Prolonged Exposure or Strenuous Activity

Caution · Extreme Caution · Danger · Extreme Danger

Figure 10.3 Heat index

(National Weather Service/ National Oceanic and Atmospheric Administration)

www.weather.gov/images/safety/heatindexchart-650.jpg

www.weather.gov/images/wrn/social_media/2017/heat_index.jpg

Classification	Heat Index	Effect on the body
Caution	80°F – 90°F	Fatigue possible with prolonged exposure and/or physical activity
Extreme Caution	90°F – 103°F	Heat stroke, heat cramps, or heat exhaustion possible with prolonged exposure and/or physical activity
Danger	103°F – 124°F	Heat cramps or heat exhaustion likely, and heat stroke possible with prolonged exposure and/or physical activity
Extreme Danger	125°F or higher	Heat stroke highly likely

Figure 10.4 National Weather Service heat index severity classification and expected effects on the body

www.weather.gov/ama/heatindex

when planning for events, especially those in hot locations, such as Saudi Arabia during the Hajj [25, 42, 63]. One way to determine the impact of heat-related illness is by using wet-bulb globe temperature (WBGT), a validated empirical index of heat stress that is based on a combination of ambient temperature, relative humidity, the heat-load impact of solar radiation, and the cooling power of wind [30, 39, 42].

Heat-related illnesses are a spectrum of symptoms and can be classified according to severity. Heat exhaustion, typically the least severe, is characterized by a core temperature between 100.4 to 104 °F (38 to 40 °C) and is associated with discomfort, thirst, nausea, and vomiting. Conversely, heat stroke, the core body temperature is greater than 104 °F (40 °C) and is associated with severe neurologic symptoms including confusion and seizures and is a medical emergency that requires prompt identification and treatment [3, 8, 11, 25]. Water and climate control are essential to minimize and treat heat-related injury. If patrons are restricted from bringing water, it should be provided to them, preferably for free, and shelters from heat and sun and cooling stations should be readily available. Absence of free water can double the patient presentation rate and lack of climate control can triple the patient presentation rate [49, 62]. In an attempt to quench their thirst, some patrons may consume alcohol to excess, which can lead to exacerbation of dehydration and increase rates of alcohol-related injury and illness [62]. In addition, crowd density, especially during summer months at outdoor venues, should be a factor that is considered when planning a mass gathering event. A high crowd density can contribute to heat-related illness, as the higher the density of the crowd, especially toward the front of the venue, the harder it is to access shade and water, especially if water bottles are restricted as they tend to be used as projectiles [55]. Many factors need to be considered by event organizers when planning, as a poor plan can inadvertently contribute to weather-related illness. During a rock concert in Denver, there was an increase in heat-related illness after a protective black tarp was placed on a field, increasing the temperature from 90 to 120 °F (32 to 48 °C) [55, 62]. Indoor events with inadequate air conditioning and ventilation may be equally affected by high temperature and heat index resulting in increased rates of heat-related illness [70].

Heat-related deaths have been reported in marathon runners despite cool conditions just as hypothermia can occur in the desert if clothing is saturated and temperatures drop or there is a breeze or wind. Overall, cold weather usually leads to lower injury rates than hot weather, and does have different injury patterns, particularly frostbite and hypothermia [55, 62].

Heat is not the only factor that contributes to injury or illness at mass gathering events. There have been mass-casualty incidents related to other adverse weather conditions. Precipitation in the form of rain can be problematic when it is unexpected or begins midway through an event. Not only does it saturate clothing, but the associated drop in temperature during a rainstorm can result in hypothermia. At the 1994 Woodstock festival, there was an increased number of orthopedic injuries from slipping and falling, and multiple "wet, exposed citizens" that required rewarming tents after the temperature dropped 30 °F [19, 55]. Inclement weather can strike suddenly and often with little to no warning. On July 15, 2012, a lightning strike at an outdoor Toronto food festival injured seventeen people. The storm that resulted in the lighting strike developed rapidly over the event site [89]. On March 12, 1988, in Kathmandu, Nepal, a sudden severe hailstorm during a soccer game triggered a human stampede resulting in the death of ninety-three people as thousands of soccer fans surged into locked stadium exits [90]. Despite the current capabilities of weather prediction, conditions on a particular day are variable and may change necessitating anticipation of the unexpected by considering the range of expected weather conditions in a particular region during a particular season [70]. The planning process needs to include a response to inclement weather, especially thunderstorms, which can produce lighting, hail, and tornadoes. The most recent data from the National Weather Service regarding tornado lead time shows that smaller tornadoes, F0–F1 classification, have a lead time of eight minutes whereas larger tornadoes, F2 to F5,

have a lead time of approximately fourteen minutes [88]. The 30–30 Rule for Lightning Safety is a method that has been used to determine when it is safe to return to the open [34, 65]. However, it is not reliable because of the inherent difficulty of associating the proper thunder to the corresponding flash. It is recommended to establish a lighting action plan that includes trained spotters and detection equipment and that they be intimately familiar with the Lightning Action Plan, including the "warning" signal and when to activate it, the evacuation plan, designated safe areas, and use of the "all clear" signal. Monitoring for the threat of lighting may need to begin days ahead of the event and should be addressed in the event planning [77]. When developing the event plan, the data and experiences from previous years should be utilized, including response delays in austere environments and during severe meteorological conditions [44].

Event Characteristics

When trying to determine if an event should be considered a "special event," addressing the following questions may help:

(1) Is the event out of the ordinary or nonroutine?
(2) Does the event place a strain on community resources?
(3) Does the event attract many people? How many?
(4) Does the event require special permitting or additional planning, preparation, and mitigation efforts by local agencies?

There are a variety of mass gathering events that occur annually and it is crucial to understand the details that need to be included in the event planning. An event can be as simple as a small local celebration or festival and as large and complex as the Hajj, the Muslim Pilgrimage to Mecca, Saudi Arabia [2, 61, 54] or the Kumbh Mela, the Hindu religious pilgrimage festival, considered to be the largest mass gathering event in the world with an attendance of approximately 120 million pilgrims from all over the world for up to two months [1]. Each event poses its own inherent challenges and has its own characteristics that must be addressed. Even events with a low number of attendees may overwhelm the local resources. However, the concepts of planning and preparation should be uniform across the spectrum to minimize any variations in the process.

Determining the type of event to be held is crucial for the planning process to begin. Patient presentation rate (PPR), average patient presentation rate per 1000, and the Medical Usage Rate (MUR), the number of patients treated per 10,000 attendees, can vary depending on the type of gathering. Classical music concerts stereotypically attract a different patron as compared to an electronic dance music concert, where the use of illicit substances is expected [22, 23, 51] or a rock concert where mosh pits and crowd surfing are common occurrences [27, 47, 56, 62]. Sporting event attendance, especially at the collegiate level, can have in the tens of thousands of spectators both within the confines of the stadium and outside in the parking lot as tailgaters. The fans are usually hyped up for the event and there is often alcohol consumption [5, 6, 33, 46, 49, 55, 56].

The type of event may also influence the number of traumatic injuries treated. When compared, concerts had a higher MUR compared to baseball and football games, and American football games had a MUR than baseball games, at which getting hit by a foul ball was a main source of injury while physical altercations were most common at football games [26, 56]. Rock concerts are fraught with unique injury patterns occurring secondary to moshing, crowd surfing, and missiles thrown from the crowd, often water bottles [56, 62].

To assist with the planning process, mass gathering events can be divided into four classes or types that can help determine needs for the provision of medical care (Table 10.1).

Table 10.1 Categories of mass gathering events
Auerbach P. S., Cushing T. A., and Harris N. S. *Auerbach's Wilderness Medicine E-Book*. Oxford: Elsevier Health Sciences; 2016.

CLASS	CHARACTERISTICS
I	Spectators are seated for a set period of time or for the duration of the event (e.g., Stadium sporting events and concerts)
II	Spectators are mobile and may become participants in the events (e.g., Golf tournament, festival celebrations, EDM concerts)
III	Large geographic area and participants often outnumber spectators (e.g., Charity walks, bicycle rides, marathons, and triathlons)
IV	Highly variable/ extreme outdoor events that pose unique challenges in providing medical support (e.g., Adventure races, endurance events)

Bounded events are those with defined boundaries and access points into the venue, for example a stadium or fenced in area. Conversely, unbounded events are those that are open that allow for easy mobility of the attendee to move freely in and out of the event area. These may be referred to as "extended events," not restricted to a single location, like a marathon or bike race such the "Tour De France." If people are bounded inside the event as opposed to being at an open venue, there may be a higher likelihood of medical care provided on scene due to the organized nature of the event with a predetermined medical treatment area and ease of access to medical care [5]. One study found that unbounded events have a PPR almost three times greater than bounded events [49].

In unbounded events, people may be more likely to seek care in a hospital rather than on scene at the event [17]. An additional challenge of unbounded events is the inability to determine the number of attendees, which can substantially impact the preparation and response to an emergency [46]. Whether attendees are seated or mobile influences crowd control efforts and presentation for medical care, with higher risk of injury for those who are mobile [23, 49]. One study compared the 1984 Summer Olympics, a largely seated event, with a rave, a scout camp, a rock festival, and a marathon, traditionally mobile events. The PPRs were significantly higher at the mobile events: the PPR was 1.6 per 1000 spectators at the Olympics, 9 at the rave, 10 at the scout camp, 17 at the rock festival, and 28 at the marathon [33, 62]. Therefore, if planning an event, it is highly suggested to have boundaries and if possible, arranged seating.

Event duration does not seem to contribute to an increased MUR. However, it may contribute extended environment exposure, exhaustion, and spread of disease, especially those with prolonged incubation periods. Furthermore, some patrons may decide to come early, camp out and depart late, thus impacting the local resources even after the event has terminated [55, 62].

The People (Crowd Demographics)

As previously alluded to, certain events might appeal to a particular demographic. Rock concerts and electronic dance music festivals often attract a younger crowd, whereas, classical music concerts or religious gatherings, attract an older demographic. Inherent to each demographic are characteristics that may have an impact on event planning. For instance, research has shown that there are more likely to be traumatic injuries from uninhibited behaviors like crowd surfing or joining in a mosh pit at a rock concert and American football games, especially if alcohol or drugs are consumed [20, 26, 47, 55], whereas medical problems may be more prominent at a religious gathering given the predominance of an older demographic, for example, elderly and those with chronic illness were more likely to be affected by heat-related illnesses at the Hajj, in Saudi Arabia [3]. Crowd size, however, does not appear to play a significant role in patient frequency, at least for basketball and football games, and there is a weak correlation during rock concerts [16]. Taking these factors into account facilitate the planning process.

Event planners continue to have challenges regarding mass gatherings. One theory why this continues to occur, is due to a lack of definitions of mass gatherings that have sufficient depth to support researchers and clinicians in their efforts to further define, describe, and explain the effects of mass gathering health. Subsequently, a basic population model of mass gatherings was proposed to help facilitate research and event planning. The main variables included in the model are: (1) the number of people in the host community (NHC); (2) the number of people attending the event (NEv); and (3) the number of patients who present to medical care (NPP) [50]. In their model, these variables or groups are nested, meaning that taken together, they comprise the total population of the community during the event, and each exists in relation to the others [50]. They each represent the people and it is the interplay between them that must be better understood to enhance the planning and preparation process.

The host community is usually the geographic or municipal jurisdiction in which the event is held and NHC represents the size of the host community or communities, as in a multi-jurisdictional event, like a marathon. To evaluate the potential risk to the community and the resources that will be needed, it is imperative to define the size of the host community and to determine specific details about the community. For example, what resources will be needed if an event will temporarily quadruple the number of people in a given community [50].

Determination of the PPR and ability to classify the size of and potential risks of a mass gathering event is dependent on defining the event population (NEv). In its simplest terms, the event population consists of the attendees. However, depending on the type of event, the event population may expand to include not only the spectators, but the participants, and those working at the event. It may be difficult to obtain consistent numbers for Nev, as depending on the event type, people are in flux and there may be variables such as spectators who are provided complimentary access and do not get reported on attendance rosters [50].

Populations are dynamic over time, as people come and go prior to, during, and after the event. When planning for a mass gathering, it is vital that planners focus on these variables with attention paid to the nesting of the populations, the interface between the populations, and the shifting nature of those interfaces. To better understand risk as it relates to an event, it is imperative to analyze population movement and the contact between population groups for each phase of the event, for example, an analysis of the interaction of attendees at the Olympic games, which attracts an international crowd to a specific community, prior to, during, and post-event [50, 76].

When people gather in crowds, they may become influenced by the people around them. Most people are just observers, the spectators of the event. However, during crowd influenced activity, some of them may become cheerleaders and stir on the activity, while others become the active core, the actual participants in the activity [79, 85]. Crowds can be classified according to type, for example, they can be ambulatory, just walking around; expressive, and just enjoying the event; or can be dense and turn aggressive and violent [10, 38]. Crowd mood can be assessed and can be classified as passive, active, or energetic. The mood of the crowd, which can be altered by their interactions with event staff, can contribute to medical workload [38, 73, 74]. The main issue of concern for planners is to try and prevent undesirable behavior. In the literature, two common factors have been attributed to undesirable crowd behavior. First, there must be a "seed," an individual or small group who incites and attracts the people in the group. Second, is engagement with the seed, resulting in the abnormal crowd behavior. For people to engage in the activity, they must modify their existing norms and have a shared sense of identity. Aberrant crowd behavior is the result of two groups, an in- and out-group, who differ in their norms or what is seen as "right." An example of this is rival sports team supporters who exchange verbal insults which may deteriorate into physical violence [74]. The preparation and planning should include a risk assessment to focus on identifying at-risk crowds, like those consuming excessive alcohol or displaying aggressive behavior [73], and monitoring for seed behavior, in order to mitigate crowd engagement, according to clearly established guidelines, with the purpose of preventing a problematic scenario from developing. To accomplish this task, there must be education for security personnel to learn how to assess and monitor crowds, development of tools and techniques to identify and manage seed behavior, and mechanisms put in place to limit crowd engagement [74].

When planning for an event, it is helpful to understand the psychological dimension of crowds. In 1895, Le Bon proposed that when people are "submerged" in a crowd, they tend to lose their sense of individual identity and rationality. Therefore, they become followers and there is a tendency for crowd behavior to become more uncontrolled [36]. This behavior change is observed during riots with looting, mosh pits, and during crushing incidents, like that occurred at the Hajj in 2015 [93], and more recently in Houston, Texas, at the 2019 and 2021 Astroworld concerts [13, 80, 81].

Current theory, however, suggests that people in a group do not lose personal identity, but rather transition to a social identity; what makes the group distinct compared to other groups, for example pilgrims at the Hajj or fans rooting for the same team at a sporting event. There are two shifts that may occur when in a group setting. The first is the normative shift, where people start to adopt group-based beliefs and values and do whatever is good for the group. The second is a relational shift, people define themselves in terms of a social identity and believe that others in the group share this identity as well, resulting in a more cohesive group [36]. These shifts can result in intense positive emotion [35], and group members may become more cooperative, respectful, trusting, and supportive of each other [48, 71].

Group norms may impact health practices and well-being and result in a person presenting for medical care. The group may affect the value placed on personal health and result in a person not taking their daily medication, believing instead that a higher power will provide them with health. At the Kumbh Mela, in India, pilgrims strive to transcend the materialistic world where the body is merely a vessel and is deemed insignificant [36, 52, 67]. Determining what is an appropriate action may also be swayed by the group dynamics. At the Magh Mela, pilgrims bathe in and sip water from the sacred, but heavily polluted Ganges River. This of course has resulted in numerous cases of diarrheal illness which in turn can lead to dehydration [78]. In other instances, people will persevere and endure despite their inability to do so. This behavior is reinforced by the collective need to complete the task as a group. A true sports fan may attend every game regardless of the weather, participants in endurance races will push to finish, and pilgrims at the Hajj will endure to completion, all despite the potential personal harm that may be incurred. Conversely, group membership may prove to be a positive experience as it may also contribute to improved mental well-being and reduce stress due to the social support from the shared group identity [24, 29].

To be able to communicate effectively with a group of people so that they will listen to important messages concerning their health and well-being, planners must have a knowledge of group culture, group psychology, and the social identity process. In addition to the standard multidisciplinary team of planners, inclusion of social anthropologists, historians, and other cultural experts will be beneficial to ensure a detailed and thorough plan has been developed [36, 37].

When preparing for a mass gathering, it is crucial that planners appreciate the population that they will be caring for. It is important to have clear and concise definitions and descriptions of the host community, the event, and the populations of people present, so that there is a better understanding of the medical needs and impact on the populations of interest, to facilitate improved operational planning, health promotion, and injury and illness prevention [50].

Security and Safety Issues

To ensure that those attending mass gatherings will be safe, it is best to prevent incidents from occurring. A key element of the planning process must address security and safety issues. During the planning phase, intelligence gathering should be conducted to perform a thorough threat assessment and a hazard analysis of the event. A threat assessment should address plans for anti-terrorism, the actions to mitigate effects of an attack, and counterterrorism, actions taken to prevent an attack. The ultimate authority responsible for canceling an event must be determined in the planning stages to minimize any arguments. The response to any incident must be planned and vulnerabilities assessed and addressed prior to the start of the event. If the event is bounded, that is a physical barrier is to be erected around the event, adequate quantity and the appropriate materials must be available and erected according to guidelines and code. The stage and associated structures must be solid and well-constructed and adhere to the local building codes. There must also be a plan in place to prevent and to respond to a fire, especially when pyrotechnics are going to be used. Most importantly, there must be a cooperative relationship between the planning team, first responders, law enforcement, event security personnel, some of whom may be off duty police officers, and personal security agents, should they be required. FEMA ICS form 208-SAFETY MESSAGE/PLAN can be used to guide safety planning [53, 79, 85].

The United Nations International Strategy for Disaster Reduction (UNISDR) defines a hazard as "a dangerous phenomenon, substance, human activity or condition that may cause loss of life, injury or other health impacts, property damage, loss of livelihoods and services, social and economic disruption, or environmental damage." A list of typical risk and hazards follows in Table 10.2 [79]. If the hazardous event exceeds the capabilities and abilities of the allocated resources it is defined as a disaster. Thorough analysis of a proposed event begins with potential hazard identification and is followed by a hazard analysis, an assessment performed to determine the frequency distribution, or likelihood of occurrence, for each type of hazard identified. The frequency distribution can be assessed in terms of cycles, hours, or years. Using historical and analytical data, as in the Zeitz method [72], a severity rating is assigned to each hazard identified which quantifies the damage expected from a specific hazard [20]. The hazards can be ranked in a table which can be used to guide resource utilization, see Tables 10.3 to 10.7 [79].

The Global Center for Mass Gathering Medicine (GCMGM), established in 2010 in Saud Arabia, plays a key role in ensuring the proper application of the standards of conducting mass gathering events through collaboration with other mass gathering organizations and WHO-affiliated groups, coordinating policies and procedures, and bringing awareness

Table 10.2 Listing of typical risk and hazards Federal Emergency Management Agency (FEMA). Special Events Contingency Planning Job Aids Manual. March 2005 (Updated May 2010) P. 2

Abandoned vehicles	Hurricane
Airplane crash	Intentional chemical release
Airspace encroachment	Kidnapping
Assault	Landslide
Avalanche	Loss of utilities (water, sewer, telephone)
Biological incidents	Lost child
Bomb threat/suspicious package	Lost and found
Building inspection	Media relations
Cancellation of event	Motorcades
Civil disturbance with demonstrations	Mudslides
Communications	Parking
Credentials	Permitting
Crowd control	Power failure (sustained)
Cyber attacks	Radiological release
Dam failure	Security
Demonstrations	Structural collapse
Dignitary protection	Subsidence
Drought	Terrorism
Earthquake	Ticketing
Epidemic or other public health concern	Tornado
Evacuation of area	Traffic control
Explosive materials	Train derailment
Fire	Tsunami
First aid matters	Urban conflagration
Flood	Volcanic eruption
Food handling violations	Wildfire
Food waste disposal problems	Winter storm
Hazardous Materials release	
Hostage without terrorism	
Human waste disposal problems	

to the management of mass gathering events. The "SALEM tool" (Table 10.8), a seventeen-factor mass-gathering risk assessment tool, was introduced by the GCMGM with the purpose of evaluating health risk at mass gathering events. The SALEM tool was developed using international special event guidelines related to health, medical, and safety planning. Mass

Table 10.3 Hazard assessment
https://emilms.fema.gov/is0015b/curriculum/1 .html. Lesson 3:
Risks and Hazards to Consider

Frequency of occurrence	• How often does this hazard occur?
Magnitude and potential intensity	• How bad could this hazard get?
Location	• Are some areas of the jurisdiction more likely to be affected by this hazard than others?
Probable spatial extent	• How much of the jurisdiction is likely to be affected?
Probable duration	• How long is the hazard likely to pose a threat?
Seasonal pattern	• Is the hazard more likely to occur during certain months of the year?
Speed of onset and availability of warning	• How fast would an incident involving this hazard threaten lives and property? • If the hazard does not threaten lives and property, what degree of disruption could it cause? • Is there a way to warn against this hazard?

Table 10.4 Hazard Vulnerability Assessment Frequency Distributions Federal Emergency Management Agency (FEMA). Special Events Contingency Planning Job Aids Manual. March 2005 (Updated May 2010) P. A-55

Exposure	Frequency
Highly likely = 3	The potential for Impact is very probable (near 100 percent) in the next year.
Likely = 2	The potential for impact is between 10 and 100 percent within the next year, or There is at least one chance of occurrence within the next 10 years.
Possible = 1	The potential for impact is between 1 and 10 percent within the next year. or There is at least one chance of occurrence within the next 100 years.
Unlikely = 0	The potential for impact is less than 1 percent in the next 100 years.

gathering events are graded based on a cumulative score of all seventeen factors to determine whether the event is a low, medium, or high-risk (Table 10.9). Based on the risk stratification, event planners can develop a plan with the goal of decreasing morbidity and mortality [43].

To determine the type and extent of security services required, the event planning should attempt to answer the following questions [79]:

(1) Which type of security will be appropriate for the event?

(2) Who will be the appropriate security firm to be contracted?

(3) Is special security being provided? YES / NO

(4) If YES, who is providing it?

(5) If NO, is it considered necessary? YES / NO

(6) Is the provider licensed to provide the service? YES / NO

(7) Event security START and END dates?

(8) What will be the role of security?

(9) Have relevant police departments been contacted in relation to security? YES / NO

(10) If yes, what will be required of the police?

(11) When will a briefing/debriefing be held involving police, security, bar staff and licensing personnel? (Date before Event) (Date after Event)

(12) Will a briefing of all personnel and officials be provided regarding helping patrons with amenities and services?

(13) Who will pay for event security costs, including overtime?

It is also important when planning to address the event access and egress for patrons and emergency services. The following questions will assist in plan development [79].

(1) What provisions can be made for patrons to access, move around, and leave the event venue without excessive queuing, or crushes (for example, gate control, pathways, free space)?

(2) Will patrons be able to access toilets, food and bar areas, and entertainment sites without difficulty? YES / NO

(3) In an emergency, will patrons be able to leave the venue or move to other areas within the venue in reasonable safety? YES / NO

(4) Are road access and egress suitable? YES / NO

(5) Are road access and egress suitable in all weather? YES / NO

(6) Are road access and egress adequate? YES / NO

(7) Will special traffic control be required? YES / NO

Table 10.5 Hazard vulnerability assessment severity ratings
Federal Emergency Management Agency (FEMA). Special Events Contingency Planning Job Aids Manual. March 2005 (Updated May 2010) P. A-56

Population/Property Level of Severity	Definition
Catastrophic = 3	Multiple deaths. Complete shutdown of critical facilities for 30 days or more. More than 50 percent of property is severely damaged.
Critical = 2	Injuries and/or illnesses result in permanent disability. Complete shutdown of critical facilities for at least 2 weeks. More than 25 percent of property is severely damaged.
Limited = 1	Injuries and/or illnesses do not result in permanent disability. Complete shutdown of critical facilities for more than 1 week. More than 10 percent of property is severely damaged.
Negligible = 0	Injuries and/or illnesses are treatable with first aid. Minor quality of life lost. Shutdown of critical facilities and services for 24 hours or less. No more than 1 percent of property is severely damaged.

Table 10.6 Hazard rating worksheet
Using the severity and frequency distribution definitions, the planning team should identify potential hazards for the event and rank them in the Rating Worksheet. Federal Emergency Management Agency (FEMA). Special Events Contingency Planning Job Aids Manual. March 2005 (Updated May 2010) P. A-57

Hazard	Frequency (Likelihood)	Potential Impact on Population	Potential Impact on Property	Level of Coverage in EOP	Point Total
	0 = Unlikely 1 = Possible 2 = Likely 3 = Highly Likely	0 = Negligible 1 = Limited 2 = Critical 3 = Catastrophic	0 = Negligible 1 = Limited 2 = Critical 3 = Catastrophic	0 = None 1 = Limited 2 = Sufficient 3 = Comprehensive (annex)	
	0 1 2 3	0 1 2 3	0 1 2 3	0 1 2 3	
	0 1 2 3	0 1 2 3	0 1 2 3	0 1 2 3	
	0 1 2 3	0 1 2 3	0 1 2 3	0 1 2 3	
	0 1 2 3	0 1 2 3	0 1 2 3	0 1 2 3	
	0 1 2 3	0 1 2 3	0 1 2 3	0 1 2 3	
	0 1 2 3	0 1 2 3	0 1 2 3	0 1 2 3	
	0 1 2 3	0 1 2 3	0 1 2 3	0 1 2 3	
	0 1 2 3	0 1 2 3	0 1 2 3	0 1 2 3	
	0 1 2 3	0 1 2 3	0 1 2 3	0 1 2 3	
	0 1 2 3	0 1 2 3	0 1 2 3	0 1 2 3	
	0 1 2 3	0 1 2 3	0 1 2 3	0 1 2 3	
	0 1 2 3	0 1 2 3	0 1 2 3	0 1 2 3	

(8) Is sufficient suitable off-road parking available? YES / NO

(9) Will emergency services have continual access and egress? YES / NO

(10) In the event of a major emergency, do access and egress allow for emergency services? YES / NO

(11) Have emergency management plans been prepared? YES / NO

Table 10.7 Hazard worksheet

Using the information from the Rating Worksheet, the planning team should complete the Profile Worksheet to assess each hazard. Federal Emergency Management Agency (FEMA). Special Events Contingency Planning Job Aids Manual. March 2005 (Updated May 2010) P. A-58

Hazard Profile Worksheet

Hazard —————————————————————————————————

Potential Magnitude

- Catastrophic: Can affect more than 50 percent of the jurisdiction.
- Critical: Can affect between 25 and 50 percent of the jurisdiction.
- Limited: Can affect between 10 and 25 percent of the jurisdiction.
- Negligible: Can affect less than 10 percent of the jurisdiction.

Areas Likely to be Most Affected (by sector) —————————————————————

Probable Duration —————————————————————————————

Potential Speed of Onset

- More than 24 hours' warning probably will be available.
- Between 12 and 24 hours' warning probably will be available.
- Between 6 and 12 hours' warning will be available.
- Minimal (or no) warning will be available.

Existing Warning Systems ————————————————————————————

Complete Vulnerability Analysis with local/State emergency management agencies?*   YES/NO

* Note that some hazards may pose such a limited threat to the jurisdiction that additional analysis is not necessary.

Table 10.8 Factors for risk scoring in the Saudi SALEM tool

Khan A. A., Sabbagh A. Y., Ranse J., Molloy M. S., Ciottone G. R. Mass Gathering Medicine in Soccer Leagues: A Review and Creation of the SALEM Tool. *International Journal of Environmental Research and Public Health.* 2021;18(19):9973–9989

1	The category of the event (music festivals, exhibitions, sports competitions, etc.)
2	The expected number of attendees
3	The criteria of attendees (families, sports club fans, community support groups, international stars, or VIP)
4	The nature of attendees' movements (static audience, young children who need constant monitoring, people with motor disabilities, people who require personal assistance)
5	The age group of attendees
6	The site of the event (open area, specific walled area, inside a building, spacious or narrow area)
7	Available health resources (district hospitals, public hospitals, small hospitals, mobile clinic)
8	The distance to the nearest public or reference hospital
9	Time for the nearest general or reference hospital
10	Duration of the event per day
11	The number of days for the event
12	possibility of drugs misuse
13	The time of the event
14	The expected temperature at the venue of the event
15	Types of Activities in the event (high-risk activities, high competition among participants (ex: wresting), the interaction between the attendees (for example the final matches), presence of cars or vehicles, including offers or race, presence of fireworks, presence of firearms of flames)
16	Accidents that occurred in previous activities or the same place or expected accidents
15	Food catering services (applying and controlling the specified standards for food catering services, municipality approval is obtained, and valid food catering services are provided)

Table 10.9 Risk classification and preparedness of Saudi SALEM tool
Khan A. A., Sabbagh A. Y., Ranse J., Molloy M. S., Ciottone G. R. Mass Gathering Medicine in Soccer Leagues: A Review and Creation of the SALEM Tool. *International Journal of Environmental Research and Public Health*. 2021;18(19):9973. P. 10.

Low-risk events	Events categorized as low severity recommend risk communication (at the population level), improved monitoring and surveillance, and medical care for the event
Medium-risk events	Medium severity events recommend risk communication (dedicated to the event), active surveillance, medical care for the event, and protective measures for the event (personal protective equipment, handwashing)
High-risk events	High-risk events recommend reducing the number of guests/visitors, adjustment of the crowd flow and seating arrangements, and reducing communication between participants, regulators, and service providers
Severe-risk events	Events with risk recommend restructuring the event, changing or moving the event site, postponing or rescheduling the event, or canceling the event

(12) Have contingency plans been prepared? YES / NO

    a. If NO, are they necessary? YES / NO

    b. If they are necessary, who will coordinate the preparation?

The following examples will highlight the importance of detailed planning and preparation for security and safety-related issues. On November 5, 2021, ten people were killed at the Astroworld 2021 Festival held at NRG Park in Houston, Texas because of a crowd crushing incident causing accidental compressive asphyxiation. Eight people died on the night of the concert, and two more died in the hospital over the following days. One of the deaths was also associated with the toxic combination of drugs and alcohol [13]. Overall, 25 people were hospitalized, and more than 300 people were treated for injuries at the festival's field hospital. Approximately 50,000 people attended the event which seemed fraught with challenges from the beginning as was suggested by the preliminary reviews and interviews with medical providers. The event was staffed by ParaDocs, a contract medical team of approximately seventy providers. According to the ParaDocs CEO, at one point, "the medical team had to attend to 11 simultaneous cardiac arrests," quickly overwhelming the team and resources [92]. Radio communication with the Houston Fire Department (HFD) was not possible as the medical team received radios from the event planners and could only contact HFD via cell phone [92, 98]. Guidance on proper communication coordination is available from FEMA Incident Command System (ICS) form 205-Incident Radio Communications Plan [53].

A novel and simplified concept, protect the "3Ps: Pocketbook, Patrons, and the Performers" [13], was recently presented and can assist event planning teams in their efforts to assure that an incident like that which occurred at Astroworld 2021 does not happen again. This concept is particularly useful when planning promoted mass gathering events [13]. As an example, if the event is going to be bounded with physical barriers, then the material used should be properly selected, well-constructed, and there should be an adequate amount to secure the venue. At Astroworld 2021, numerous gate breaches, including approximately 300 at one VIP entrance and approximately 4,000 unscanned patrons at another entrance, tallied more than $1 million of lost revenue to the event promoters. This also posed a significant security risk as those unscanned patrons entered without adequate screening. At the 2014 Miami Ultra Music Festival (UMF), a large electronic dance music gathering that attracts more than 100,000 people, a security guard was trampled and critically injured by fence crashers without tickets and later sued the organizers of UMF for $10 million [13, 80, 81]. Prior to the start of the event, the organizers were advised by the Miami Police Department that there was inadequate fencing, but no changes were made [79, 80]. Inadequate perimeter security can also lead to trespasser injury. Shortly after a gate breach of the secondary checkpoint the morning of Astroworld 2021, approximately thirty minutes prior to gates opening, HFD records show that four individuals needed medical attention. Additional injuries occurred later that day at the same location because of a large group attempting to go over a fence. Fortunately, more people were not seriously injured in the numerous security breaches [13, 79, 80].

Protecting the patrons is ultimately the main goal of planning. Assuring the presence of adequate and well-trained security should deter any mischievous behavior and ensure that everyone who enters the venue is screened, vetted, and accounted for. This allows for an orderly, safe, and equitable process for all patrons. However, it must be stressed that those acting in the role of security are well trained and knowledgeable professionals. In 2014, an Ultra Music Festival patron was beaten by event security, who happened to be off duty Miami police officers, and as a result, he was awarded $400,000 in damages paid by the insurance company for UMF [94]. With the stress of the situation at Astroworld 2021, security guards were seen shoving some gatecrashers. If the trespassers had been injured by security, there could have been additional revenue lost due to lawsuits. Security must often also protect the patrons from themselves particularly during crowd surfing attempts and mosh pits [13]. Physical barriers, for example, a T-shaped barricade at the front of the crowd, can be used to separate the audience and prevent lateral movement [13, 79]. The ideal physical barrier must be designed to sustain a certain amount of flex to prevent the crushing of spectators and it must be sufficiently solid so that it will not collapse and cause injuries. Unfortunately, fences installed as stage barriers fail to meet this requirement [79]. It is also suggested to have someone trained in crowd dynamics to assess the crowd and prevent unwanted activities from occurring [79]. Thus, to protect the pocketbook and ultimately and more importantly the patrons, there must be an investment in adequate security and safety measures.

Security measures must be balanced, otherwise if too extreme or lacking, they can negatively affect the safety of the patrons [13]. In February 2003, at the Station nightclub in West Warwick, Rhode Island, 100 people died and more than 200 were injured when fire caused by non-approved stage pyrotechnics engulfed the club [95]. The fire was able to spread rapidly through non-fire-retardant foam used as sound proofing and patrons were trapped because of inadequately marked fire exits, one that was hidden by a foam-covered door that also became engulfed in flames, blocking egress. In 2004, 194 people died and over 1,000 injured when a fire erupted at the República Cromañón (Cromagnon Republic) nightclub in Argentina after flares were set off by the audience at the request of the band performing. The club reportedly had the appropriate permits, however, more than 4,000 people packed into a space intended for just 1,500. In addition to the lack of fire extinguishers, working emergency exits, and non-flammable walls, the club doors were locked to prevent trespassers from accessing the club [13, 99, 100]. Again in

January 2013 at the Kiss nightclub, Santa Maria (Rio Grande do Sul), Brazil, a fire started by pyrotechnics engulfed the club and killed 242 people and injured 168 [102]. Poor planning and lack of preparedness ultimately contributed to these tragedies.

Fire safety has become an integral part of emergency planning and lessons can be learned from previous tragedies. It seems that these incidents have similar attributes that emergency planners need to consider when planning for a mass gathering:

1) Several emergency exits should be made available at any planned event. 2) Emergency exits should be free from obstruction, not blocked and functioning properly, with appropriate signage. 3) Adherence to fire safety protocols is key including prevention of overcrowding of venues, 4) Event employees should be allotted specific duties to be performed in the event of the fire, with regular fire drills held on the premises, and 5) Full site fire evacuation plans are essential. These could include signage to evacuation points. [66]

Threats to safety not only come from patrons but also from unfamiliar surroundings and can include stage hazards like gaps or holes or unstable structures like scaffolding and stage supports. In 2017, during the Atmosphere dance music festival in Esteio, Brazil, a DJ performing was killed by scaffolding that collapsed under the force of strong winds from a developing storm [13, 97]. On August 14, 2011, during a fair in Indiana, a severe rain and hail storm with 70mph winds, resulted in the death of five patrons and injured forty-five more, after a stage collapsed only minutes after a safety announcement was given [65, 91, 96]. A review of the incident revealed that there was a failure to share National Weather Service predictions about the approaching storm, reluctance of the band to delay its performance, and a stage structure that was too weak to resist the wind force [65, 91, 96]. These examples highlight the importance of considering factors outside the control of the safety team, like the weather, during the planning process and utilizing the risk intelligence to perform risk assessments based on events and weather patterns from previous years [13, 79].

Security charged with protecting the performer or dignitary are under a great deal of scrutiny by the public. Most of their workload occurs prior to the start of the event as they work collaboratively with the event planning team to develop the safety and security plan. During a dignitary visit, such as the

Pope [21, 32, 55, 58, 64] or a Head of State, the agencies tasked with security will take lead and guide all responses [12].

If the President of the United States is visiting, it is commonplace for the United States Secret Service to perform security sweeps of a venue prior to the event and this is a habit that both personal and event security should adopt. This practice allows them to assess, take control of, and become familiar with the areas traveled by the performer or dignitary. Additionally, when planning dignitary events, it is vital to remember that the primary duty of the protective team, including the dedicated medical unit, is the safety and survival of the dignitary. The event plan must therefore address what the response will be to medical needs that arise. For example, if a motorcade police officer gets injured or a spectator falls ill. The lead agency has total command and control over the event and will determine what they deem to be the most appropriate course of action at the time. It is recommended that a "shadow" unit be assigned to step in to cover the primary unit should it be incapacitated, such as during a terrorist attack, or occupied if directed to provide care to the injured or ill [12].

In May 2017, a terrorist attack during a music concert at the Manchester Arena in England, resulted in the death of twenty-two people. Despite the tragedy, some good did come from it. In the Manchester Arena Inquiry Volume 1: Security for the Arena [13, 101], it was concluded that it would be beneficial if employees with a "Protect Duty" were "trained in first aid relevant to injuries of the type caused during the Attack on 22nd May 2017" [13, 101]. Furthermore, "Protect Duty-holders are required to ensure that employees are trained in first aid relevant to injuries which are particularly likely to occur during a terrorist attack." As a result, in October 2021, the Security Industry Authority (SIA), the regulatory body for the United Kingdom's private security industry, added first aid training to its licensing requirements for some security guards [13, 101].

Based on the conclusions of the Manchester Arena Inquiry and after review of numerous mass shooting events and life-threatening incidents at mass gatherings, it makes sense that security officers or those tasked with "Protect-Duty" be trained at the very least in basic First Aid and Cardiopulmonary Resuscitation (CPR) or basic life support (BLS). Additional focused training in hemorrhage control would also be beneficial. After the 2012 mass shooting at Sandy Hook Elementary School in Newtown, Connecticut where twenty children and eight adults were killed, the American College of Surgeons Committee on Trauma developed the "Stop the Bleed" program to teach civilians and nonmedical people how to control bleeding using tourniquets, pressure dressings, and wound packing [82]. This program is an extension of the military Tactical Combat Casualty Care program that trains soldiers in multiple basic life-saving skills with strong emphasis on tourniquet application and hemorrhage control.

Conversely, medical personnel staffing the event should at the minimum be certified as emergency medical technician (EMT-Basic) with preference for advanced life support paramedic level of training [27]. The quality of the medical provider is important, and it is recommended to choose highly skilled and trained providers over a larger number of non-skilled volunteers. On-site medical care should always be provided by health professionals [44].

Public Health

Public health is a significant concern when large groups of people come together. This has been even more evident since the COVID-19 pandemic began in March of 2020 when government regulations in multiple countries restricted large gathers due to the risk of spreading the disease [103]. Depending on the event, different aspects of public health need to be considered as part of the event medical plan. The characteristics of each specific event will dictate which of these presents a more pressing need for the event's success, however there are common themes that must be considered in all mass gatherings as outlined in Table 10.10.

Most communicable diseases spread at increased rates when in close contact with an infected vector. This is especially true of respiratory infections. The development of the COVID-19 pandemic has placed

Table 10.10 Key public health concerns

Key Public Health Concerns
Communicable disease transmission
Sanitation concerns
Environmental concerns and exposures
Presence of intoxicants (alcohol and other substances)
Potable water

this issue in the forefront of many events and event planners. While these concerns existed prior to this pandemic, it was unheard of for an event to be cancelled due to influenza. The political landscape surrounding the COVID-19 pandemic has called even greater attention to public health and personal liberty where certain restrictions are imposed for the greater good [68]. The purpose of this section is not to challenge personal liberty or suggest any part of the pandemic was handled inappropriately, but to provide an outline of common public health themes to consider in mass gatherings.

Since 1998, due to the discredited work that associated autism spectrum disorders and the MMR vaccine, there has been a tremendous rise of the "anti-vax" movement [9]. As a result, numerous other illnesses must be part of public health planning that would not have needed to be considered. On such example is measles. Once declared eliminated from the United States in 2000, its resurgence can be directly tied resistance to accepting the MMR vaccine [18, 83]. One recent event in the United States that highlighted this was the 2019 World Scout Jamboree, held in West Virginia [84]. The confounding part of the plan was not that US-based scouts would introduce the disease to the population, but that a scout from a country where measles remains endemic would carry it onto the property and infect an ever-growing unvaccinated population.

Mass gatherings must also plan for nonrespiratory diseases than can cause an outbreak at their event. Enteric pathogens can also create significant incidents at mass gatherings. Whether it's due to lack of hand washing or a lack of sewage disposal infrastructure, these pathogens have the potential to overwhelm event medical services and the surrounding healthcare system. A unique example of enteric pathogens impacting an event was the 2013 Kumbh Mela, a fifty-five-day long Hindu religious pilgrimage in India that involves prolonged bathing in a river. This specific year resulted in an outbreak of Cholera at the site, despite significant public health activity around sanitation, surveillance, and medical treatment facilities. Specifically, this event was exacerbated by a cultural norm to engage in open defecation and urination that quickly resulted in the river developing hazardous levels of bacteria [75]. In fact, this event is notorious for its public health implications year after year. One of the most unique examples was in 2015 when gathering was complicated by the emergence of antibiotic-resistant bacteria in the river.

The presence of intoxicants independently increases the risk injury and illness at an event. The physical characteristics of many intoxicants, such as their ability to inhibit one's compensation to extreme temperatures as well as their ability to cause dehydration absent exertion or high heat index creates a high-risk situation. Pair this with the characteristics of an intoxicant's ability to diminish one's critical thinking and decision-making capacity, and we have the perfect storm [22, 51]. While some intoxicants are more likely to be present at recreational gatherings (such as alcohol or ecstasy at a concert), some intoxicants may also be used at religious gatherings (such as peyote or other hallucinogens) [60]. The characteristics of the gathering and the manner in which intoxicants will be used need to be considered in the planning process. For example, for a concert in an area by a pool, the water may need to be roped off after a certain hour, or additional lifeguards must be staffed to ensure attendees are safe in the area even beyond times when the pool is no longer officially open.

During preplanned mass gatherings, food safety is a primary public health concern. Most of these events fall under the jurisdiction of local laws, ordinances, or regulations governing food service, but that does not mean that those planning a mass gathering do not have to consider the implications. Planning must account for the time necessary to establish food serving areas, whether it's a free-standing, pop-up facility, or a food truck, and the time for the area to be inspected, ensuring it is up to code. Planning teams must also consider what additional steps must be taken to allow a food service vendor to operate at their site – will there be an additional license required for the event? Will the planning team require additional items above local code? For example, if the local health code does not require it, will the organization require something similar to ServSafe® to operate on site to ensure the safety of participants?

The primary goal of these public health interventions on food preparation is preventing foodborne illness. Foodborne illnesses come in two forms: organism-mediated and toxin-mediated. Generally, organism-mediated illness requires ingestion of the organism which then colonizes within the GI tract causing the well-recognized symptoms of foodborne illness, including, cramping, flatulence, nausea, vomiting, and diarrhea. Toxin-mediated infections can certainly be caused by an organism colonizing in the intestines of the patient, however toxin-mediated

Table 10.11 Examples of foodborne illnesses

Examples of foodborne illnesses	
Organism-mediated	Toxin-mediated
Campylobacteriosis	Scrombroid
Cryptosporidiosis	Shiga-toxin (ETEC)
E. coli (EHEC)	C. perfringens
Giardiasis	S. aureus
Listeriosis	B. cereus
Norovirus	
Salmonellosis	
Shigellosis	
Vibrio	
Yersiniosis	

illness can also result when bacteria has colonized poorly handled/prepared food products, produced the toxin, and the patient ingests the preformed toxin. These illnesses have a much more sudden onset than traditional organism-based infections and are sometimes referred to as foodborne intoxication [57]. Some common examples of foodborne illnesses are found in Table 10.11.

One key logistical concern directly related to public health is the presence of sewage management systems. As illustrated in the 2013 Kumbh Mela example above, the lack of use of provided sewage management systems created a significant public health crisis in the region. Event planners need to consider whether the site should be supported by permanent facilities or supported by temporary systems, such as trailers or a commercially available portable toilet. Considerations need to be made if organizers opt for commercially available portable toilets so that sanitation pumping vehicles can access the area to replenish each stall. If the event is using existing sanitation systems, organizers should check that local infrastructure is sufficient to support the increase in volume.

A highly controversial issue since the COVID-19 pandemic has been the requirement for vaccinations to attend mass gathering events. While things like public schools have had vaccination requirements, it is not typical to have such requirement for mass gathering events. Many cities, states, and countries have had executive orders in place to require proof of vaccination to attend concerts, gyms, or indoor restaurants, let alone true mass gatherings [104]. In deciding whether an event should include vaccination requirements, organizers must consult local, state, and federal authorities to determine their abilities to require such items. Some jurisdictions have created rules, via legislation or executive order (i.e., Texas

Executive Order GA 40, Oct. 11, 2021) that would prevent anyone from creating a vaccine mandate. Organizations need to weigh these local and regional rules with the overall objective and beliefs of the hosting organization to determine the need for such restrictions.

Perhaps the single, most impactful public health consideration has to do with weather. Regardless of if the mass gathering is a spontaneous protest, a planned concert, or religious event, the weather has an overarching influence on the outcome of the event, especially when the event is held outdoors. Large sporting events with indoor arenas are usually able to avoid significant morbidity due to the weather, however, large open are events are subject to the influence of mother nature. A meta-analysis published in April of 2014 identifies the extremes of weather as positive correlates to increased rate of medical usage. If an event is planned to take place during an extreme, say high heat index, organizers need to take into consideration mitigation techniques to prevent a surge in patients that will overwhelm event and area medical resources [4]. Mitigation techniques include changing the time, moving the event to a shady/covered area, use of cooling stations, increasing the frequency of hydration stations, and increasing the on-site medical staff so that mild and moderate heat casualties can be cared for on-site without being transported.

Public health consideration to mass gatherings present an expansive list, many of which will be specific to the geography and specific event and cannot be translated universally. The above themes serve as a starting point on items to consider for each event. Organizers should engage local experts in prehospital and disaster medicine, public health, and event medicine for further assistance with each of these areas.

Resources/Production

Support of mass gatherings involves a complex, multidisciplinary team ranging from production personnel and public safety personnel to hospitality vendors and security. Planning for mass gatherings should start early and involve all stakeholders [45]. More information on this can be found in *FEMA's Special Events Contingency Planning Job Aids Manual (Updated May 2010)*. As the plan is designed, FEMA ICS forms should be utilized to ensure uniformity in communications between organizations.

The logistical support of a mass gathering is going to differ based on the type of event. Organizers need to take into consideration all aspects of the event to provide for contingency planning. As discussed in the public health considerations, potable water is vitally important to ensure a healthy event. If potable water needs to be brought into a location for a planned mass gathering, arrangements need to be made delivery, set up and continuous replenishment of the drinking water. This ongoing process will need to involve measurements of consumption and reporting back to appropriate personnel to ensure that the correct amount is ordered. Other logistics need to involve the ordering and delivery of supplies needed to set up the event, such as chairs, tables, tents, food service equipment (if not subcontracted out), electronics, computers, and more.

Most mass gatherings will need a radio system to support their operation. The location and size of the event will dictate whether this is a repeated public safety system or a smaller line-of-sight system. Additional considerations should include interoperability between organizations and encrypted frequencies. Specifically around law enforcement, but it can also be true for any public safety organization, encrypted radio frequencies add to operational security, but they have limited interoperability and can result in having to purchase additional hardware or software to ensure operations at the event will happen without any disruption. Organizers also need to identify whether there is cell service on site. The absence of cell service will significantly hamper one's ability to communicate with anyone who does not have a radio. At times, temporary infrastructure can be installed to support mass gatherings to ensure there is cellular or Wi-Fi coverage for participants and organizers. If communications are unique in the environment where the event is, ICS Form 205 and 205A should be used to communicate this with all stakeholders.

During event operations, it is imperative that all stakeholders have come together to create a unified command structure [45]. This is an area where NIMS should be used for organizations. Most mass gatherings, especially planned ones, would benefit from a Unified Command structure. Maintaining unified command will allow for the event to quickly pivot in the event of an emergency or evolving crisis. The size of the organization structure will depend on the specifics of the event. For example, a one-day protest likely does not need a Finance or Logistics branch,

and likely would not need a Planning branch either, however, as events evolve, these branches can be added to support event.

Medical support of mass gatherings is vitally important. Numerous studies have sought to identify average medical usage rates (MURs) at these events and have found varying values. The biggest predictors are the type of event, the weather, and the presence of intoxicants [56]. In determining what types of medical facilities to put on site, event organizers need to communicate with local public safety officials and local healthcare leaders. Depending on the needs of the event, an onsite medical tent resembling a temporary ED or field hospital can be set up. For larger, longer events, such as the National and World Scout Jamborees, military support can be requested, and true field hospitals can be constructed to support the success of the event. The level of care provided on scene should be considered based on the amount of and distance to local healthcare facilities. Additionally, staffing medical tents on site of a mass gathering can become quite costly if the model involves physicians and advanced level of care.

Medical tents need to be set up in a conspicuous area that they can be found by those when needed, but also need to be set up in an area that allows for easy egress and ingress of emergency vehicles and resupply or logistical support vehicles. Medical personnel should be in easy to identify uniforms so they can easily be identified when they are needed. Planning for on-scene medical support must occur early as supply chain constraints can make it difficult to acquire needed materials and substitutions may be needed.

As we have identified previously, each mass gathering event is unique and specific to itself. Because of this, each event will have specifics needs, but any large gathering needs liaison officers for key outside agencies. One example could be a hospital liaison or emergency management liaison to help coordinate where patients are transported, their status and condition, or to provide streamlined communications with the 911 dispatch center if there are additional responding units.

Agencies involved in care of patients as mass gathering events should examine their protocols and determine what, if any, adaptations are needed for the event. If using EMTs and paramedics, some jurisdictions allow treat and release, whereas others require consultation with a medical command physician. If working with a team of physicians, advanced practitioners, nurses and technicians, the event medical director needs to determine necessary treatment protocols for all patients, such that minor injuries and illness can be seen by nonphysician staff to expedite their throughput and leave advanced medical services available for the most critical patients.

The final thing to consider when planning a mass gathering are any local regulatory obligations. Large events, such as concerts, religious retreats are all subject to inspection by various regulatory bodies. For example, the stage may need to be approved by construction officials, lighting approved by electrical inspectors, and crowd ingress and egress routes approved by fire officials. Local ordinances governing noise pollution need to be considered. Lastly, organizers need to take ensure that any limits on crowd capacity are adhered too. Lessons have been learned from prior disasters like the Coconut Grove Fire and the Happy Land Fire in 1942 and 1990, respectively, that have strengthened building codes, but also created and strengthened the Life Safety Code. Organizers should work with local officials to ensure

the only headlines are positive and not about disastrous outcomes due to poor planning [69].

Mass gathering medicine brings with it inherent challenges. Caring for people on a large scale can be daunting. To alleviate the challenges, an organized and thorough process for planning should be undertaken by a multidisciplinary team with expertise in various fields to include, but not limited to, security and law enforcement, medical care, and public health. Understanding the common themes across mass gatherings, (1) location and geography of the venue and the associated weather patterns (especially temperature and humidity); (2) type and scope of event, (3) the people (crowd demographics and population modeling); (4) security and safety challenges posed; (5) public health concerns; (6) resources required and production elements; and (7) regulatory issues and the logistics of the gathering, will hopefully facilitate the development of a robust event plan that will assure the safety, security, and well-being of all those in attendance and those employed at the event with the goal of decreasing morbidity and mortality. The following schematic (Figure 10.5) highlights the process that

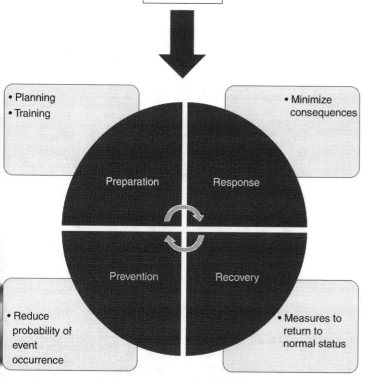

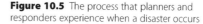

Figure 10.5 The process that planners and responders experience when a disaster occurs

Khan A. A., Sabbagh A. Y., Ranse J., Molloy M. S., Ciottone G. R. Mass Gathering Medicine in Soccer Leagues: A Review and Creation of the SALEM Tool. *International Journal of Environmental Research and Public Health.* 2021;18(19):9973. P8.

planners and responders experience when a disaster occurs. With thorough preparation and response, consequences can be minimized, and the focus can transition to learning about and developing an improved plan of prevention and action for the next event.

References

1. Aggrawal V., Dikid T., Jain S. K., et al. Disease Surveillance during a Large Religious Mass Gathering in India: The Prayagraj Kumbh 2019 Experience. *International Journal of Infectious Diseases.* 2020;**101**:167–173. doi:10.1016/j.ijid.2020.09.1424

2. Alaska Y. A., Aldawas A. D., Aljerian N. A., Memish Z. A., Suner S. The Impact of Crowd Control Measures on the Occurrence of Stampedes During Mass Gatherings: The Hajj Experience. *Travel Medicine and Infectious Disease.* 2017;**15**:67–70.

3. Alkassas W., Rajab A. M., Alrashood, S. T., et al. Heat-Related Illnesses in a Mass Gathering Event and the Necessity for Newer Diagnostic Criteria: A Field Study. *Environmental Science and Pollution Research.* 2021;**28**:16682–16689.

4. Alquthami A. H., Pines J. M. A Systematic Review of Noncommunicable Health Issues in Mass Gatherings. *Prehospital and Disaster Medicine.* 2014;**29**(2):167–175.

5. Arbon P., Bridgewater F. H., Smith C. Mass Gathering Medicine: A Predictive Model for Patient Presentation and Transport Rates. *Prehospital and Disaster Medicine.* 2001;**16**(3):150–158.

6. Arbon P. Mass-Gathering Medicine: A Review of the Evidence and Future Directions for Research. *Prehospital and Disaster Medicine.* 2007;**22**(2):131–135.

7. Auerbach P. S., Cushing T. A., Harris, N. S. *Auerbach's Wilderness Medicine E-Book.* Oxford: Elsevier Health Sciences; 2016.

8. Baird M. B., O'Connor R. E., Williamson A. L., et al. The Impact of Warm Weather on Mass Event Medical Need: A Review of the Literature. *American Journal of Emergency Medicine.* 2010;**28**:224–229.

9. Benoit S. L., Mauldin, R. F. The "Anti-Vax" Movement: A Quantitative Report on Vaccine Beliefs and Knowledge Across Social Media. *BMC Public Health.* 2021;**21**; 2106. doi:10.1186/s12889-021-12114-8

10. Berlonghi A. Understanding and Planning for Different Spectator Crowds. *Safety Science.* 1995;**18**:239–247.

11. Bouchama A., Knochel J. P. Heat Stroke. *New England Journal of Medicine.* 2002;**346**(25):1978–1988.

12. Cahill J. Special Events: Detail-Oriented Details. *Domestic Preparedness Journal.* 2010;**6**(1):10–11.

13. Campbell K. The Dangers of Not Protecting The "3Ps". *During Events. Domestic Preparedness Journal.* 2021;**17**(11):6–11.

14. Delir Haghighi P., Burstein F., Zaslavsky A., Arbon P., Krishnaswamy S. The Role of Domain Ontology for Medical Emergency Management in Mass Gatherings. *Bridging the Socio-technical Gap in Decision Support Systems: Challenges for the Next Decade.* 2010;**212**:520–531.

15. DeLorenzo R. A. Mass Gathering Medicine: A Review. *Prehospital and Disaster Medicine.* 1997;**12**(1):68–72.

16. DeLorenzo R. A., Gray B. C., Bennett P. C., Lamparella V. J., Effect of Crowd Size on Patient Volume at a Large, Multipurpose, Indoor Stadium. *The Journal of Emergency Medicine.* 1989;**7**(4):379–384.

17. DeMott J. M., Hebert C. L., Novak M., Mahmood S., Peksa G. D. Characteristics and Resource Utilization of Patients Presenting to the ED from Mass Gathering Events. *American Journal of Emergency Medicine.* 2018;**36**(6):983–987.

18. Dimala C. A., Kadia B. M., Nji M. A. M., et al. Factors Associated with Measles Resurgence in the United States in the Post-Elimination Era. *Scientific Reports.* 2021;**11**:51.

19. Dress J. M., Horton E. H., Florida R. Music, Mud & Medicine. Woodstock 94: A Maniacal, Musical Mass-Casualty Incident. *Emergency Medical Services.* 1995;**24**(1):21–32.

20. Erickson T. B., Koenigsberg M., Bunney E. B. Prehospital Severity Scoring at Major Rock Concert Events. *Prehospital and Disast Medicine.* 1996;**12**(3):195–199.

21. Federman J. H., Giordano L. M. How to Cope with a Visit from the Pope. *Prehospital and Disaster Medicine.* 1997;**12**(2):15–20.

22. FitzGibbon K. M., Nable J. V., Ayd B., et al. Mass-Gathering Medical Care in Electronic Dance Music Festivals. *Prehospital and Disaster Medicine.* 2017;**32**(5):563–567.

23. Friedman M. S., Plocki A., Likourezos A., et al. A Prospective Analysis of Patients Presenting for Medical Attention at a Large Electronic Dance Music Festival. *Prehospital and Disaster Medicine.* 2017;**32**(1):78–82.

24. Gallagher S., Meaney S., Muldoon O. T. Social Identity Influences Stress Appraisals and Cardiovascular Reactions to Acute Stress Exposure. *British Journal of Health Psychology.* 2014;**19**:566–579.

25. Gauer R., Meyers B. K. Heat-Related Illnesses. *American Family Physician.* 2019;**99**(8):482–489.

26. Goldberg S. A., Maggin J., Molloy M. S., et al. The Gillette Stadium Experience: A Retrospective Review

of Mass Gathering Events from 2010 to 2015. *Disaster Medicine and Public Health Preparedness.* 2018;**12** (6):752–758.

27. Grange J. T., Green S. M., Downs W. Concert Medicine: Spectrum of Medical Problems Encountered at 405 Major Concerts. *Academic Emergency Medicine.* 1999;**6**(2):202–207.

28. Grange J. T. Planning for Large Events. *Current Sports Medicine Reports.* 2002;**1**:156–161.

29. Haslam S. A., O'Brien A., Jetten J., Vormedal K., Penna S. Taking the Strain: Social Identity, Social Support, and the Experience of Stress. *British Journal of Social Psychology.* 2005;**44**:355–370.

30. Havenith G., Fiala D. Thermal Indices and Thermophysiological Modeling for Heat Stress. *Comprehensive Physiology.* 2016; **6**:255–302.

31. Hewitt S., Jarrett L., Winter B. Emergency Medicine at a Large Rock Festival. *Journal of Accident and Emergency Medicine.* 1996;**13**:26–27.

32. Hnatow D. A., Gordon D. J. Medical Planning for Mass Gatherings: A Retrospective Review of the San Antonio Papal Mass. *Prehospital and Disaster Medicine.* 1991;**6**(4):443–450.

33. Hodgetts T. J., Cooke M. W. The Largest Mass Gathering: Medical Cover for Millennium Celebrations Needs Careful Planning. *BMJ.* 1999;**318** (7189):957–958.

34. Holle, R. L., López R. E., Zimmermann C. Updated Recommendations for Lightning Safety: 1998. *Bulletin of the American Meteorological Society.* 1999;**80**:2035–2042.

35. Hopkins N. P., Reicher S. D., Khan S. S., Tewari S., Srinivasan N., Stevenson C. Explaining Effervescence: Investigating the Relationship Between Shared Social Identity and Positive Experience in Crowds. *Cognition and Emotion.* 2016;**30**:20–32.

36. Hopkins N., Reicher S. Adding a Psychological Dimension to Mass Gatherings Medicine. *International Journal of Infectious Diseases: IJID: Official Publication of the International Society for Infectious Diseases.* 2016;**47**:112–116.

37. Hopkins N., Reicher S. D. The Psychology of Health and Well-Being in Mass Gatherings: A Review and a Research Agenda. *International Journal of Epidemiology of Public Health.* 2016; **6**(2):49–57.

38. Hutton A., Zeitz K., Brown S., Arbon P. Assessing the Psychosocial Elements of Crowds at Mass Gatherings. *Prehospital and Disaster Medicine.* 2011;**26**(6):414–421.

39. Hutton A., Ranse J., Gray K. L., Turris S. A., Lund A., Munn M. B. Environmental Influences on Patient Presentations: Considerations for Research and Evaluation at Mass-Gathering Events. *Prehospital and Disaster Medicine.* 2019;**34**(5):552–556.

40. Jaslow D., Yancey A., Milsten A. Mass Gathering Medical Care. *Prehospital Emergency Care.* 2000;**4**:359–360.

41. Jung H., Chung, K. Ontology-Driven Slope Modeling for Disaster Management Service. *Cluster Computing.* 2015;**18**:677–692.

42. Kakamu T., Wada K., Smith, D. R., Endo S., Fukushima T. Preventing Heat Illness in the Anticipated Hot Climate of the Tokyo 2020 Summer Olympic Games. *Environmental Health and Preventive Medicine.* 2017;**22**(1):68.

43. Khan A. A., Sabbagh A. Y., Ranse J., Molloy M. S., Ciottone G. R. Mass Gathering Medicine in Soccer Leagues: A Review and Creation of the SALEM Tool. *International Journal of Environmental Research and Public Health.* 2021; **18**(19):9973.

44. Koski A., Kouvonen A., Sumanen H. Preparedness for Mass Gatherings: Factors to Consider According to the Rescue Authorities. *International Journal of Environmental Research and Public Health.* 2020;**17**(4):1361. doi:10.3390/ijerph17041361

45. Koski A., Kouvonen A., Nordquist H. Preparedness for Mass Gatherings: Planning Elements Identified Through the Delphi Process. *International Journal of Disaster Risk Reduction.* 2021;**61**:102368. doi:10.1016/j.ijdrr.2021.102368

46. Leonard R. B. Medical Support for Mass Gatherings. *Emergency Medicine Clinics of North America.* 1996;**14**:383–397.

47. Levens L. K., Durham J. E. Pop-Music Festivals: Some Medical Aspects. *BMJ.* 1971;**1**:218–220.

48. Levine M., Prosser A., Evans D., Reicher S. Identity and Emergency Intervention: How Social Group Membership and Inclusiveness of Group Boundaries Shape Helping Behaviour. *Personality and Social Psychology Bulletin.* 2005;**31**:443–453.

49. Locoh-Donou S., Yan G., Berry T., et al. Mass Gathering Medicine: Event Factors Predicting Patient Presentation Rates. *Internal and Emergency Medicine.* 2016;**11**:745–752.

50. Lund A., Turris S. A., Bowles R., et al. Mass-gathering Health Research Foundational Theory: Part 1 – Population Models for Mass Gatherings. *Prehospital and Disaster Medicine.* 2014;**29** (6):648–654.

51. Lund A., Turris S. A. Mass-gathering Medicine: Risks and Patient Presentations at a 2-Day Electronic Dance Music Event. *Prehospital and Disaster Medicine.* 2015;**30**(3):1–8.

52. Maclean K. *Pilgrimage and Power: the Kumbh Mela in Allahabad, 1765–1954.* Oxford: Oxford University Press; 2008.

53. Margolis A. M., Leung A. K., Friedman M. S., McMullen S. P., Guyette F. X., Woltman N. Position Statement: Mass Gathering Medical Care. *Prehospital Emergency Care*. 2021;**25**(4):593–595.

54. Memish Z. A., Stephens G. M., Steffen R., Ahmed Q. A. Emergence of Medicine for Mass Gatherings: Lessons from the Hajj. *Lancet Infectious Diseases*. 2012;**12**(1):56–65.

55. Milsten A. M., Maguire B. J., Bissell R. A., Seaman K. G. Mass-Gathering Medical Care: A Review of the Literature. *Prehospital and Disaster Medicine*. 2002;**17**(3):151–162.

56. Milsten A. M., Seaman K. G., Liu P., Bissell R. A., Maguire B. J. Variables Influencing Medical Usage Rates, Injury Patterns, and Levels of Care for Mass Gatherings. *Prehospital and Disaster Medicine*. 2003;**18**(4):334–346.

57. Nyachuba D. G. Foodborne Illness: Is It on the Rise? *Nutrition Reviews*. 2010;**68**(5): 257–269.

58. Paul H. M. Mass Casualty: Pope's Denver Visit Causes Mega MCI. *JEMS*. 1993; **18**(11):64–75.

59. Perron A. D., Brady W. J., Custalow C. B., Johnson D. M. Association of Heat Index and Patient Volume at a Mass Gathering Event. *Prehospital Emergency Care*. 2005;**9**(1):49–52.

60. Prince M. A., O'Donnell M. B., Stanley L. R., Swaim R. C. Examination of Recreational and Spiritual Peyote Use Among American Indian Youth. *Journal of Studies on Alcohol and Drugs*. 2019;**80**(3):366–370.

61. Rahman J., Thu M., Arshad N., Van der Putten M. Mass Gatherings and Public Health: Case Studies from the Hajj to Mecca. *Annals of Global Health*. 2017;**83**(2):386–393.

62. Moore R., Williamson K., Sochor M., Brady W. J. Large-Event Medicine: Event Characteristics Impacting Medical Need. *The American Journal of Emergency Medicine*. 2011;**29**(9):1217–1221.

63. Sarofim M.C., Saha S., Hawkins M. D., et al. Temperature-Related Death and Illness. In: *The Impacts of Climate Change on Human Health in the United States: A Scientific Assessment*. US Global Change Research Program, Washington, DC; 2016.

64. Schulte D., Meade D. M. The Papal Chase: The Pope's Visit: A "Mass" Gathering. *Emergency Medical Services*. 1993;**22**(11):46–479.

65. Soomaroo L, Murray V. Weather and Environmental Hazards at Mass Gatherings. *PLoS Currents*. 2012;**4**.

66. Soomaroo L, Murray V. Disasters at Mass Gatherings: Lessons from History. *PLoS Currents*. 2012;**4**:RRN1301.

67. Sridhar S., Gautret P., Brouqui P. A Comprehensive Review of the Kumbh Mela: Identifying Risks for Spread of Infectious Diseases. *Clinical Microbiology and Infection*. 2015;**21**:128–133.

68. Savulescu J. Good Reasons to Vaccinate: Mandatory or Payment for Risk? *Journal of Medical Ethics*. 2021;**47**(2):78–85.

69. Teague P. E., Farr R. R. Supplement 1, Case Histories: Fires Influencing the Life Safety Code. In: NFPA 101 ® Life Safety Code®, 2009).

70. Turris S. A., Lund A., Hutton A., et al. Mass-gathering Health Research Foundational Theory: Part 2 – Event Modeling for Mass Gatherings. *Prehospital and Disaster Medicine*. 2014;**29**(6):655–663.

71. Wakefield J. R., Hopkins N., Cockburn C., Shek K. M., Muirhead A., Reicher S., van Rijswijk W. The Impact of Adopting Ethnic or Civic Conceptions of National Belonging for Others' Treatment. *Personality and Social Psychology Bulletin*. 2011;**37**:1599–1610.

72. Zeitz K. M., Zeitz C. J., Arbon P. Forecasting Medical Work at Mass-Gathering Events: Predictive Model Versus Retrospective Review. *Prehospital and Disaster Medicine*. 2005;**20**(3):164–168.

73. Zeitz K., Bolton S., Dippy R., Dowling Y., Francis L., Thorne J., Butler T., Zeitz C. Measuring Emergency Services Workloads at Mass Gathering Events. *Australian Journal of Emergency Management*. 2007;**22**(4):24–30.

74. Zeitz K. M., Tan H. M., Grief M., Couns P. C., Zeitz C. J. Crowd Behavior at Mass Gatherings: A Literature Review. *Prehospital and Disaster Medicine*. 2009;**24**(1):32–38.

75. Memish Z. A., Steffen R., White P., et al. Mass Gatherings Medicine: Public Health Issues Arising from Mass Gathering Religious and Sporting Events. *Lancet*. 2019;**393**(10185):2073–2084.

76. Zielinski A., Pawlak B. J. Toolbox for Implementation of Surveillance at Mass Gatherings: Surveillance During Mass Gatherings. 2013. www.rki.de/EN/Content/Prevention/React/Work/wp4/WP_4_ToolBox.pdf?__blob5publicationFile. Accessed January 10, 2022.

77. Zimmermann C., Cooper M. A., Holle R. L. Lightning Safety Guidelines. *Annals of Emergency Medicine*. 2002;**39**(6):660-A1

78. The Kumbh Mela Public Health (KMPH) team. Public health at the Kumbh Mela. Harvard School of Public Health. http://fxbkumbh.wordpress.-com/. Accessed January 20, 2022.

79. Federal Emergency Management Agency (FEMA). Special Events Contingency Planning Job Aids Manual. March 2005 (Updated May 2010).

80. www.youredm.com/2014/03/29/ultra-music-festival-fa n-stampede-tramples-security/. Accessed January 15, 2022.

81. www.rollingstone.com/music/music-news/ultra-festi val-guard-in-extremely-critical-condition-after-gate-crash-246582/. Accessed January 15, 2022.

82. www.stopthebleed.org/. Accessed January 20, 2022.

83. www.cdc.gov/measles/about/history.html. Accessed January 18, 2022.

84. www.whsv.com/content/news/WVa-officials-plan-for-measles-at-World-Scout-Jamboree-510037791 .html. Accessed January 18, 2022.

85. https://emilms.fema.gov/is_0015b/curriculum/1 .html. Accessed January 27, 2022.

86. www.weather.gov/ama/heatindex. Accessed January 27, 2022.

87. www.weather.gov/images/safety/heatindexchart-650 .jpg. Accessed January 27, 2022.

88. https://weather.com/storms/tornado/news/2021-04-05-tornado-warning-nws-accuracy. Accessed on January 27, 2022.

89. www.cbc.ca/news/canada/toronto/17-injured-in-ligh tning-strike-at-ontario-food-festival-1.1129795. Accessed on January 27, 2022.

90. www.latimes.com/archives/la-xpm-1988-03-13-mn-1 821-story.html. Accessed on January 27, 2022.

91. www.reuters.com/article/us-usa-indiana-fair-accident/e rrors-cited-in-deadly-indiana-stage-collapse-idUKBR E83B1NQ20120412. Accessed on January 27, 2022.

92. www.ems1.com/astroworld-festival/articles/astroworld-staff-treated-11-cardiac-arrest-patients-at-once-para docs-ceo-said-AMMyjJefTmxEvj1X. Accessed January 27, 2022.

93. www.nytimes.com/interactive/2016/09/06/world/mi ddleeast/2015-hajj-stampede.html. Accessed January 27, 2022.

94. www.miaminewtimes.com/news/ultra-music-festival-pays-400-000-to-man-beaten-by-off-duty-miami-cops-in-2011-6545190. Accessed January 27, 2022.

95. www.cbsnews.com/news/the-station-nightclub-fire-rhode-island-what-happened-and-whos-to-blame/. Accessed January 20, 2022.

96. www.mikesmithenterprisesblog.com/2011/08/hor ror-in-indianapolis.html. Accessed January 27, 2022.

97. www.npr.org/sections/therecord/2017/12/18/5716 40549/stage-collapse-at-dance-music-festival-in-brazil-causes-death-of-dj. Accessed January 18, 2022.

98. Astroworld 2021 Event Operations Plan (EOP). https:// s3.documentcloud.org/documents/21100364/cnn-astroworld-operations-plan-redacted.pdf. Accessed January 27, 2022.

99. https://en.wikipedia.org/wiki/Rep%C3%BAblica_ Croma%C3%B1%C3%B3n_nightclub_fire#cite_not e-:0-3. Accessed January 18, 2022.

100. www.theguardian.com/world/2011/apr/21/ argentinian-band-the-callejeros-convicted-nightclub-fire. Accessed January 18, 2022.

101. https://manchesterarenainquiry.org.uk/ report-volume-one. Accessed January 15, 2022.

102. www.buildingcontrol-ni.com/assets/pdf/Kiss_Nigh club_Presentation_Fire_Safety_Panel_2014.pdf. Accessed January 27, 2022.

103. www.governor.pa.gov/newsroom/wolf-administra tion-announces-targeted-mitigation-efforts-in-resp onse-to-recent-covid-case-increases. Accessed January 16, 2022.

104. https://coronavirus.dc.gov/sites/default/files/dc/site s/coronavirus/page_content/attachments/2021-148 %20Vaccination%20Requirement%20for%20Entra nce%20into%20Certain%20Indoor%20Establishme nts%20and%20Facilities.pdf. Accessed on January 15, 2022.

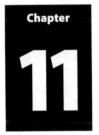

Chapter

11

Mass Gathering Events: Youth, High School, Collegiate, Olympic, and Professional Sporting Events

Korin Hudson, Matthew Sedgley, and Aaron J. Monseau

Introduction

From a road race with tens of thousands of runners, to a youth sports tournament welcoming hundreds of teams, to the Super Bowl and the World Cup, sporting events are often by definition mass gathering events. While many sporting events are staged primarily for the entertainment of fans, these competitions are also demonstrations of incredible athletic performance which carry inherent risk of serious injury to the participants. And though injuries may be anticipated in athletics, planning for the medical care at these events requires careful consideration and special preparation.

Sporting events and other mass gatherings are often held in the same or similar venues. The high school stadium that hosts football games in the fall may also be the venue for a graduation ceremony in the spring, and the arena that is home to an NBA team may also host concerts and political rallies. While the care of the spectators attending these events may be similar, it is important to consider the differences that do exist related to proper planning for the participants on the stage, court, rink, or field. Proper emergency action planning and coordination between various resources can help prepare for common emergencies such as musculoskeletal injuries, concussions, lacerations, and illnesses, as well as for critical conditions such as cardiac arrests, spinal injuries, heat stroke, and mass casualty events.

Defining the Event

As with any event, planning begins with first considering the nature, size, and scope of the event. For sporting events, consideration often begins with the nature of the sport itself which can be a predictor of the medical needs that may arise both for the

participants and for the spectators. For example, an elementary school one-mile fun run on a cool fall day in a suburban township is likely to have different medical needs than a remote, endurance, obstacle race on a hot summer day complicated by the availability of alcohol, with thousands of spectators.

Sports and activities may be classified based on the risk of contact with other participants or objects, and by the force and frequency of such contact. By doing so, we may classify sports as *collision, contact, noncontact,* or *extreme.* Table 11.1 lists examples of sports in each category. *Collision sports* include sports in which athletes intentionally and/or frequently impact each other, other objects, or the ground, often with significant force. In *contact sports,* athletes routinely come into contact with another player or with an object, the ground, or water, though typically with less force than that which is seen in collision sports. Some sports may also be designated as "limited contact" where player-to-player or player-to-ground contact is unintended, but still somewhat frequent while in *noncontact sports,* any contact with another person or object (including the ground) would be rare or unexpected. So-called *extreme sports* are activities that often involve significant height, speed, and a high level of physical exertion and often highly specialized gear. While the definition of extreme sports is not universally accepted, it is generally agreed that one must possess considerable physical skill and ability to execute the activity and that the activity itself poses considerable risk of serious physical harm if poorly executed (Figure 11.1). Each of these classes of sports may be played at various levels including youth, high school, college, professional/elite, or international/Olympic. However, younger athletes may be discouraged from participation in some collision and high-risk extreme sports.

Table 11.1 Classification of sports: representative examples of sports in each category; note: this is not meant to be an exhaustive or comprehensive list.

Collision	Contact	Non-Contact	Extreme
* American Football	**Full Contact:**	* Tennis	* Bungee jumping
* Rugby	* Soccer	* Running	* Hang gliding
* Ice Hockey	* Basketball	* Golf	* Mountain biking
* Men's Lacrosse	* Diving	* Shooting	* Snocross
	* Gymnastics	* Archery	* Whitewater rafting/kayaking
	* Downhill Skiing	* Rowing	
	* Snowboarding		
	* Women's Lacrosse		
	* Field Hockey		
	* Surfing		
	* Skateboarding		
	Limited Contact:		
	* Volleyball		
	* Softball		
	* Baseball		

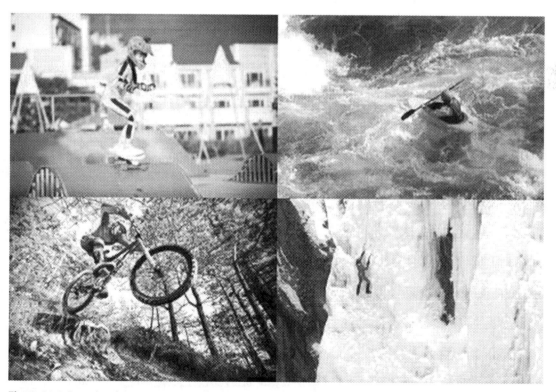

Figure 11.1 Examples of extreme sports – clockwise from top left: skateboarding, whitewater kayaking, mountain biking, and ice climbing

It is also important to consider sporting activities that may carry additional risks of injury due to the nature of the sport itself such as in motor sports, and equestrian events. *Motor sports* is a global term that includes a large group of competitive sporting events that use motorized vehicles for racing and nonracing competitions. These include road racing and off road or motocross events, two-wheel/motorcycle events as well as both open wheel (e.g., Formula One and Indy Car) and closed wheel (e.g., stock car/NASCAR) events. *Equestrian sports* is an equally broad category of activities including English and Western riding, rodeo, harness, and polo. Table 11.2 summarizes some of the key venue and staffing considerations for each of the types of events listed here.

Defining Roles: Medical Providers at Various Levels of Athletics

In order to support and care for the athletes involved, various medical and training staff are required. At higher levels of competition, this staff may become quite large and complex. Many of these professionals are not typically encountered in other event medicine venues, but all should be considered when creating an Emergency Action Plan (EAP), also referred to as an Incident Action Plan (IAP). In most cases, these medical providers will care for the athletes but not the spectators, though this should be clarified during the planning and preparation for the event. Additional and separate resources may be required for the general public as described below.

At nearly all levels of sporting events, you are likely to find athletic trainers (also known as ATC: athletic trainer, certified, or CAT: certified athletic trainer). Though this role may not be a well understood role outside of sports medicine, it is important to recall that these professionals typically hold a graduate degree and have extensive knowledge of anatomy, exercise physiology, biomechanics, and are very familiar with the assessment and treatment of athletic injuries, and the provision of sideline care. For many sports and teams, these athletic trainers attend every practice and competition with their teams and have in-depth knowledge of the athletes, sport, and equipment that are invaluable in an emergency scenario.

At the youth or club sports level, there may be no specific requirement for sports medicine or event medicine coverage at regular games. Event organizers may opt to rely on municipal emergency medical services (EMS) in case of an emergency; expecting that a coach, administrator, or spectator will call emergency dispatch (e.g., 911 in the United States or 999 in the United Kingdom) if needed. However, larger tournaments and events may be better served by having one or more athletic trainers or EMS units on site to manage injuries and/or emergencies that arise. When considering how to plan for medical coverage, event organizers and medical directors should consider the number of participants, spectators, duration of the event, weather forecasts, and data from prior years' events (if available) to predict need for medical staffing.

In the United States, and elsewhere around the world, sports are predominantly performed at high school level. With more than 24,000 high schools in the United States, there are hundreds of thousands of competitions each year. State and local laws often define the requirements for medical coverage, in many (but not all) cases requiring an athletic trainer on site. High schools are more likely to have athletic trainers and/or EMS on-site for competitions in collision sports such as football or hockey, and they may be present or available for contact sports such as basketball as well. However, noncontact sports such as volleyball, cross country, and baseball are less likely to have specific medical coverage onsite for each practice and competition. These teams may rely on coaches or other persons to provide first aid in the event of an injury or emergency until an athletic trainer can be summoned or while EMS is called. High schools may have a designated team physician, though it is unlikely that the physician is present for more than the highest risk competitions (e.g., home football games).

In the United States there are currently approximately 5,300 colleges and universities, and approximately 1,200 of these schools have athletics programs. These programs represent a wide range of resources. Some of the wealthier institutions may have monies but do not spend them principally on athletics while other schools may dedicate significant resources to their athletic programs. Smaller institutions may not have as many athletes or teams per capita, but this rule is not universal. A few small schools have large athletic programs, or particularly renowned programs in certain sports. These programs benefit from large alumni endowments which allow for robust resources in terms of facilities, staff, and equipment. There is likely a heterogeneity to resource dispersion between sports even within a single institution.

Table 11.2 Venue and staffing considerations for various types of sporting events

[1] Additional Resources may be required for: prolonged or multiday events, events that are remote or distant from hospitals or other medical resources, events where there are anticipated: extremes of temperature or weather events, and/or events where alcohol is served or where other drug use is anticipated

[2] At least one EMS team (2 BLS/ALS providers and 1 ambulance) should be dedicated to the athletes and field/court/track, etc. Separate EMS and First Aid resources may be required for spectators.

	Youth/Club	High School	College	Professional/ Elite	International/ Olympic
Noncontact Sports	· Parents or Coaches should have phone access to emergency services · Large tournaments or events may require additional resources[1]	· Emergency Action Plan should be reviewed and rehearsed annually · Parents or Coaches should have phone access to emergency services · Large tournaments may require additional resources[1]	· Emergency Action Plan should be reviewed and rehearsed annually · Athletic training staff should be available if not directly on site · Coaches should have access to phone to call emergency services · Large events may require additional resources[1]	· Emergency Action Plan should be reviewed and rehearsed annually · Athletic training or EMS staff should be available · Staff trained in CPR and first aid should be on site at all times · Staff should have access to phones to call emergency services if needed · Large events may require additional resources[1]	· Emergency Action Plan should be reviewed and rehearsed before each event · Athletic training or EMS staff should be available · Staff trained in CPR and first aid should be on site at all times · Staff should have access to phones to call emergency services if needed · Large events may require additional resources[1]
Contact Sports	As above	· Athletic training staff should be available if not directly on site	As above with the following additions: · Athletic training staff should be on site · Physician coverage on-site or on-call/available · EMS on-site[2]	As above with the following additions: · Athletic trainer(s) should be on-site · Physician coverage on-site · EMS on-site[2]	As above with the following additions: · Athletic trainer(s) should be on-site · Physician coverage on-site · EMS on-site[2]
Collision Sports	As above with the following addition: · Athletic training staff or EMS should be available	As above with the following additions: · Athletic training staff should be on site · Physician coverage either on-site or on-call/available · EMS should be available or on site[2] if response times are prolonged	As above with the following additions: · Physician coverage should be on-site	As above	As above with the following additions: · Dedicated Physician roles may be required (Orthopedics, Primary Care, Emergency "Airway" Physician, etc.)
Extreme Sports	As above with the following additions: · Athletic training and/or EMS should be available or on-site if response times will be prolonged	As above with the following additions: · Emergency Action Plan should be reviewed and rehearsed prior to each event	As above with the following additions: · Emergency Action Plan should be reviewed and rehearsed prior to each event.	As above with the following additions: · Emergency Action Plan should be reviewed and rehearsed prior to each event	As above with the following additions: · Emergency Action Plan should be reviewed and rehearsed prior to each event

Table 11.2 (cont.)

	Youth/Club	High School	College	Professional/Elite	International/Olympic
	• Emergency Action Plan should be reviewed & rehearsed before each event	• Athletic training and EMS should be on-site[2]	• Athletic trainer(s) should be on-site • Physician coverage should be on-site • EMS on-site[2]	• Additional resources or personnel may be required for remote or austere environments	• Additional resources or personnel may be required for remote or austere environments
Equestrian Sports	As above for collision and extreme sports	Most high schools do not have organized equestrian programs though adolescents may participate in youth competitions as noted here • Emergency Action Plan should be reviewed and rehearsed prior to each event • Parents or Coaches should have phone access to emergency services • EMS should be available	Most colleges do not have organized equestrian teams, though students may participate in club sports or other competitions as noted here • Emergency Action Plan should be established and reviewed prior to each event • Athletes, Staff, and Coaches should have phone access to emergency services • EMS should be available	Emergency Action Plan should be reviewed and rehearsed prior to each event • EMS on-site[2] • Physicians should be on-site (preferred) or on-call and immediately available	Emergency Action Plan should be reviewed and rehearsed prior to each event • EMS on site[2] • Physicians should be on-site
Motor Sports	Venue should have an Emergency Action Plan that is reviewed and rehearsed prior to each event • EMS should be, at a minimum, available, and preferably on-site, for these events	Most high schools do not have organized motor sports teams though adolescents may participate in youth competitions as noted here • Venue should have an Emergency Action Plan that is reviewed and rehearsed prior to each event • Athletic training and/or EMS should be on site available at these events, especially as speed and level of competition increase	Most colleges do not have organized motor sports teams though some students may participate in organized competitions. • Venue should have an Emergency Action Plan that is reviewed and rehearsed prior to each event • Athletic training and/or EMS should be on site at these events, especially as speed and level of competition increase	Venue should have an Emergency Action Plan that is reviewed and rehearsed prior to each event • EMS on-site[2] • Must include fire/rescue teams with expertise in vehicle extrication should be available and/or onsite • Aeromedical evaluation teams should be notified and/or on-site if transport to trauma center is likely to be delayed or prolonged	Venue should have an Emergency Action Plan that is reviewed and rehearsed prior to each event • EMS on-site[2] • Must include fire/rescue teams with expertise in vehicle extrication should be available and/or onsite • Aeromedical evaluation teams should be notified and/or on-site if transport to trauma center is likely to be delayed or prolonged

All colleges and universities should have athletic trainers present for collision and contact sports and available for all varsity athletes and athletic activities. EMS is likely to be required by league rules for certain competitions and tournaments as well. Most colleges and universities will have one or more designated team physicians. However, these physicians may or may not be present on campus for routine visits and their presence at competitions may be defined by conference requirements; often for collision, contact, and other high-risk sports only.

By contrast, at the Olympic, international, and professional levels of athletics, medical care teams are diverse, and include not only athletic training staff and EMS, but also physicians from a variety of specialties including orthopedics, primary care, emergency medicine, ophthalmology, cardiology, otolaryngology, dentistry, and others. These teams will also have physical therapists and strength and conditioning staff, and may have psychologists, clergy, and private security as well. Many of these staff members will be present for training as well as competition and some will travel with the team as well. Most, or all, of these professionals will be on-site during a sporting event and in an emergency or mass casualty event, and each will likely play a role in patient care.

Roles of the Home and Visiting Medical Teams

Most leagues and conferences will define requirements for host medical teams for both regular competitions as well as for tournaments and championships. Certain professional leagues also have players' associations that may negotiate that specific medical standards must be met for practices and/or competitions. For regular competitions, each event will likely have a home, or host, team/institution and a visiting team (or teams). The home team medical staff should be licensed or credentialed in the locality where the competition will occur, and should be familiar with the surrounding area, including local hospitals, imaging centers, EMS agencies, and pharmacies. They should also know the venue well including the location of key equipment such as automatic external defibrillators (AEDs), the location of on-site EMS teams, and points of egress. These host medical staff should also be familiar with the EAPs for the venue and for the event and should have all of the relevant emergency contact information at hand.

Visiting medical staff traveling to cover an event or team at an "away" venue, whether across town or in another state or country may encounter challenges related to unfamiliarity with the site and/or surrounding area. This could potentially complicate or slow care for even the most commonly seen injuries and medical conditions. For this reason, visiting team staff should coordinate with the home or host staff, and the host staff/institution should provide ample information to visiting teams including emergency action plans, maps, and local resources.

Event Planning

As in any other event, large or small, the use of an incident command structure (ICS), with well-defined roles, responsibilities, and reporting structure, is crucial for success; refer to Chapter 7 for Incident Command Structure discussions. Pre-event planning and discussions regarding these roles and assigned duties are essential. For any large sporting event such as a road race, large tournament, or multiday event, this includes developing a comprehensive list of roles, job descriptions, and personnel including both paid and volunteer staff. The medical team for a sporting event may differ widely based on the nature and size of the event (see Defining the Event above), and coordinating the providers for the athlete, home team, visiting team, host site, venue, EMS, and so on in a critical situation can be difficult. It is crucial that each team member understands his/her role in an emergency so that critical steps are not missed and so that confusion/disagreements on patient care do not occur. It is particularly important to predetermine who will be directing care for which groups of patients, which protocols will be followed, and when and how hand offs will occur. In particular it is important to define how hand offs will occur between athletic trainers and EMS in situations where athlete care is involved, especially in venues where no physician is present on scene.

Communication

Before, during, and after a sporting event, communication among members of the sports medicine and event medicine team is a central aspect of success. Specifically, these groups must coordinate regarding planning, staffing, and event logistics. For example, when planning a large multiteam college basketball tournament, it must be clear who is responsible for

Table 11.3 Medical timeout: key components

Key EAP Components to Be Reviewed	Key Contact Information to Be Shared
• Advanced Cardiovascular Life Support (ACLS) algorithms	• Athletic Trainer(s)
○ role/designation in the event of a cardiac arrest	• Team Physician(s)
• AED placement on the sidelines	• EMS Lead
○ also other locations in the venue	• Designated transport hospital
• Backboard/Spinal Motion Control	• Designated trauma center
• Protocol for Face Mask Removal	
○ Review of available tools	
• C-Spine injury protocol	
• Environmental risk status (e.g., heat, lightning, cold)	
• Procedure for exertional heat stroke	
○ Cool prior to transport & location of ice tubs (if needed)	
• Lightning plan	
• Hemorrhage control kit, locations	
• Evacuation Plan and MCI plan	
• Any other site or event specific information, potential risks or threats	

coordinating EMS coverage. Will this be arranged through the venue/arena? Or by the host institution? Likewise, who will decide if on-site X-ray technicians are needed? And if so, how will they be contracted? And how will their equipment be sourced? If tournament organizers determine that laboratory resources are needed (e.g., testing for COVID, strep throat, or influenza) this may require specialized licensing for the venue and may require the presence of specially credentialed staff and/or laboratory technicians. How will all of this be arranged? Communication regarding such issues must start months before a planned event. In person meetings, video/conference calls, and e-mail communication in conjunction with shared files, spreadsheets, lists, and protocols help keep all necessary medical team members informed and up-to-date.

In addition, pre-event email communications, webinars, and video chats can be effectively utilized to provide event personnel with "just-in-time training" regarding EAPs and other key information they will need for the event. In some cases, in-person conferences or day-of-event briefings may also be used to share important details and to review critical protocols and procedures. One such pre-event briefing is the so-called "medical time-out." While emergency action planning is a core component of sporting

event safety, it is still not enough without some pre-event communication and practice. This brief interaction allows the staff to introduce themselves and their roles and there is a discussion and review of the EAPs, on-site resources, hospital transport destinations, and any potential threats or perceived risks specific to the day. Essential components of the medical time-out are reviewed in Table 11.3.

Pre-Event

Coordination with Local Resources

Many sporting events will require coordination and communication with civil authorities and the local municipalities, including Fire, EMS, Police/Public Safety, and possibly a government permitting office as well. Many events will rely on private EMS and/or security groups in addition to municipal services. Depending on the event, participants, and potential threats, the inclusion of state or national assets may also be appropriate. It will be important that the private, municipal, and any state/federal government resources are all coordinating with regard to equipment, logistics, staffing, protocols, and command structure. For large or multiday events, notification of local hospitals is also appropriate as this will help their administrators and emergency planners prepare for a possible surge in patient volume through their own pre-event planning and staffing models.

During Event

Depending on the size of the event, one or more people should be designated to a command center (or lead role if no formal command center exists) and should track the number and severity of patient contacts, ambulance transports, and equipment and staff resources. Documentation and patient care records may be electronic or paper-based depending on the complexity of care, location, and type of event, but should be maintained in a manner similar to any other EMS medical record. The status of equipment, staff, and transport units should be known in real-time so that additional resources can be requested or requisitioned if there is any risk that they will be required.

During the event, real-time event discussions and dispatch of personnel within the event commonly occurs through forms of communication such as radios or mobile phones. In larger events, separate, dedicated radio channels for fire, EMS, police, and administration can simplify communication. In addition, in large running events and multi-field tournaments, newer technologies with internet-based group chat and direct messaging are becoming more common. With these technologies, the manner in which the members of the care team communicate can be structured in a way to help clarify communications. In addition to technology-based communication methods, it is also important to consider low-tech methods such as ham-radio for large events, remote situations, or disaster scenarios where cellular and radio signals may be lacking, or may fail entirely.

During sports competitions, communication between the team staff and the EMS/venue care providers may be wholly separate. Team medical staff will manage most injuries and illnesses without interaction from onsite venue care medical staff. However, in the event that an athletic injury occurs that requires emergency care, a simple hand signal from the athletic trainer on the field may indicate that additional personnel and/or equipment is required. Some groups use different hand signals to demonstrate the type of emergency and to indicate the specific equipment and response type requested. These signals should be arranged and rehearsed in advance and should be reviewed during the medical time out. EMS teams responsible

for field or court coverage should ensure that they have direct site lines to the athletic trainer. If direct site lines cannot be guaranteed, a radio or other back-up method should be used. Staffing plans should account for a backup EMS team to backfill into the on-field position if the primary team must leave to transport an injured athlete. This secondary team must be equally aware of all on-field protocols, hand signals, and should also be part of the pre-event medical time-out, if possible.

Post-Event

The post-event review is a critical, and often overlooked, part of the event cycle. During post-event analysis, in person or video conference may be used in conjunction with surveys or informal "comment cards" to debrief and consider possible improvements for future events. It is here that the entire process is reviewed with a critical eye to what worked and what did not. The total number and types of patient interactions is reviewed to consider whether changes are needed to staffing models or equipment plans for future events. Were there any unforeseen problems? Were they handled well? Why or why not? Is any additional training indicated before the next event? This is also a good time to review equipment for any used, broken, or missing equipment that will need to be replaced before the next event.

Specific Considerations at Sporting Events

Venue Considerations

When considering planning and logistics for any venue it will again be important to consider both athletes and patrons. How many of each will be present? As noted elsewhere in this text, the needs for medical staffing at an event can often be considered with regard to the age of the attendees? What is the duration of the event? What considerations are needed if alcohol is served? Are there different needs whether it is an indoor versus an outdoor event? If outdoors, what is the predicted weather for the event? If available, data regarding medical needs from prior year events or similar events in other locations can also be helpful in planning staffing needs.

It is often important to dedicate resources to the athletes that are separate from the resources designated to the spectators. This means defining which

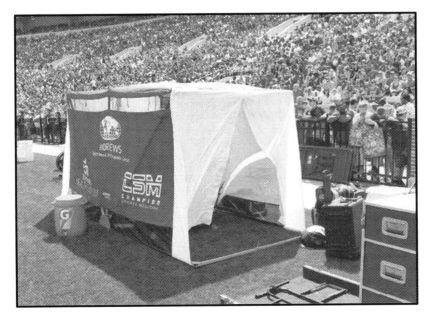

Figure 11.2 Sideline tents at some sporting events provide a temporary area where a patient may be examined in relative privacy

medical staff will care for who and which facilities will be open and available to which group. Will there be separate transport/ambulance pools? Will the transport destinations differ? In many cases this is dictated by the sport's governing body, which may require that EMS providers, physician(s), athletic training, and other resources be dedicated specifically for the athletes on the field (court, ice, etc.). These staff are not expected to respond to calls for assistance or emergencies that occur in the stands or crowd except in rare or extenuating circumstances.

In most cases, athlete care is separate from first aid rooms and mobile facilities, such as tents which are set up specifically to provide medical care for patrons. Depending on transport availability and community medical resources, spectators are often transported according to standard EMS protocols to the closest appropriate facility with capacity to provide care. Athletes however may instead be transported to the facilities affiliated with their team physicians or sponsoring medical groups in order to maintain continuity of care.

Though there are no widely accepted guidelines for medical staffing for sporting events, EMS and physician staffing ratios used for other mass gathering events should be used as they apply to spectators. However, additional staffing should be provided for the athletes with attention paid to: number of athletes, likelihood of injury, duration of event, and likelihood

that medical staff will be traveling with the teams. That is to say that a tournament of six-year-old soccer players probably requires less medical coverage because even though they are unlikely to travel with their own athletic trainers or team physicians, they are also less likely to sustain serious injury. On the other hand, a college lacrosse tournament is more likely to require medical coverage because even if the teams do have their own athletic trainers and physicians traveling with them, they are also more likely to sustain significant injuries. Adequate emergency medical equipment should be available on-site for the management of the most likely and most critical emergencies including such as cardiac arrest, heat illness, respiratory emergencies, anaphylaxis, head and spine injury.

On-Site Training Room Facilities

It is often the goal of large events and professional teams to keep patient care on-site at the venue both for reasons of convenience and privacy, and to avoid overwhelming local hospitals during sporting events. Initial evaluation of athletes will often begin in a sideline area and in some cases a tent or curtained area may be used for privacy (Figure 11.2). In addition, many schools, arenas, and sporting venues will have an athletic training room facility and/or doctor's office on site that allows for the care of many minor illnesses and injuries. Some collegiate and professional sports venues may also have x-ray, ultrasound, even CT scan and/or MRI available in or adjacent to the facility to help facilitate rapid access to imaging and treatment, making on-site care an excellent option for athletes.

Athletic training rooms provide a quiet and relatively private space for medical evaluations before, during, and after a competition. While initial triage often occurs on the field/court or on the sideline, once an immediate life threatening injury has been ruled out, it may be prudent to perform a secondary evaluation in this setting. The familiar setting also offers a convenient opportunity for athletes to share concerns without the distraction of ongoing competition or the intrusion of media or spectators. In addition, athletic training rooms often stock many of the supplies that medical staff require to promptly address concerns during a sporting event such as splinting supplies, IV fluids, over-the-counter medications, and wound care and epistaxis supplies, including sutures. When severe injuries occur, the training room may offer a place for acute stabilization while the medical staff makes a determination regarding transport.

Multiteam/Multisite Events

Tournaments, showcases, and festivals often include multiple teams and take place across several fields or courts across a large venue or multiple facilities. These large events may have dozens of courts or fields spread out across great distances or within a large single venue such as a convention center. Adequate staffing and supplies must be provided so that responses to an emergency situation are equal to (or better than) municipal EMS response times for similar emergencies. EAPs should also account for multiple simultaneous emergencies, especially at large events. Bike teams, all-terrain vehicles, or other modes of rapid transportation may be necessary to move staff and patients between sites, and special attention must be paid to accessibility of each site (e.g., streets, sidewalks, grass, fields, hills, track) as many are not accessible by standard cars.

Event planners and medical directors must determine the necessary staffing as well as the quantities and types of equipment needed to achieve this goal. For example, when planning for events in which exercise-associated heat illness is a concern, or where heat stroke may affect spectators, the medical equipment

cache must include an adequate number of thermistors for core temperature monitoring and a method for cold water submersion or another form of rapid cooling prior to transport. Staffing must be adequate so that response to a collapsed athlete or spectator with possible cardiac arrest should be no more than five minutes in non-austere settings and should include an AED with trained emergency personnel. Furthermore, the medical team must decide how all emergency equipment and staff will be deployed so that resources are available to provide necessary care to athletes/patrons who may sustain illness/injury at any of the various venues. In most cases, aid stations and medical tents should be placed as centrally as possible or at least every 5 kilometers for very large venues/events, so as to minimize response times to each location and medical staff should be provided with radios, cell phones, or other devices for rapid communication. Figure 11.3 shows an example of how resources may be deployed to cover multiple fields for a large event.

Environment

Certain sporting venues carry with them specific challenges and concerns. For example, ice hockey requires specific training and EAPs to care for injuries and plan for safe extrication of the injured athlete from the slick playing surface. The combination of dangerous skate blades and the slippery playing surface poses a risk to rescuer safety as well. Similarly, if a gymnast is injured in a foam pit the very equipment in place to protect the gymnast is now a hindrance to extraction. If performed incorrectly, rescuers are likely to sink further and deeper into the foam well, complicating an already high-risk scenario. As many as eight rescuers will be needed to extricate even a small gymnast. Finally, if a swimmer has a cardiac arrest or a diver sustains a spinal injury, they will require stabilization and urgent extrication from the pool for emergency care. In this scenario, coordinating care between lifeguards, ATC, EMS, and team physician is paramount in safely caring for and moving the athlete. Each of these rescuers has specific expertise and a skillset they bring to the emergency event that is critical to the success of the rescue. Extreme sports, remote venues, and motorsports in particular have their own specific venue considerations which are likely to be unique to the sport and event. Each should be reviewed and rehearsed at least annually and then again discussed during the

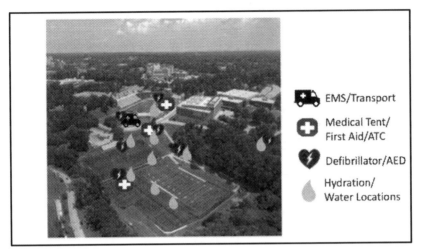

EMS/Transport

Medical Tent/
First Aid/ATC

Defibrillator/AED

Hydration/
Water Locations

Figure 11.3 This diagram demonstrates how a college campus will be used for a large, multifield lacrosse event that will take place across several days in the summer. The medical team has developed a plan that denotes the location of medical tents, athletic training staff, EMS, hydration stations, and defibrillators.

Courtesy of Kellie Loehr, ATC, US Lacrosse.

medical time out immediately prior to the event with specific roles described and assigned in case of such an emergency.

Nationally Syndicated Events

Some sporting events are organized such that the same, or similar, race or fundraising event may occur in cities around the country. In these cases, there may be an overarching organization that manages logistics and helps with permits, equipment, and supplies. However, the local medical director will likely still be responsible for staffing and coordinating with local hospitals, EMS, and law enforcement. Furthermore, the local group may be responsible for providing some medical supplies which will then be added to the cache to be used in future events. In events such as these, it is even more important to communicate and coordinate well with the larger organization because the local medical director may not be responsible for all of the supplies, but needs to be sure they know what supplies are coming and what they will need to provide.

International Venues

In the case of international sporting events such as the FIFA World Cup or the Olympic Games, qualifying rounds and various events may take place across hundreds of miles at venues in different cities. In these cases, while there must be a cohesive and overarching plan with consistent medical protocols for the entire event, each city and each venue must also have protocols specific to the site. Hosts should be identified for each site, and materials should be available for all visiting teams that clearly define the host and describe what services are available on-site including physicians, radiology, pharmacy, translators and so on. In addition, the host should provide maps and describe the locations of the closest hospitals, EMS, and venue-specific information including the locations of AEDs, ambulances, emergency egress routes, and so on. Specific information about game day emergency action plans, including a mass-casualty plan, should be defined/described as appropriate. A list of key contacts and critical phone numbers should also be provided. Details below are discussed regarding the Olympics, but similar considerations apply to any large international competition.

Olympics

The Olympic Games are a massive international event with delegations from all over the world convening on one central location for about two weeks of events. The 2018 Winter Olympics in Pyeongchang hosted nearly 3,000 athletes and the 2020 Summer Olympics in Tokyo (held in 2021 due to the COVID-19 pandemic) welcomed over 11,000 athletes. At each event, the Olympic Village serves as the central hub where the majority of athletes reside during their stay in the host country. It has amenities such as cafeterias and restaurants, exercise facilities, entertainment spaces, and a medical clinic among other conveniences.

The central medical clinic at the Olympic Village is a fully functional clinic with capabilities for evaluation for all common medical complaints, including imaging, laboratory testing, and treatment modalities. Imaging modalities are available at the clinic and should include plain radiographs, ultrasound, CT scan, and MRI. Medicinal treatments should be available with an attempt made to accommodate different medical systems around the world to the extent that is permissible in the host country. Finally, a rapid process for obtaining a therapeutic use exemption should be available at the medical clinic in the Olympic Village.

While this clinic is staffed by licensed medical professionals from the host country, most delegations will also bring physicians to help care for their athletes. As a courtesy, the host country should have a process to grant temporary privileges for the visiting physicians so that these physicians may be allowed to take part in this process. The type of medical care that visiting physicians will be permitted to provide and degree to which they will be permitted to practice will differ for each host country. Still, all medical professionals should feel empowered to offer care in an emergency situation without concern for repercussions from the host country.

The outlying venues should also have access to convenient medical care, either a venue specific clinic or a clinic in a setting such as an "Olympic Park" where several venues are in close proximity. During the planning stages, the events which will be contested in each venue should be discussed as well as the frequency with which each event has needed medical care in the past. International governing bodies for the different sports can offer advice regarding the most common medical conditions encountered, equipment requirements, and any other sport-specific needs. Events with historically high utilization of medical care such as combat sports should be given priority for hosting a larger medical clinic inside the venue.

The host medical group will be able offer insight regarding the expertise and ability of local hospitals, pharmacies, and other resources to provide the different services that may be necessary for both medical problems and traumatic injuries. The hosts should offer each country the opportunity to establish a contact and form a plan with local hospitals for members of their delegation to access care if needed. This access should not be hampered by insurance or payment issues at the time of care. The relationships formed during the planning stages should be communicated to all members of the delegation before arrival in the host country.

Finally, all medical clinics both inside the Olympic medical system and in the local hospitals should be prepared for patients who speak every language in the world. The 2020 (2021) Tokyo and 2018 Pyeongchang Olympics had athletes from 206 and 93 countries respectively. The medical clinic in the Olympic Village should make an attempt to have a large team of interpreters who are adept at translating in the medical setting. Live interpreters are preferred over telephonic or video/internet-based interpretation services whenever possible, though this may not be feasible for outlying clinics to have such a large roster of interpreters. However, it may be possible to predict the most likely nationalities and languages for the largest number of competitors and support staff given historical data for each event. Based on this, certain languages could be selected for in-person translators while remote, telephonic, or internet-based translators remain available for the others.

Other Special Considerations

Therapeutic Use Exemptions

One of the interesting challenges in caring for athletes is that medications that may be considered standard care for most patients may be restricted for use in certain athlete groups due to concern that they may confer an unfair competitive advantage. Some medications and treatments may be banned outright (e.g., anabolic steroids) while others may be restricted only in certain leagues or sports (e.g., beta- blockers, prohibited in archery, darts, freediving, and certain other sports) or in certain concentrations (e.g., pseudoephedrine, prohibited by the World Anti-Doping Agency, WADA, when the concentration in the urine is greater than 150 micrograms per mL).

Certain medications are permitted, but only with a therapeutic use exemption (TUE), documentation from a physician confirming the prescription, providing medical justification, and defining the anticipated duration of use. For example, the NCAA may consider medications such as albuterol for asthma or methylphenidate for attention deficit disorder (ADD) to fall into this category though the latter may require a formal evaluation by a psychologist and/or psychiatrist to confirm diagnosis and treatment plan for ADD prior to use of a stimulant medication. This TUE can alleviate the athlete's concern and reassure them that their medically necessary treatment is "legal." It is also widely agreed that medically necessary treatments do not confer an unfair competitive advantage.

However, these TUE considerations are generally intended for nonemergency care. Though athletes may ask whether any medication, IV fluid, or other medical treatment is permissible, emergency care is by definition exempt when used for true emergency and life-saving situations. For example, treatment with a stimulant or sympathomimetic may generally be prohibited, but when required for a life-threatening condition, such as anaphylaxis, epinephrine is absolutely permitted and a retroactive TUE may be filed. In short, physicians providing venue care should be aware of restrictions that exist regarding the use of certain medications in athletics and should not routinely offer treatments without careful consideration. But, in emergency situations, standard life-saving protocols should be followed.

League and Players' Association Guidelines

As noted above, in some cases, there may be specific guidelines from the event, venue, league, or the players' association (union) that inform medical guidelines and/or reporting systems. For example, World Athletics may set specific guidelines for the management of race-day emergencies for the marathon. These may differ from local EMS or hospital protocols and are intended to be used by the medical staff on site at the event. The National Football League (NFL) and the National Hockey League (NHL) both have specific requirements for an on-site airway physician at every game, a role that is unique and that differs from traditional sideline event coverage. The NFL also requires an independent neurological consultant for the evaluation and management of head injuries and a visiting team liaison who specifically manages host duties for the visiting team, separately from the medical staff for the home team. These physicians are present specifically to assist in the management and care of injured athletes and are present in addition to the orthopedists, primary care physicians, athletic trainers, and other medical staff. Emergency action plans for these events and venues must include these specialists in these roles in order to be successful.

VIP Care

In certain elite and professional sports environments, it is not uncommon for personnel associated with the athletes to seek care from the medical team at the sporting venue. Because the athlete/team has direct access to high quality medical care, this care may be extended to coaches, support staff, family members, and the ownership group. At times, affiliates or other business associates are referred to the medical team as well. In such instances, it is appropriate for the medical staff to assess the need for immediate care versus a referral for appropriate consultation. It is imperative to recall the importance of ethical priorities such as privacy and to maintain appropriate medical records in situations when care is provided – which may be challenging in these settings. However, emergency care should never be withheld when it is required.

HIPAA (Health Insurance Portability and Accountability Act) Issues Related to Media and Agents

Members of the media are ubiquitous in sporting venues. Athletes themselves are often "influencers" with social media accounts and entourages, posting their own accounts of what is happening around them at all times. Many of the people you encounter in the sports setting will seek to gain information about athletes, their illnesses, and injuries by interviewing players or staff, including members of the medical team. It is critical that the medical team maintain strict confidentiality and provide no specific information regarding any medical condition. This includes commenting on conditions which are already "public knowledge" and includes any comments on severity, or projected duration of recovery as even the most benign sounding comment can be construed many ways. Furthermore, in the digital media, a comment made is a comment that cannot ever be fully retracted. All communication should be through the athlete, the team, or the athlete's agent (with the athlete's permission). No member of the medical or venue staff should comment on any medical care provided to athletes, staff, or other patrons.

Bystanders

In a true emergency or critical situation, an athletic trainer and other medical staff members may need assistance when caring for an athlete or other patients at an event. Though a call for emergency services is often appropriate, there may also be an offer of assistance from the crowd. This may prove to be helpful, especially if the offer is for something that requires little skill, such as crowd control, or an offer to call emergency services. Accepting such an offer is low risk. However, if the offer involves patient care that requires certification (e.g., basic life support), accepting this offer may carry additional risk. This must either be addressed by standing protocol or these offers should be considered on a case by case basis, which must be done quickly, taking into consideration the nature of the emergency, the number of patients, the type of care offered, and the stated qualifications of the person offering.

Minors

In many medical event settings involving athletes, the patients involved may be minors. At large events involving high schools and so-called elite or "travel" teams, these young athletes may be traveling with their coaches and team, but without their parents or guardians. Unless emergency care is required, obtaining permission from parents or guardians prior to rendering care is the accepted standard. Gaining this permission in writing prior to sports event, may be appropriate. Otherwise, in most non-emergency cases, healthcare providers should not administer medications, obtain imaging, or undertake other medical care, without parental permission. In certain circumstances it is acceptable to assist the minor in the use of a medication that has been prescribed by their own healthcare provider (e.g., albuterol for exercise-associated bronchospasm). However, in the event of a serious or potentially life threatening emergency (e.g., cardiac arrest or spine injury), it is acceptable to provide standard emergency care without waiting for parental permission, particularly if waiting would cause irreversible harm. In each of these cases, appropriate documentation should be completed, and a conversation with the parents/guardians should take place at the earliest possible opportunity.

References

1. Anderson J. C., Courson R. W., Kleiner D. M., McLoda T. A., National Athletic Trainers Association Position Statement: Emergency Planning in Athletics. *Journal of Athletic Training.* 2002;**37**(1):99–104.

2. Khan A. A., Sabbagh A. Y., Ranse J., Molloy M. S., Ciottone G. R. Mass Gathering Medicine in Soccer Leagues: A Review and Creation of the SALEM Tool. *International Journal of Environmental Research and Public Health.* 2021;**18**(19):9973. doi: 10.3390/ijerph18199973. PMID: 34639274; PMCID: PMC8508246.

3. Tajima T., Takazawa Y., Yamada M., et al. Spectator Medicine at an International Mega Sports Event: Rugby World Cup 2019 in Japan. *Environmental Health and Preventive Medicine.* 2020 Nov 24;**25**(1):72. doi: 10.1186/s12199-020-00914-0. PMID: 33234126; PMCID: PMC7684143.

4. Korey Stringer Institute. https://ksi.uconn.edu/prevention/sports-medicine-policies-procedures/. Accessed April 11, 2022.

5. The Kyle Group. www.kyle-group.com/friday-night-medical-time-out/. Accessed April 10, 2022.

6. The World Anti-Doping Agency 2022 Prohibited List. www.wada-ama.org/en/news/wada-publishes-2022-prohibited-list. Accessed April 12, 2022.

Mass Gathering Events: Music Concerts and Festivals

W. Michael Bogosian, Gerald W. (Jerry) Meltzer II, and Paul E. Pepe

Introduction

In developing the specific mass gathering medical plan for large-scale musical events, the medical needs will vary dramatically based on a series of both relatively unrelated and interdependent variables as well as other unique factors that will impact planning, responses, and the hurdles to be overcome during the event. To begin, a thorough understanding of the structural and shifting anatomy of the mass gathering itself will guide the practitioner in terms of optimally developing a complete and effective mass gathering medical plan. In addition, all factors that can modify that plan need to be addressed as well. Ultimately, coordination and communications with security teams and event organizers need to be closely aligned, particularly in the event of a sudden evolving or definitive threat such as a sudden explosion, fire, crowd crush, stampede incident or some other multiple casualty occurrence, including a terroristic attack [1–6].

Therefore, in this chapter, the authors take a closer look at the unique characteristics of music-related mass gatherings and the various considerations that could influence the overall mass gathering medical plan. Recommendations will be made with the understanding that music-related mass gatherings, especially multiday, migrating festivals, can be unexpectedly challenging and efforts to achieve the most optimal mitigation can be facilitated through some of the lessons addressed within this discussion.

Basic Premises of Mass Gatherings Applied to Music Concerts and Festivals

As described throughout this publication, mass gathering events can vary greatly in their focus, complexity, and behavior of the crowd [7, 8]. Nonetheless, the fundamental considerations for building an effective mass gathering medical plan still remain the same for most events, including many of the tenets laid out in both earlier and subsequent chapters. Among other recognized foundational pillars [9, 10], basic planning considerations can be categorized by a PEER SOP acronym (Table 12.1).

Population/demographics: There should be a consideration of whether or not the event, artist(s), or entertainment will attract older persons, younger children, or will it bring on an additional cadre of disabled persons or youthful imbibers or hallucinogenic drug experimenters – will any of the likely attending populations have track records in terms of predilections for intoxicants or event violence?

Event Type: What is the type of event, be it sporting, convention, concert, religious, public celebration. Each of these attract different demographics, different behaviors, different durations and sometimes geographical differences and ability to rapidly provide medical care.

Environmental Factors: Will the specific event (or related events) take place in indoor or outdoor venues, or both? What are the predicted weather/climate conditions, air quality threats, insect/zoological risks, or endemic public health or security threats? The environmental considerations could also include local issues such as traffic concerns, endemic civil unrest considerations, distances to appropriate skilled hospital facilities (or even availability of such in some venues).

Researched findings: What are the known historical risks for the same (or similar) events and what were the previously tabulated or documented occurrences from those prior similar events and what are current intelligence sources now sensing or reporting particularly those related to security or public health issues?

Table 12.1 The first tier basic risk assessment considerations for planning medical support, resource and personnel needs for any mass gathering event can include the elements of the "PEER SOP" acronym for population demographics, environment, event-type, researched historical and current intel findings, site/structure, organizers' expectations, and consideration of all potential/conceivable risks, even if less likely.

- **P**opulation/Demographics (e.g., older persons, young children, disabled persons, youthful experimenters or any attending populations with predilections for intoxicants or violence)
- **E**nvironmental Factors (e.g., indoor or outdoor venues, weather/climate, air quality, insects, endemic public health, civil unrest or security threats, traffic, distance from hospital facilities)
- **E**vent Type (e.g., sporting, convention, concert, religious, public celebration)
- **R**esearched Findings (i.e., what are the known historical risks and tabulated/documented occurrences from prior similar events – or what are current intelligence sources reporting regarding public health, civil unrest, or potential security threats)
- **S**ite/Structures (i.e., arena, stadium, open/closed, field, hillside, beach, waterside, multiple stages, numerous simultaneous events shifting with migrating crowds)
- **O**rganizers expectations (i.e., be it private entities, contracted parties, governmental agencies, or hybrid combinations) along with local regulatory requirements for medical care)
- **P**otential/Conceivable Risks (i.e., identify all conceivable medical risks and relative risks, including credible external or sociological threats, structural collapses, stampedes/crush events, latest street drugs, politics, or risk of terrorism and violence, explosions or fire, etc.)

Site/Structures. Where is the event being held? Is it an established arena or stadium? If so, is it open or closed or a shell with both roofed and open air sections? Is it to be on a large field or park, a hillside, a beach, a waterside setting, a farmland, a desert, an austere environment, a lakeside or a racetrack and will there be multiple stages and/or numerous simultaneous events or ones that shift from site to site with migrating crowds? Will the structure(s) be portable, or built up de novo from the ground up? What will the stage(s) look like and how many moving parts will be involved?

Organizers' expectations. What are the organizers expecting, be they private companies/corporations, contracted parties, governmental agencies, or a hybrid combination of these various entities? Who is contracting whom regarding medical aspects and, if applicable to health and safety concerns, what do contract riders stipulate? Expectations should be made clear, particularly with respect to identifying chains of command and whether that reporting system will shift if the event becomes a security challenge or if a multiple casualty event evolves requiring the governmental agencies to take over the event medically and/or security-wise. What are the insurance and government regulatory requirements for providing medical care for mass gatherings (such directives can be in statute in some countries for certain events)? Furthermore, what are the licensure and practice statutes/regulations for physicians, nurses or paramedics working on-site in such settings? What are the practitioners' malpractice and liability policies covering? These requirements should be known, understood and respective compliances ensured [8].

Potential and conceivable risks. While perhaps less likely to occur, the mass gathering medicine planner should still identify all *conceivable* medical risks and relative risks. Some of the most benign types of events have become the target of terrorists or deadly drug distribution [4, 11–13]. Considerations may include external or sociological threats, potential for wind gusts and structural collapses, false alarm stampedes or crowd crush events, a novel street drug with behavioral impact, local politics, or even the risk of accidental explosions, fire, flooding, or sudden lightning strikes prompting rushed evacuations. Foodborne illness, severe sunburn, hypothermia, and communicable disease spread do not always come to the top of many lists, yet they are potential risks in some settings [14, 15].

Regardless of the type of mass gathering event, those base considerations become the backbone for the effective mass gathering medical plan, but where they may differ significantly is more dependent on the considerations of specific variables, emphasized by the COLD BREW acronym (Table 12.2).

Crowd size: The size of the crowd (i.e., 5,000 versus 50,000 versus 150,000 persons) will, of course, overall predict the expected relative volume of work. However, crowd size and the accommodating space also affect crowd density. In turn, crowd density also affects rapid access to potential patients. Dense crowds can not only compromise rapid identification, accessing and retrieval of patients in the crowds, but it also affects the degree of resources required, the number and placement of intrasite or cross-venue medical aid stations. All those considerations impact the staffing and medical care space capacities (and limitations) on-site. For similar reasons,

Table 12.2 When considering the nuances of music-related mass gatherings, additional important considerations include various multifactorial and often interactive risk dynamics as delineated by key elements of the "COLD BREW" acronym.

- **C**rowd size (i.e., 5,000 versus 50,000 versus 150,000 will overall predict relative volume of work as well as access to care issues including rapidly finding, retrieving and transporting patients)
- **O**ccupancy and crowd density issues (i.e., physical space and geographical layout, including how crowds will be dispersed – across established venues or full-site de novo build-outs with unknown structural integrity – or challenges of open space fields versus large, elongated venues with multiple sites within one event – or multiple types of seating charts or general audience containment zones within the same event and also the popularity of one intra-venue site versus another at different time points or artist-driven)
- **L**ocale (i.e., urban versus rural versus austere settings – delayed evacuations may occur at either locale, either due to traffic or physical distance to medical facilities; local medical support could be strong or could be less optimal, less resourced or less experienced)
- **D**uration (single evening, single day, or multiple-day (with or without internal on-site camping)
- **B**arriers and access set-ups (i.e., pathways for more rapid access to persons becoming ill or injured with concomitant mechanisms for facilitating their extrication within any part of the event as well as cleared pathways for the most expeditious rapid evacuation and exiting from the site)
- **R**esources (what are the local community assets being provided and/or what are the organizers providing – and what is the actual competency (experience, skills, and equipment) of the assigned medical care providers – and can required additional resources still be acquired as risk assessments evolve?)
- **E**vent-specific medical considerations (e.g., decibel levels prompting headache treatment and hearing protection requests, endemic drugs, endemic air quality issues or there may be many elderly fans or many disabled or special needs populations, heat illness due to predicted climate, excess foot lacerations at a beachfront/shoeless event, slips and falls in muddy venues, falls from heights in multilevel arena)
- **W**ary-worthy behaviors and crowd influencers (e.g., age-related behaviors, history of artist-related behaviors and provocations, potential political speakers/protesters' crowd influencer, frank civil unrest locally/history of violence events or adverse crowd behaviors (mosh pits), and, more recent claustrophobia/psychological panic concerns)

crowd size, crowd density, and structural factors can impact the proximity to ambulances and the timeliness of evacuations to skilled, designated medical facilities. In general, and depending on some basic demographic distributions, such as a disproportionate number of elderly or disproportionately younger persons, the average municipality can roughly expect one true critical emergency for every five to fifteen thousand residents in the population over a twenty-four-hour period, such as a significant heart attack, cardiac arrest, or stroke, most commonly between noon and midnight [16–17]. Therefore, even if stretching over a four- to five-hour period, an event with 50,000–100,000 attendees in an afternoon or evening should be associated with one or more of these critical illnesses as just as a matter of chance. In the case of music-related events, there usually is a preponderance of younger age groups attending such events, thus altering that statistic to a much lesser risk. However, the stressors of such events and comorbid conditions such as heat, crowds, noise din, and the simple excitement of the event could re-elevate that risk for both younger and older persons alike. Adding in drug overdoses, falls, and intoxications, that risk continues to increase.

Occupancy and crowd density issues: A key ingredient in risk assessment is the physical space and/or geographical layout of the event, including how crowds will be dispersed, be it across established venues or if they will be compacted into makeshift de novo build-out settings with unknown structural integrity. There are additional logistical challenges when the event is held in open-space fields or in large, elongated venues with multiple sites or stages set up within one event. Even in an established structure, multiple types of seating configurations or general audience containment zones within the same event can affect medical response. If the medical incident occurs at an upper stadium seat in the middle of a row of fixed seats, there are challenges, not only in terms of retrieval but movement through crowded stairwells. In a multisite event, the popularity of one intra-venue site may change at different time points or depending on the artists (singer, band, disc jockey) performing at each of several stages. Crowd movement can affect crowd density and the associated increased risks for incidents and the greater compromises to rapidly identify and access patients.

Locale: Whether it is in an urban, rural, or austere setting, mass gatherings can delay evacuations, either due to intra-city traffic or physical distance to medical facilities [8, 18]. Also, nearby medical support and facilities could be less optimal, lesser resourced, or less experienced, depending on the locale.

Duration: Music-related events can be the typical single evening, single artist performance or a multiple-day festival with numerous varieties of artists and it is important to appreciate if there will be internal camping on the on-site grounds – and everything in between. Multiple-day musical events create great challenges and require special medical resources and preparations as detailed later in this discussion.

Barriers and access set-ups: Particularly at musical events, audiences are often packed closely together, especially in general audience areas near the stage (Figures 12.1, 12.2). While many arena and stadium venues have designated spaced seating for football matches, basketball games, or rugby tests, during music concerts, the field of play is usually taken over by large contingents of audience members, sometimes with folding chairs separating them, but more often with packed crowds vying to be as close as possible to entertainers on-stage. Conditions can be quite crammed with audience members unable to move very well or be seen by others, let alone be retrieved from the crowd if they become ill or injured (Figure 12.1). On-scene evaluations of those persons, especially among drunken audience members,

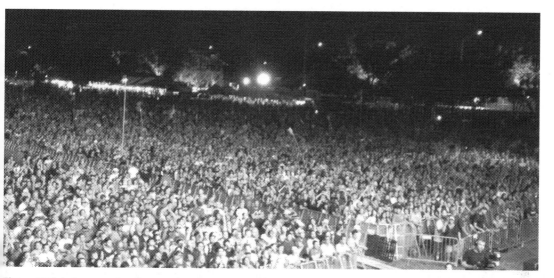

Figure 12.1 In the general audience setting of many musical festivals and events, thousands of audience members will be packed in tightly and as close as possible to the stage. This frequent scenario enhances medical risk, but it also makes it very difficult for any ill or injured person to alert anyone for help, particularly in terms of the generally darkened lighting (as seen here in the far stretches of the venue, stage right) and also because of exceptionally loud din of the cheering/singing crowd combined with the high-decibel amplified music being produced at this festival rock concert. Not does this situation inhibit the locating of patients, but also gaining access to them and extricating in a safe and timely manner as needed

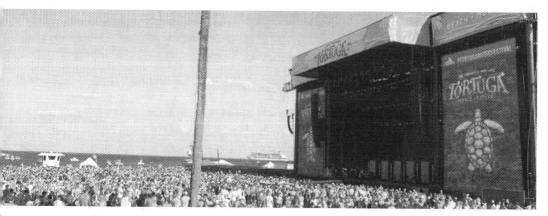

Figure 12.2 Beachside and waterside festivals add additional threats such as broken beer bottle lacerations to the toes and soles of barefooted attendees and even water-associated threats ranging from jellyfish stings to near-drowning events, all exacerbated by intoxication, celebratory dancing, and hallucinogens

particularly those taking videos of the incident, can be exceptionally difficult. Therefore, ample numbers of barriers and fencing must be in place to allow rapid movement of medical personnel and their retrieved patients along pathways created by those barriers. Barriers are primarily set up to help with crowd management, but they also should be considered to have a secondary benefit as a "safety corridor" for medical evacuation. Accordingly, the rapid access to persons becoming ill or injured must be accompanied by concomitant mechanisms for facilitating their extrication either through intermittent (guarded) fence or barrier openings or tools to safely lift persons quickly over the barriers without straining/injuring rescuers or causing significant discomfort to the patient(s). Likewise, medical personnel should help to clear pathways where barriers are not present deep within the crowds. Of greatest concern is to prospectively construct the ability to rapidly but safely funnel persons out in a widened evacuation pathway.

Resources: If the medical practitioner is contracted or part of a team, he or she must understand the local community assets being provided (e.g., local team of city or county paramedics staffing the event and the optimal area receiving hospitals) [8]. They should also know what resources the organizers or the venue are providing, be it a private company, hospital-based team or what mechanism is used to comply with local, state, or even national regulations for mass gatherings. At the same time, it is important to know the actual competency (experience, skills, and equipment) of both the venue and the assigned medical care providers in order to be better positioned to request additional resources as health risks and risk assessments evolve.

Event-specific medical considerations: In the case of music festivals, risks can range from decibel levels prompting headache treatment and hearing protection (e.g., earplug) requests, endemic drugs, endemic air quality issues. There may also be many elderly fans attending to see their long-standing favorite musical stars of days gone by or many disabled or special needs populations for parallel reasons. Other considerations include the usual suspects of heat illness exacerbated further by stifling humidity (Figure 12.3), but also, in some settings, one can expect cold temperature illness during a very wintry wet day [7–9].

In shoreside settings, one can expect jellyfish stings and even near-drownings as well as a multitude of toe and foot lacerations at a shoeless beachfront event in which broken beer bottles or unrecognized broken shells are culprits (Figure 12.2). Slips, falls, sprained ankles, and wrist fractures can occur in wet or muddy venues. For various reasons, there may also be falls from heights in multilevel arenas. One can also expect to see the random occurrence of the usual routine seizures, overdoses, and cardiac arrests to which EMS crews respond on a day to day basis throughout any community. However, for a myriad of reasons, the event itself may heighten the risk and increase the likelihood of encountering such life-threatening cases.

NWS Heat Index — Temperature (°F)

Relative Humidity (%)	80	82	84	86	88	90	92	94	96	98	100	102	104	106	108	110
40	80	81	83	85	88	91	94	97	101	105	109	114	119	124	130	136
45	80	82	84	87	89	93	96	100	104	109	114	119	124	130	137	
50	81	83	85	88	91	95	99	103	108	113	118	124	131	137		
55	81	84	86	89	93	97	101	106	112	117	124	130	137			
60	82	84	88	91	95	100	105	110	116	123	129	137				
65	82	85	89	93	98	103	108	114	121	128	136					
70	83	86	90	95	100	105	112	119	126	134						
75	84	88	92	97	103	109	116	124	132							
80	84	89	94	100	106	113	121	129								
85	85	90	96	102	110	117	126	135								
90	86	91	98	105	113	122	131									
95	86	93	100	108	117	127										
100	87	95	103	112	121	132										

Likelihood of Heat Disorders with Prolonged Exposure or Strenuous Activity

☐ Caution ☐ Extreme Caution ☐ Danger ■ Extreme Danger

Figure 12.3 The *National Weather Service* (NWS) matrix chart for determining the heat index, what the ambient temperature feels like when combined with humidity readings

*From the *National Oceanic and Atmospheric Administration*, US Department of Commerce (US Government Agency)

Certain regional animals, or certain irritating or poisonous plants could affect a given site. For example, a thorough medical plan for sites in tropical or subtropical climates should include preparations to treat illnesses and injuries associated with snake bites, poisonous spiders, and other indigenous threats. In a desert climate, music event sites can experience extreme heat during the day and then extreme cold at night. Attendees can experience true hypothermia, occasional cold-induced Raynaud's syndrome, and even frostbite. Others may start fires with the attendant risk for burns.

Wary-worthy behaviors and crowd influencers: There is no question that misbehavior will occur in younger generations and particularly in adolescent and young adults who are most likely to attend musical festivals and most likely to take risks (e.g., drinking, drug-taking, jumping, diving, unclothing, and brawling). But beyond attendee age-related behaviors, a history of artist-related behaviors and provocations must also be recognized. Some political speakers, protesters for a sociological cause, and or other types of crowd influencers, including celebrities, may induce or even prompt civil unrest at certain music events, even those established for a beneficial cause. A history of violent events with certain artists or types of music can create adverse and risky crowd behaviors (e.g., mosh pits) or it can be complemented by the more recent escalations of reactionary claustrophobia, psychological panic eruptions, and occasional stampedes or crowd crush events [1–5].

Cultural differences also affect crowd dynamics and behaviors. In one country or region, audience members standing in a general audience section of a rock concert may respectfully stand behind a two-inch wide line of yellow tape placed on the stadium floor without budging for the entire show. In contrast, audience members in other nations may routinely attempt to breach barricades, dance without clothing, or throw objects at performers!. However, even in polite cultures, there will still be certain outliers with which to contend including international visitors arriving at the event.

The categorization provided here of the basic planning considerations (PEER SOP) and the variable factors focused around musical events are somewhat arbitrary constructs and they even overlap to a large degree. In fact, music-related events span a large spectrum of mass gatherings that have many different and unique challenges. Nonetheless, this proposed constructs still help to build a pyramid foundation and additional pragmatic check lists outlining important considerations for the mass gathering medicine practitioner altogether.

Each Factor Affects the Other Factors, and Vice Versa

Each of the cited basic considerations and variable factors will often influence one or more of the other factors. In some mass gatherings, variables and their effects can be dynamic and ever-changing such as a multiday, multisite festival with on-site overnight camping where many features and influences are in flux throughout the event.

In contrast, for many other types of mass gatherings using the same venue, most of the variable factors will typically remain consistent in the way they influence each of the other factors. For example, at a professional football game, the teams and the contest will always occur in one place, on the football field in a stadium. The crowd size and occupancy density will invariably be consistent and the event-specific medical considerations will be relatively predictable and consistent. In most cases, the crowd will focus their attention on the game and with the exception of toilet breaks, they will not move about the venue space very much, thus reducing some of the inherent medical risks observed with mass movement of large crowds. Although the typical excess in alcohol consumption can increase risk for deleterious events to a certain degree, that variable still remains relatively predictable. Therefore, medical resource needs will likely be predictable and operating policies will be practiced consistently for each game. In short, many mass gatherings, based on their structure, programming, and frequency, exhibit predictability among the variable factors. Problems are relatively uncommon due to such familiarity and regularity.

In contrast, however, music-related mass gatherings tend to be quite the opposite in terms of predictability and they are often quite complex when compared to most other types of mass gathering events. They also can vary country to country [19–21]. Even for the same type of set-up or seemingly similar line-up of artists, certain variable factors can change the dynamic of the whole event and those can also be further influenced by other changing factors. For example, a multiday music event with a myriad of stages or festival activities that would be ongoing throughout several days, one might experience different crowd influencers throughout each of the different days, especially when considering the time of day (early afternoon versus late evening attendees), different migrating crowd densities depending on the show, artist, or music being featured, and different weather influences from day to day (heat, humidity, breeze) or even changes from day time to evening time. In turn, all of these variables can influence event-specific medical considerations (differing heat indexes each day, different intoxications, different age groups), crowd densities (increased/lower medical service demand), and crowd influences (different types of programming or different types of artists). This complex of fluctuating variables can create a very dynamic environment that can alter medical demand significantly at different intervals throughout each day and throughout the duration of the event. It also implies the need for rotating shifts of medical care providers who must be well-trained, well-coordinated, and well-integrated with the production management and security teams.

Again, one factor can significantly affect the others, even in real-time. The combination of the size of the crowd, the type of crowd, the crowd barriers, geographical logistics of the event and crowd density can have all affect the consequences of a sudden and unexpected "crowd influencer" coming from the audience itself. In such a scenario, a specific visual or very loud popping sound can suddenly prompt a well-intended, "crowd-influencing" warning that can incite attendees, without proper information, to trigger stampedes, crowd crushes, and subsequent multiple casualties[3].

For example, in September of 2018, during the Global Citizen Festival in Central Park, New York City, a rapid unplanned large crowd movement occurred that resulted in a number of trauma-related injuries even though it was launched by a well-intended "false alarm" [3]. In this exemplary incident, a cardboard water container was purposely stomped on and popped in such a manner that it created a very loud sound that was interpreted by some in the crowd as being a likely gunshot. A group of guests immediately reacted by shouting "shots fired, shots fired." This shout-out not only led to a crowd rush in the immediate area, but it also "triggered" a massive police response into the crowd. A panic chain reaction then occurred for the many other guests who had not even heard the noise or "shots fired" shout, but saw the frightened crowd movement and massive police deployment. Interpreting the happenings around

them as something clearly dangerous, the panic continued to amplify and that accelerated the crowd dispersal. At that point, the unintended the crowd dispersal had destabilized with attendees running in all directions trying to seek apparent safety from a vector unknown to most of them. The result was ensuing trampling, crushing, falls, and subsequent physical and psychological injury for many.

Only minutes later, announcements were made from the stage telling the guests that there was no danger, but the crowd energy increased so quickly that a number of injuries occurred almost simultaneously. The medical response was not only compromised by having to penetrate the unorganized rambling crowd itself, but also by the breadth and spread of patient scatterings. Fortunately, although there were multiple patients calling for medical care, the swift intervention by police and security teams to identify that there was not a threat, did stabilize the crowd and that did reduce the number of potential injuries and even the potential severity of those injuries.

Of note, in this scenario, the crowd reacted in a very disorganized manor with each guest developing their own reaction based on the available information at hand, which likely is uniformed conjecture or nothing at all. Overall, such disorganized movement creates rapid changes in the crowd energy and impacts the flow of movement that predictably results in injury. When a crowd reacts in a disorganized manor, it is incumbent upon the event organizers to have a plan for managing these movements. One consideration is to place plans in motion that they would use for rapid evacuations in a true panic situation such as that for an explosion, fire, terrorist, or even tornado [1, 5, 6].

For all of these considerations, as explained below, time and space are the key elements. Questions to be addressed are whether the time needed to move the crowd to safety is sufficient to allow attendees to get from point A to point B safely and whether the space through which the crowd is to move is large enough and designed in a way to safely allow the mass movement of the crowd size and density. If these two components are not sufficient, the density of the crowd can rapidly amplify. As the density increases, an individual's ability for free movement decreases and that can cause even more panic, creating a vicious cycle. When persons are pushed and collapse (and often trampled and unable to get up), crowd movement is further compromised. In essence, wide enough spaces, multiple exits, and directives to optimally channel the crowd should be in place. Regardless, medical personnel must be prepared for such random-occurrence responses and include them in medical planning considerations.

Veritable Varieties of Variables

Clark County, Nevada, experienced a horrific tragedy on October 1, 2017, at the Route 91 Harvest Festival [6]. This mass casualty, occurring less than a year before the Global Citizen Festival event, was medically complicated by many of the same crowd panic and dispersal factors experienced in Central Park, but, this time, the threat was quite real [3, 6]. This music-related mass gathering event was largely a country music festival. As one of the featured artists was performing on-stage, a sniper using automatic weaponry shot hundreds of persons from an high-rise hotel located quite a distance from the actual venue. As discussed in more detail in Chapter 20, the sudden slaughter of dozens and dozens of persons created a chaotic challenge for medical care providers attempting to provide on-scene triage and evacuation. What carried a particular medical distinction in this case was that the crowd was largely standing on a paved area allowing bullets hitting the ground to ricochet and cause further injuries leading to a higher number of persons injured and a higher proportion of critical injuries as a result. In most multiple casualty incidents (MCIs), most persons are either killed outright or only moderately injured with only 5–15 percent typically being critically injured [22]. In this setting, however, with the weaponry, the hidden unknown assailant source and trajectory, the darkened show environment, and the specific audience setting (pavement, not grassy field or turf), hospitals were quickly overwhelmed with a very large percentage (40+ percent) of very seriously injured patients [6, 23]. Again, in the panic, persons were also trampled or pushed to the ground on the hard surface resulting in additional injuries.

Also of note, because of the chaos, many persons sought makeshift medical transport mechanisms such as rideshare providers (LyftTM, UberTM) or private vehicles or taxis [6, 23]. The rideshare programs ironically provided some advantage because of their geographical positioning applications that expedited the finding of the prospective riders or their pick-up locations.

These alternative (nonambulance) transports complicated traditional triage plans. In the end, on-site care providers did not have an optimal grasp of how many patients were going to hospitals and to which facility they went. This raises the issue of ensuring that mass gathering medicine practitioners have real-time ongoing communications with all of the likely receiving hospitals to gauge their degree of saturation and current capabilities [22–24]. Hospitals can be overwhelmed at one moment but under control again, sometimes within a matter of minutes, when it is ascertained that many of the arriving injured were found to be relatively stable [22]. This music festival gone awry also brings up the reality of how all the many variables are interwoven and how risk must be assessed and reassessed accordingly, particularly for future events.

Risk Assessments for Medical Needs, Planning, and Funding Justifications

The prior examples raise the question of how medical professionals can better address and account for potential changing circumstances and evolving medical demand in a music-related mass gathering event. The short answer is to implement in-depth, multifaceted planning in conjunction with security, production teams, and local emergency medical services teams and hospitals. For the mass gathering medicine clinician, this process can begin with application of an analogous multifaceted matrix for medical risk assessment such as use of the Event Risk Scoring Matrix (ERSM) for both security and medical risks (Figure 12.4).

A medical risk assessment is a process in which the medical practitioner first examines all the base considerations (such as the PEER SOP) and then analyzes the more variable (such as the COLD BREW) factors (Tables 12.1 and 12.2). The ERSM helps to quantitate a risk score for a specific factor based on the probability of that risk occurring. It also helps to predict the impact that the risk being scored would have on the overall medical plan (and applicable resources). Once the probability score is determined and the likely impact of that medical risk is identified, the two numbers are multiplied together to determine the overall risk.

As a relatively simple example, by using the ERSM, the relative medical risk and relative demand for medical services associated with heat-related illness at an outdoor event with 50,000 people attending can be scored. Prior to that event, the ten-day forecast predicts high temperatures of 88 degrees Fahrenheit (31°C) with 80 percent humidity on the event day which

EVENT RISK SCORING MATRIX

I M P A C T

	Insignificant 1	Minor 2	Moderate 3	Major 4	Severe 5
Almost Certain 5	**LOW** Overall Risk Score 5	**MODERATE** Overall Risk Score 10	**HIGH** Overall Risk Score 15	**HIGH** Overall Risk Score 20	**HIGH** Overall Risk Score 25
Probable 4	**LOW** Overall Risk Score 4	**MODERATE** Overall Risk Score 8	**MODERATE** Overall Risk Score 10	**HIGH** Overall Risk Score 16	**HIGH** Overall Risk Score 20
Possible 3	**LOW** Overall Risk Score 3	**LOW** Overall Risk Score 6	**MODERATE** Overall Risk Score 9	**MODERATE** Overall Risk Score 12	**HIGH** Overall Risk Score 15
Unlikely 2	**LOW** Overall Risk Score 2	**LOW** Overall Risk Score 4	**LOW** Overall Risk Score 6	**MODERATE** Overall Risk Score 8	**MODERATE** Overall Risk Score 10
Rare 1	**LOW** Overall Risk Score 1	**LOW** Overall Risk Score 2	**LOW** Overall Risk Score 3	**LOW** Overall Risk Score 4	**LOW** Overall Risk Score 5

P R O B A B I L I T Y (vertical axis label)

Overall risk score is calculated by multiplying the probability score by the impact score.

Figure 12.4 The Crowd Management Event Risk Scoring Matrix (ERSM)*, used to determine the overall level of risk for certain threats that might be anticipated for mass gathering events, includes: (1) the probability of the type of medical threat actually occurring, especially anticipating the volume of attendees; and (2) the impact that such a threat would impose on medical resources and capabilities. The multiple of risk probability and risk impact predicts the overall level of the risk calculation

*provided with permission from Crowd Management Consultants of Maine (USA) for whom the first and corresponding author is the both founder and principal (and also the ERSM designer).

creates a heat index of 106 degrees Fahrenheit (41°C), generally rated as a danger level (Figure 12.1). Therefore, the probability of medical practitioners specifically treating heat-related illness during that event is very likely and scored as "probable." Under these conditions (heat index 106), the "probable" risk score (4) predicts that the practitioner will treat many cases of heat-related illness with an outdoor-exposed crowd of 50,000 persons. Depending on the audience demographic, this threat could be augmented if there are many persons such as older persons with higher risks for certain comorbidities or if they are taking medications or drugs exacerbated by the heat. At the same time, the most common "comorbidities" typically encountered at music festivals and concerts include alcohol intake and relative dehydration, most often seen with younger healthy persons. An overwhelming number of these cases could require multiple treatment

modalities, diminish supplies, and lead to extended need for care severely straining the on-site medical operation. Therefore, the impact from such a scenario would be major (risk score 4), not only based on the medical plan, but the event overall. Using this example of a probability score of 4 multiplied by an impact score of 4, the overall score for heat-related illness alone provides a final Risk Score of 16 categorizing heat-related illness as a High Risk for this event using the ERSM (Figure 12.4).

This predicted high risk impact on medical resources, of course, would have been less threatening if only a few cases were to be encountered and if the event was actually held later in the evening with a much smaller crowd attending seated in a well-shaded, well-ventilated, less dense crowd (such as a shell arena). However, in the scenario presented, it is very reasonable to expect that there will be many people needing treatment for heat illness with crowd of 50,000 attending in an outdoors setting with direct sunlight, densely packed crowds (allowing little ventilation despite an existent breeze), and limited ability and likelihood to leave their position in the crowd and get water frequently.

While the high-risk score calculated in this scenario may seem neither surprising nor counterintuitive to veteran event managers and medical professionals, the scoring system does provide a semi-quantitative tool that can be used to help to justify the rationale for funding more resources. Such resources, in this case, could be the justification for stocking additional heat-related care equipment from ice baths and intravenous fluids to plentiful large fans and air-conditioning, including generator-powered and air-conditioned stand-alone medical tents in some circumstances.

Of course, there are also other less probable threats such as the sudden appearance of a new "recreational" drug du jour being distributed at the event or the unanticipated terrorist attack such as that occurring at music festivals such as the Route 91 Harvest Festival incident [6, 11–13]. While probability scoring will be relatively lower compared to heat illness in a given upcoming event, those potential threats still add to the justification and planning for medical resources. Even with a probability score of 2 (= unlikely), when appropriately combined with a severe impact score (i.e., 5), this still leads to a score of 10 (moderate risk) overall. That risk score elevates those profiles for budgeting, planning, and preparations.

Translating Assessments into Risk Reduction, Contingencies, and Planning

How can risk scoring help to develop and execute an optimal medical plan? Beyond the heat and terrorist examples, the medical practitioner will need to identify all POTENTIAL medical risks centered around the base factors (e.g., PEER SOP) and the variable factors (e.g., COLD BREW). Based on the severity of each risk, the practitioner can then:

- **Identify ways to reduce the risk**

  For example, with a severe risk of heat-related illness, the medical planner may recommend additional cooling tents and large-scale, multisite free water distribution along with increased preemptive public service

announcements through mass and social media as well as on-site communications and large-scale messaging about heat-related illness prevention. These messaging systems can include strong emphasis on staying hydrated and recommending what to wear (such as the three L's of light-colored, light-weight, loose fitting clothing) [8, 25]. In terms of diminishing bad outcomes when they do occur, risk reduction efforts helps to better plan the stocking of advanced life support therapies such as IV fluids and ice baths (as indicated) including use of circumferential coverings (Thermal Emergency Management Patient bags) constructed like body bags and fill with ice water, to prevent deaths and morbidity [21].

- **Develop contingency plans**

  Contingency plans are those preparations developed to appropriately deal with any escalating or anticipated risks, ranging from worse than expected climate conditions, errant novel drugs du jour, stampedes and crowd crush incidents, falls from heights, outbreaks of violence, or even purposeful attacks on the crowd. These finite concerns would warrant more medical staff, increasing IV supplies, oxygen, sedation, and other medications and tools to manage toxicological emergencies, cardiac arrest, and impending heat stroke, let alone a large supplement of hemostatic devices and tools (e.g., tourniquets) in case of multiple casualties. Local hospitals should be notified a priori of the potential for numerous transports and they also should be provided early alert if there are steadily increasing and near-overwhelming escalations in patient volumes due to rising numbers of heat-illnesses, overdoses, or other types of insidious challenges.

- **Develop care plans**

  As discussed in other chapters, ensuring an appropriate level of medical care for each person needing it will be largely determined by the volume of attendees, the various risks, and the logistics and geography of the event. Accordingly, the medical care plan may call for staffing multiple on-site medical facilities staggered at different levels of a stadium or strategically positioned at various stretches along an elongated beach shoreline or the elongated promenade of a large waterside park festival in other scenarios, it might involve at least one centrally located, but easy to find and access, medical facility that could be a large tent, portable building, or large on-site trailers, with a number of beds/cots, staff, and supplies to mitigate all potential calls for service in a timely manner. Experiences such as the medical facilities established for both the Las Vegas and Orlando productions of the Electric Daisy Carnival have been quite successful using these tactics despite the challenges of large geographical acreage, constantly migrating and imbibing crowds of over 100,000 attendees per night, and typically high-heat locales (e.g., Las Vegas Speedway) or high-humidity, microburst-predisposed locales (Orlando) [21]. Developed steadily over the years, these on-site, well-stocked treatment centers have consistently protected the local medical systems, particularly with their well-funded, aggressive stocking, expert staffing, high coordination with security, and significant high-level preparations for severe heat illness and drug overdoses and other intoxications [21, 26].

Location, Location, Location in Music-Related Mass Gatherings

Music mass gathering events happen in spaces of all different shapes and sizes. Many occur in established venues with built-in set seating while others are built de novo on an empty stretch of land. Based on the prior discussion and many of the elements described in Chapter 4 and subsequent chapters, the type of event space, its geographic location, and its associated local climate can have a pivotal impact on the medical plan. In essence, there is no standard plan for all music-related events per se, but an analysis of differences in various types of music-related events can be insightful.

The Established Venue

Spaces in established venues (stadium, arena, auditorium) tend to be the easiest to understand and manage as they may be climate-controlled, weather-protected and they typically have established on-site medical facilities. Moreover, they often have several first aid stations on various floor levels of an arena or stadium. Beyond the clinical infrastructure, there usually are longstanding established memoranda of understanding (MOUs) or set contract riders with local ambulance providers along with participating medical staff from affiliated institutions or contracted or sponsoring medical facilities. Accordingly, music events at established venues, especially indoor arenas (protected from the elements) are the simplest music-related events to plan and the least complicated to execute.

Many of these established venues also have established actual seating (e.g., folding chairs) on the event

floor, an abundance of access pathways to audience seats, and, in turn, they avoid the crush of general audiences packing near the stage and allow for more rapid identification and seat location of patients.

Nonetheless, any new practitioner, agency provider, or emergency medical services (EMS) medic assigned to provide care should be familiar with the entire structure, locations of various levels, sections, rows, and seats and be familiar with event level location-finding terminology such as "stage-left" and "stage right," "front of house consoles" and "back of house." They should have knowledge of the entire "house" and conduct a focused site survey to better understand the capabilities of the space and location of medical assets prior to developing a cogent medical plan. This mental inventory includes knowledge of sections, rows, and seat numbering, both along the rising stairwells and on the event floor.

When recruited to provide medical support, basic considerations when dealing with established venues should include (and address) the following queries:

- Is there an established medical facility on-site?
  - If so, how many are there and what are the relative capabilities/locations?
  - How large is the facility overall and how many levels?
  - Are there established medical clinics with some degree of diagnostic tools within the facility?
- How far away is the closest hospital and how far away are appropriate destination hospitals based on condition (e.g., closest trauma center, stroke center, pediatric center, or STEMI-capable center)? [8]
- Will there be accessible and sufficient ambulance staging near or within the facility and who is providing that service (private, municipal, or other service)?

Outside the Established Entertainment Venues

Stepping away from the well-established structure venues (arenas, stadiums, auditoriums), other music concert or festival settings can be much less familiar and much more challenging. For some of the very large-scale mass gathering events involving musical performances, the entire event site can be built entirely de novo from the ground up and involve specialized master builders akin to an army corps of engineers with generator-powered services, self-contained internet access, and immeasurable water supplies, large-scale cafeterias for production crews, and much more.

Compared to the mass gathering events occurring in arenas and stadia, this type of venue imposes many special challenges for the medical practitioners and, in turn, it will require significant advance planning. It is important for the clinical practitioner to be engaged enough in the site design phase to ensure that the on-site medical facilities are built to a specification that is adequate and appropriate for mitigation and treatment of the risks identified during the risk assessment. It is worthwhile to note that, in most large musical festivals, several easy-to-locate medical facilities are typically spread across the site, but often with one "main medical" facility and multiple smaller satellite sites such as well-positioned medical tents.

Over the years, large mass gathering music events have been conducted and managed medically on a large area of diverse terrains. As previously alluded, from stretches of beaches (Figure 12.2) or farmlands to cruise ships, city streets, or parks, each type of location poses its own associated risks and nuances. In some instances, such as an urban environment, twenty-four-hour security and surveillance of the medical facility may be indicated (possible needle/drug/generic theft). In rural areas, such as farmlands or so-called "green field" sites, it may be more difficult to get an optimal medical infrastructure in place. Site failure may be due to extreme rainy conditions or wintry mixes that can make a site unstable or impassable for response vehicles. This not only makes it a challenge for medical teams to respond or provide continuity of care, but it also impedes on-site response and intra-site retrieval of patients. Coastal locations have been known to run the risk of high winds and flooding. This can set up hazards such as swaying and collapsing speaker towers, falling large stage objects and other forms of objects potentially hitting production crews or attendees. However, recent experiences at the 2023 Burning Man festival demonstrated that there is a potential for high winds and flooding anywhere, including an inland desert. These are just a few examples of why it is important for the medical practitioners to anticipate and identify such risks associated with the physical space and why they should work to prevent or plan how to mitigate those risks as part of the medical risk assessment tasks.

Long Duration Events That Augment Medical Contingencies

Obviously, the duration of the mass gathering music event directly influences the medical plan and there is direct correlation between event duration and the number of interactions for medical assistance. Intuitively, the longer the event, the more calls for service, but the authors' experience has also shown that participants can gradually fatigue, further dehydrate, become less rested (or nonrested) and testier, and, overall, less safety-vigilant. All of these factors can lead to medical calls requiring higher levels of care. For future planning or even real-time modifications and mobilization of resources, these trends should be identified, logged, and reported to organizers.

Public and personal hygiene issues also worsen. Even independent of that concern, there is a greater risk of communicable disease exposures especially with closely mingling, loudly singing participants and intoxication-driven shouting, physical contact, and also vomiting and defecation that remain unremoved from the site where they were deposited [9, 10, 14, 15].

When an event includes on-site camping that spans multiple days, demands for medical services can quickly become akin to operating a twenty-four-hour medical urgent care program for an entire small city. It should be expected, for example, that aside from event-related risks, patients will also present with exacerbation of their preexisting medical conditions, the severity of which can range from relatively benign to critical. While most of the participants at such events are typically young and healthy overall, the event itself cannot only contribute to exacerbating those underlying conditions for the subgroup of young and old with existing conditions, but as previously described, depending the locale and conditions, there are so many other potential health threats even to the young and healthy. Also, those with evolving illnesses may be more apt to seek help late in the evening and not necessarily during performances or socializing hours. Particularly when they have problems sleeping due to illness or injury, this may trigger the late night visit for medical help.

Therefore, the most feasible strategy in developing a medical plan for such a multiday camping-included event should indeed be analogous to setting up an urgent care facility or free-standing emergency center for a small city including:

- The presence of at least one qualified physician on-site at all times around-the-clock should be prioritized [8]. Preferably, staffing could be implemented using overlapping shifts for nursing, physician, and paramedic personnel assigned and the overall numbers of staff would be determined according to anticipated event volumes for each assigned shift, including surges 2 to 3 days in.
- The plan should involve a cadre of rotating event medicine doctors who are appropriately trained and experienced in evaluation procedures akin to emergency department (ED) medical screening exams (MSEs) [8]. Their related expertise, knowledge of regulatory issues, and also their understanding of the pragmatism of sparing in-hospital resources from a potential onslaught of otherwise manageable cases on-site is invaluable to the event and the community at large. Not only would they be capable of managing the acutely ill or injured as indicated, but they can also serve to appropriately determine and direct any necessary treatment and transportation protocols for the on-site medical teams.
- Most major events will have a lead physician at any given time alongside numerous others. While physician assistants are often well-versed in such triage and MSEs, the unpredictable nature of these events, certain regulatory stipulations and even the organizer's contractual and insurance riders may indicate the presence of locally licensed qualified doctors to assume these duties.
- Assurances that facilities will be adequately staffed, resourced, and stocked enough to manage all medical responses ranging from all minor requests for care to the ability to immediately stabilize critically ill or injured patients while designating and facilitating their expeditious transport to the nearest appropriate hospital for the indicated critical condition. In essence, the on-site facility will provide twenty-four-hour round-the-clock coverage and it will be able to perform at the highest level of care expected for such urgent care centers.
- Plans to have adequate (if not excess) supplies that can ensure management of all potential risks identified in the medical risk assessment such as naloxone and other opioid antagonists, but also to include a large supplemental stock for mass casualty situations including a considerable supplies of hemostatic devices (e.g., tourniquets and pressure dressings).

- A plan and protocol for managing on-site deaths including required actions for forensic examination, medical examiners' needs, and law enforcement oversight as indicated. They should also include plans for appropriate and compassionate notifications to next of kin, loved ones, and friends as indicated.
- High-level coordination and communications with incident commanders, organizers, security teams, receiving facilities, and transporting agencies as discussed in great detail in Chapters 4 and 20.
- As also indicated in Chapter 4, the role of accompanying friends, companions, or family members can be invaluable assets starting with eye-witness reporting about what happened to the patients and particularly those with altered mental status. They may also be of great value in terms of providing information about underlying conditions, medications, and past medical history let alone sociological information such as the patient's home location, next of kin, and contact information. In some cases, they can provide trusted reassurances to keep the somewhat altered patient calm and compliant with the care being received. They can also keep closer attention on the treated patient who is now only being monitored, freeing up the staff. Accordingly, arrangements for bedside seating, be it a stool or chair, should be considered. Of course, some companions can also be very confrontational, but most will be quite cooperative, especially when that friend or family member is treated with respect and provided appropriate reassurances and expectant timelines for the treat and release phases. Therefore, practical accommodations and/or a safe, nearby waiting areas for these companions should be routinely considered and built into the facilities.

Additional Special Risks for Long Duration Music-Related Events

Needless to say, guests at camping-related festivals will be living on-site for as many as four days or more [19–21]. During this time, they are not simply listening to music and then sleeping, but they are also consuming food, drinks, and, in some cases, consuming illicit drugs made available to them on-site despite questionable content, potencies, and formulations.

As mentioned previously, issues of compromised hygiene, sleeplessness, and dehydration can also compromise immunity and constitutional resilience. Food sources can be left out in heat and humidity without proper refrigeration by vendors (or others) or even arrive on-site under-refrigerated after traveling long distances. Foods brought in and not refrigerated as indicated can carry similar risks. Multiday outdoor events can increase and even accelerate those risks.

In that respect, it should be understood that as the duration of the event increases, the potential for widespread illness due to foodborne contamination and communicable disease is very possible [14, 15]. Despite promises of being fully compliant with the jurisdictional public health department stipulations, it takes only one popular food vendor to serve enough servings of tainted food to create a rapidly developing "multi-casualty" incident (MCI) that will place tremendous strains on the medical resources if not anticipated as a probable contingency.

This same "bad batch" concept is true for drug consumption. One bad consignment of illicit drugs can suddenly wreak havoc during a long duration event [11–13]. This frequent occurrence can even result in multiple patients suddenly presenting, almost simultaneously, to the medical team in respiratory or even cardiac arrest. Occasionally, early "word on the street" hearsay anecdotes about the available drugs on-site may have indicated good reviews and even accompanying encouragements to partake. Those socially driven peer recommendations can then prompt many others to indulge over ensuing days with the resulting proportional increases in the numbers of susceptible persons experiencing complications. Either way, a whole new batch of substances can also arrive at a later stage and the ingestion or inhalation of some undisclosed new "product" can also turn out to be near-deadly (or even deadly) for many attendees. Accordingly, practitioners should develop contingency plans to address a sudden drug mass casualty and this plan should include a reporting of this to event security and local law enforcement and event organizers for potential messaging. It also can include preemptive public services announcements and social media messaging in real-time when serious events are being detected either on-site or in the community.

Caring for Production Teams

For many music events, be they in traditional spaces or sprawling fields, medical coverage may be needed for days, or even weeks, before the actual entertainers or audience arrives on-site. Specifically, there are many high-risk jobs and tasks associated with transporting in and building the components of a music-related event. As part of an overall safety plan, medical coverage should be specifically requested for the assembly/construction and load-in phases of production as well as the disassembling phases. Some of the considerations and personnel involved include:

- Rigging workers who are typically working for lengthy periods from a position of height. Especially with high winds or high heat indices or prior related injuries, there is a potential for falls or for very serious medical emergencies that would require immediate attention to best prevent a deleterious outcome. In many circumstances, considerations for such contingencies might include specialized medical staff such as a cross-trained emergency medicine technician (EMT) firefighter who has confined rescue training (and experience) as well as high-rise rescue training and experience.

- The "steel" team, the workers who bring in and build the typical stage's backbone components. Similar to riggers, they may be working from a position of height as they assemble heavy steel structures, but also handle heavy parts with potential for crushing, impaling or blunt force trauma as well as inducing falls. Again, specialized heavy rescue personnel crossed-trained with medical capabilities are a key component for protecting those producing the mass gathering event.

- Backstage, back-line (under-stage), and back-of-house elements (as well as front of house consoles and lighting structure personnel). These various crew members can range from audio monitoring personnel, videographers, digital and electronic artists, information technologists, carpenters, lighting element persons, and the like. Even when working out of direct sunlight, some are still working in closed booths or under the stage in poorly ventilated areas. Such persons can become unsuspecting victims of a high-heat environment or trapped with an inadvertent structural collapse. As such, for all these personnel from riggers, steel, and back of house crews, "buddy systems" are strongly advised in addition to the usual high viz (high visibility) vests and hard-hat requirements.

- All crews members from the production office, promotion office, cafeteria, laundry, transporters, and all other "back of house" personnel can present with any type of ailment from sore throats, urinary tract infections and conjunctivitis to large carbuncles and abdominal pain. Despite these various afflictions or symptoms, many crew members are so dedicated to their respective jobs, that they are resistant to go off-site to seek treatment in these building phases, especially if there is a lengthy distance to medical care at a clinic or emergency department. Therefore, on-site physicians teams would be a much preferable route to manage this pre-festival phase. An alternative could be advanced level practitioners (nurse practitioners or physician assistants) who can perform or prescribe certain therapies or who are quite capable of reaching to appropriate physicians by telemedicine tools. Most of the time, however, actual on-site visits by a qualified physician are the usual norm.

- Especially during pre-event rehearsals or night-before sound checks, there may be the artist (or artists) on-site for whom expert medical consultation could be requested. The extraordinary nuances of dealing with such evaluations and visits with "VIPs" are detailed later in Chapter 14.

- Again after a performance, the disassembling (load-out) process may be even more tedious and risk-generating among exhausted production teams. As a result, some of this process may not even begin until the next day (or several ensuing days), thus extending the period for potential medical coverage.

- Similar to precautions for COVID-19 and other contagious diseases, medical personnel can also serve as public health officers or even as testing supervisors in such circumstances (as seen during the COVID-19 pandemic). Additional tasks can include recommending protections from cross-contamination in food lines (e.g., providing hand sanitizers, gloves for handling ladles) and other preemptive measures.

Clearly, having the proper personnel, necessary gear, equipment, and plans (such as hospital destinations) for these pre- and post-event tasks can be considered a very important aspects of mass gathering medicine in modern times.

Efficient On-Site Coverage Versus Contingency Planning

When developing the medical plan for music-related mass gathering events, the clinical practitioner should understand the total operational period as well as "system status management" staffing concepts. For example, it may require only two (or more) paramedics or cross-trained EMTs who understand and are trained in rescue operations during stage set-up phases and the same early on the day of the event (i.e., to attend to the production crews, caterers and arriving venue staff). One would *then* expect to have staggered and augmenting increases in medical staffing, including on-scene physician oversight on the day (or days) of the event prior to signaling of "doors" (opening the gates/doors to the event to the public). Depending on the event, the entire crowd may begin to enter at the same hour that the doors and gates open or the attendees may arrive over time with gradual increases accelerating steadily over the hours, peaking with featured performers in the evening. In those latter cases, as crowds increase and the day wears on, one can often expect much more medical traffic and staffing should be parallel and accommodate the expected medical traffic and response. The larger component should likely stay until very late hours but then it could taper off after crowds have departed. Also, using the medical risk schema, this staffing pattern may be accelerated if unusually hot and humid conditions are expected at an outdoor event during the daylight hours or if guests will be arriving en masse early in the day or if the nature of the event poses additional risks and especially considering the previously described additional risks posed in the latter days of a multiday event. Factors such as crowd behavior and crowd influence can certainly skew the actual resource needs disproportionately. As recommended, careful pre-event research should be conducted to determine any factors, new or old, that may skew the need.

Whatever phasing-in and phasing-out staffing configuration is determined, contingencies and back-up staffing plans need to be in place in case of sudden unexpected threats ranging from drug-related outbreaks, weather-related microbursts, and errant earthquakes to explosions, panic stampedes, and actual terrorist attacks. Furthermore, the concept of "it ain't over till it's over" is, historically, quite applicable to music-related events as evidenced by the May 2017 Manchester (UK) arena bombing of the departing Ariana Grande concert audience [4, 24, 27]. Many violent attacks or untoward incidents have occurred long after the performances have ended and entertainers have departed. Such malicious events can occur even when *most* (but not all) of the crowds have departed (see Chapter 20) [4, 24, 27]. Therefore, medical staffing needs will not end when the music's over.

Beyond the various risk injuries from inebriated departing attendees (falling or fighting) or blatant attacks upon outgoing crowds, there are still the remaining crews on-site who may be rapidly disassembling and moving out equipment, steel, and rolling storage boxes during load-out, another high-risk period for injuries. At the very least, regardless of the requested or contracted pre- and post-event coverage, adequate medical team support has to be available on-site from the time the guests arrive until the time the last guest leaves the space.

In terms of contingencies, there are multiple strategies including having many additional extra medical staff on-site who can attend and enjoy the main entertainment itself but still are "on-call" and prepared to respond as needed (i.e., not drinking and constantly monitoring their texts or other alert systems amidst the noise of the event). These medical personnel can be remunerated for their stand-by time or, more often, these top clinicians can be allowed to enjoy the music festivities at no cost as a guest of the production including the privilege of bringing a companion guest, be it a spouse, son or daughter, or, preferably, another medical colleague.

Plan B would be to place and maintain numerous other qualified medical personnel in the community in a similar "on-call" stand-by mode, but, in this case, they would not be on-site. The likely limitation with that approach is the potential for limited access if a yet-to-be-secured violent situation has occurred, if there are significant obstructions to access with peri-event traffic, or if the on-call teams lack the specialized credentials for the event. These credentials would therefore have to be issued ahead of time. Optimally, these back-up team assignments would include those who could arrive in their own response vehicles or those who could be prospectively assigned with EMS crews who could respond. There could also be a combination of plan A and B, but having additional high-level medical staff credentialed and on-site, ready to go to work is optimal. This approach is not only much preferred, but it is even better if the on-site physician(s) include the local jurisdictional medical authorities (physician medical directors) for the responding EMS ambulance system (i.e., 999, 911, 112, 000, 111, etc.) who can help to oversee ambulance routings, on-site MCI management, or help organizers with specialized information about best destinations/options for their artists, crews, and others who may need some type of specialized care or prescriptions.

Typical Experiences in Various Music-Related Mass Gatherings

As alluded to, every music event has event-specific factors that can impact the medical plan. Again, the type of music event can have major impacts on the scope of the medical operation and on the types of medical risks the practitioner should expect to encounter. Different genres of music bring with them different cultures and these cultures bring different medical risks. Electric dance music (EDM) fans typically espouse the "Love, Peace, Unity and Respect" philosophies and, in general, they follow directions and even abide by most safety policies. Not only is brawling very uncommon, but they rarely rush the stage and they typically do not consume a lot of alcohol. There is, however, a huge drug use culture with electronic dance music. A majority of the medical calls for service are directly related to consumption of various drugs ranging from hallucinogens to dangerous narcotics mixed with worrisome stimulants. Medical risk assessments of this event-specific factor will consistently identify drug-related illness, including life-threatening overdoses, among the highest risk. Medical responders, both those at the aid stations and those responding in the crowd, should carry appropriate antidotes and/or indicated treatment modalities.

Certain country music events lie at the opposite end of the spectrum. Alcohol consumption is typically excessive and related behaviors and sequelae are quite common and consistent. Brawling is common and the "projectiles" can also include frequent vomiting. Syncope from alcohol exacerbated by hot settings is frequent. In that respect, medical plans for a country music event may look moderately different from EDM plans. In either case, close coordination with police/security teams is key as well as allotment of special spaces for detoxification and possibly laceration repair and splinting.

Likewise, certain artists will attract specific age demographics and the behaviors and medical risks associated with that age group. An event featuring a 60s pop star will bring in an older demographic which in turn may present less risk related to intoxicant consumption, but perhaps an increased risk related to the individual's past medical history, disabilities, and mobility. Likewise, some music-related mass gatherings will attract a particularly younger demographic and gender. The majority of those attending a "boy band" concert would likely be young girls and women. While not a particularly risky group of attendees medically, the excitement of being in front of pop stars can, commonly, trigger syncopal episodes, hyperventilation, and anxiety-related conditions. Certain heavy-metal or punk rock groups can invoke traditional errant behaviors including mosh pits. Crowd crush incidents may have a certain degree of risk predictability for security and medical planners based on some historical factors with the type of event or artist. At the same time, a predictably low-risk event like the indoor Ariana Grande concert and its relatively benign attendee demographic can still experience an unexpected terrorist attack. In that respect, perhaps the most benign types of indoor arena events with a very young, healthy, and relatively well-behaved audience can be considered the very group terrorists might target (Chapter 20).

The Importance of Tracking All Requests for Medical Assistance

Most persons requesting aid will come to medical aid stations. In many situations, attendees may just ask for hydration (even just water bottles) for some dizziness or over-the-counter (OTC) medications for headache (e.g., acetaminophen) or even earplugs. When otherwise very busy with truly ill and injured persons, these requests may not need to engender a full medical assessment and report. However, medical providers rendering support and advice should still tabulate or annotate such requests to help inform future stocking needs, relevant logistics and planning, and even funding and risk management considerations for future events. Naturally, advice about where to get food or find a toilet does not fall within the specific realm of medical advice, but these frequent interactions should still be anticipated and managed with a knowledgeable, courteous, public service orientation as part of the overall positive experience being provided to guests attending.

The Unique Logistical Challenges of Responding in the Crowd

One unique challenge for the mass gathering medicine specialist is how to find, manage, retrieve, and transport persons becoming ill or injured in the crowd. In music events, it is usually quite dark during showtime

and there are thousands of cheering, shouting audience members amidst exceptionally loud entertainment and, of course, packed crowds with ill-defined locations (no defined section, row, or seat) in a general audience event on a field or stadium grounds. This creates great difficulty for a prospective patient or their accompanying companions or adjacent bystanders in terms of alerting security or medics about the incident amidst the encompassing throng and excessively loud entertainment. Responders finding them under these circumstances is the next challenge.

Many of these concerns are addressed in much greater detail in Chapter 4 including strategies for locating patients and retrieving them by using tools ranging from the implementation of new tracking applications (apps) and well-positioned spotter personnel. It also includes guidance on dealing with the ethical and practical concerns of interacting with superfans falling ill or becoming injured. After fainting or having a brief seizure or some other illness or minor injury, many devoted fans who have decision-making capacity will not concede to leaving their coveted positions in the audience for this long-awaited and special opportunity to see their favorite artist live.

In large crowds or more austere locations, standard mobile phones texts or internet use may be slow or inoperative altogether [18, 28]. More recently, specialized apps for geospatial locators have been introduced in some locales such as utilization of mobile apps such as the "What3words" app to assist rescuers in terms of pinpointing potential patients across widely dispersed sites [29]. These apps may have some of the potential limitations of standard texting in large audiences or austere conditions [18, 28]. Nonetheless, when these apps have been used, they have been shown, to date, to be capable of geolocating individuals within a three-meter square zone and do so almost anywhere on the globe using only three words. But even if located, incoming responders still need to reach those ill or injured persons under the same obstacles of packed crowds, loud noise, and/or distances from medical aid centers.

As noted, most patients present themselves to medical aid stations or are brought in by companions while others will be identified by bystanders or event staff. In some settings, designated event staff have been used as "spotters." Dedicated spotters can be particularly helpful, especially during musical festivals that allow on-site camping or events with high patient volumes such as those crowded events involving exceptional levels of alcohol consumption and those taking place over several days of high heat and humidity. Although usually nonmedical personnel, these spotters can assist with the medical reconnaissance and should also be trained to provide basic first aid with immediate lifesaving interventions, including hemorrhage control, CPR, choking procedures, and automated external defibrillator (AED) use. Protocols can be used to enable these individuals to support the medical staff when they identify potential patients, pinpoint their precise location, and begin basic first aid. They would also be knowledgeable about the location of the closest AED or bleeding control kits. Spotters may even fall under the auspices of embedded law enforcement or tactical teams that are already scanning and observing the crowd for suspicious behaviors and even possible criminal activities. Spotters should be strategically positioned, usually at an elevated position to have a wide view of attendees, while also being close enough to directly see the potential patients. Spotters can also be embedded within the crowd depending on audience density and event type. In all circumstances, spotters should be protected from the elements, including protection from precipitation, and provided with appropriate heating or cooling strategies.

Even before the event or doors opening, consideration should be given to patients located outside of the immediate event area or venue. Medical teams should preferably monitor for and identify patients in parking lots or in event queues. Long-awaited events will often be preceded by lengthy outdoor queues and sometimes these can extend for several days in a variety of challenging climates and without access to food and water. Therefore, event staff, spotters, or even medical personnel should also be positioned external to the event venue in areas where attendees are expected to congregate many hours, if not days, in advance. In certain unbounded events, external areas may involve significantly large geography. Mutual aid agreements between local jurisdictions and event personnel should be established a priori.

Protecting the Patients

As mentioned, many guests identified as having a potential illness or injury will be adamantly opposed to leaving their coveted spot in the audience or be taken away from any part of the entertainment. Especially when attendees paid dearly for premium passes or tickets and traveled from afar to attend a long-awaited evening with their favorite band, the resolve to decline care and even defer a standard medical evaluation will be strong. While understandable in many respects, this scenario can lead to difficult and often frustrating decision-making for medical professionals. This is additionally difficult in somewhat intoxicated persons who still have distinct capacity for decision-making. Also, evaluations can be difficult in the din of the event and when serious underlying medical conditions are not disclosed, especially in that public forum. As noted in earlier chapters, these psychological and emotional aspects of crowd demographics and dynamics have even become their own discipline of study. Be it modesty, impatience, or embarrassment, most of these patients will insist that he or she is "just fine." Receiving medical attention in public places is often rejected, especially when it involves a one-time-only cherished event. This reality should not only be well-understood and recognized, but appropriate tactics should be in place to compassionately manage these challenges and include sensitive strategies to enhance privacy, minimize the embarrassment and yet gain trust, while also keeping in mind that many of these interactions may be videoed by others. Again, such tactics are discussed in some detail in Chapter 4.

In contrast, if patients are successfully extricated from the scene, every effort should be made to shield patients from direct sunlight, opportunistic videographers, and any other elements including rain, sleet, and snow as well as taking care to avoid a rough transport over the given terrain.

Responding to Needs and Requests of the Artists and Crews

One particular challenge for the mass gathering medicine clinician is the need to respond to a medical need of the artists themselves or perhaps crew members. This unique nuance of music-related mass gathering medicine is well discussed in more detail in Chapter 14 discussing "VIPs," but some highlights are worth reinforcing within the context of the musical world.

First of all, local medical personnel will often be relied upon to provide recommendations for hospitals or clinics, including specialty care centers, or other healthcare resources, ranging from trauma, stroke, and cardiac care centers to endodontists, ophthalmologists, or otorhinolaryngologists of the highest quality and discretion. Accordingly, these identified resources need to be vetted and established well ahead of time with all efforts at discretion being maintained.

Above all, if asked to attend to the artist directly, one should sensitively assess the comfort level of the "VIP" who is now being evaluated by an unfamiliar person. Even if the responding clinician is a renowned and respected medical professional within the medical community at large, VIP encounters will often entail an entirely different realm of culture and expectations including the presence of others being in attendance as well. During the evaluation, the VIP may not be entirely open about underlying conditions and their chiefs of staff, publicists, family members may all insert themselves into what typically would be a private assessment between a clinician and a patient. It is therefore incumbent upon the local medical professionals to have patience, sensitivity, and situational awareness during each encounter and to adjust their level of engagement based on the VIP's comfort level, the acuity of the medical condition, and the understanding that the clinician's index of suspicion for undisclosed conditions needs to be high.

The medical professional should also be aware of typical reticence to concede to a hospital transport or even recommendations to receive further evaluation at the time of the event. Beyond personal stoicism or wanting to avoid disruption to tight schedules, transport will be perceived as something that will engender embarrassing news stories and social media speculation in this era of mass communication and optics. Therefore, one needs to first be patient, gain trust, and not attempt to use scare tactics to coerce the principal into accepting transport but rather use a more patient demeanor of diplomacy and perhaps some reliance on others to help with informed decision-making and encouragement as indicated.

Beyond the overriding protective, discretionary, and "optics" concerns for the principal involved, there are also similar attendant issues within the accompanying entourage. Declination of care or transport is also common among those serving the artists such as a longstanding touring crew member working for a popular entertainer and assigned to a pivotal task for the band. Unyielding loyalty will often override what would otherwise be appropriate standards of care and medical decision-making. Discussions on how to manage such scenarios are outlined in detail in Chapter 14. Such situations are not infrequent, and they can be unsettling and even angering for a prudent medical professional, but compassion and appreciation for the dedication to mission should still be respected.

Professional Standards and Ethical Challenges

Some artists, staff, or family members may request to see a medical professional for atypical or fad-promulgated treatment such as certain vitamin or hormone injections or unusual intravenous infusions. The practitioner may be asked to give some alternative therapy, pain medications, intimacy related pharmaceuticals, or anxiety/depression medications. Such medications may even have been prescribed by other doctors or a primary care physician either in the country of the event or in their home nation. Often, the requests may be filtered through surrogates (e.g., personal assistants). This circumstance is an unusually awkward situation for conscientious medical professionals when direct access to the requesting patient is not being permitted. Without the standard professional interaction, communication and evaluation regarding medical need and necessity, such second-party requests are not the norm in prudent medical case management and in most professional conduct codes.

Naturally, medical professionals wish to please every patient and none would want to disappoint any patient, let alone a famous person. Nonetheless, maintaining ethical standards and maintaining one's integrity in medical decision-making should always predominate. There are strategic and compassionate ways to communicate the reason for not granting the request when coupled with willingness to help in another way. Alternative solutions such as contacting the person's usual physician or referral to an appropriate local specialist may be suggested. In the end, one should consider the wise premise about whether or not they would administer the requested therapy to his or her own family members – and, pragmatically, also consider if their medical licensure (and source of livelihood) could be in the balance. Regardless of these ethical and philosophical issues, discretion and confidentiality is also always paramount. The mass gathering medicine professional must avoid any interaction with the media – or anyone else, including medical colleagues for that matter, if they are not directly involved in the case. If explicitly asked to make a public statement by the patient, their empowered family, or the patient-authorized representative, media commentary should always be provided with the explicit approval of what could be revealed. Again, suggested tactics are provided in Chapter 14 and in other commentary [25].

As a final comment, mass gathering medicine is an ever-evolving practice and many of the numerous concerns and tasks for clinicians have been well-outlined in this discussion even though it reflects only one special subcategory (music-related events). There are a myriad of other types of mass gatherings ranging from a spectrum of major professional sports events, high school crew regattas, and public holiday celebrations to mass gatherings associated with religious pilgrimages, massive refugee shelters, and large political protests, just to name a few. The incumbent threats will require an expertise that comprise a whole new level of competencies well-beyond the traditional "rock doc" image of old. These professional competencies may eventually require specialized training and mentoring akin those necessitating accredited fellowships and subspecialty board certifications now required for disciplines like sports medicine, EMS, and toxicology within the specialty of Emergency Medicine [9, 30]. Event medicine is clearly maturing as indicated by this textbook. The discussions in this chapter and throughout the other chapters clearly indicate, repetitively, an entirely new set of competencies, knowledge, and skills requirements for the medical practitioner. Specialized expert training and veteran clinical experience in this realm will clearly benefit the public at large and it will also better ensure the health, medical security, and safety needs for the many millions of persons attending mass gathering events each day worldwide [8].

References

1. de Almeida M. M., von Schreeb J. Human Stampedes: An Updated Review of Current Literature. *Prehospital and Disaster Medicine*. 2019;**34**(1):82–88. doi: 10.1017/S1049023X18001073 Epub 2018 Nov 27. PMID: 30479244

2. Macaya M., Mahtani M., Wagner M. (CNN). The Latest on the Deadly Astroworld Crowd Surge. November 8, 2021. www.cnn.com/us/live-news/astroworld-houston-crowd-surge-travis-scott-11-08-21/index.html. Accessed September 21, 2023.

3. CBS news report. Chaos, Stampede at Central Park Concert After False Alarm of Gunshots. September 29, 2018. www.cbsnews.com/news/global-citizens-festival-central-park-stampede-chaos-today-2018-09-29/. Accessed September 21, 2023.

4. Craigie R. J., Farrelly P. J., Santos R., Smith S. R., Pollard J. S., Jones D. J. Manchester Arena Bombing: Lessons Learnt from a Mass Casualty Incident. *BMJ Military Health*. 2020;**166**(2):72–75. doi: 10.1136/jramc-2018-000930. Epub 2018 Apr 6. PMID: 29626139

5. Lowe S., Tremlett G. Eta Bomb Scare Clears Madrid Stadium as Real Play Basques. *The Guardian*. December 12, 2004. www.theguardian.com/world/2004/dec/13/football.spain. Accessed September 21, 2023.

6. Lombardo J., et al. Las Vegas Metropolitan Police Department Report of the October 1 (2017) Mass Casualty Shooting (event number 171001–3519). August 2, 2018. pp 1–187. www.reviewjournal.com/crime/homicides/read-the-final-report-from-las-vegas-police-on-the-oct-1-shooting/. Accessed September 21, 2023.

7. Locoh-Donou S., Guofen Y., Welcher M., Berry T., O'Connor R. E., Brady W. J. Mass-Gathering Medicine: A Descriptive Analysis of a Range of Mass-Gathering Event Types. *American Journal of Emergency Medicine*. 2013;**31**(5):843–846.

8. Pepe P. E., Nichols S. Event Medicine: An Evolving Subspecialty of Emergency Medicine. In: *2013 Yearbook of Intensive Care and Emergency Medicine*. Vincent J. L. (ed.) Springer-Verlag: Berlin Heidelberg; 2013; pp. 37–47.

9. Yancey A., Luk J., Milsten A., Nafziger S. Mass Gathering Medical Care Planning: The Medical Sector Checklist. Publication of the National Association of EMS Physicians; 2017; pp 1–74. https://ncw-herc.org/wp-content/uploads/2020/09/NAEMSP_MassGatheringsChecklist-D1-.pdf. Accessed September 21, 2023.

10. Margolis A. M., Leung A. K., Friedman M. S., McMullen S. P., Guyette F. X., Woltman N. Position Statement: Mass Gathering Medical Care. *Prehospital and Emergency Care*. 2021;**25**(4):593–595.

11. The Recovery Village. Drugs at music festivals. April 23, 2022. www.therecoveryvillage.com/teen-addiction/drugs-music-festivals/. Accessed September 21, 2023.

12. Ridpath A., Driver C. R., Nolan M. L., et al. Illnesses and Deaths Among Persons Attending an Electronic Dance-Musical Festival – New York City, 2013. *Morbidity and Mortality Weekly Report* (MMWR) December 19, 2014;**63**(50):1195–1198.

13. Lin R. G., Hamilton M. These are the Stories of 29 Rave-Goers Who Died of Drug-Related Causes. *Los Angeles Times* July 5, 2017. www.latimes.com/local/california/la-me-rave-deaths-snap-htmlstory.html. Accessed September 21, 2023.

14. Abubakar I. P., Gautret P., Brunette G. W., et al. Global Perspectives for Prevention of Infectious Diseases Associated with Mass Gatherings. *The Lancet Infectious Diseases.* 2012;**12**(1):66–74.

15. Memish Z. A., Stephens G. M., Steffen R. P., Ahmed Q. A. Emergence of Medicine for Mass Gatherings: Lessons from the Hajj. *The Lancet Infectious Diseases.* 2012;**12**(1):56–65.

16. Curka P. A., Pepe P. E., Ginger V. F., Ivy M. V., Sherrard R. C., Zachariah B. S. Emergency Medical Services Priority Dispatch: *Annals of Emergency Medicine.* November 1993;**22**:1688–1695.

17. Levine R. L., Pepe P. E., Fromm R. E., Curka P. A., Clark P. S. Prospective Evidence of a Circadian Rhythm for Out-of-Hospital Cardiac Arrests. *JAMA.* June 3, 1992;**267**:2935–2937.

18. Bledsoe B., Songer P., Buchanan K., Westin J., Hodnick R., Gorosh L. Burning Man 2011: Mass Gathering Medical Care in an Austere Environment. *Prehospital and Emergency Care.* 2012;**16**(4):469–476.

19. Maleczek, M., Rubi, S., Fohringer, C., et al. Medical Care at a Mass Gathering Music Festival. *Wien Klin Wochenschr.* 2022;**134**:324–331. doi:10.1007/s00508-021-01856-5

20. McQueen C., Davies C. Health Care in a Unique Setting: Applying Emergency Medicine at Music Festivals. *Open Access Emergency Medicine.* 2012;**4**:69–73. doi: 10.2147/OAEM.S25587. PMID: 27147863; PMCID: PMC4753976 www.ncbi.nlm.nih.gov/pmc/articles/PMC4753976/. Accessed September 21, 2023.

21. Carlo P. The Electric Daisy Carnival: What It's Like to Provide Medical Coverage for a 400,000 Person Rave. *US Acute Care Solutions* publication. December 10, 2018. https://theshift.usacs.com/the-electric-daisy-carnival-what-its-like-to-provide-medical-coverage-for-a-400000-person-rave/. Accessed September 21, 2023.

22. Pepe P. E., Anderson E. Multiple Casualty Incident Plans: Ten Golden Rules for Prehospital Management. *Dallas Medical Journal.* November 2001:462–468.

23. U.S. Department of Health and Human Services (DHHS), Assistant Secretary for Preparedness and Response (ASPR) Technical Resources, Assistance Center, and Information Exchange (TRACIE). Mass casualty trauma triage: paradigms and pitfalls. July 2019; pp. 1–59. https://files.asprtracie.hhs.gov/documents/aspr-tracie-mass-casualty-triage-final-508.pdf. Accessed September 21, 2023.

24. Heaphy T. J., Garney T. T., Dine K. C., et al. Final Report: Independent Review of the 2017 Protest Events in Charlottesville, Virginia. *Hunton and Williams, LLP* report: pp. 1-207.

25. Pepe P. E., Pepe L. B., Davis R. M., Mann P., Whitmeyer R. EMS Physicians as Public Spokespersons. Chapter 15, Volume 2; Section II: Clinical Leadership and Oversight: Emergency Medical Oversight: In: *Emergency Medical Oversight: Clinical Practice and Systems Oversight*, 2nd Edition. Cone D. C., Brice J. H., Delbridge T. R., Myers J. B. (eds). Hoboken, NJ; Wiley and Sons, Inc.: 2015; pp. 146–159. Companion Website: www.Wiley.com\go\Cone\NAEMSP

26. Inverse. EDC Orlando Was a Win for the Harm Reduction Movement. www.inverse.com/article/23690-electric-daisy-carnival-orlando-first-hospital-edc-harm-reduction. Accessed July 23, 2022.

27. Pepe P. E., Metzger J. C. It Ain't Over Till It's Over: The Unfortunate Evolving Experience with Active Shooters. *Journal of Emergency Medical Services.* 2018;**43**:43–48 (special supplement on 2017 *Lessons Learned*).

28. Lund A., Wong D., Lewis K., Turris S. A., Vaisler S., Gutman S. Text Messaging as a Strategy to Address the Limits of Audio-Based Communication During Mass-Gathering Events with High Ambient Noise. *Prehospital and Disaster Medicine.* 2013;**28**(1):2–7.

29. https://what3words.com/products/what3words-app

30. Metzger J. C., Eastman A. L., Benitez F. L., Pepe P. E. The Life-Saving Potential of Specialized On-Scene Medical Support for Urban Tactical Operations. *Prehospital and Emergency Care.* 2009;**13**(4):528–531. doi:10.1080/10903120903144940

Mass Gathering Events: Motor Sport Events

Paul A. Kozak, Jeff Grange, and John Aguilar

Introduction

Motorsports is a broad term used to encompass use of motorized vehicles for racing or nonracing competition. Although motorsports are commonly thought of as several types of auto racing, they can also include motorcycles, go-karts, snowmobiles, boats, airplanes, trains, drones, hovercraft, lawn mowers, radio-controlled models, trucks, or any other motorized vehicle. Nonracing competition includes, but is not limited to, drifting, demolition derby, motorcycle trials, gymkhana, freestyle motocross, and tractor pulling. It is important to also recognize that motorsports will increasingly involve autonomous vehicles without traditional "race car drivers" in the future [1].

Motorsports medicine encompasses a unique body of knowledge and a skill set that is not currently available in other medical subspecialty training [2–4]. Since motorsports medicine generally involves care in the austere uncontrolled prehospital environment, it is considered a subspecialty of Emergency Medical Services (EMS) which is itself a subspecialty of Emergency Medicine. Motorsports medicine includes much of the field of EMS with the addition of the unique aspects of dealing with motorsports related injuries, illness, venues, and events. The evolving subspecialty of motorsports medicine includes but is not limited to the following:

○ Clinical Aspects

- Planning for all aspects of medical care (personnel, equipment, supplies, etc.) with an emphasis on initial treatment of emergency medical conditions with limited resources in an uncontrolled setting such as on a racecourse or in grandstands or in the middle of an off-road desert race

- Evaluation and management of participant injuries and illness
- Evaluation and management of spectator and other injuries and illness
- Organizing appropriate (BLS, ALS, CCT, etc.) transportation (ground, air, boat, etc.) of critical patients to appropriate facilities for definitive care
- Rehabilitation of injuries
- Preventive medicine to prevent injuries

○ Medical Oversight of System

- Coordinating with local hospitals, EMS, and public safety agencies
- Coordinating with sanctioning bodies and motorsports venues
- Supporting evidence-based motorsports safety equipment
- Post-crash investigations
- Negotiating and implementing a business plan
- Risk management
- Dealing with the media
- Educate and integrate other healthcare providers, racers, and others
- Participating in motorsports safety and medical research
- Optimizing/customizing the local healthcare infrastructure

Motorsport medicine is a unique version of Emergency Medicine. If the medical provider has been asked to participate in a motorsport event, he/she will be dealing with traumatic injuries, large crowds, and weather issues in a location that will be remote from the hospital. All the principles discussed will have a bearing on whatever form of motorsport that will be encountered, with some modifications.

Providing care at a motorsport event has changed drastically over the past few decades. Expectations are higher, bad outcomes more visible, and technology is pushing drivers to the limits of their endurance. In the past, medical care was an afterthought by most event promoters. Now, proper medical coverage and protocols need to be in place prior to most high profile motorsport events or "the show will not go on." This strategy does require planning ahead of time and this section will assist in preparation for this approach.

Motorsport racing has been a testing ground for technology since its inception. Innovations would appear first on the track and then show up in the civilian world.

Some examples of this include:

Four-wheel disc brakes

Hydraulic shock absorbers

Low pressure (balloon) tires

Torsion bar springing

Fuel injection

Turbocharging

Independent wheel suspension

Tire compounds

Synthetic oil and lubricants

As these innovations improve the vehicles' performance, the speeds have also increased. With an increase in speed has come a concomitant increase in kinetic energy. Over time, safety innovations have also advanced to protect the drivers. The very first winner of the Indianapolis 500, Ray Harroun, used the first rearview mirror in 1911.

We will discuss our safety considerations by breaking them down into:

1. Driver safety
2. Vehicle safety
3. Track safety
4. Spectator safety

Driver Safety

We can break down some driver safety issues by looking at:

1. Driver compartment
2. Firesuit
3. Head and neck restraint device
4. Driver physiology
5. Competency to drive

Driver Compartment

The driver compartments in Indy Car and in Formula 1 racing have the best conformation. The drivers can sit down in a bag of beads to get a seat that conforms exactly to their body. Because of this configuration, energy loads are dispersed across a larger surface area not just a few contact points. They have good lateral torso and shoulder support and good head impact protection. Stock car compartments have the driver in a more upright position and close to the steering wheel. There is less lateral support and seat designs have been improving the shoulder support. A carbon fiber seat has been made for a stock car configuration that resembles the Indy car tub and is now common. Extrication teams need to be familiar on how to remove the driver from these seats and will need access to carbon fiber cutting tools. Racing that involves jumps will put an axial load on the spine. There is controversy regarding increasing padding on the seats in this case versus having belts come loose in a rollover and has a been driver preference decision so far.

In the job of a track physician, it is highly recommended to inspect whatever vehicle will be on the track. Specifically, consider passenger impact areas. Where is the gear shift knob and is it able to hit the thigh? Is there netting or seat modifications to restrain the helmeted head? If not, cervical spine injuries are a concern. Seat belts need to be inspected and changed. Nylon belts will stretch 15 percent while polyester will stretch only 5 percent. With a significant impact, the stretching will weaken the belt. A two foot nylon belt will stretch an additional three and a half inches. The greater the stretch, the more the body will move out of position and increase possible injury. Most NASCAR

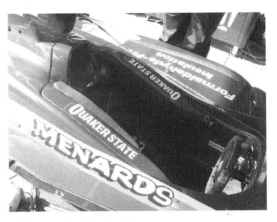

Figure 13.1 Indy Car Cockpit

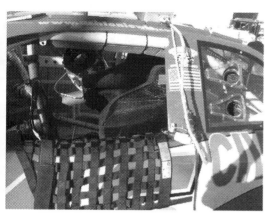

Figure 13.2 NASCAR Cockpit

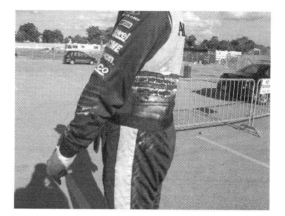

Figure 13.3 Fire damage to a driver's fire suit

Cup teams will change the belts every two to three races [5]. In a more grassroots, lower budget race circuit, the medical provider can anticipate longer periods of equipment use prior to replacement. Belts can melt from the friction energy of an impact and in-car video of crashes shows that belt stretch is a significant concern. Dumping of a belt occurs when there is a severe or asymmetric impact that separates and tears the belt fibers in a catastrophic failure.

If the medical provider is covering a motorcycle event, then a driver compartment does not exist. Attention needs to be directed to adequate safety gear on the driver and to what they would potentially strike on the track. Use of hay bales is common, and a driver can get lost in a fractured hay bale especially if it is on fire from a hot engine or brake part.

Firesuit

The firesuit is designed to protect its wearer from a flashover fire. It is not a superhuman skin that will allow a person to stand in a fire for prolonged periods of time. Suits are rated by the SFI Foundation in California for their Thermal Protective Performance (TTP). They are subjected to a "standardized fire." Each suit then has a patch on it to describe its rating. The higher the rating, the longer the fire exposure can be. Keep in mind, we are still dealing in fifteen to thirty seconds of time only. The best way to avoid injury is to never be in the fire in the first place. Multiple layers of a firesuit will trap air which will offer better protection. Just because the skin is not in direct contact with the fire does not mean injury is not possible. What can happen is the driver's sweat can become superheated and cause a steam burn. Any driver involved in a fire

needs to remove the firesuit to look for these burns as well as careful attention for any inhalation injury of fire, smoke, or fire extinguisher material.

Head and Neck Restraint Device

Head and neck restraint systems are currently mandated by Formula 1, Indy Racing League, and NASCAR. NHRA mandates them for their higher speed competitors. The purpose of the device is to limit the flexion and extension of the neck during a crash. This configuration is especially important as the head is weighed down with a helmet. Basilar skull fractures are caused by neck tension. The threshold for a basilar skull fracture is 4000N (Newtons – one pound of force = 4.448 Newtons). Sled testing has shown a significant reduction in these forces when a device is in place. One test developed 7000N of force in an unrestrained dummy and 1000N of force with a restraint device [6]. These devices are also evaluated and certified by SFI. Racing leagues do not usually recommend a certain device but do mandate standards that SFI tests for. Some examples of these devices would be the HANS or the Hybrid devices. When a race is in progress, it is important to examine what the drivers are using so the medical provider is familiar with removing them in the event of a driver extrication. Some drivers use a foam collar around their neck; this collar is for comfort only to support helmet weight and does absolutely nothing to protect the neck.

Driver Physiology

Many arguments have been made about whether drivers are athletes and books have been written on

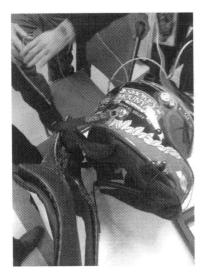

Figure 13.4 HANS device and helmet

the subject. One of the things that makes motorsport racing so popular is that we can all identify with driving. What we cannot identify with is driving at 200 mph, inches from other equally fast vehicles for hours at a time. The racing environment is truly brutal and high level competitors are gifted in their abilities.

Internal car temperatures of 120 degrees are not uncommon. Experiencing such heat for three hours while wearing a firesuit is very fatiguing and will produce dehydration. Conservative estimates of one liter of fluid loss per hour raced are very realistic. In-car rehydration systems are especially important during endurance races such as the 24 Hours of Le Mans. The tradition of drinking milk at the end of the Indianapolis 500 came from the fact that the driver was thirsty and hungry after four hours of driving. It is important to impress upon the competitors the importance of prehydration. They should be drinking more fluids for two to three days prior to the race. What is NOT recommended is prerace intravenous fluids. This treatment is commonly requested as the drivers feel it will prevent dehydration. Drivers have been known to be given letters from private physicians in other countries imploring medical staff to give their driver/patient a prerace IV. Ask the driver to imagine what his veins will be like after multiple punctures over multiple years. The analogy of "you can't fit more gas into your tank if it's already full" seems to work as well. If the competitor is ill with vomiting, diarrhea, and is tachycardic, then that is

a different situation. Watch for heat illness after long races in the summer months.

Vibration will also take its toll on a driver. It will result in muscle fatigue as well as mental fatigue. Many drivers relate that keeping in top aerobic physical condition will assist them with dealing with this fatigue. Telemetry testing during race conditions has shown heart rates in the 140–180 range. This tachycardia will occur for extended periods during the race only coming down for pit stops and race cautions. Each corner taken at race speed at the Indianapolis Motor Speedway will subject the driver to 4Gs (four times the force of gravity) of force. As they fight to turn against these forces, get progressively dehydrated, deal with the extreme heat coming off the pavement and their engines and the stress of driving at high speed in a pack of cars, it will get progressively harder just to pump blood into their head during a 4G turn.

Carbon monoxide has been a concern in closed-cockpit cars, but testing has not shown it to be an issue unless there has been considerable body damage to the vehicle during the race. At the end of a race, when a driver presents confused and injured after a crash, the medical provider must consider concussion, heat injury, and carbon monoxide in the equation.

Competency to Drive

At some point in time, the driver must prove that they can get on the track and have enough proficiency not to crash into other cars around them. "Rookie" driving tests will take them through laps at ever increasing speeds until the director of competition feels that they are ready to race. Prior to granting their competition license, every major sanctioning body has the driver get an annual physical. These physicals are usually provided by the driver's personal physician. This evaluation is done for liability reasons as the sanctioning body does not want to get into the health care business. Changes from year to year need to be discussed. At lower tier levels, there are many more drivers, so it is difficult to keep up on these changes. The Sports Car Club of America has a list of requirements. They have a medical board that will go over the physicals and have a form which they will send out to the driver's physician. A copy of this form can be seen at www.scca.com/assets/Physical.pdf. Diabetics need to prove tight glycemic control; seizure disorder patients need to be compliant with their medications and seizure free for a year; and drivers on warfarin need to know that they run a risk every time they strap on a helmet. Some organizations have let drivers on warfarin race, but for most upper-level racers, this treatment would be a contraindication to participation. Finding out that a driver is on warfarin should prompt contact with the sanctioning body. Any injuries over the previous year should be addressed to see if they have impaired the driver's ability on the track.

The most controversial of these injuries is the concussion or Traumatic Brain Injury (TBI). There is no clear cut pathway to evaluate concussion and best practices algorithms are continuously being revised. One method that has been helpful has been neuropsychological testing. Forms of this test that have gotten a lot of use have been the ImPACT (Immediate Post-concussion Assessment and Cognitive Testing) test (http://impacttest.com) and the King-Devick test (used by NASCAR). These can be done trackside rapidly on a laptop computer or smartphone application and are extremely helpful in assisting physicians with correlating the driver's clinical picture with some objective test. Ongoing research will hopefully help us to determine when staying out of competition is the only safe option. One site for up-to-date information on TBI is the Centers for Disease Control and Prevention website [7].

While discussing the subject of competency, we need to be certain that we as track physicians do not adversely affect the driver. Drivers and crew present with a myriad of various medical complaints when they come through the medical center, usually colds, allergies, or bad food from the constant traveling. Nondrowsy medications have been a great help. Always ask crew members if they will be over the wall during the race as making them drowsy from medication can result in serious preventable injury.

Vehicle Safety

Vehicle safety is a dynamic topic that technology keeps pushing forward. Every severe crash now leads to an examination of how we can do things better and make the sport safer. The concepts can be broken down into:

1. Car construction
2. Performance in a crash
3. Type of fuel
4. Speed of vehicle

Car Construction

The Indy Car chassis is a mid-engine vehicle with a normally aspirated V8 engine producing about 650–700 horsepower. The skin is mostly carbon fiber. The vehicle has three separate areas connected by high sheer strength aviation grade bolts and weighs about 1,550 pounds (driver and fuel not included). The tub with the driver compartment is what is entered into the race (as other parts have been known to fall or rip off in practice and qualifying). These three sections are designed to break apart during an impact to carry kinetic energy away from the driver. Video of crashes in the early 1900s show an intact, usually burning vehicle barrel rolling down the straightaway. The driver received the full brunt of the kinetic energy of the crash and often did not survive. In front of the driver's compartment, the nose cone provides a crush zone prior to reaching the driver's legs. In earlier models, the feet were in the nose and many foot and ankle injuries resulted. The driver sits in front of the engine. Behind the engine is an attenuator to absorb energy from a rear end impact. In the driver's compartment, the head surround is designed to limit head travel and absorb impact. The tub also conforms to the driver's body to spread out the force of impact.

The NASCAR chassis is a front engine vehicle with a V8 engine supplied by a four-barrel carburetor. It is a steel tube frame chassis with a steel skin and a minimum weight of 3,400 pounds (driver and fuel not included). Some lower tier levels will have

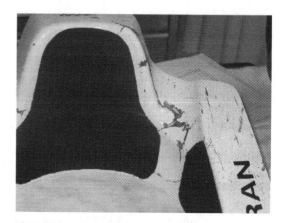

Figure 13.5 Damaged head surround from a rear impact

a fiberglass skin instead. The driver is more upright than his Indy Car or Formula 1 colleagues. The seat has been reinforced to provide more support to the shoulders and the head. Head containment straps or webs are used to keep the helmet from getting outside the seat structure to prevent neck injury. Both chassis rely on the steering wheel to stop forward motion of the head. NASCAR has attached tethers to the hood, trunk, and wheel assemblies to prevent them from becoming projectiles into other competitors or into the stands. IRL and Formula 1 have similar wheel tethers as well.

Belts have already been discussed but these are checked by the sanctioning body during prerace car inspection. Improper mounting and worn belts will be extremely dangerous for the occupant in a crash. Fuel cells will have a Kevlar bladder in them to help prevent puncture during a crash. Fire extinguishers in the trunk (by the fuel cell) and in the driver compartment will help with fire suppression giving the driver more time to extricate themselves. NASCAR has mandated energy absorbing foam in the vehicles side panels, moved the driver more centrally in the car, and enlarged the greenhouse to increase safety. Roof flaps will push the vehicle down if it is in a spin to prevent it from flipping.

Performance in a Crash

As mentioned above, the race vehicles are designed to break apart during a severe crash to disperse kinetic energy. Crash analysis and vector force measurements with accelerometers have given engineers a better appreciation for what happens in a crash and have been instrumental in advancing safety features. "Black Boxes" in the cars are accelerometers attached to the frame that measure "G" forces in the X, Y, and Z axes. One "G" is the force of gravity. It is a measure of force on an object. It was the first measure looked at to determine the severity of an impact. Another measure is the Delta "V" which represents "G" force over time. A body can sustain an exceedingly high "G" force impact without too much damage if it is over a short period of time. Impacts of 120Gs have been recorded to drivers without significant injury. Impacts over 50Gs have a higher likelihood of causing damage. If the G force is applied to the driver over a longer period, it results in a higher delta V and a higher probability of injury. The car's impact can have vastly different consequences depending on how it strikes the wall. A rear impact for a NASCAR vehicle is usually not a damaging event for the driver. The trunk provides a deep crush zone before forces reach the driver. In contradistinction, for the Indy car, a rear impact drives the engine into the back of the driver's seat. This mechanism will result in spinal injuries as the driver is vectored up into his heavy helmet compressing the spine. A front end impact for the Indy car has the nose cone to crush before reaching the driver's legs. The NASCAR front impact drives the engine into the driver compartment with a limited crush zone. Rallycross cars coming over a 130 foot jump need to preferentially land with either front or rear wheels first. If all four hit at once, the suspension (three to twelve inches depending on the series) rapidly bottoms out sending an axial shock wave through the driver's spine.

At the Daytona 500 on February 18, 2001, Dale Earnhardt got turned and crashed into the wall of Turn Four. As he turned, his belt ripped, and he was driven forward into the dash. His head was moved to the right and down and his left posterior head was felt to have hit the steering wheel in the occipital area causing a basilar skull fracture. The car hit at a 55–59 degree angle which did not allow for much deflection by rotation. The full brunt of the impact went into the car. It was a 47G force over 80 milliseconds for a Delta V of 42–44 mph [8]. This amount of energy corresponds to driving a car into a brick wall at 44 mph and having it come to a complete stop. Dr. Dean Sicking from the University of Nebraska and Delphi reenacted this event on a crash sled. The neck tension needed to create a basilar skull fracture is 4000N (Newtons). This Delta V can create the 4000N force. A HANS device on the crash test dummy in the same crash reduces the force to 1000 N [6].

NASCAR safety engineers made some recommendations that evolved into the "Car of Tomorrow." The car a has larger greenhouse with more support, wing changes were made to slow the car down, the seat was moved more centrally, and energy absorbing foam was placed in the side walls.

Type of Fuel

Methanol is the fuel used in Indy cars, gasoline in NASCAR. When an Indy car crashes, the visible fireball results from the oil and not from the fuel. Methanol burns with a clear flame that is about six foot high. The boiling point is 64.7 degrees Celsius (148.46 °F). These physical properties mean that the fuel turns to vapor on the hot pavement. Since the vapor is heavier than air, it moves out along the pavement until a spark ignites it. It is miscible in water, so a methanol fire is contained and extinguished by diluting it in water [9].

If PPK powder or CO_2 is used to extinguish fire, it will put out the initial flame, but another spark will reignite it. Medics and physicians who respond on track must be in firesuits to protect the rescuers. They look for the heat shimmer of the invisible methanol flame, bubbling paint, and if the driver is swatting at invisible flies – it is probably because he or she is on fire. One Indy driver cared for noticed that the electric wires on his control panel caught fire on the straightaway during practice for the Indy 500. He stopped the car and flipped up his visor to get some air. He then realized he was in a methanol fire, there was no air, so he flipped down the visor and barrel rolled out of the cockpit. He sustained some thermal burns to his hands and face. The pressure release valve on the engine behind him, popped off and sprayed methanol up in the air, down into the cockpit.

Gasoline is a more familiar fuel. The biggest issue seen at the track is that racing octane is higher than normal fuel and very irritating to the skin. NASCAR gas men usually wear heavy reflective metal surfaced aprons to protect them from the gas. If the gas gets on the firesuit and soaks into the skin, it causes a severe chemical dermatitis. The crew member usually ends up in the med center stripping down because his thighs feel like they are on fire. Soap and water debridement, Vaseline or bacitracin ointment, and ibuprofen are usually the answer. Splashes in the eye require Morgan Lens lavage and a soothing ophthalmic ointment.

Speed of Vehicle

As technology pushes the envelope on how fast the car evolves, the driver evolves at a much slower pace. This imbalance in safety evolution was really made evident when the Firestone Firehawk 600 race at Texas Motor Speedway was cancelled by CART medical director Dr. Steve Olvey in 2001. The drivers were noted to be dizzy after extended practice laps in the car. They were hitting speeds of 230 mph but the speed, in combination with the degree of banking, was subjecting the drivers to sustained combined G forces of about 5Gs for two-thirds of a lap [10]. Man had reached the crossroads of either slow the cars down or put the drivers in compression G suits. It was a tough but necessary decision for Dr. Olvey to make. He probably saved someone's life that day.

Track Safety

As we devise ways to make the cars safer, we can also look at ways to make what they drive on safer as well. Looking at track safety, we can discuss track construction, safety personnel, and communications.

Track Construction

The greatest leap forward was the fence. In early motor racing and currently at rally racing, there was/is no barrier between the race and the spectators. A pit wall was not put in at Indy until 1938. Remember, the first race there was in 1911. The most recent great advance has been the SAFER wall. The Steel and Foam Energy Reduction (SAFER) barrier was developed at the Midwest Roadside Safety Facility at the University of Nebraska-Lincoln by a team of engineers led by Dr. Dean Sicking. It was first installed at the Indianapolis Motor Speedway in 2002 [11]. It consists of rows of rectangular steel tubes welded together and backed by pyramids of polystyrene foam. At first glance, one might think that the foam absorbs the energy, but that is not so. The weight of the steel absorbs the energy, and the foam just helps it get back into shape so we can resume racing. Consider it as a heavy, moveable elastic wall before coming in contact with the immovable concrete one behind it. The best representation of its effect is in the comparison of two NASCAR crashes at Richmond International Speedway a year apart. In 2003, Jerry Nadeau crashed into the outside wall between Turns 1 and 2 suffering head, lung, and rib injuries. The crash ended his racing career with a 140G impact recorded by the car's accelerometer [12]. A year later, the SAFER barrier was installed at the RIR track. Jason Keller hit the wall going the same speed at a comparable angle but walked away without a scratch. The accelerometer reading revealed that the kinetic energy of the Keller crash was half that of the Nadeau crash (personal communication with Steve Peterson-NASCAR crash investigation team). The SAFER barrier was installed at Phoenix International Speedway (the lead author's track) in 2004. It will not prevent all fatalities at a racetrack, but it has had a remarkable "history" since its inception.

The catch fence is also an important piece of safety equipment. Its job is to reflect debris back onto the racing surface and away from paying customers. It is reinforced by heavy steel cables to support the weight of a car and should have the web fencing on the inside of the supports not the outside. If it is the reverse, not

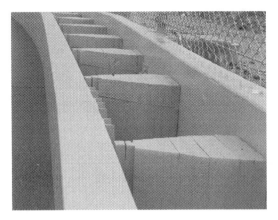

Figure 13.6 SAFER barrier

only will the race car get stuck on a support if it hits it, but the metal twist ties are also the only thing keeping the car out of the stands. Any gate out onto the racing surface needs to be reinforced to sustain an impact. At Bristol Motor Speedway at a NASCAR Busch Series practice in August 2002, Mike Harmon struck a gate that was not completely secured and ripped his car apart. He miraculously walked away with only a bruised right side, but it is now common practice to have someone to check every gate prior to any on-track activity as a result [13].

The track surface must be seasoned prior to an event. The down force of the cars creates a suction effect underneath them which, when combined with the friction forces of the tires above, can pull chunks of asphalt up. This track damage happened at the Las Vegas Motor Speedway during a Professional Sports Car event when the cars were driving over one-week-old new pavement and tearing it up. The condition of the track has put races in jeopardy several times over the years with widening heat cracks, ground water leaks, or from melting from a fire directly overhead. At the February 2012 Daytona 500, Juan Pablo Montoya's car crashed into a jet dryer that was cleaning the track during a caution lap. The crash tore a hole in the fuel tank, spewing burning jet fuel all down the track. It took two hours to clean up and determine that the track (which was new) was safe to race on [14].

Stand construction can come into play as well. Nice wide aisles are easy to move people back and forth. An exit ramp at the back of the stand as well as bottom can make it much easier to evacuate spectators in the event of a piece of car getting into the stands or incoming tornado. No parking under the

stands can be allowed in the post-9/11 world which has changed large event planning as well by bringing the introduction of daily sweeps by bomb sniffing dogs. Spectators need someplace to get out of inclement weather or to cool off in sweltering heat. Mist machines and fans to move air as well as tents for shade can help achieve this. One hot summer Brickyard 400 race at Indy had patients in air-conditioned buses to cool off. This addition was a great idea until one fan vomited in the enclosed space making it essentially unusable. Tents with cooling stations have worked out better.

Safety Personnel

There are an army of people behind the scenes at a race, who contribute to its safe and smooth running.

Approach to Medical Care

Every motorsport event is different. The approach to setting up medical care for a particular event depends significantly on the type of event/race, the location, the expected weather, the anticipated spectator and other attendance, the construction of the vehicle, unique safety equipment, the age and health of the participants, the presence or absence of human racers, proximity to trauma centers, etc. For instance, planning for a 1,000-mile-long race through the desert and open public roads such as the Baja 1000 versus planning for a race at a fixed motorsports venue with state-of-the-art barriers to protect spectators is extremely different [15]. The fixed motorsports venues typically have all the modern accoutrements with proximity to major trauma centers while the Baja 1000 has limited or no preexisting emergency medical services with transportation times to a major trauma center measured in hours and sometimes days. While racers are typically at highest risk for severe injury at major motorsports venues, the opposite is true for races held in the less controlled settings such as off-road races where the spectator is at the most risk for death and injury.

The approach to setting up medical care for a motorsports event is typically two-pronged. First, the spectators, crews, and other nonracers must be prevented from injury whenever possible. Much of the planning for medical care of spectators and others is analogous to many mass gatherings and depends on the crowd size, weather, type of venue, etc. [16–19]. Particular attention and planning, however, must focus on keeping race vehicles and/or parts separate from the spectators. Numerous spectators have been killed at motorsports events when they have been hit by vehicles and/or debris from race vehicles [20–22]. Major motorsports venues are able to plan and build permanent barriers to minimize the chance of spectator injuries but may not eliminate these risks entirely. Races held in the desert or other uncontrolled settings are not able to mitigate these risks to the same degree necessitating different approaches to planning.

Second, a detailed plan for a rapid response to a crash site with immediate provision of an advanced level of emergency medical care for racers is critical. Since procedures beyond the scope of practice of other healthcare providers (e.g., surgical airways, amputations) may be required, a board certified emergency or EMS physician is preferred when available. The nature of any motorsports event medical action plan varies depending on the facilities (if any), on-site response vehicles, medical staffing, and other unique issues.

Facilities at a motorsports event vary significantly. For instance, a permanent motorsports facility that routinely hosts sanctioned races by NASCAR, IRL, NHRA, Formula 1, and so on, will typically have a designated Infield Care Center with highly trained emergency personnel and state-of-the-art equipment. Such facilities are usually staffed with emergency medical technicians (EMTs), paramedics, nurses, and emergency physicians with the equipment, medications, and supplies typical of most large hospital-based emergency departments. The National Fire Protection Agency publication, NFPA 610: Guide for Emergency and Safety Operations at Motorsports Venues offers an excellent detailed map for planning at such venues [23].

Considerations for Care of Spectators

The primary objective in planning for on-site medical care at a motor sports event is to prevent overwhelming the transport capabilities of local EMS agencies and the resources of local hospitals by providing the capabilities to treat minor injuries on-site [24]. This important objective is accomplished by anticipating and preparing to treat the most commonly encountered injuries of spectators at motor sports events and appropriately triaging patients for transport for further work-up and management in the emergency department. If an event is a recurring one, it is often helpful to base preparations on prior after-action reports or event summaries to have an approximation of anticipated patient volume, patient acuity, common diagnoses, and medical supplies utilized at prior events.

An additional variable that should be considered when planning for patient volume and acuity at a motor sports event include considering weather effects for events held outdoors. Extremes of weather and a higher heat index can produce hazardous results to spectators at an outdoor event increasing patient presentation rates at on-site medical care facilities. Some recommended mitigation plans include adequate preparation for the extremes of weather (i.e., ice baths and cooling stations for hot weather, warming stations for colder weather, etc.). It is unknown exactly how the presence of alcohol influences the patient presentation rates at an on-site medical facility, but it has been seen to increase patients' needs. Should alcohol sales be present for the event it is recommended to allocate an appropriate space and resources to allow patients to achieve sobriety in a monitored though private area [25, 26].

A five-year retrospective analysis of patient presentations of an outdoor race circuit that averaged nine events annually with approximately 41,800 in attendance demonstrated that 21 percent of the patient presentations consisted of spectators. The three most common complaints treated were insect envenomation (i.e. wasp stings), lacerations, and soft tissue injuries [27]. In comparison in another retrospective review of the Indianapolis 500 mile race, over 8 consecutive races that had an estimated 400,000 people in attendance had intoxicated patients, lacerations, and acute exacerbations of preexisting conditions as their three most common presentations [28]. Some more rare though unique and catastrophic patient presentations of spectators at a motor sporting event may include isolated trauma secondary to an on-track accident.

In addition, for anticipating routine medical care of minor injuries one should consider the potential for a mass casualty incident involving the racetrack and surrounding area. Potential mass casualty incidents unique to a motor sports events can include the potential for trauma secondary to stray debris from an on-track crash, an uncontrolled vehicle into the crowds, a grandstand collapse, or inappropriate ventilation for indoor events leading to accumulation of toxic gases.

Spectators come to large events in various levels of preparation. Some know what to expect and come prepared ... others do not. Some wear multiple layers of appropriate clothing ... others do not. Some keep hydrated with large amounts of nonalcoholic fluids ... others do not. Some tracks care for spectators as well as participants. Crowd size is one variable that one needs to consider. Phoenix Raceway will have about 125,000 visitors pass through its gates on a race weekend. The Indianapolis Motor Speedway may have in the ballpark of 250,000. The logistics of managing these numbers is very impressive. Everyone needs a place to sit, something to drink, a hot dog, and somewhere to go to the bathroom. Think about it for a minute. Where do we let a good sized city park their cars for a day to enjoy the event? The number of support staff will change depending on the crowd size. It will never cease to be amazing regarding the sheer size of the crowd and how everyone gets home at the end of the day. Alcohol will certainly increase the number of patient contacts. Weather also has an impact. One race resulted in dealing with 90 degree Fahrenheit heat during the day while practice sessions were going on with spectators dropping like flies from the heat. A rain shower passed through, and spectators were dancing in the rain in relief. Then the sun went down resulting in a rush of wet hypothermia patients by the end of the night. Severe weather presents a more pressing problem. One Indy 500 ended with an announcement of tornadoes in the area and evacuation of anyone left in the stands. Most of the local fire safety crews for the track raced off to rescue patients from a nearby nursing home whose roof got ripped off. Fortunately, it was after the race had ended and most spectators had already cleared the stands. One of the authors watched a funnel cloud pass north of the track while observing from Turn 2. Sturdy metal stands will offer some shelter from heat, rain, and hail but not a tornado. That requires a meteorological early warning system and evacuation. Wood seats have been a bane in the past. Usually found in temporary stands, the medical team will be digging large splinters out of the back of spectator's thighs as they slide down to make room for someone else. Traffic control is another factor that can make or break a track's reputation. The track physician is there to help everyone have a safe and enjoyable time – an asset to the track. If someone got a gust of dust in the face, they may just need an SVN and a place to sit for a while so they can go back and enjoy the rest of the day. Track physicians provide organization, first aid, and early resuscitation. Lab work and radiographs need to go to the hospital. We do what we can for the teams and officials in the infield who spend most of their time on the road. I will put in sutures for a crew member who catches his hand on sheet metal with the expectation that my counterpart at next weekend's race will take them out. Blood pressure or chronic medication refills (not narcotics) are part of this service as well. This service is not offered to spectators so they can access their usual medical follow-up. They go home after the race. If the injury was caused by something at the track (like the splinters), we will transport to the infield medical center to care for it as best we can.

September 11, 2001, changed all our lives forever and large event planning is no exception. Any large gathering of people, especially on live national TV, can be considered a potential terrorist target. Recall the World Series in Phoenix when President Bush threw in the first pitch. There were F-16s circling overhead and manhole covers welded shut in the street. We have had updates by local police authorities to keep us up to date on Homeland Security issues. Airspace control is important as a crop duster over the stands could create a panic to rival any soccer match or "The Who" concert even if it were spewing water not a toxin. A car in the stands could also create an accidental disaster. A small area of packed stands holds many people in a vulnerable position as they cannot move quickly out of the way. The track physician will need to work in concert with local authorities and have a disaster plan in place. Hold practice disaster drills out at the track. If it were to happen, would we shut down the race or let the show go on? There have been arguments that out of respect for any injured spectators, the race should be shut down. I vehemently disagree. It is necessary for the other spectators to remain in their seats, not obstructing roads that require being open to allow resources in and injured patients out to the trauma center.

Medical Staffing

Planning for medical staff at motorsports events should focus on two primary issues: (1) the ability to provide the highest level of care as soon as possible following a major trauma and (2) preventing unnecessary patient transfers to hospitals to prevent overwhelming the local EMS system. While EMTs, paramedics, and nurses are invaluable toward meeting these goals, most regulatory authorities require at least one board certified emergency physician or EMS physician on-site to provide medical care and system oversight. At least one prospective study at a large motorsports event demonstrated an 89 percent reduction in hospital transports with on-site physicians [29]. Medical personnel at a track are usually going to be practicing Emergency Medicine physicians and nurses. Surgeons with trauma experience are also seen. The Medical Director should, however, match that description. The reason is that, for the weekend, the track physicians are caring for a good-sized city of 50,000 to 200,000 persons with all their usual illnesses. Add some alcohol and trauma, it can get challenging. Past scenarios have involved pediatrics ("Little Johnny is all floppy, we took him out of the Peds ICU for his asthma to watch the race, but he will not respond to the SVNs we have given him in the stands"); obstetrics ("My water broke with 50 laps to go but I didn't want my dad to have to leave since I bought him tickets and flew him out for the race"); cardiology (at least one transport or code per weekend); endocrinology (thyrotoxicosis, hypoglycemia); neurology ("He was cooking fries on the deep fryer when he had a seizure and hit his head on the side of the fryer … he was lucky he didn't land face first in the oil"); gastroenterology (bad burrito versus cholecystitis); dermatology ("What's this rash? I've had it since the Daytona race" (three months ago)); ophthalmology (metal grinding in the garage); and even entomology ("I drank my soda and swallowed a bee. It bit me on the tongue"). Emergency Medicine practitioners are also familiar with disaster drills and interacting with prehospital personnel, fire, security, and law enforcement. Each track needs to be individualized to meet local needs. Weather in the Poconos dictates a ground transport backup for the helicopter, location around an Army chemical depot means a decontamination plan at the Talladega track. Daytona is adjacent to an airfield which mandates strict airspace control. Milwaukee is less than a mile from a Level One Trauma Center. Each track has its own challenges. How far away is the transport time? Is it more logical to scoop and run to the closest trauma center or put the chest tube in first if the flight time is over forty-five minutes?

Helicopters

Helicopters have been employed to provide medical support at larger motorsport events for many years [30]. Although there is no standard or uniformity of approach to such use in the medical literature, many case reports have advocated for helicopters at any high-risk motorsport events if transport times to a trauma center can be significantly decreased. The prolonged transport times may be related to either traffic congestion surrounding large events or the prolonged distance to a trauma center. At least one ten-year description of motorcycle racers injured at the Isle of Man demonstrated decreased mortality with the use of helicopters [31]. The costs of helicopter coverage have skyrocketed. Initially, the company would stage at the track, so they got national TV coverage every time the camera panned over the infield. Now it can run upwards of $100,000 for the weekend. It will become rarer to have a helicopter staged at an event for this reason but may require being requested for the reasons mentioned above.

Considerations for Care of Drivers

Planning for provision of on-site medical care at a motorsports event requires knowledge and anticipation of certain unique challenges faced that are distinct to the sport. These unique challenges are apparent when considering how to provide medical care for drivers on a race circuit. One of the initial primary considerations is scene safety given the many different hazards that could be present. These include but are not limited to other drivers continuing the race, instability of a damaged vehicle, potential for fire, electrocution, and exposure to other hazardous materials (i.e., oil, toxic fumes). The possibility for these hazards to be present stresses the importance of having appropriate resources available to aid in managing an incident alongside medical providers. An additional consideration is the substantial risk for a mass casualty incident with on-track accidents given the high speeds and proximity in which drivers will be racing [3, 32]. It is recommended that a triage system be established to facilitate the identification of the driver who needs the most immediate medical attention should an accident involve multiple vehicles.

Once an injured driver is identified the next hurdle to address is how to gain access and extricate the patient from the driver compartment. In some accidents the driver will be able to self-extricate from the motorized vehicle. If they are unable to self-extricate, extrication efforts will need to be performed. The relationship between the on-site extrication team and the medical team should be seamless to facilitate providing the best medical care as quickly and safely as possible. It is imperative for the on-site medical providers to have some familiarity with the driver compartments before the race begins. This knowledge aids in anticipating challenges to extrication and in predicting certain injuries based on the configuration of the driver compartment.

Primary trauma assessments and management should be immediately initiated once a healthcare provider gains access to the patient. It should be noted that patient assessments (i.e., continuous pulse oximetry) and certain treatments (i.e., oxygen, intranasal medications, selective spinal immobilization) can be initiated during the extrication process should it be safe to do so. These assessments and treatments should be performed in communication with the extrication team to not impede their efforts. Due to the mechanism of injury of a high speed motor vehicle collision the most concerning injuries involve head trauma and cervical spine injuries. It is imperative to understand the implications of the gravitational forces at play and their propensity to cause intracranial and cervical spine injuries [33, 34, 35]. Historically burns from vehicle fires were a common cause of morbidity and mortality at motor sports events. With the implementation of new safety regulations and technology an improvement in preventing these injuries has been seen, though it is recommended to keep these injuries in consideration when assessing a critically ill driver. Other considerations that may factor into care for a driver on the race circuit, though in the ideal world should not affect patient care, can include the potential for a livestream of the race where the care provided is being recorded or the driver wanting to continue the race or make the appearance of walking off the field.

Track Response

Rapid response to injured racers and spectators at motorsports events is necessary to minimize morbidity and mortality at motorsports events. Accessing injured racers in a timely manner frequently requires customized vehicles when a standard fire truck and ambulance is unable or inappropriate to quickly access a racing incident. Examples of such vehicles include modified 4WD ambulances, UTVs, ATVs, rail buggies, snowmobiles, boats, and so on. The track physician also needs to be ready to respond out on the track. Any medical staff that will respond onto a "hot track" should also be extensively trained and outfitted with all appropriate safety gear such as a firesuit, boots, ear and eye protection and so on to

protect them from injuries. Analysis of crash response has made a significant impact on track procedures. A fatality that occurred at the track during a practice session at Phoenix International Raceway in February 1996 is one such event. Looking at the footage revealed a lot of mistakes that have been acted upon. First off, the physician was resuscitating the patient in a polo shirt and jeans. Firesuits are now mandatory for anyone on the track surface after that event. The resuscitation was during a qualifying session and was performed on the track holding up tarps to shield the spectator's view. Now we transport immediately to the care center to clear the track and get safety personnel back to a safe area. The TV footage from the long lens went through the front window of the ambulance where it was obvious that CPR was in progress. Media has eyes everywhere and the patient should be out of the photo lens during a time like that. Now, when the physician is called out onto the track a whole ballet is initiated. The physician, now in a firesuit, will respond in a specially designated vehicle to the scene. The doctor has a jump kit/difficult airway kit with them in case the need arises. Each kit should match what the physician is comfortable with. The doctor is in constant radio contact with the race dispatcher who is watching from the control tower. That way, if an unsafe condition arises or more help is needed, it can immediately be called in. Everyone who sets foot on the track surface should be in radio contact with the control tower for those same reasons. The doctor gets an on scene report from the paramedic who called for them and the patient gets transported from the track surface while resuscitation is commenced. Once at the helipad or infield care center, IV access and the airway are secured prior to transport. After the helicopter has lifted or ambulance has cleared the track, the track doctor will call the trauma center to give a report to the trauma team. While this notification is happening, the track will make sure the patient's family is informed and can get to the hospital. We provide a police escort to the freeway if needed. Officials from the race sanctioning body are notified of the patient's condition (all drivers sign HIPPA forms to allow the race officials to be notified of the driver's condition). The car is impounded by the sanctioning body so a crash investigation can be started. The coroner would be notified to be available in case of a fatality. At the end of the day, a briefing will take place with all officials, track safety, and medical personnel to examine the event and discuss what could be done to make things smoother in the future.

Jump Kit Contents

No brand endorsement is made. This list is just one example from Phoenix Raceway [5].

Each kit should be tailored to the individual physician's practice

ILMA-Intubating Laryngeal Mask Airway

IGel obturator airway #4

Surgical cricothyrotomy kit (#11 scalpel, skin hook, Trousseau dilator, hemostat, various

Shiley trach tubes or cuffed pediatric endotracheal tubes

Bougie

Oral airway

SOFTT tourniquet

EZ IO intraosseous infusion system

etomidate

lidocaine

succinylcholine

Deaths

Motorsports is a high-risk endeavor and inevitably can lead to tragic injuries and death. On-track deaths can create public spectacles if a plan is not in place with the local coroner or regulatory agency. Although it is unlikely that any driver would be pronounced dead rather than being resuscitated and transported, the possibility of an obvious death such as a racer being incinerated or decapitated must have a plan. Planning meetings must include local representatives with authority to move a body to prevent such spectacles and to be respectful of the injured or dead while protecting any investigations in the future. It may also be important to have a plan regarding who can cancel a race due to such incidents with the understanding that cancelling a race may do more harm than continuing the event to allow emergency response to the incident to continue rather than create gridlock from ending the event.

The medical director should make it a point to get to know the medical examiner that has jurisdiction at the track prior to any event.

Concept of Traveling Doctors

What about the model of a traveling safety team with doctors, nurses, and paramedics? Well, it is comforting for the drivers to see familiar faces. Most sanctions do have some form of medical team liaison that are familiar with the drivers and their issues. It is impossible however, to have personnel licensed to practice in every state and/or country that a sanctioning body holds a race in. NASCAR has 100 races in its top 3 tiers alone, often racing in different tracks on the same weekend. The other issue addresses the need for actively practicing medical personnel. If the NASCAR paramedic has spent the last year traveling from race to race and has not placed an IV since, is that the best person to be handling an IV on a Level One Trauma patient? The local doctors, nurses, and medics are needed to know the contacts and vagaries of the local system and they need to be good at what they do daily. They do need some form of orientation to the track. NASCAR comes to the track to put on a course to get safety personnel up to speed on issues such as where to park the rescue truck during a crash, to always keep two persons on the stretcher so it does not run down the embankment into another race car on national TV, what are some of the latest safety equipment that that will be encountered, and so on. We have periodically held training at the track for fire suppression and using the hydraulic tools (Jaws of Life). All our Safety team members are actively working firefighters although it has not always been that way. It takes a balance between local talent and the national race sanctioning body to make everything work seamlessly together.

Communications

Everyone with their feet on the track surface needs to be on a headset with direct radio contact to the race control dispatcher. Radio control and communication are also essential with other medical personnel stationed around the track. We have physicians stationed on the outside of the track to give assistance to spectators. They are on a different radio frequency than the people on the racing surface so as not to clog up the airways. A command center monitors these calls and assists getting the correct resource to fix the problem. That way anyone can call in for maintenance, suspicious package, or a lost child. Not all tracks will care for spectators. They have a system where each call gets an ambulance dispatch just as if they sprained their ankle on the street. My personal feeling is that caring for spectators is a good risk management move. It provides a contact point for the track to know if someone did sprain their ankle, is there a pothole the track needs to fix now before someone else gets hurt? Any traumatic spectator injury at the Indianapolis Motor Speedway gets a visit from Risk Management with everything taken down by a court stenographer as soon as medical care has been completed.

Communications is also important on a more global scale. Many meetings take place before a race to ensure resources are in place. A small city of people will be overwhelming the race venue on race weekend. Race traffic will need to be planned for to ensure the people who live nearby do not become hopelessly entangled in traffic delays. Helicopter access to the track for the times just before and after the race when roads are too clogged for even an ambulance to get through for a medical emergency needs consideration. Before the race, the hospitals involved are made aware of the event and a public relations contact person is nailed down. A discussion with the sanctioning body to make sure we are prepared even to the point of sending in a roster of physicians who will be covering at the race happens a few weeks prior to each major event. The county coroner is made aware of the event and kept in the loop as a nationally visible fatality will certainly make national news. It is good to know who has authority at the track as some tracks cover more than one county line. If celebrities or political figures are at the race, is extra security needed? Will the Secret Service be there? The airspace around the track needs to be secured so only expected air traffic is in the area. Homeland Security may have intelligence that will be useful to the track's security and the local police, fire, and sheriff's departments that will be assisting at the race. At our track, the local fire department services the 911 calls that come through our command center. The RV camping area stretches out over a mile beyond the track and is an active place days before and a few days after the actual racing takes place. The command center can coordinate medical 911 calls as well as requests for a police presence. One track has paramedic bike teams to get to ill persons as they can quickly navigate congested areas better than an ambulance and pass easier through a crowd.

Each morning that cars are on the track, we have a safety team group meeting including the paramedics, the doctor responsible for responding on track, firefighters, the towing and cleanup crews. We

will discuss procedures, radio frequencies, and any driver issues. Issues can be addressed such as a driver that is recovering from a fractured foot and may need more assistance getting out of the vehicle. Sometimes a driver will have a different form of safety equipment that we need to familiarize ourselves with. It is also a suitable time to evaluate what went wrong or right from the day before.

Injury Patterns

Depending on what form of motor sport covered, the injury patterns will be different. The authors have covered NASCAR, Indy, USAC, Motorcycle, NHRA drags, off-road racing, rallycross, sports car, and air races and each will have differences and similarities. Racers are subject to crash trauma, fire, heat injury, and chemical exposure. Indy car participants are subject more often to leg injuries, vertebral spine injuries, and head injuries because of the chassis design (reclining driver position) for reasons previously mentioned in this chapter. Motorcycle road racing has a high incidence of clavicle fractures and head injuries. Rallycross cars have jumps and tend to have more impact along the "Z" axis and rollovers. Any spine pain to palpation needs imaging to rule out vertebral compression fractures.

The NASCAR 2003 season had the following injury list as shown in Table 13.1.

There has been a marked improvement ever since.

Table 13.1 Injuries sustained by drivers during the 2003 NASCAR season*

No fatalities.

Diagnosis	Season Total
Extremity pain (Upper, Lower, Ribs, Coccyx, Thoracic Spine)	28
Concussion	14
Cervical Strain	14
Skeletal fractures	11
Medical complaints (non-trauma)	8
Burns	5
Heat issues	4
Dental	4
Severe Closed Head Injury	1
Tinnitus	1

*Note that this list is from the end of the era prior to SAFER walls and mandatory head and neck restraint devices.

Other Planning Issues

Certain types of motorsports events necessitate specialized planning. For instance, races that utilize rocket fuel powered vehicles such as land speed racers on dry lake beds may be exposed and become toxic to monomethylhydrazine which is in the rocket fuel. Such acute exposures are rare but can cause seizures, coma, and death. Since high-dose intravenous pyridoxine is the treatment, this approach should be part of a plan for motorsports events involving the use of rocket fuel [36].

A unique consideration for planning medical support of autonomous vehicle races includes the use of "kill switches" to deactivate or turn off any race vehicles either remotely or by pushing a switch on the vehicle in a standardized form and location since there is no actual racer to control the vehicle. This feature was first used at the DARPA Grand Challenge autonomous vehicle race and should be considered for any future autonomous vehicle motorsports events.

More recently, there have been electric vehicle races. Formula E raced in 2021 in New York with electric motors in Formula 1 type bodies. Nitro Rallycross were due to introduce electric vehicles in the 2022 racing season. Protecting crashed drivers and extrication crews will require precautions to prevent electrocution if the battery is compromised.

Closed head injuries (CHI) are a big frontier for not only racing but the entire sports community. During the lead author's time as a NASCAR medical liaison, a basic guideline for CHI based on the American College of Sports Medicine recommendations (see the Appendix) was utilized. It is still an elusive subject. The first step is diagnosing it. If the driver is unconscious after an impact, the diagnosis is not always certain. There have been instances where the in-car camera revealed the racer had a syncopal episode as he was not immediately unconscious from the impact. Other racers have amnesia, nausea without a loss of consciousness. If the driver comes in from the track, the medical provider must consider heat injury, carbon monoxide exposure, or plain orneriness for their behavior. One USAC Silver Crown driver came in mad as a hornet, had no complaints and he left the med center with me thinking he was the biggest jerk I ever met. His crew chief brought him back a half hour later because he was perseverating. He later wrote me the only apology letter I have ever received from a driver. He recovered from his concussion and is a standup guy. The biggest change in my practice has been using provocative tests. If I suspect a CHI and the physical exam is normal, the patient can do exercise to get their heart rate up to 140 (sit-ups, push-ups, or running in place). Any concussion symptoms such as headache, nausea, vision change that are elicited while the pulse is elevated are a reason to sit out of competition. Neuropsychological testing (mentioned in the Competency to Drive section) has been immensely helpful in monitoring drivers and has shown good results in Indy Racing League, Formula 1, NASCAR, and the National Football League. As research proceeds, the next piece of safety equipment that needs improvement will be the helmet. In its current form, it provides protection from penetration but does nothing for shock absorption.

A more uncommon list of racing injury follows. Rear end impacts before SAFER walls, head and neck restraints, and attenuators in Indy racers led to shearing of their nasal nerves at the cribiform plate and anosmia. Purtscher's retinopathy is another uncommon injury. First described in 1912 as a syndrome of sudden blindness associated with severe head trauma it also has nontraumatic causes such as pancreatitis, vasculitis, fat, or amniotic fluid embolus. Lymphatic extravasation causes cotton wool spots and endothelial injury causes microvascular occlusion [37]. Usually it will result in vision loss within two days of the trauma and has no proven treatment. Vision will usually return within months. There were two cases seen in NASCAR drivers and they both improved within a few weeks.

Clinical Vignette: Putting It All Together

You are at your first event as a track physician at XYZ International Raceway. An Indy Car race is underway, and you are in the infield medical center monitoring the race on the infield track TV feed. Suddenly, over the radio, you hear, "Yellow, yellow, yellow … Two cars into the wall Turn One. The pace car has the field. Safety One, Ambulance One, Go, Go, Go." The feed moves over to the demolished cars. One car has spun and rear-ended into the wall. The other has right side damage and has drifted down to the grass on the infield apron. As you ready yourself, you notice both drivers are removing their steering wheels. You feel relieved realizing that they are both conscious and alert enough to start self-extricating from the car. The driver on the apron is already out of the vehicle standing next to it. The other driver is having difficulty getting out and the safety team is waving in the medics. The safety team has members at the front and back of the car with water bottles in hand for fire suppression. You know that Indy cars carry methanol which can ignite on hot pavement and fire suppression is with water which dilutes the fuel. Your seasoned medic team is looking for bubbling paint and the driver swatting at the air indicating that there is a six-foot tall methanol fire that is invisible to the eye except for a heat shimmer. The driver is removed on a backboard, his helmet and neck restraint removed, and he and the other driver are brought into the medical center for evaluation. You move to the driver on the backboard as the other driver walks to a seat nearby. The medic hands you the helmet and HANS device the driver was wearing and starts his report. "Heavy rear end impact outside of Turn One, Doc. The red light was on the dashboard [indicating a 50G or harder hit]. He was awake and alert but is complaining of back pain, so we had to help him out of the car." Your patient verifies that his back hurts as you start going through your trauma assessment. As you carefully remove his firesuit, he is describing the accident to you. Airway-good, Breathing-good, Circulation-good. A look at the helmet does not reveal any cracks and the head and neck restraint device also appears intact. Neck is supple and nontender. Chest has equal breath sounds with no bony tenderness and abdomen is soft and nontender. You run your hands over each joint and long bone of his body and find no deformity or tenderness. With assistance from the nurses and medics, you log roll him to examine his back. He has tenderness but no crepitus or skin lesion at the upper portion of his lumbar spine. "That's a little sore, doc but it's OK, I'm fine." What is the most appropriate course of action? The wife and car owner want to see him. The media wants an interview outside. The driver wants to go see his car.

Since you have read this chapter on becoming a savvy motor sports physician, you realize that this driver had a heavy impact collision. The engine struck the wall and was driven forward into the driver's seat. In his reclining position, the seat was forced upward into the heavy helmet. This mechanism put a compression force on his spine. Due to the adrenaline rush, the driver may not feel much pain for another few minutes or an hour. You have the wife and owner see the patient and you inform them all that you are sending the driver in to the nearest Trauma Center to image his spine.

An hour and a half later, the trauma surgeon calls you back to inform you that his CT scan revealed a burst fracture of L1. Twenty-five more laps to go, let's see what else happens … This scenario by the way … really happened.

Appendix 1

Motor-Sports Concussion Guidelines

CONCUSSION SIGNS AND SYMPTOMS

Amnesia	Nausea
Balance Problems	Poor Concentration
Confused	Ringing in Ears
Clumsy	Seeing Stars
Dazed	Slowed Reactions
Dinged	Sluggish
Disoriented	Unsure
Dizzy	Unsteady Gait
Foggy	Vacant Stare
Headache	Visual Problems

COGNITION

Driver should recall:

Day/date

Track name

What happened

Area/turn where wreck occurred

Which lap

Who was leading race?

Series points leader

Winner of last race

Driver should be able to:

Recall four random numbers and repeat backwards

Repeat days of the week in reverse

Recall four random objects at zero and five minutes

PHYSICAL EXAM

Alert and normally conversant

Strength normal bilaterally

Gait normal

Coordination normal

Finger-Finger/Finger-Nose

Eyes closed single leg stance

Straight line heel-toe walking

PROVOCATIVE TESTS

(Done only if all above normal)

Exercise to get heart rate to 140

Sit-ups

Push-ups

Deep knee bends

Run in place

RECOMMENDATIONS

ANY loss of consciousness, amnesia or memory abnormalities

OR

ANY motor or sensory signs or symptoms

OR

ANY abnormal findings on physical or cognitive exam

OR

ANY recurrence of symptoms with provocative testing

INDICATES need for further testing and clearance before return to racing

Appendix 2

Suggested Medications: Infield Medical Center

ASA 81 mg

ASA 325 mg

Acetaminophen 325mg

Ibuprofen 400 mg

Ibuprofen 600 mg

Silver sulfadiazine topical cream

Bacitracin topical ointment

Cyclobenzaprine 10 mg

Ketorolac inj 30 mg

Ketorolac inj 60 mg

Cimetidine 400 mg

Odansetron ODT 4mg

Odansetron inj 4 mg

Promethazine 25 mg

Promethazine inj 25 mg

Prochlorperazine 10 mg

Cephalexin 500 mg

Penicillin VK 500 mg

Levofloxacin 500 mg

Ciprofloxacin 500 mg

Azithromycin 250 mg

Trimethoprim/sulfamethoxazole 160/800 mg

Neo-synephrine nasal spray

Loperamide 2 mg

Oral glucose

Loratidine 10 mg

Diphenhydramine 25 mg

Diphenhydramine elixir

Diphenhydramine inj 50 mg

Pseudoephedrine 60 mg

Viscous xylocaine

Aluminum hydroxide/magnesium hydroxide liquid

Simethicone 80 mg

Furosemide inj 40 mg

Famotidine 20 mg

Clonidine 0.1 mg

Pantoprazole 40 mg

Pantoprazole inj 40 mg

Methylprednisolone sodium succinate inj 125 mg

Prednisone 20 mg

Dexamethasone 4 mg

Albuterol MDI inh

Albuterol SVN 0.083%

Ipratropium SVN

Epinephrine 1:1000 SQ inj

Tetracaine ophthalmic 0.5% soln

Sulfacetamide buffered ophthalmic 10% soln

Gentamicin ophthalmic 0.3% soln

Ciprofloxacin ophthalmic 0.3% oint

Tetanus booster (for officials/crew who travel)

Rapid Sequence Intubation medications

Code medications on the ambulance

Appendix 3

NASCAR Recommended Equipment for Infield Medical Center from NASCAR 2012 Medical Verification Form

Rooms	1 required / 2 suggested
Beds	3
Resuscitation bed	1
Radio communication	2
(One for Med Center, One for On Track Physician)	
Decontamination shower	1
Closed Circuit TV	1
(for on track activities)	
Internet access	recommended
Shredder	recommended
Separate driver exam room-recommended	
Separate family waiting room-recommended	
Phone line	1
(with long distance capability)	
Fax phone line	1
Separate drivers/ambulance entrance-recommended	
Break room for medical staff	recommended
Locked cabinet for meds	recommended
Professional attire for medical staff	recommended
Security dedicated to med center during on track activity-required	
Golf cart to transport drivers. crew to garage	1
Transport vehicle for med center transport	1
Nasal cannula	5
Non-rebreather mask	5
Bag valve mask device	2
Oropharyngeal airways assorted sizes	3
Nasopharyngeal airways assorted sizes	3
Oxygen bottles and regulators	2
Pulse oximeter(may be part of CO monitor)	1
Suction machine	2
Yankauer suction catheter	4
Nasopharyngeal suction catheters	4
Intubation Kit	2
Cricothyrotomy kit	2
Rapid Sequence intubation capability	strongly recommended
Carbon monoxide monitor	recommended
Crystalloid solution (liter)	24

(cont.)

Central venous access kit	2
Peripheral venous access kit	8
Chest tube kit	2
Chest tubes assorted sizes	required
Chest tube drainage system	2
Scalpels assorted sizes	required
Suture kits	4
Dermabond wound glue	recommended
Large burn dressing	2
Small burn dressing	4
Wound Dressings assorted sizes	required
Cervical collars assorted sizes	6
Backboard	1
Splinting devices	4
Cardiac monitor	2
(may be included in Defibrillation unit)	
Defibrillator	1
12 Lead EKG	1
Advanced Cardiac Life Support Medications in accordance with AHA	
or local Emergency Services guidelines	
Drinking water	25 bottles
Isotonic solution for drinking	25 bottles
Crutches-recommended	
Eye irrigation system	required
Slit lamp	recommended
Tetanus	recommended
Antihistamine (include non-drowsy option)	recommended
Antiemetic (include non-drowsy option)	recommended

References

1. Davies A. The Autonomous-Car Chaos of the 2004 DARPA Grand Challenge. *WIRED* 2021. www.wired.com/story/autonomous-car-chaos-2004-darpa-grand-challenge. Accessed November 28, 2021.

2. Grange J. T., Bock H., Davis S. Motorsports EMS: An Evolving Specialty. *Journal of Emergency Medical Services* 2004;**29**(5):92–114.

3. Grange J. T., Cotton A. Motorsports Medicine. *Current Sports Medicine Reports* 2004; **3**:134–140.

4. Grange J. T. Motorsports Medicine. In: *Sports Injuries and Emergencies, A Quick Response Manual*. Rubin A. (ed.). New York: McGraw-Hill; 2003 331–335.

5. Kozak P. A. (2014) Motorsports Medicine in Challenging Environments. In: *Mayo Clinic: Medicine in Challenging Environments for Apple iOS (Version 7.1)*. Stepanek J., Johnson R., Cocco D. (eds.).

6. Sicking D., et al. Official Accident Report: Car No. 3. autopsyfiles.org. 2001.

7. www.cdc.gov/traumaticbraininjury/.

8. www.nascar.com/SPECIAL/er/download/index.html.

9. http://pubchem.ncbi.nlm.nih.gov/summary.

10. http://sportsillustrared.cnn.com/motorsports/news/2001/04/30/fish_olvey_q_a/.

11. http://journalstar.com/news/local/education/unl-center-key-player-in-motorsports-safety/article_74d866f2-55fc-5841-84e9-bfc7e8c00705.html.

12. http://blog.ctnews.com/takeonlife/2010/03/11/jerry-nadeau-a-human-ghost/.

13. www.stockton99speedway.com/99%20Articles/2001-3articles/MHarmonWreck.html.

14. www.sbnation.com/nascar/2012/2/27/2829676/daytona-500-crash-video-juan-pablo-montoya-jet-dryer-fire.

15. Romero S. SCORE Air Rescue: Improving the Safety Factor. *SCORE Journal*. 2015:66–73. http://read.uberflip.com/i/539275-score-journal-issue-6-2015/65?. Accessed November 28, 2021.

16. Grange J. T., Baumann G. W. The California 500 – Medical Care at a NASCAR Winston Cup Race. *Prehospital and Emergency Care*. 2002;**6**:315–318.

17. Grange J. T. Planning for Large Events. *Current Sports Medicine Reports: An Official Journal of the American College of Sports Medicine*. 2002;**1**:156–161.

18. Jaslow D., Yancey A., Milsten A. Mass Gathering Medical Care. National Association of EMS Physicians Standards and Clinical Practice Committee. *Prehospital Emergency Care*. 2000;**4**(4):359–360.

19. Milsten A. M., Maguire B. J., Bissel R. A., Seaman K. G. Mass Gathering Medical Care: A Review of the Literature. *Prehospital and Disaster Medicine*. 2002;**17**(3):151–162.

20. Valencia N., Johnston C. California Off-Road Race Crash Kills 8. *CNN*. 2010. www.cnn.com/2010/US/08/15/california.racing.deaths/index.html. Accessed November 28, 2021.

21. Three Race Fans Killed at Michigan Speedway. 2009. A&E Television Networks. www.history.com/this-day-in-history/three-race-fans-killed-at-michigan-speedway. Accessed November 28, 2021.

22. Three Deaths Confirmed at 2016 Baja 500 Including 8-Year-Old Spectator. *Jalopnik*. 2016. https://jalopnik.com/three-deaths-confirmed-at-2016-baja-500-include-8-year-1780670922. Accessed November 28, 2021.

23. Oates J. H., Wilkinson C. L., et al. Guide for Emergency and Safety Operations at Motorsports Venues. *National Fire Protection Agency 610: Safety at Motorsports Venues*.

24. Brown J. F., Smith J. G., Tataris K. Medical Management of Mass Gatherings. In: *Emergency Medical Services Clinical Practice and Systems Oversight: Vol. 2 Medical Oversight of EMS*. Cone D. et al. (eds.). West Sussex: Wiley & Sons Ltd; 2015; pp. 264–271.

25. Locoh-Donou S. et al. Mass Gathering Medicine: Event Factors Predicting Patient Presentation Rates. *Internal and Emergency Medicine*. 2016;**11**(5):745–752.

26. Delany C., Crilly J., Ranse, J. Drug and Alcohol Related Patient Presentations to Emergency Departments During Sporting Mass-Gathering Events: An Integrative Review. *Prehospital and Disaster Medicine*. 2020;**35**(3):298–304.

27. Chesser T. J. S., Norton S. A., Nolan J. P., Baskett P. J. F. What Are the Requirements for Medical Cover at Motor Racing Circuits? *Injury: International Journal of the Care of the Injured*. 1999;**30**:293–297.

28. Brock H. C., Cordell W. H., Hawk A. C., Bowdish G. E. Demographics of Emergency Medical Care at the Indianapolis 500 Mile Race (1983–1990). *Annals of Emergency Medicine*. 1992;**21**:1204–1207.

29. Grange J. T., Baumann G. W. On-site Physicians Reduce Ambulance Transports at Mass Gatherings. *Prehospital and Emergency Care*. 2003;7:322–326.

30. Spencer-Jone R., Varley G. W., Thomas P., Stevens D. B. Helicopter Transfer of Trauma Patients: The Isle of Man Experience. *Injury*. 1993;**24**(7):447–450.

31. Grange J. T., Corbett S. W. Helicopter Event Medical Support. In: *Principles and Direction of Air Medical Transport*. Blumen I., Davidoff J., et al. (eds.). Salt Lake City: Air Medical Physician Association; 2015.

32. Gorove L. Motorsports Injuries, Current Trends and Concepts. In: *Sports Injuries*. Doral, M. N. et al. (eds.). New York: Springer-Verlag; 2012; pp. 1113–1119.

33. Deakin N. D. et al. Concussion in Motor Sport: A Medical Literature Review and Engineering Perspective. *Journal of Concussion* [Internet]. October 6, 2017 [cited December 2021]; available from: https://journals.sagepub.com/doi/full/10.1177/2059700217733916 doi: 10.1177/2059700217733916

34. Kreinest M., Scholz M., Trafford P. On-Scene Treatment of Spinal Injuries in Motor Sports. *European Journal of Trauma and Emergency Surgery*. 2017;**43**(2).

35. Kaul, A. et al. A Revolution in Preventing Fatal Craniovertebral Junction Injuries: Lessons Learned from the Head and Neck Support Device in Professional Auto Racing. *Journal of Neurosurgery: Spine*. 2016;**25**:756–761.

36. Nguyen H., Chenoweth J. A., Bebarta V. S., et al. The Toxicity, Pathophysiology, and Treatment of Acute Hydrazine Propellant Exposure: A Systematic Review. *Military Medicine*. 2021;**186**:e319–e326.

37. https://pubmed.ncbi.nlm.nih.gov/31194324. Accessed November 28, 2021.

Chapter 14

VIP and Executive Medicine Considerations at Mass Gathering Events

Asa M. Margolis, Glenn H. Asaeda, C. Crawford Mechem, and Paul E. Pepe

Introduction

The involvement of dignitaries within mass gathering events can often impose several difficult levels of complexity, both during the planning phases and throughout the event itself. Whether the dignitaries are the reason for the mass gathering or they are on location as additional special attendees of the event, so-called "very important persons" (VIPs) such as celebrities, royalty, or major political figures can affect the planning and preparations for medical management contingencies as well as the operational aspects of such events [1–3]. Beyond the typical challenges of mass gathering medicine and protective security aspects, the concepts and practice of executive medicine, concierge medicine, or "protective medicine" pose unique and often unfamiliar and uncomfortable adaptations in terms of delivering medical advice and care. Medically, there is often limited access and reticence to expose the VIP to unfamiliar practitioners. Requests for medications or therapies in the absence of directly seeing the patient is more common. There is also an expectation that the medical care provider will come to see the VIP at the site and not at an off-site medical facility.

On occasion, due to national security, political, or publicity concerns, there is an extreme need for privacy, discretion, and considerations for strategies to achieve rapidly earned trust when a medical professional is called upon. There will be experiences with alternative medical care in many cases and the experienced health professional's recommendations are not always taken as a given nor are they accepted for nonmedical reasons. This level of complexity is further amplified when the dignitaries are from other nations or other cultures and they have their own state or private security entourage and, in some cases, their own medical personnel of variable expertise and backgrounds accompanying them.

Most importantly, for all medical professionals at the event, security factors can affect medical decision-making and dispositions independent of the medical care providers' recommendations. They can also affect access and egress of medical resources and also supersede the medical needs for others in attendance (Figure 14.1). Beyond direct issues affecting the event venue activities and logistics, mass gatherings involving dignitaries can have protracted impacts on

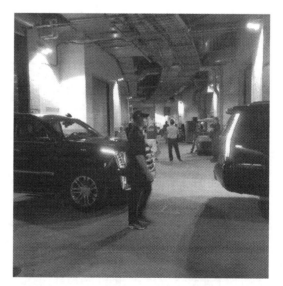

Figure 14.1 Locked-down and impassable zones of security as well as secured zones for stand-by motorcade readiness are common incursions when VIPs and dignitaries are in attendance at mass gatherings. Officials or dignitaries may require rapid secure evacuation from the site as well as large protected areas that can buffer them from the crowd and even venue staff. Particularly when there are multiple heads of state or dignitaries involved, these protected zones can cutoff the most direct routes for medical professionals' response to an emergency. They may also result in displaced, and often more distant, staging areas for ambulances standing by on-site for the general attendees.

Photograph (June 25, 2017) taken and provided with the permission of Dr. Paul Pepe regional traffic, airspace, local hospital operations, and the community at large, particularly with multi-day activities.

VIPs and Mass Gatherings

Public events are an inherent obligation for many dignitaries, be they the focus of the gathering or a special attendee at such events, especially those activities requiring national or international coordination and higher-level security needs, let alone the local jurisdictional coordination always required. As such, the greatest challenges can occur during a high-profile, ongoing series of events that extend over many days such as the Olympics, Super Bowl, United Nations in session, economic summits, and political conventions. These high visibility multiday mass gatherings become more complex when they involve numerous dignitaries and protectees who will have multiple movements within the larger event over several successive days.

In some scenarios, the prime minister of a given nation may be in attendance to see and even "meet and greet" a famous performing entertainer or perhaps a visiting Pope or a fellow head of state who may be in attendance. In another situation, heads of state may even be seated together while attending the Olympics, a Summit of Nations, or even a state funeral for another world leader. Again, they may also be moving and regathering from one subevent location to another, all involving their own mass gatherings or crowd-lined avenues between those sites such as that seen in the celebration of the platinum jubilee of the seventy-year rule of England's Queen Elizabeth II in June 2022. The security elements, perimeter of access to the principals involved, boundaries to vehicles, and equipment movements can all impose restraints to typical medical responses, not just to the "protectees," but to all others in attendance.

As alluded previously, such dignitaries of special concern can include heads of state, presidents, prime ministers, royal family members, religious leaders, government officials, ambassadors, entertainment celebrities, noted athletes, high-ranking business officials, and other such "VIPs," particularly those whose sudden illness or injury can have wide-ranging consequences and impact. However, it is less so the dignitary who will be impacted by the event but rather the crowd itself who will be compromised by the logistics.

Given such consequences, the presence of dignitaries at mass gathering events often requires more sophisticated medical planning strategies which are separate from those ordinarily established for other event participants including the event principals themselves such as the athletes or entertainers performing at "center stage." In turn, early, preemptive medical advance work, including interagency cooperation and direct communications for many months beforehand, are critical to ensure the safety and welfare of both the dignitary and the general public at large while also minimizing any negative impact, not only for the event itself, but also for the entire local jurisdiction affected by the mass gathering. At the same time, there may be more unanticipated and spontaneous events such as a state funeral or a visit to grieving families after a tragedy that may preclude prospective planning. Understanding the likely dynamics to be addressed in this discussion may still help to facilitate more effective medical operations.

Planning and Contingencies

As has been discussed throughout this textbook, a mass gathering event is either a scheduled or spontaneous event that brings together a very large number of people who may range from spectators, attendees, or the public at large to the featured athletes, dignitaries, press corps, performers, and their attending entourage and crews. It can place a strain on a community's ability to both meet its routine public safety, public works, and public health needs as well as its ability to respond should a large-scale emergency occur, either at the event or elsewhere in the community [1]. Accordingly, many national, state, and local jurisdictions have rules and regulations in place mandating minimum requirements for medical coverage for such mass gathering events. As such, mass gathering medicine practitioners need to be familiar with those policy and regulatory factors.

For example, the Commonwealth of Pennsylvania in the United States requires the submission and approval of a special event emergency medical services (EMS) plan that addresses: (1) the nature of the event; (2) its location, duration, and anticipated attendance; (3) medical direction and EMS personnel staffing; (4) a description of on-site treatment facilities; (5) communications capabilities; (6) a contingency plan for mass-casualty incidents and other disasters; (7) contingencies and response to weather emergencies; (8)

venue evacuation; (9) pre-event and real-time communication with attendees and the public; and (10) the numbers of available ambulances. In addition, the plan will include hospital destination contingencies for various scenarios along with the mechanisms for communications and coordination with those receiving facilities. In that respect, coordination with local EMS response leadership and their medical directors needs to be established ahead of time.

Similar to recommendations for other jurisdictions noted in other sections of this textbook, mass gatherings and asset requirements may even be regulated by government. For example, in the US state of Pennsylvania, events that will attract more than 5,000 participants are also categorized according to expected attendance and event type and requirements are adjusted accordingly. For example, an event can be classified as being a stationary and stable entity, such as sporting events and concerts, or can be dynamic or fluid entities such as marathons, bicycle races, certain music festivals and parades, where the events move along from one location to another. While such categorization may determine placement and logistics of medical resources, overall the level of medical staffing is guided by the anticipated attendance, increasing incrementally from that example base of 5,000 participants. In Pennsylvania, if more than 55,000 attendees are anticipated, then three ambulances and minimal staffing for emergency responses must be stationed on-site and those numbers may be augmented as indicated [1]. Nonetheless, the special needs of the performers, athletes, or other competitors will impose supplemental needs and these specifications can become tremendously more complex when political figures and dignitaries are also participating.

Supplemental Planning and Considerations for VIPs

The presence of dignitaries often requires a supplemental medical plan separate from that prepared for event attendants. That dignitary plan may include a detailed medical threat assessment (MTA), incorporation of security considerations, preselection of destination hospitals based on their capabilities, dignitary evacuation contingencies accompanied by strict confidentiality and operational security. The location, duration, and nature of the event are important factors in those contingencies as are the dignitary's baseline

health and potential need for extraordinary specialty care. Multiple local, state, and federal agencies may be involved in the gathering and thus interagency pre-planning, cooperation, and communication are therefore mandatory to ensure the safety and welfare of the dignitary, particularly in very large and relatively uncontrolled mass gathering events.

Some additional considerations and challenges that arise in VIP situations include the reality that dignitaries commonly are surrounded by an extended entourage inner circle of family, staff, and advisors. If called in to attend such a VIP, the presence and influence of these family members, staff, and "personal advisors" may hinder the usual doctor–patient relationship by imposing either a large sense of entitlement in terms of giving directives beyond the patients themselves or, more often, behaving and interacting with a very strong posture of protectiveness [3, 4]. Be it with the patient, the family, or staff, immediate trust building is critical. Clinicians who are asked to attend, advise, and care for dignitaries should therefore possess a skill set that includes the ability to interact with their patients with a high degree of tolerance and patience in a variety of settings and contexts while also maintaining and assuring a high degree of strict privacy. There should also be the understanding that the patient, family, publicists, and staff may not be entirely forthcoming with underlying medical problems, drug use, medications, and other conditions that they would go to great lengths to avoid disclosing to anyone.

In that respect, confidentiality and discretion in dealing with any medical event involving a protectee goes well beyond the privacy notions that healthcare professionals typically encounter. As alluded, prior history or certain key medically related details that might otherwise be pivotal in providing optimal assessments and medical care treatment plans may not be revealed to an unfamiliar clinician who has been asked to evaluate and treat a dignitary and also asked to do so usually in a matter of minutes. Moreover, transport decision-making for hospital transport may also be preset well in advance and even involve security personnel posted at one designated hospital that has been vetted and secured for all issues. More often, ambulances will often not be the vehicle of transport if a transport occurs at all.

At the same time, despite those limitations and frequent lack of historical disclosures, clinicians should also possess the same necessary skills for initial emergency management and resuscitation under such compromised circumstances and exude a sense of confidence and control in executing them just as EMS personnel do on a day to day basis. They must also be prepared to function and behave similarly in the outpatient, inpatient, and emergency settings [5, 6]. Also, the clinical care can often entail a combination of recommendations for preventive interventions, acute care, and management of chronic health conditions which can have an impact and opportunity for subsequent continuity of care. Nonetheless, such specialized skill sets for dealing with dignitaries and VIPs are typically outside of the realm of routine medical training and standardization for such practices are also generally lacking.

Specialized Training for Providing Executive and Protectee Medicine

Day-to-day, clinicians who are asked to provide this specialized level of "executive medicine" or medicine for special protectees will come from a variety of medical backgrounds, often with little standardized training to guide them through the special nuances of these encounters. Using a modified Delphi methodology, Mobarak et al. identified a set of skills for clinicians who are asked to provide dignitary medical care as a mechanism to address, to some degree, the lack of a uniform initial training curriculum as well as techniques for continuing education in this growing field [7].

While some physicians and other categories of clinicians are assigned to provide executive medical care as part of their job duties such as the White House Medical Unit, professional football club team physicians, or National Basketball Association trainers, those day-to-day medical care providers overseeing mass gatherings may also be asked to step in and provide medical management of VIPs and thus they need to recognize the need to adapt accordingly. Moreover, they need to know their limitations, sociologically, logistically, ethically, and even regulatory-wise, in the case of dignitary protection.

Statutes and Regulations for Special Security Events That Affect Clinicians

A very unique type of dignitary-affected mass gathering in the United States may be one carrying the designation of National Special Security Event

(NSSE). In May 1998, the Presidential Decision Directive 62 (PDD-62) was issued, formalizing and delineating the roles and responsibilities of federal agencies in the development of security plans, including medical care, for major events. In December 2000, the Presidential Protection Act of 2000 became law and included an amendment to Title 18, USC § 3056, which formally codified PDD-62 [8].

Prior to the establishment of the US Department of Homeland Security (DHS) in January 2003, the President determined what events of national significance were to be designated as NSSEs. Since the establishment of DHS, the DHS Secretary, as the President's representative, has held the responsibility to designate NSSEs. The decision to designate an NSSE is based on several factors, which include anticipated attendance by US officials and foreign dignitaries, event size, and the significance of the event [8].

As examples, previous NSSEs have included presidential inaugurations, summits of world leaders held in the United States, presidential nominating conventions, presidential State of the Union addresses, and major sporting events of great notoriety (e.g., Olympics and Super Bowl). PDD-62 also names several federal departments and agencies that will provide the lead oversight for the NSSE [9]. Mass gathering medicine health care professionals assigned to such events, be it in a routine position at the venue for day-to-day events, or a specially assigned task for an NSSE, all need to be aware of these regulated elements that may impact what would otherwise be considered best practice medical care under more ordinary circumstances.

When an event is designated by the US Secretary of Homeland Security as an NSSE, the United States Secret Service (USSS) assumes the role of lead agency for the design and implementation of the operational security plan, which will include specialized medical care contingencies. In that respect, the USSS maintains a core strategy to carry out security operations. This strategy relies heavily on established partnerships with law enforcement and public safety officials at the local, state, and federal levels [10]. Other US agencies that will play other key roles include the Federal Bureau of Investigation (FBI), the Federal Emergency Management Agency (FEMA), the US Department of Defense (DOD), and US Department of Health and Human Services (HHS). This framework is essential as it allows for effective multiagency integration and cooperation that bridges all levels of government. Similar counterpart matrices will be operational in other nations for such occasions and sometimes entail even more complex and detailed plans for medical evaluation, care, and transport.

Even if a particular event does not receive the NSSE designation, the impact on the local, regional, and state jurisdiction could be very significant and may still require coordination and special planning, including medical care contingencies, among the many partners noted above if it entails a very large mass gathering. A Special Event Assessment Rating (SEAR) event is one that is perhaps similar to an NSSE, but not of the same magnitude or significance. One example would be a large National Football League (NFL) game during the regular season of contests.

Besides national significance, differentiating an NSSE from SEAR events includes the expected number of dignitaries and overall anticipated event size [11]. SEAR events are classified into five categories based on the level of support needed, with SEAR 1 events requiring full support of the federal government and SEAR 5 events generally requiring only state or local support. In any case, the Secretary of Homeland Security appoints a Federal Coordination Team (FCT) for all SEAR 1 and select SEAR 2 events [12].

Special Credentialing and Clearances for VIP Involved Events

For the purposes of medical care providers, these NSSE and SEAR designations become important in that security clearances and associated credentialing become critical elements in the coordination and implementation of the overall security plan for many events. All medical support staff at the event may need to have special credentialing approved regardless of their task or station of duty.

For the individual clinician, the duration and exclusiveness of the vetting process will be unique to the event and can vary significantly. Background checks for NSSE credentials, similar to those implemented for standard Presidential and Vice Presidential visits, are conducted by the USSS and similar vetting is conducted in other nations. For these types of head of state events, only those participants who have a relevant and defined role, responsibility, and/or function, will even be afforded a credential application [13]. At large mass gathering events, however, the sheer numbers of medical

staffing personnel can be significant and can extend the credentialling process. Even at non-NSSE events, while both the credentialing and background check processes may not be as exclusive or in-depth, they may still be conducted with some significant scrutiny.

Again, depending on the event, the length of time to obtain a credential can vary greatly. It is important for the supporting entities and medical teams to have a realistic understanding of those timeframes if they want to ensure that all essential personnel can get the required credentials well before the event. Again, this applies to all first aid station personnel and roving paramedics, let alone backstage stand-by units or clinicians asked to attend the dignitaries, their aides, or family members.

Considerations Beyond the Typical First Aid Station

As would be inferred here, medical planning for these unique special events can become a very challenging undertaking. The plan must address the specific needs of the dignitaries as well as contingencies involving attendees, participants, employees, public safety personnel, and even the public-at-large. Beyond the event, routine calls for help to 911/999/112/000 (or equivalent) emergency numbers continue to be made across the surrounding community. That call volume may even be amplified because of factors related to the event itself and the augmented populations of visiting attendees that it creates. Therefore, successful event management must include a thorough understanding of the local host public safety infrastructure and integration of key existing emergency healthcare and public health resources. These resources include, but are not limited to, emergency medical services agencies, acute care hospitals, specialty hospitals, resource health systems, and public health authorities.

Depending on the magnitude and expected volume of attendees, some events involving dignitaries will have planning committees and subcommittees that convene months or even a year or more prior to the start of the event. For US NSSEs, for example, the very large Health and Medical Subcommittee (HMSC) is the primary entity responsible for medical planning. Smaller scale events will also have specific committees dedicated to out-of-hospital and hospital medical care. These committees bring together agencies and individuals with similar background who will often have overlapping and complementary roles during the event. Additionally, these committees help to build strong relationships among agencies and their leadership personnel proactively. Such preemptive interactions and relationships prove to be invaluable in terms of addressing unforeseen issues that might often arise during an event ranging from sudden severe weather, fire, and public health threats to unexpected stampede events, terroristic threats, active shooter(s), or structural collapse. Tabletop walk-throughs and other drill exercises involving all of these moving parts can be helpful in advance, especially if each primary agency for a given scenario takes a turn at playing out a challenge that is specifically dealt to them, be it primarily a medical issue, or primarily a traffic issue, or primarily a law enforcement issue, and so on. This clever strategy allows each agency to see each other's specific roles and interactions and how they would fit in to support the primary lead under those varying situations.

The impact that security measures can have on the local jurisdiction range from minimal to very significant, depending on the scope of the event. The impact of security-driven factors on operations are not entirely obtrusive for events with high-level dignitaries alone, but that can become a dynamic in any major mass gathering, especially if it involves attendant celebrities (entertainers, athletes) or league commissioners, and owners. Nevertheless, in the case of dignitaries, security-driven elements are generally more restrictive, particularly when multiple high-level protectees are involved. Regardless of the level of security, initial planning must consider several points of impact upon the community, the regional public safety agencies, and even the impact on businesses and public services. Beyond the imposition placed on general vehicular traffic and public transportation in that community, such events may also make it difficult for public safety responders and particularly EMS/fire operations to respond, not only to the event, but also any other emergency within the affected community. Motorcade and evacuation lane closures amplify those impositions (Figure 14.1).

In particular, the impact of secure zones on EMS access to patients within and around the venue as well as secured zones for traveling to and from the hospitals should be considered a priority. Such secure zones and their relation to rapid vehicle access/egress need to be mapped out specifically with law enforcement and security teams, well beforehand. Also, redundancies should be built into the plan. Multiple ingress and egress points or alternates should be identified, not only for unexpected events blocking one area (fire, bombing, protestors, active shooter), but also for simultaneous removal of multiple high-level protectees, especially those who have been injured in a multi-injury incident.

Depending on movement of the dignitary (or dignitaries), previously identified routes of travel for EMS may be closed for an undetermined amount of time with little to no warning. Also, if a hospital or regional referral center is designated and established to be within a secure perimeter, accessibility and modifications in drop-off points for ambulances and for patients who arrive by means other than EMS, need to be addressed ahead of time. In addition, areas for secondary triage at the hospital itself should be considered within that plan in case of a multiple casualty incident (MCI) either in the community or at the event itself such as that experienced at the 2017 Route 91 Harvest Festival mass shooting event in Clark County, Nevada.

In that respect, area hospitals will need to consider supplementing their staffing and bed assignments within their emergency departments, surgery theatres/operative areas, and imaging and catheterization laboratories. This stand-by supplementation will often have the consequence of decreasing the pool of medically trained personnel to help work at the actual event and often conducted at additional cost without remuneration [14]. It will also create uncompensated use of budget for those facilities as well, perhaps balanced by the recognition for their public service. Regardless, these considerations must be part of the planning.

Finally, and not least of all, one of the most important considerations at the time of the event is establishing clear, rapid, secure and redundant mechanisms for maintaining ongoing communications to ensure safety and privacy for the dignitary in addition to ensuring the safety and health of all who attend the event.

Due to the background noise of the event, such as music, crowd cheers, fireworks, engines and other auditory confounders, texting and other nonverbal mechanisms are becoming more useful (see Chapter 4), but they also must be configured for encryption or privacy in the case of the VIP or public figure.

Formally Designating Medical Support Teams

For the mass gathering medicine practitioner, it is also important to recognize that many of the local, state, and federal agencies may also specifically provide support using their own personnel, including deployment of a formalized medical support team (MST) or series of MSTs [15]. Such MSTs can play an essential role in delivery of care to the agencies supporting mass gatherings, particularly for events where maintaining security is paramount. Similar to tactical operators such as special weapons and tactics (SWAT) teams on the law enforcement side, the MSTs generally are mobile, and they are given specialized security access permitting their medical response to personnel at all assigned posts of duty. Additionally, these MSTs may also play a special role in providing care to dignitaries attending the event. The MSTs can be comprised of prehospital personnel such as emergency medical technicians (EMTs) and paramedics who may or may not be paired with advanced practice providers or physicians.

The individuals who make up these teams should understand the unique considerations of providing medical care to a wide variety of individuals, including law enforcement personnel and dignitaries, as well as the core principles of maintaining operational security (OPSEC). As such, the specialized training previously discussed should be part of the preparations and planning for mass gatherings.

The medical equipment cache plan, also known as the "medical loadout" items to bring along, is optimally configured to address common "sick call" ("not feeling well") type of medical complaints for force health protection internally, but it should also proscribe capabilities for managing all other routine and emergency conditions [16]. Also, these MSTs do not replace or supplant the activation of routine EMS response as required by the nature of the incident.

Interagency and Community Coordination and Collaboration

The ability to coordinate all of these potential responses becomes one of the main objectives of the multiagency HMSC, which should be in operation long before these major events occur. As previously indicated, this committee is responsible for developing a comprehensive plan that will address all aspects of public health and medical response for the designated events. The resulting compendium of information extends well beyond the basic elements comprising a standard MSA for dignitary events and it forms the backbone of information that will drive

successful coordination of these events. As previously discussed, in addition to federal partners, to optimize coordination through the planning committee, representation from local, regional, and state public safety, hospitals, and public health entities is necessary. Preferably, those representatives will be the actual personnel likely to be in leadership roles on-site at the actual event. Establishing relationships and familiarity far in advance enhances and expedites response effectiveness .

Planning must also ensure that the local emergency healthcare infrastructure is able to meet the ongoing medical need demands of the community while maintaining the ability to also respond to unexpected events, such as a public health threat, violent demonstrations, or a terror attack, let alone the routine responses augmented by additional populations and activities brought into the local community.

Inside the Entourage and Circle of Trust

As noted previously, some dignitaries travel with their own medical team. The "team" may just be an individual or it may be several layers of clinicians. As such, it can vary in size and capability depending on the distance, duration, and location of the event. While some of these medical teams will remain at a staging location, other teams will often directly accompany their "principal" and be staged nearby whenever and wherever possible. As a general rule, the dignitary's medical team will dictate the medical care whether or not they are licensed to practice medicine in that country/jurisdiction. Nonetheless, local EMS medical directors, EMS physicians, and other out-of-hospital clinicians providing oversight and onsite medical care for events involving dignitaries may be called upon to provide initial stabilization, assist in the care, or even assume oversight of treatment altogether. In situations where the dignitary is traveling abroad, local medical personnel will often be relied upon to provide recommendations of hospitals, including specialty care centers, or other healthcare resources ranging from trauma, stroke, and cardiac care emergency centers to specialists such as endodontists, ophthalmologists, or otorhinolaryngologists of the highest quality and discretion. In this case, these identified resources need to be vetted and established well ahead of time. Also, when language barriers are encountered, credentialed medical translators should be used if available. Alternatively, use of translation applications may be necessary while initiating care.

Above all, if asked to attend the dignitary directly, sensitivity and special attention should be given to assessing the comfort level of the dignitary in being evaluated by unfamiliar persons. Even if the consulted doctor is a renowned and respected medical professional within their own nation's medical community, VIP encounters are very different domains. If not an outright emergency manifested by loss of consciousness, severe dyspnea or worrisome injury, some dignitaries may prefer the initial medical interaction to be a simple, discrete conversation with just one individual practitioner who is often asked to leave medical equipment behind. It should be anticipated that security personnel and other confidantes of the VIP will likely be in attendance as well and the patient should at least give verbal consent to have the others listen in.

For similar issues of discretion, medical assets, equipment, and supplies may need to be deployed in nontraditional manners, such as use of typical luggage bags or plain "civilian" back packs [17]. In essence, there must not be any overt indication that any medical care is needed or will be needed. In fact, to avoid any public perception that the dignitary or VIP has an illness or injury, the principal or staff may avoid requesting medical care altogether or delay an evaluation well beyond what would seem appropriate. The dignitaries, their staff, or family members can be concerned about political rivals taking advantage of any revelation of a new or chronic health condition. On occasion, exploitation of a possible condition has indeed been used to gain a political advantage including the use of exaggerated misinformation, innuendo, and rumored speculation.

For similar reasons, medical personnel asked to evaluate or stand-by a dignitary should consider wearing "plain clothes" (no white coat or scrubs) and blend in as a general (nonmedical) part of the entourage. They should anticipate engaging the VIP in a discrete location and a low-key, more informal manner, one to first ascertain and develop an initial level of trust and confidence. If it is determined that the individual will require additional medical care or evaluation outside that immediate area, the focus will then transition into one that asks if and how it is possible to discretely and safely transport the individual. As previously noted, if transport is elected, the transport route should have been preplanned. Even if ambulance

transport itself is not determined to be necessary, such emergency care vehicles could still be staged, as indicated, to allow for ongoing care should it be needed. At times, the protective limousine, and not the ambulance, may be the conveyance with the medical care provider providing care and monitoring within those secure vehicles.

Beyond the overriding protective, discretionary, and "optics" concerns for the principal dignitary, there are also similar attendant issues within members of the accompanying entourage. Declination of care or transport is also common among those serving the dignitary, be it a chief of staff for a prime minister or a longstanding touring crew member working for a popular entertainer and assigned to a pivotal task for the lead singer. Terse loyalty to the mission can often derail what would otherwise be logical and appropriate standards of care and medical decision-making. A pervasive stoic mindset, in which such individuals believe they would be abandoning a critical mission, can readily override personal concerns, even with respect to possible life-threatening conditions. In such circumstances, extraordinary contingencies may need to be entertained for these dedicated support persons who are reluctantly, but also adamantly, declining evaluation and transport.

One potential accommodation would be the assignment of a dedicated medical professional to provide close individualized stand-by monitoring and observation of that person for as long as needed during the event. Hopefully, when that loyal member is eventually feeling free or relieved of their related obligations, they will then be willing to receive proper evaluation and treatment. Such situations are not infrequent, and they can be unsettling and even (internally) angering for a prudent medical professional. Nonetheless, compassion, understanding, and respect for the mission first mentality should still be applied to such persons assuming they are deliberating their own fate with full capacity.

Moreover, it is very common for any human being, regardless of demographics, to feel embarrassed about needing medical attention following an unclear and transient medical event, particularly one occurring in a public setting. It could be a young healthy women having a very brief, unexplained, and yet uncomplicated syncopal episode on a trans-Atlantic flight when getting up from her seat or an elderly and proud veteran of foreign wars whose family called for help when he seemed to have a momentary loss of speech at a restaurant. In both cases, the most common and predictable iteration will inevitably be, "I'm okay – really – I'm okay." Furthermore, most persons will also strongly avoid the embarrassment (in their mind) of being transported by ambulance crews in full view of others and especially with sirens blaring. In essence, the psychological aspects of receiving medical attention in public places, particularly when it involves conscientious persons in the middle of performing their duties and obligations, should be well understood as a typical human reaction and appropriate tactics should address strategies to enhance privacy, minimize the embarrassment, and gain persuasive trust, always with a compassionate, appreciative demeanor.

Medical Standards and Ethical Challenges

It must also be recognized that some VIPs and family members may request to see a medical professional for what may be questionable treatment requests such as vitamin injections or special intravenous infusions. The event physician may be asked to provide some alternative therapy, pain-killers, or anxiety/depression medications outside the usual scope of practice. Sometimes these non-traditional requests may be communicated through surrogates without providing direct access to the patient for prior evaluation of the medical need and necessity. Most physicians have a natural inclination to want to please their patients, celebrities or not. However, maintaining one's integrity and ethical standards in medical decision-making should always take precedent, especially if the practitioners medical licensure could be in the balance. There are sensitive and strategic ways to communicate the reason for not granting the request. For example, being able to personally decline the request, but also communicating a willingness to help in another way is a good start. Providing an alternative solution such as offering communication with their usual physician or referral to an appropriate specialist may be suggested as well as the offer to reach out to that alternative. In the end, one should always ask themselves, if this were my family member, what would they want the attending physician to do.

Again, discretion, confidentiality, and avoidance of embarrassment is paramount. If involved in medical care of the VIP, the mass gathering medicine professional still must avoid any interaction, even "off the record" commentary or speculations with other medical personnel not involved in the case, let alone the media or anyone else.

If explicitly asked to talk to media by the patient and/or their family or other patient-authorized persons in the dignitary's chain of command such as a publicist or chief of staff, any and all media commentary should always be done with that explicit approval of the patient or their appointed advocates. This approval should involve delineation of what could or should be revealed. It should be seen as part of an overall media communication from the patient and/or entourage members. The medical professional should always speak the truth, but the communication should be concise and avoid too many unnecessary details or anything that begs another question [18]. At the same time, there should be enough information to mitigate speculation and it should be expressed in a compassionate and human manner balanced by sense of "business as usual" for an experienced medical professional. For example, if asked about if specific worrisome conditions were present (e.g., "Did she have a stroke?", responses may include, "There is no clear indication of that at this time, but, as we always do for any patient, we will still conduct a thorough evaluation of all potential threats and will let you know. What I *can* tell you, she's in the best of hands right now."

Ultimately, each situation involving the care of a dignitary by medical personnel who is unfamiliar to that individual will be quite unique and often driven by the comfort level of the dignitary and the acuity of their condition at that time. Again, the individual may not be entirely open about underlying conditions and their chiefs of staff, publicists, family members may all insert themselves into what typically would be a private assessment between a clinician and a patient. It is therefore incumbent upon the local medical professionals to have patience, sensitivity, and situational awareness during each encounter and to adjust their level of engagement based on the dignitary's comfort level, the acuity of the medical condition, and the understanding that the clinician's index of suspicion for undisclosed conditions still needs to be high.

In addition, one might anticipate a clear reticence to concede to a hospital transport or recommendations to receive further evaluation. Beyond a personal sense of stoicism, such extraordinary attention will be perceived as something that will engender embarrassing

Asa M. Margolis, Glenn H. Asaeda, C. Crawford Mechem, and Paul E. Pepe

news stories and social media speculation in this era of mass communication and optics. In that sense, one needs to first be patient, gain trust, and not attempt to use scare tactics to coerce the principal into accepting transport but rather use a more patient demeanor and diplomacy as well as explore potential support from those close to the principal under evaluation.

Dignitary Protection Units

In the spirit of avoiding unfamiliar actions and to address some of the nuances of dealing with VIPs, many local prehospital systems and law enforcement teams have now designated specialized a Dignitary Protection Units (DPU). DPUs have been established particularly for events involving dignitary participation and are most often in place in highly trafficked large cities for VIPs or national capital city regions. To become part of the DPU, medical providers first undergo vetting and security clearance by law enforcement. They then go through specialized training to understand how their roles as medical providers blends into the overall security plan. The role of the DPU team may simply be transportation of the dignitary with the dignitary's imbedded medical team to the most appropriate receiving emergency department or specialized facility or it may be used to provide emergency care as indicated.

As such, it is essential that the DPU personnel understand their roles and responsibilities if providing care alongside the dignitary's medical team. Training includes understanding the logistics of standard operations in which the dignitary may be located at one specific type of venue for a prolonged period of time. This essentially places the DPU crews into a prolonged "standby" mode. At the same time, ongoing vigilance is important as there may be sudden rapid movement when the dignitary is suddenly on the move from one location to another entirely different type of setting.

In that sense, it is also essential to identify where in a motorcade the DPU ambulance will be located or where it will be staged at a given location. Most often, the DPU ambulance is hidden or placed toward the end of the motorcade during movement of the dignitary but security leads will dictate those positionings in given circumstances. Additionally, the DPU members must be trained and have knowledge of their permitted roles and capabilities during a true medical emergency as many dignitaries may have severe underlying medical conditions and their personal medical teams may still feel responsible for leadership. As previously noted, adding to that complexity is the potential that foreign dignitaries may use medications that are unfamiliar to the event care provider, especially the name or formulation. They may also have their own vaccination and public health requirements that may be different from the nation visited. Learning about these issues ahead of time should be part of the planning, assuming such information can be obtained.

Protective Medicine and Harmful Threats

Attendance at large public events is an inherent obligation for many dignitaries, but these events can also pose many multifaceted threats to the dignitary and create complex steps for medical preparations. For the dignitary, attendance at mass gathering events can create many types of worrisome exposures, including environmental, sociological, physiological, or intentional harmful threats. Jet lag, stress of the event, political pressures, and accompanying compromise to sleep, exercise, and diet can have physiological impact. Other threats can come from difficult climates, endemic infections, and public health threats whose control may vary by culture and by traditional diplomatic manners and protocol. For those assigned to protect the principal from harm, the usual protective plans and security logistics immediately face compromise and need to adapt if an injury or illness occurs. In these cases, injury can result from active shooters, bombs, and other terrorist threats. Knowledge of how to best manage all of these various threats should be part of the portfolio of all event medicine and crowd medicine practitioners.

Summary

Physicians practicing event medicine need to appreciate the complexities and nuances of managing VIPs. While one ideally treats all patient with the same level of compassion and caring, the protection of the dignitary's privacy, safety and public image may impact the assessment, treatment and disposition of the medical concerns encountered, be it for such individuals or a member of their entourage. As such, high level security concerns may create obstacles to care for others. Due to external forces and even governmental regulations, the medical planning for the dignitary generally takes on predominant role in the overall protective plan for the event, even when the planning of care for tens of thousands of others is the most likely need. Accordingly, training, credentialing, protocols, and resources must be planned well in advance and be dedicated to ensuring that responders are prepared to manage all types of emergencies, including VIPs as needed. Similarly, the successful execution of these unique events involving these VIPs is reliant upon the ability for multiple agencies throughout all levels of government to work in a complementary fashion and have established cooperation well in advance.

As such, early identification of all stakeholders impacting the medical care is necessary and regular prospective communication among these stakeholders is key. Due to the scope and nature of these mass gathering events, planning often begins months, if not a year or more, in advance. Security considerations that accompany the presence of a dignitary (or dignitaries) will have a major impact on the EMS planning process and event operations overall, including expeditious patient access and evacuation. The presence of the dignitary also affects the public and local community in close proximity to the event location(s), routine emergency medical response, and the operations of potential receiving facilities. All of these factors and issues must be part of medical care planning for mass gathering events involving such VIPs.

References

1. Margolis A. M., Leung A. K., Friedman M. S., McMullen S. P., Guyette F. X., Woltman N. Position Statement: Mass Gathering Medical Care. *Prehospital and Emergency Care.* 2021;25:593–595.

2. www.pacodeandbulletin.gov/Display/pacode?file=/secure/pacode/data/028/chapter1033/chap1033toc.html&d=reduce. Accessed October 26, 2021.

3. Groves J. E., Dunderdale B. A., Stern T. A. Celebrity Patients, VIPs, and Potentates. *Primary Care Companion to the Journal of Clinical Psychiatry.* 2002;4:215–223.

4. Guzman J. A., Sasidhar M., Stoller J. K. Caring for VIPs: Nine Principles. *Cleveland Clinical Journal of Medicine.* 2011;78:90–94.

5. Maniscalco P. M., Dolan N. J. Dignitary Protection. *Emergency Medical Services.* 2002;31:126–128.

6. Smith M. S., Shesser R. F. The Emergency Care of the VIP Patient. *New England Journal of Medicine.* 1988;319:1421–1423.

7. Al Mulhim M. A., Darling R. G., Sarin R., et al. A Dignitary Medicine Curriculum Developed Using a Modified Delphi Methodology. *International Journal of Emergency Medicine.* 2020;13(1):11.

8. https://sgp.fas.org/crs/homesec/R43522.pdf. Accessed October 26, 2021.

9. Presidential Decision Directive 62 is classified. The White House issued a fact sheet abstract about it, and the Federation of American Scientists has posted an "unclassified abstract" said to be "derived from" PDD 62, available at www.fas.org/irp/offdocs/pdd-62.htm. Accessed October 26, 2021.

10. https://asprtracie.hhs.gov/technical-resources/85/Mass-Gatherings-Special-Events/0. Accessed October 26, 2021.

11. https://homeport.uscg.mil/Lists/Content/Attachments/2718/Users%20Manual%20for%20NSSE%20Job%20Aid.pdf. Accessed October 26, 2021.

12. www.dhs.gov/sites/default/files/publications/19_0905_ops_sear-fact-sheet.pdf. Accessed October 26, 2021.

13. www.secretservice.gov/protection/events/credentialing. Accessed October 26, 2021.

14. Mechem C. C., Laster J., Baldini C., Kohn M. D. Prehospital Medical Planning for the 2015 Philadelphia Papal Visit. *Prehospital and Emergency Care.* 2016;20:695–704.

15. Tang N., Margolis A., Woltman N., Levy M. Force Protection Medical Support at National Special Security Events: Experience from the 2016 Republican and Democratic National Conventions. *Journal of Special Operations Medicine.* 2016;16(3):72–75.

16. Levy M. J., Tang N. Medical Support for Law Enforcement-Extended Operations Incidents. *American Journal of Disaster Medicine.* 2014;9:127–135.

17. Stair R. G., Polk D. A., Shapiro G. L., Tang N. *Law Enforcement Responder: Principles of Emergency Medicine, Rescue, and Force Protection.* Burlington, MA: Jones & Bartlett Learning; 2013.

18. Pepe P. E., Pepe L. B., Davis R. M., Mann P., Whitmeyer R. EMS Physicians as Public Spokespersons. In: *Emergency Medical Oversight: Clinical Practice and Systems Oversight,* 2nd Edition. Cone D. C., Brice J. H., Delbridge T. R., Myers J. B. (eds). Hoboken, NJ: Wiley and Sons, Inc.; 2015; pp. 146–159. Companion Website: www.Wiley.com\go\Cone\NAEMSP

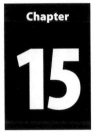

Chapter 15

Mass Gathering Events: Community Events

Ana M. Romero-Vasquez and K. Sophia Dyer

Introduction

Plans are worthless. Planning is essential.
Dwight D. Eisenhower

Community events can have several definitions depending on context. For legal definitions, the determination of a community event might have specific use of space, public or private for gathering, either public or nonprofit. This might change based on the local regulatory definitions. Other broader consideration of a community event is an event with a gathering of people, sometime defined as more than fifty for a multitude of purposes. Concert, protest, festival, graduations, street-block parties, celebrations (such as religious, weddings, marking a holiday), for fund raising, or unplanned events such as social protest (for example the many protests and marches after the death of George Floyd or in support of Ukraine after the Russian invasion). Community events have benefits to the community, social connection, support for groups and individuals for whom the event was planned and financial benefit for community-based both municipal and private business. More longitudinal benefit to the community can come from publicity about the event and the community for tourism events outside of the confines of the event days.

Planning is an enormous part of any community gathering. This holds true even for events that were unplanned, for example, a spontaneous celebration or protest. If a community engages in longitudinal planning for events, they will be better prepared to respond to events they develop with little warning, like protests.

Whether a community event is public or private, involving community space or private space, any community event can have an impact on the location, even if unintended. For example, a celebration can have an impact on road traffic and first responder resources, or even an impact on utilities such as power and water.

The process should be a comprehensive identification of stakeholders. Stakeholders could be municipal leaders' municipal government municipal services, volunteers, and other first responder agencies such as private emergency medical services (EMS), municipal regulators, public health, hotels and lodging facilities, food and other supply vendors as well as the local health care system.

Planning Considerations for Community Events

Pre-event planning is important in order to determine which resources are readily available and accessible to use during community events and which need to be brought in or privately contracted. The extent of planning will vary depending on the scale of the event but will always have the goal of anticipating and preparing for the management of different types of illnesses, injuries, medical emergencies, and mass casualty incidents that could arise during these events [1]. Medical action plans must be prepared with the purpose of ensuring the health and safety of all in attendance. In the National Association of EMS Physicians (NAEMSP) Mass Gathering Medical Care Planning documentation, it is encouraged for medical action plans to be completed thirty days prior to the event [2].

There are a number of variables that must be taken into consideration when planning a community event. These variables will change depending on the type and extent of the event as well as any incidents that could unfold during the day of the activities. Events are described by the nature of the event, time of year, location and venue, duration, expected

Table 15.1 Pre-event planning variables

Event location	Urban, suburban, rural, remote setting, water versus land, indoor, outdoors
Degree of planification	Planned versus unplanned
Type of event	Festivals, concerts, sporting/athletic event, political rally, parades, fixed versus moving
Season/Weather	Summer/fall/winter/spring, extremes of temperature, heat waves, storms
Attendees	Age of attendees, special needs, predicted medical needs, intent at event
Presence of substances	Alcohol, controlled substances, illicit substances
Access to weapons	Firearm, explosives, combat weapons, sharps
Activities	Extreme sports, vehicle races, fireworks
Surrounding healthcare system	Close proximity/remote, ground/air transport
Transfer system	Preplanned transfers, unexpected transfers, transfer and acceptance agreements with hospital systems, access to medical care sites, ingress and egress routes, evacuation sites
Public Health	Toileting, access to water and food, food safety, cost considerations, communicable diseases, terrorist threats or attacks, MCI planning

References: [3, 4, 5]

attendance and attendee demographics, activities, involvement of alcohol and illicit drugs, and event history if it is a recurring event [1, 3, 4, 5, 6, 7]. Table 15.1 lists all these variables and their categories. Based on these variables, medical needs at mass gatherings can be anticipated to a degree and expectations for resource demand can be set [3].

However, in many instances EMS, medical, police, and fire department resources are run by local and state agencies. Event planners and coordinators need to keep in mind that the goal of creating medical action plans is to reduce the burden that the increased population density from the event would bring to the already existing teams, agencies, and hospital systems. Event managers and medical directors will need to coordinate with volunteer groups, private groups, and contracted groups to create teams that will oversee day-of activities and have local agencies serve as backup if needed.

Location of Event: Community events can take place in numerous locations. These can be generalized into urban, suburban, rural, and remote. Each of these locations have specific benefits as well as challenges that must be accounted for when planning mass gathering events. The type of location, access to hospital systems, and access to event-specific teams as well as public EMS, law enforcement, and fire department teams will be fundamental in determining the type of resources available and need for resource allocation during the event.

For all events, managers and coordinators will need to make an assessment of the event type and venue and identify geographical and structural barriers that would disrupt the flow of the event and will need to devise a plan to work around these. Event managers will need to create a map of the space being utilized for the event and determine where to set up base operations, where to establish fixed medical care sites, and create dispatch areas for mobile units.

Urban and *suburban* settings are those with moderate to high population densities and at times encompass large geographical areas [1]. These settings typically have more accessibility to resources such as hospital systems, law enforcement, fire departments, EMS, and other private and public agencies. In these settings, local resources will be readily available as backups for event teams if the additional help were needed. Another benefit associated with these settings is their robust communications infrastructure. This is fundamental during the planning process as any failure in communications during the event can be detrimental to the safety of those in attendance as well as the chain of operations. Lastly, another consideration when organizing community events in an urban and/or suburban setting is the capabilities of the setting to sustain increased pedestrian and vehicular traffic. During these events, roads are often blocked to direct flow so as to avoid overcrowding situations as well as traffic standstill. It is important to have alternate routes set up for exclusive use by mobile care units and EMS to prevent breaks in event flow and ensure patient care is not affected.

There are, however, some contrasts between urban and suburban settings. Resources at *suburban* settings may not be as readily available as they would be in an urban setting. Thus, it is important for event managers and medical directors to consider these limitations during the pre-event planning process and coordinate acquisition of or privately contracting out the services that would be needed. Transportation both for the event and for patient care will likely not be as robust and might require one or more agencies working together so as to have the required number of units available to safely run the event. Receiving medical facilities will be farther away and will require longer transport times in cases where more definitive care is needed. There could be more geographical barriers when compared to urban settings. Traffic flow will be different and will not necessarily be as constrained as in an urban environment, but plans need to be made to manage the influx of vehicles and pedestrians to these areas during the event. Event planners and managers will need to determine where to set up parking lots for those attending the event and set up routes for pedestrians to reach the main sites where the event will take place.

Rural and *remote* settings are those with low or lower population densities and greater transport times to surrounding hospital systems [1]. In this type of setting, resources are constrained and oftentimes not available. When planning community events in these settings it is imperative for event coordinators to methodically plan for all services to be brought in for the execution of the event. Given the distance from bigger towns and cities, rural and remote settings will require more coordination to create a robust transportation system. The addition of air medical transport teams should be considered for extrication of patients from scenes that are otherwise not easily accessible and for faster transport to hospital systems for definitive care. Local law enforcement agencies as well as EMS and FD agencies often are smaller and run by volunteers, thus, event coordinators will need to privately contract agencies from other locations to provide the services needed as the influx of patients presenting to these settings can very easily overwhelm local agencies. Communication strategies known to work in urban and suburban settings might not work as well in rural and remote settings and thus incorporating alternate communication systems and infrastructures should be considered during the planning process. Lastly, preparing and having a plan of action for mass casualty incidents and extrication protocols is imperative in these settings given the lack of quick access to care.

Most community events tend to occur on land. However, there is a subset of events that take place on water and for these there are special considerations to have. While on land, most providers and event staff have easy access to attendees and medical care sites. Water events carry a higher level of complexity in that personnel involved in the day of activities will need to have additional skill sets and credentials as they must be able to practice while on water – be it swimming, diving, or navigating vessels. Event managers and coordinators will need to take into consideration the dangers, threats, and injury patterns that are inherent to water events and adjust medical action plans to be prepared for these.

Unplanned Events versus Planned Events: Most mass gathering events that take place are meticulously planned with time in advance. However, unplanned events have become more and more popular in recent years in light of the social, political, and ethical climate. Unplanned events are any unexpected and spontaneous events that can rapidly unfold with little to no planification or organization. Because of this, unplanned events often result in the need to rapidly create teams to cover logistics and management of medical care, security, transportation, and communications. Events such as anniversaries, protests, marches, and rallies have been the most common unplanned events in recent years. Examples of these are rallies for female reproductive rights, the insurrection at the United States Capitol in 2021, Black Lives Matter movements across the United States during the summer of 2020, the Unite the Right Rally in Virginia in 2017. All these event have a common theme of a more rapidly developing event, including the need for sudden coverage needs for security, communications and medical care.

It will be difficult to prepare for risk management and mitigation during unplanned events [1]. Authorities will need to rapidly develop plans to cover fire safety, security, overcrowding and crowd control, medical preparedness, access points, ingress and egress. During unplanned events, local resources can become saturated and this in turn increases the burden on surrounding hospital systems. Local and state agencies should be prepared with preemptive and ready-to-deploy assets who are pretrained in crowd management and riot control (if needed). There should be an established team who would be able to rapidly set up a unified command center which in turn will aid with communication between heads of departments (security, law enforcement, fire, EMS, medical support) and gathering intelligence. Heads of departments should attempt to work with group organizers to better understand the intentions and to be able to gain control of the event with the goal of ensuring safety.

Injuries commonly seen are related to anxiety and panic attacks, stampedes, overcrowding, crush events, asphyxiation, violence, and involvement of weapons. It is of extreme importance to have a group of people working on gathering intelligence days prior to these unplanned events (if possible). As the event unfolds to better understand crowd intentions and the degree or extent of coverage that will be required (medical, EMS, security/law enforcement, public health, etc.) to better prepare and staff the event [3, 8]. Teams could look at social media publications, communications, and trends to better understand the demeanor and intent of the event.

Medical preparedness during any type of event is of great importance and the type of medical care needed and staffing levels will depend on the extent of the event. Planned and recurring events are much more predictable than their counterparts. Over the years, researchers have been able to create equations to better predict future resources at recurring events [1, 7]. The type of medical care needed and staffing requirements can be extrapolated from historical data from recurring or similar events. The Medical Usage Rate (MUR) or Patient Presentation Rate (PPR) calculates the percentage of visits or patients per 1,000 or 10,000 persons in attendance. Transport To Hospital Rates (TTHR) calculate the number of patients from the event that are transported to local or regional hospitals per 10,000 attendees. Both these calculations are used to predict resources at community events [1, 7].

Type of Event: There are an infinite number of types of community events that occur every year. These can be sporting and athletic events, religious events, political rallies, holiday celebrations, parades, the list goes on and on. The characteristics and goals of the event and the environment around it will also determine the risk associated with the event. Events can be fixed or mobile, recurring or once in a lifetime, single day or several days to weeks. Some events will require that there be barricades present or street closures to confine the attendees to certain perimeters while others have vast open spaces for attendees to walk through. Regardless of the characteristics and goals of any event, public safety should remain the number one priority for everyone.

Because of all the moving variables that define an event, it is difficult to predict with certainty the risks associated with the event and how to prepare for them. However, over the years, specialists in mass gatherings have come up with risk stratification tools that help determine the needs and resources required to properly prepare for events of different magnitudes.

Hartman et al. suggested a classification system where they allocated points to the following categories: weather (heat index >90° versus <90° without climate control versus climate controlled), number (<1,000 versus 1,000–15,000 versus >15,000) and demographic (younger versus mixed versus older) in attendance, presence of alcohol (none versus limited versus significant), and crowd intentions (calm versus intermediate versus animated). They then use this scoring model to stratify events into minor, intermediate, and major events. In their study, they state that this classification system helps predict the need for BLS versus ALS crews, the amount of limited and full evaluation contacts, the number of resources needed, and the number of transports needed. In their study, they found that minor events often require one BLS and one ALS provider; intermediate events require one to two ALS providers, one to six BLS providers, and two transport units; and that major events vary but oftentimes require multiple ALS and BLS providers, specialized equipment, and the presence of an on-site physician [3].

Another tool produced by the state of Minnesota risk stratifies mass gatherings to identify their potential to generate medical events that would in turn need EMS response [4]. They created a matrix where they add scores from six categories: weather for outdoor events (heat index, wind chill, climate control shelter), peak attendance (<1,000 versus 1,000–15,000 versus >15,000), alcohol consumption (significant, limited, none), crowd age (older, younger, mixed) and intent (animated versus intermediate versus calm), and transport time to hospital (>30 min versus 20–29 minutes versus <20 minutes). They stratify events into lower risk, intermediate, and higher risk events and give recommendations on resources needed for each. They state that lower risk events need BLS onsite care with consideration of incorporating a BLS care ambulance. Intermediate risk events need a BLS on-site medical aid station and an ALS care ambulance with the caveat that the amount of staffing, aid stations, and addition of mobile teams is contingent on event characteristics. Lastly, they state that for higher risk events, they would recommend ALS on-site medical aid station(s), ALS on-site ambulance, mobile teams with the added consideration of having an onsite physician [4].

Knowing the type and characteristics of an event will help managers prepare in advance for event-specific injuries or medical presentations that can be associated with activities that take place during the events. For example, it can be expected to see problems with fluid status and electrolyte derangements during sporting and athletic events such as dehydration, heat injury, and/or stroke, hypothermia, frostbite, hyponatremia, hypoglycemia, immersion/submersion injuries. It is of great importance that all healthcare providers be briefed on how to look for and identify signs and symptoms associated with activity-specific pathologies in order to improve care and reduce transfers to hospitals when able.

Seasonal and Weather Considerations: Event managers and directors should also prepare for adverse events and weather as well as public health threats. They should have plans in place to prevent overwhelming event-dedicated and local resources (law enforcement, fire department, EMS, hospital systems) [7]. Seasonal weather trends must be followed, and teams should continuously look for day to day changes in weather leading up to the event [7]. Sudden weather changes must be taken seriously, and action plans should be established to prevent these changes from affecting event flow as well as the health and safety of those in attendance. Extremes of weather will affect all attendees, including event staff, and specific measures should be implemented in advance. In warm weather, heat illness is one big condition managers should prepare for and this can be done by increasing the amount of water available to everyone, preparing areas with shade and shelter, setting up areas with fans and cooling centers where attendees can rest and recover during the event. For events where attendees are expected to be exposed to cold weather, hypothermia and frostbite are two main conditions to prepare for and thus facilities where attendees can shelter from the cold should be set up or areas that offer re-warming options should be set up throughout the venue.

Attendees: One main determinant of risk during community events is attendee demographics. Knowing who will be in attendance for planned events is important because it will help determine age-specific needs, intentions, and potential injury/illness patterns during events. Data such as health status, predisposition to

certain injury or illness patterns, history of substance use at previous or similar events, intentions, and behavior can be used to anticipate resources needed during events. Younger populations are typically healthier, they also tend to partake in high-risk activities and behaviors including the use of alcohol and other substances. While older populations tend to be less risk-taking but are prone to suffering from medical emergencies such as heart attacks, strokes, or weather-related illness. However, these are not mutually exclusive and there can be instances where older populations partake in high-risk behaviors and younger populations are affected by medical complications.

Event Managers and Sponsors

Based on what has been previously discussed, event managers have numerous duties and tasks to complete during the pre-event planning phase. At times managers will be experienced providers or professionals who have received formal training in event management. Oftentimes, events will have a formal sponsor who will work alongside the event manager until the completion of the event. Sponsors can be professional companies who have had experiences in the past with event management, but they can also be community organizations such as schools, churches, small businesses, and even families. Event managers will need to identify what the sponsor's expectations and preconceived ideas of event planning are. They will also have to identify what the sponsor's past experiences have been (if any) and identify how much support will be required during the planning process.

Event Permitting and Interactions with Municipal Agencies

Obtaining all the necessary permits to run a community event can be a gargantuan task due to the number of offices and departments that are involved. Event managers and planners must meet with local and state authorities to discuss event regulations and requirements that are specific to the location where the event will take place. This is something that should be done with ample time in advance so as to provide enough time for local and state departments to complete the permit review process.

The Special Events Contingency Planning-Job Aids Manual created by FEMA drafts all the necessary interactions, permitting, and insurances that should be obtained during the pre-event planning process [8]. A summary of some of these tasks to verify during the pre-event planning process is located in Table 15.2.

Local governments and politicians could be contacted to obtain endorsements and potential funding for events. For this to be a possibility, event managers and planners will need to prove that hosting the event will benefit the community – be it by providing new jobs to people in the community, impacting quality of life, bringing monetary revenue to the community, or by raising awareness on certain topics or problems [8]. Permitting for structure and venue use, mass gathering, parades, sale and consumption of alcohol, food preparation and storage as well, food sales and pricing, use of pyrotechnics, must be obtained through local government offices [8]. Vendors will need to have their own licenses and certificates for food preparation and handling as well as alcohol dispensing. If merchandise will be sold at the events, vendors must have their own sales licenses. Local ordinances will need to be followed such as noise ordinances.

Event managers must partner with local public safety officials during the pre-event process to address event logistics. Discussions about security and policing and security functions, crowd control, traffic flow and direction, and road closures should be had with law enforcement [6, 8]. Fire safety inspections should be completed prior to the event by local fire departments [8]. Response measures to fire related incidents should be created and agreed on by FD and event management [1]. Local EMS should also be involved during the preplanning process to evaluate the possibility of local agencies covering patient transport versus bringing in private EMS companies to avoid leaving local agencies understaffed and underpowered. Event medical directors and surrounding hospital system medical directors should discuss indications for patient transfer and draft a protocol for those preplanned event transfers. Event managers, medical directors, hospital system administrators, and public safety officials must discuss mass casualty activation and management protocols and action plans should be drafted during this process. For high-stakes events and events that are potential targets for terrorist attacks, the US Department of Homeland Security should be contacted and strategies for disaster and security management and mitigation should be created [6].

Event managers should be responsible for ensuring that all medical personnel involved in the day of activities (on-site activities as well as transport teams) have appropriate liability coverage [1, 2]. Liability insurance should cover liability for injuries, acts or omissions, financial obligations incurred in responding to emergencies that occurred because of the event, costs of response to emergencies/venue cleanup/traffic and crowd control/policing functions [8]. This liability insurance can be covered by event sponsors, hospital systems/employer's plan, or through individual previously existing plans [1, 2, 6]. It is the event manager's responsibility to verify that all providers have active licenses and certifications to practice in the state and region where the event is taking place [1].

"Good Samaritan" laws may provide protection from medical malpractice liability in the setting of unplanned events. Any event utilizing volunteers should inquire about legal coverage in their jurisdiction. Relying on presumption of Good Samaritan protections can be a risk when providers are being compensated for the services they provide during a planned event [2].

Surrounding Health Care System and Preplanned Transfers

Mass gatherings and community events tend to create a burden on surrounding hospital systems. The purpose of pre-event planning is to create plans and put together medical teams that will help reduce the burden the event would otherwise place on neighboring healthcare systems [1]. With established medical care areas and mobile units patrolling through the event, medical professionals can triage and treat certain pathologies or injuries on scene and reduce transfer to hospital rates. The amount of providers and expertise of the providers available will also play an important role in reducing transfer rates and reducing the burden placed on surrounding hospital systems.

Event managers should meet with hospital administrators during the pre-event planning phase to discuss the resources available at their facilities and to implement transfer guidelines. Knowing the attendee demographics ahead of time will also aid with determining if specialty care will be needed based on predicted needs. Event managers will need to discuss surrounding hospital system capabilities and determine whether they need to partner with other hospital systems to ensure proper coverage of specialty care (pediatrics, trauma and burn, stroke, cardiac catheterization labs, obstetrics, toxicology, and poison control).

Delineating a clear plan in case an MCI takes place during the event should be discussed with hospital administrators as well.

Automobile Traffic Changes

Population density at the location of the event is increased throughout the duration of the event and puts a burden on local transportation and traffic flow. Concentrating large volumes of people in one area brings on challenges such as increased road and pedestrian traffic. During planning processes, multiple groups (Department of Transportation, Police Department, Fire Department (FD), event security) will need to work together to create a plan for directing traffic flow and develop alternate routes for ingress and egress from the event. It is important for event management teams to meet with local transportation authorities during the pre-event planning period as they can provide valuable information regarding predicted traffic flow which will aid with the creation of alternate routes for ingress and egress. Coordination of transfer of care for those patients who require a higher level of care will be fundamental and thus event managers and medical directors will need to communicate with administration teams from surrounding hospital systems to devise plans for day-of-event transfers. Local police department teams will likely be present at the event helping to provide order and direct traffic. Should any incidents occur and access to injured attendees is limited or complicated, fire department and EMS teams will respond to calls to gain access to these sites and provide transport to medical care sites or hospital systems. In rural and remote settings, the wilderness, as well as in settings where attendees are exposed to extremes of temperature and weather, other means of transportation will likely be needed such as helicopters, snowmobiles, four tracks, horses, jet skis, or boats.

Public Health Considerations

Public health oversight should be another field to cover during pre-event planning processes. This task is one that could be led by event managers, medical directors, or public health authorities [6]. Table 15.2

Table 15.2 Interface with local, state, and national agencies

Local Government	• Sale and consumption of alcohol
	• Food preparation and storage
	• Sale of food and pricing
	• Structure/venue fees
	• Mass gathering permitting
	• Noise ordinances
	• Community impact – quality of life and monetary
	• Funding
Local Law Enforcement	• Security coverage/Policing functions
	• Crowd control
	• Road closures
	• Traffic direction
	• MCI coverage
Local EMS	• Patient transport to hospital systems
	• Event coverage (local vs contracted)
	• Extrication/Ingress/Egress strategies
	• MCI coverage
Local Fire Department	• Fire safety inspections
	• Fire prevention
	• Fire response measures
	• Extrication/Ingress/Egress strategies
	• MCI coverage
Surrounding Hospital Systems	• Pre-planned event transfers
	• MCI activation protocols and management
US Department of Homeland Security	• Disaster and Security Management
	• Mitigation strategies
Public Health Authorities	• Access to potable water
	• Toileting and hand washing stations
	• Waste storage and management
	• Sheltering available
	• Communication stations
	• Disease surveillance
	• Behavior surveillance
	• Evacuation plans

References: [1, 8].

includes some public health measures that should always be present during event planning.

Teams should discuss access to and availability of potable water, toileting and hand washing facilities, waste storage and management (both human and nonhuman), contingency shelters, and telephone or communication stations [1, 6, 7, 8].

Food and drink vendors must meet local and state regulations when storing, handling, and selling their food products and public health officers are responsible for verifying that all vendors are following food safety codes. This is important so as to prevent the development and the spread of foodborne illness [1, 6, 7, 8].

Real-time surveillance plays an important role during events for the detection of outbreaks and gaining intelligence on development of incidents [1]. Should any outbreaks be detected, teams must work quickly to shut down the source of the outbreak and contain any attendees affected by it. In events where there is potential for crowd destabilization and development of riots, following behavioral patterns will play an important role in preventing such developments. Behavior surveillance is also important to detect any patterns of substance ingestions, intoxications, and overdoses in a timely manner for early treatment and fatality risk reduction. If there are any tips on potential warfare, criminal, or terrorist attacks, the Department of Homeland Security must be contacted, and tactical teams deployed to manage and mitigate the situations.

Public safety measures that can aid with prevention of fatalities include considering ticketing for entrance, having controlled access points where the number of attendees entering and exiting is monitored, having security checks, and having emergency exits with clear signage identifying them [1]. All these measures help control the number of people in attendance and with prevention of overcrowding and the complications associated with this. Implementing these measures while also utilizing the MUR, PPR, and TTHR tools helps predict with more certainty the amount of resources that will be required during recurring events.

Communications

Maintaining open communication during community events will be fundamental in the success of the event. Keeping constant communication to relay information will be key in the development of situational awareness. A command center must be established and should have continuous communication with external entities such as EMS agencies, law enforcement, fire departments, and surrounding hospital systems. This will help providers better prepare

for patient care and to perform in an organized and efficient way.

Medical directors must take into consideration noise in the environment and event, communication traffic and cell tower capacities, and the number of radio channels available when determining which communication strategy will be best for the event. Medical directors and event managers should plan to have redundancy in communication strategies to avoid losing communications all together – teams may consider primary dispatch frequencies, event-specific frequencies, cellular phone systems [2, 5].

In remote and austere environments, communications could be very limited and thus teams will have to consider having other forms to relay information such as designating someone as the messenger and having them drive to the nearest area with cell service [6].

MCI Planning

When gathering crowds for community events, there is increased risk for development of incidents. Medical emergencies from violence surges, inclement weather, structure collapse, and biochemical warfare can occur and can lead to response, triage, and transport surge capacity of event and local services [7]. To be able to respond in an organized and secure way, event managers and planners must perform risk assessments and hazards analyzes to prepare management plans and protocols that can be converted from general operations into MCI operations.

Event

Having planned the event with the concept of a unified command center, that area should be the hub for any decision-making and communication. That unified command center, depending on the size of the event, could be a larger designated area with complete infrastructure for joint decision-making, or if a small event, could be a small group of leaders making collaborative decisions on issues such as traffic, security, and weather response. Decision-makers could represent one or multiple agencies, depending on custom and size of the event. For small events, such a unified command center could be virtual. For example, decision-makers having a virtual platform for communication about the ongoing event and the ability to meet virtually for key decisions during the event.

Event organizers should be part of the communication plan and the command center, either in person or virtually. To be able to directly get information to workers on the ground, which could be volunteers and others responsible for crowd control, entrance queue, vendor services and so on. As discussed earlier in preplanning the ability to have a decision tree on pausing or cancelling the event will make decisions easier in the moment that leaders are faced with a situation that requires definitive action. Situations from weather, to crowd surge, threats to disrupt the event from concerning actors, to multiple drug overdoses are examples of the need to operationalize the need to pause, delay, or cancel the event. Part of that decision tree will need to include reputable data sources. Accurate early warning weather services for lightning or tornado risk assessment can be a vital tool. Ongoing connections with law enforcement or other intelligence agencies, such as a joint terrorism task force can be valuable in both a planned large community event or a suddenly develop protest. Although these might be evoked more for large community events, just-in-time communication pathways to such information might be as important if the need arises in response to a sudden protest, such as the announcement of the overturning of *Roe* v. *Wade* by the Supreme Court of the United States on June 24, 2022. After that announcement marches and protests throughout the nation occurred within hours.

Marcus et al. of the Harvard National Prepared Leadership Initiative discussed the concept of swarm leadership. Based on swarm intelligence theories, some principles of this could work very well for community events, especially when participants in the planning and day of event have prior relationships. The principals of swarm leadership includes concept of joint decisions made for the benefit of the whole including dynamic allocation of labor, evaluation of data input, and choosing among multiple options; individuals follow social cues and simple rules to coordinate complex activity. Each actor individually directs his behaviors, actions, and decisions in relation to what is going on and what needs to happen next. This behavior was observed in the response to the Boston Marathon bombing in the analysis of that event by Marcus et al. [9].

During an event interagency cooperation between all stakeholders is key. The ability to swap out or rotate decision-makers may be valuable in a multiple day event, to prevent cognitive overload of decision-makers.

Khan et al. described soccer league crush injury threats to spectators, from firecrackers to fights that precipitated a stampede. The Saudi SALEM offers a risk factor classification and preparedness tool, that moves from low severity with recommendations on public communications to severe risk with recommending restructuring of event, cancelling, changing, or moving location [10].

During the Event: Need to Incorporate Data

Having a data plan for real-time information to leaders and stakeholders should be an aspiration of any community event. This does not always require a complex system. Hourly accounts of the number of persons entering a ticketed event can be helpful for understanding crowd size; other techniques for crowd size estimation include aerial photos from drone or helicopter.

Law enforcement activity such as arrests and other encounters, occurrences of violence, and use of weapons can give the unified command center information to help inform management and screening of crowds. Findings of illicit drugs can be helpful general information for medical providers to predict what type of clinical presentations that could occur.

Medical encounters and type of encounter should be collated and feed back to the unified command center or appropriate leadership. Maintaining appropriate confidentiality consideration for the jurisdiction, type of encounter (minor medical, treat and release, or treat and transfer) can inform leadership as to the impact of the event, heat illness, intoxication, or injuries. The other component of data during the event can be volume of attendees who have self-presented to the local medical system. For more prolonged events, public health data on infectious disease reports such as COVID-19 or enteric infections can be helpful knowledge and acted on in real-time to prevent continued infection.

Traffic information, real-time, is valuable information in the event of the need to transport a patient with a critical illness or injury to definitive care. If access and egress is expected to be limited, planners should predetermine the ideal access route. Those decisions will need to be supported by traffic enforcement and re-evaluated frequently.

End of day summaries can be helpful for multiday events and offer the potential to respond to trends in injuries, illness, and other occurrences during the event. The goal of any end-of-day (or operational period) summary will be to evaluate what occurred during the period and then be responsive as an event team to correct any gaps. Gaps can include staffing and placement of staffing, equipment to address medical needs, and appropriate medications. Other more preventive functions can be found in end-of-day summaries. What trip/fall hazards or other causes of injuries can be corrected in the interval before the next operational period? One author noted a significant decrease in presentations for insect bites when a hive nest was located and contained [11]. What other hazards can be mitigated, for example road traffic accidents, overserving of alcohol, illicit substances impacting the health of participants? What communication strategies can be used to better inform event participants? Heat advisories, hydration recommendations, precautions about alcohol and substance use, information about how to access care are all possible messaging that can be useful.

Post-Event Debriefings and Considerations

A comprehensive summary and feedback from all levels of service as a post-event summary can be an invaluable source of information. Do not assume that even with good communications during the event that you are aware of all the occurrences. At the Boston Marathon, medical tent leaders are encouraged to provide near-time feedback on what happened in their area, opportunities for improvement, and gaps that need to be filled from services, personnel to equipment. Those medical tent leads then transmit post-event feedback to a cross-section of the marathon leadership.

Stakeholders for post-event after-action can include: police, traffic control, EMS, fire suppression, public health, local clinics and hospital impacted by the event, municipal services such as water, sewer, parks and public works, community members, and event sponsors/managers.

A quality management approach to post-event after action should also include data on the total number of encounters, refusals, percent of minors, and transfers to medical facilities also designated as TTHR. If possible, calculate the patient presentation rate [12].

A longitudinal review of 2011 to 2017 music festivals, published by Maleczek et al. [11], reported a median of 12 per 1,000 visitors and TTHR of 0.57 per 1,000. In this review only 5 percent were attributed to alcohol and 14 percent to recreational drugs. The number of clinical presentations increase as temperature increased [11]. In an evaluation of southeastern universities over 23 months. Presence of alcohol was not found to be a significant contributor to PPR. With heat index and percent of seats occupies was. American football games having the highest patient census [13].

Special attention should be given to any critical incidents, for example, episodes of violence, death, or serious injury to those in community or connected to an event, or accidents resulting in injury.

The demobilization of a community event also deserves attention depending on infrastructure added for the event. Event demobilization can also have potential for injury especially in workers and should be considered part of the event for medical coverage. Large shipping trucks and wide cargo departing the event grounds can have impact on the traffic patterns of a community getting back to daily life.

Conclusion

In summary, the framework of pre-event, event, and post-event steps can assist teams that are responsible for community events to have a backbone when organizing safe and secure gatherings as well as help them be able to respond to minor or more major occurrences during a community event. As the tragic events in Highland Park Parade on July 4, 2022, show, even an annual celebration in a midsize community can evolve into a situation requiring immediate action.

References

1. Brown J. F., Smith J. G., Tataris K. L. Medical Management of Mass Gatherings. In: *Emergency Medical Services: Clinical Practice and Systems Oversight*. 3rd ed. Cone D. C., Brice J. H., Delbridge T. R., Myers J. B. (eds.) Hoboken, NJ: Wiley-Blackwell; 2021; pp. 273–282.

2. Yancey A., Luk J., Milsten A, Nafziger S. Mass Gathering Medical Care Planning: The Medical Sector Checklist [eBook]. Overland Park, KS: NAEMSP; 2017. [cited June 20, 2022]. https://ncw-herc.org/wp-con tent/uploads/2020/09/NAEMSP_MassGatherings Checklist-D1-.pdf

3. Hartman N., Williamson A., Sojka B., Alibertis K., Sidebottom M., Berry T, et al. Predicting Resource Use at Mass Gatherings Using a Simplified Stratification Scoring Model. *The American Journal of Emergency Medicine.* 2009;**27**(3):337–343.

4. Special Event and Mass Gathering Medical Care Planning Guideline [Internet]. [State of Minnesota]; 2014 March [cited June 20, 2022]. https://mn.gov/boards/assets/Special%20Events%20and%20Mass%20Gathering%20Matrix%20-%202015_tcm21-28041.pdf

5. Fraley M. 7 Ways to Be Prepared Before the Mass Gathering Turns into an MCI [Internet]. EMS1. EMS1 By Lexipol; 2021 [cited June 16, 2022]. www.ems1.com/mass-casualty-incidents-mci/articles/7-ways-to-be-prepared-before-the-mass-gathering-turns-into-an-mci-HdDCR9igqgxEJv0 k/

6. Millin M. G. Mass Gatherings. In: Tintinalli's Emergency Medicine: A Comprehensive Study Guide. 8th ed.: Tintinalli J. E., Stapczynski J., Ma O., Yealy D. M., Meckler G. D., Cline D. M. (eds.) New York: McGraw-Hill Education; 2018.

7. Schwartz B., Nafziger S., Milsten A., Luk J., Yancey II A. (2015) Mass Gathering Medical Care: Resource Document for the National Association of EMS Physicians Position Statement. *Prehospital and Emergency Care.* 2015;**19**(4);559–568, doi: 10.3109/10903127.2015.1051680

8. Special Events Contingency Planning: Job Aids Manual. [Internet]. FEMA; 2010, May. [cited June 20, 2022]. https://emilms.fema.gov/is_0015b/media/261.pdf

9. Marcus L. J., McNulty E. J., Henderson J. M., Dorn B. C. *You're It: Crisis, Change, and How to Lead When It Matters Most.* New York: PublicAffairs; 2019.

10. Khan A. A., Sabbagh A. Y., Rase J., et al. Mass Gathering Medicine in Soccer Leagues: A Review and Creation of the SALEM Tool. *International Journal of Environmental Research and Public Health.* 2021;**18**:9973–9988.

11. Maleczek M., et al. Medical Care at a Mass Gathering Music Festival. *Wiener Klinische Wochenschrift.* 2022;**134**:324–331.

12. Ranse J., et al. Enhancing the Minimum Data Set for Mass-Gathering Research and Evaluation: An Integrative Literature Review. *Prehospital and Disaster Medicine.* 2014;**29**:280–289.

13. Locoh-Donou S., et al. Mass Gathering Medicine: Event Factors Predicting Patient Presentation Rates. *Internal and Emergency Medicine.* 2016;**11**:745–752.

16

Mass Gathering Events: Endurance Athletic Events

Kristin Whitney and Pierre d'Hemecourt

Introduction

A mass community-based endurance sports event has classically been defined as "a planned and organized endurance sports event, usually with over 1,000 entrants (recreational and/or elite), at a specific location, for a specific purpose, and for a defined period of time (either single day, staged or multiple stages, or several consecutive days)" [1]. Endurance sports events include one or more of the following sport types: distance running, cycling, swimming, rowing sports, cross country skiing, or mixed endurance events (e.g., duathlon, triathlon) and other similar activities that combine any of these disciplines [2]. Mass-participation endurance sporting events have grown in number and in popularity over the past several decades. Events can vary greatly in their format and scale, from smaller local five-kilometer run-walk events where participants are mostly recreational athletes to major international marathon and triathlon events including large numbers of competitive athletes and professional participants. Medical coverage for endurance events is a multifaceted responsibility that requires extensive planning and preparation in collaboration with race executive leadership and community agencies. Medical facility planning, team training, and use of treatment protocols help to ensure that medical care is administered in a standardized, high quality, and efficient manner. As always, prevention of injury and illness is the ideal, and there are many opportunities for prevention through athlete education before the event. The overall goal is safety for event participants, staff, and the surrounding community.

Pre-Event Planning and Preparation

Thoughtful preparation and detailed planning prior to an endurance athletic event is crucial and can have a tremendous impact on ensuring smooth execution of medical support services on the day of the event. A medical plan should be established in collaboration with key contributors and stakeholders, and the plan should take into account the potential risks of the event. The potential risks should be discussed, and a discerning evaluation should be made of which potential risks should be managed on-site by event medical staff, versus what types of risks would be beyond the capabilities or capacity of on-site event medical teams/facilities. Resources that should be evaluated include total number of medical team members on staff and with what specific qualifications, medical area size and bed/equipment capacity, surge capacity, specialty care personnel, and equipment available to support athletes requiring higher levels of care – for example medications, intravenous fluids [IV], or cardiac monitoring. For risks that may be beyond the capability/capacity of event medical resources, it must be determined if community medical resources would be an acceptable back-up to mitigate those risks if needed. Event planning should be multilayered, including standard preparation and protocols, as well as established contingency plans and strategic redundancies in case of any potential difficulties, so that issues that arise can be efficiently and effectively addressed. The International Institute of Race Medicine (IIRM) (www.racemedicine.org) and the National Center for Spectator Sports Safety and Security (NCS4) (www.ncs4.com) are both organizations created to provide education and resources to support those responsible for medical care at mass sporting events.

For endurance races involving swimming components, such as triathlons and open water swim races, race medical directors should have substantial input regarding the safety of the swim. Considerations will include the number of safety personnel. Water temperatures and water quality may impact planning and resource utilization.

Considerations for endurance events involving biking may include access to resources that would determine whether the race course is open or closed to traffic, with substantial implications regarding overall risk [3].

Establish a Unified Mission

Fundamental mission, goals, and scope of care should be carefully considered and endorsed by members of the medical team as well as by race organizers. Core objectives of event medical services should be clearly established and shared with all medical team members to unify the group around a core mission. Provision of medical care to support the health and safety of event participants is likely to be a pillar objective for the group. More specifically, this objective can be achieved through either one of two basic types of coverage models: either a "triage and transport" model or a "triage and treat" model.

In the "triage and transport" model, the key goal of the event medical team is to serve as a first response to event medical encounters, to stabilize, assess illness/injury severity, and facilitate transport to local emergency departments where most of the treatment and care is provided. This model can be an appropriate fit for smaller scale events with lower numbers of total participants and oftentimes less event medical resources compared to larger scale events. With a lower participant field size, there is relatively less likelihood that the volume of athletes would overwhelm the capacity of local emergency departments compared to larger events. When considering using the "triage and transport" model, it is important to communicate with local emergency departments and municipality leaders, to ensure that there are no concerns about placing excessive strain on local hospitals. Communication with local ambulance companies to relay estimated injury rate and number of anticipated transports based on past years' experiences, coordinate logistics, determine numbers of ambulances available for transport, and preestablish locations for the most efficient ambulance access near the event course will be important. It will be important to plan for any additional EMS staffing or repositioning of EMS response units that may potentially impact local EMS and hospital services for the general community. The hospitals that have been preidentified as the main medical transport centers will likewise need to plan for additional staffing dependent on the number of race participants and potential number of hospital

transports projected. Medical transport routes will need to be adjusted to accommodate for event-related road closures or event-related crowding; route planning will typically be planned in detail by ambulance services however event medical directors should have an understanding of these logistics factors when anticipating any possible delays in time-to-transport for patients in need of management at a local emergency department.

In contrast, the "triage and treat" method is the second potential model, where all nonlife threatening conditions are managed on-site at the event medical facility. If resources allow, there are some considerable advantages to this model: it is more efficient for initiating treatment, and local emergency departments are not strained by a potentially large sudden influx of patients from the event; thus freeing the emergency department to maintain their standard capacity to provide timely medical care for other medically ill or injured patients not related to the race from the surrounding community. Moreover, there can be advantages to having event-specific systems immediately available and in place to respond to the unique needs of the endurance athlete population, such as readily available ice baths for treatment of hyperthermia on-site. Doing the most to avoid treatment delay during transport or waiting during the time needed to set up an appropriate ice bath in a local emergency department setting where the specific items necessary may be less immediately available.

Preparing for Anticipated Volume

A key step in preparation for an upcoming endurance event is generating predictions on the expected total volume of medical encounters that may be held, and subsequently estimating the medical resources needed, including procurement of adequate supplies, medical area space requirements, and total number of medical volunteers needed. Review of past historical data from prior years can help inform prediction models, including estimating total numbers of medical encounters to prepare for, and any association between past year's weather conditions and the numbers and types of presenting illnesses/injuries.

Medical encounter incidence data suggests weather conditions, race length, and athlete training level all play a role in the incidence of medical encounters at an event [4]. At the Twin Cities Marathon between 1982–94, Roberts reported 19 encounters per 1,000 entrants and 25 encounters per 1,000 finishers [5]. At the Baltimore marathon between 2002 and 2005 there was a reported medical encounter incidence of 34 per 1,000 entrants [6]. Half-marathon and shorter distance road races have lower medical encounter rates than marathons [7]. Among youth marathoners, there has been a reported incidence of medical encounters among 13 per 1,000 finishers [8]. The majority of medical encounters are for minor or moderate medical problems [5]. That being said, the risk of sudden cardiac death during endurance events from half marathons to marathons ranges from 0.25 to 3 per 100,000 race entrants [9]. Previously sedentary individuals and those with chronic underlying illness are at higher risk [10, 11]. Sudden cardiac death during triathlons has been reported with a higher risk among older participants, and higher risk among males compared to females, with most deaths occurring during the swim segment [12]. Thus, on the swim segment course, there should be spotters (e.g., lifeguards, kayakers, surf boarders, paddle boarders) available to both identify swimmers in distress and perform rescues if needed – with a typical goal being one safety staff team member per twenty-five to fifty athletes [3].

Medical Planning and Team Organization

For each area of the medical team, there should be a designated leader or captain to coordinate both advanced planning as well as event-day operations. Teams may be comprised of physicians, nurses, nurse practitioners, physician's assistants, athletic trainers, and physical therapists. In some circumstances, medical teams may include trainees in limited roles under direct supervision of a fully licensed supervisor present at the event. Professional liability insurance for trainees should be verified prior to their participation, which can vary with different healthcare disciplines, levels of education, and institutions. The total number of medical staff necessary will vary depending on the length of the race and total number of athletes participating, and the level of care being delivered at the event.

Prior to the date of the event, area captains should establish a timeline for key steps in their planning, and each successive group meeting should focus on providing updates, sharing any potential challenges or setbacks so that the group can discuss and troubleshoot. Regular meetings also provide the opportunity for collaboration and streamlining workflows. Providing captains autonomy in their different areas provides a sense of ownership on behalf of the team captains and helps to bolster more familiarity and cohesiveness between medical team volunteers and their respective captains on event day. Medical teams should be made up of medical staff that should have training in caring for acute injuries and high volume emergent medical environments. It is ideal to have providers with varying skill sets including on each team: nurses, emergency medical technicians (EMTs), paramedics, Athletic Trainers Certified (ATC), medical doctors (MD/DOs), residents/fellows, and physical therapists, so that team members can offer the breadth of skills required in treatment for athletes on the event day.

Medical Protocols

As part of medical planning prior to an event, medical protocols may be developed for triage and management of athletes. Event-specific standardized protocols may cover conditions commonly presenting at each event, from management of dehydration, hyperthermia, or electrolyte derangements. Medical protocols will be based on literature-supported medical best practices, as well as practical/logistics considerations specific to each event. Protocols can be distributed to medical team members in a variety of formats, including the provision of a medical manual, to a web-based resource, and/or quick reference pocket cards for team members to carry with them on the day of the event. Event medical protocols provide a unifying point of reference for medical team members. Oftentimes medical volunteers may primarily practice at different medical institutions where practice patterns may vary slightly, and having event-specific protocols provided for all team members can help teams coordinate and standardize care and make management decision-making more efficient. Some event medical committees have begun to develop online video resources available for training personnel in advance of the event, and event medical teams may benefit from practicing together in practice simulation clinical scenarios before the event [13].

Medical Facility

Endurance athletic events should have a medical area stationed near the event finish line but not directly at the finish line, so that athletes who have just finished can have a brief period for "cool down" as their cardiovascular and respiratory systems adjust after the sudden completion of strenuous exercise, and thus oftentimes may help with avoiding unnecessary visits to the medical area. At the same time, mobile "sweep" teams of medical volunteers equipped with wheelchairs should be stationed not only at the finish line but also in the post-finish line areas and beyond to help athletes who may decompensate after they have already moved beyond the medical tent location. These teams should be equipped with automatic external defibrillators (AEDs) and radio communication equipment to communicate centrally regarding appropriate transport destinations.

The floorplan of an event's medical area can have a substantial impact on overall flow and efficiency. First, near the front entrance, a triage area should be established, where medical professionals can briefly assess, and athletes and support staff can check vital signs and record demographics. It also can be helpful to have a table set up near the front entrance stocked with accessible "self-care" items commonly in demand at endurance events, including petroleum jelly, pre-wrap, gauze, and athletic tape.

For athletes who subjectively do not feel well but otherwise have appropriate vital signs, cognitive status, and are ambulatory, a separate observation area should be set up with chairs and access to appropriate snacks and fluids available as needed during recovery.

Each facility's major medical area is intended for substantial medical problems that warrant further evaluation and treatment. Cots are typically set up and subsectioned into small pods, well-marked with numbered signage to facilitate efficient transport from the triage area. A small area for rapid lab testing should be located near this area.

Near the major medical area, a separate area for critical care should be set up, staffed by an intensive care physician and critical care nurses. The intensive care section should be nearby both the main medical area and an accessible exit area, to facilitate rapid transport between locations if needed. A specific area should be established specifically for management of hyperthermia, with ice immersion tubs and rectal thermometers available for core temperature monitoring. This area should be set up such that tubs can be easily drained into a collection system appropriate to accept potentially contaminate water (e.g., a sewer drainage location) and the tubs can then be cleaned in between treating patients.

A communications area located in the medical facility will be staffed by a team using radios and/or a special network communication via messaging. These communication tools are necessary given lack of reliability for cellular communication in highly populated areas and/or in case of emergencies. The communications area team will be essential to help monitor communications from along the event course or finish line about incoming patient transports, and to communicate with the Unified Command Center and local hospitals if needed.

A separate area for massage and soft tissue modality treatments may be staffed by massage therapists, chiropractors, and physical therapists. An area specifically for podiatric and dermatologic issues can be established as well and having this dedicated area for these issues can help streamline workflow and ensure availability of specific dressings and procedural tools if needed.

A waiting area for families should be established, separate from the aforementioned medical treatment areas. Family members may be worried about their loved ones and may require periodic updates regarding an athlete's status or plans to transport to a local hospital. Social workers and psychologists can be helpful in counseling families in this area. A family relations staff member may be available to help connect families with any resources needed and transportation coordination. It is important for family members to remain outside of the medical treatment areas for reasons of privacy and confidentiality for other patients, and to prevent scenarios of crowding in the medical area which can interfere with care delivery.

A separate exit from the medical tent should be set up, typically at the opposite side of the tent from the entrance in order to streamline flow of traffic through the facility. Athletes should "check out" at the time of exiting the facility, and many events are starting to implement electronic trackable check-in/check-out systems to assist in tracking athletes' status and to allow for leadership to monitor volume in the medical facility and thus anticipate any needs based on resource availability [14, 15].

Course Medical Operations

Medical care provided along an endurance event course can range from first aid to significant medical intervention. Every course should have aid stations set up along the entirety of the course, either overlapping with or separate from hydration/nutrition stations. Aid stations should be equipped with at least basic first aid supplied, ice, fluids, an AED, and communication devices. Communication devices selected for the event may include cellular phones, two-way radios, satellite phones, tablets, and/or computers. Communications tools will be selected based on considerations including availability of cellular signal or Wi-Fi along the course, and potential consideration of back-up communications options in the event that one communications signal or infrastructure were cut-out or temporarily lose signal during the event. They should be staffed by at least one physician, at least one nurse, and may also include EMTs, nurse practitioners, physician's assistants, and athletic trainers.

Separately, secondary medical tents may be set up along the course in addition to standard course aid stations. These secondary medical tents typically have similar capabilities as the main medical area but on a smaller scale. These can be useful particularly in large-scale events with longer courses so that athletes can receive medical care without requiring transport to the main medical tent, thus reducing potential delays in initiating treatment related to travel distance and potential road closures.

Along the course, bike medical teams, marked with GPS and equipped with a radio, can be used to quickly respond to athletes in distress. Commonly, bike medics are first responders for initial evaluation followed by ambulance response and further care/transport. EMS ambulances should be stationed along the length of the course at aid stations, any secondary medical tents, and at the finish. Higher risk areas should have secondary ambulances ready to fill to maintain continuity of coverage, should the first available ambulance need to transport a patient.

The finish line is typically the busiest area for medical coverage at endurance events. A finish line medical team comprised of physicians, EMTs, and paramedics should be stationed directly at the finish line as well as strategically distributed in small groups spread out along the final portion of the race course, given that it has been shown that most sudden cardiac arrests occur within the last quarter mile of a race. Finish line groups should be equipped with wheelchairs or stretchers, AEDs, and radios [16, 17]. The finish line is a high traffic area and may be busy with both race operations staff and media presence, however positioning of the medical team specifically in these high traffic areas is crucial for time-sensitive provision of emergency care and this should be reinforced at all race planning meetings. There should be a direct and unobstructed path between the finish line and the medical treatment area.

In the event that an athlete requires EMS transport, a specific protocol should be established and disseminated to medical volunteers. For all other EMS transports from locations along the course, a person assigned to the Unified Command Center (UCC) from the transporting entity should convey this information to an EMS liaison in the UCC. Athletes who are transported from the finish area or picked up from along the course route should be entered into an emergency tracking system that records their bib number and cell phone number. EMS personnel are then advised to notify the hospital emergency department staff upon arrival if they have transported a patient from the endurance event, and the receiving hospital staff can then update the emergency tracking application to track the patient's arrival at the hospital.

Medical Documentation

Accurate documentation of each medical encounter is an important aspect of care for each athlete, including recording presenting problem, vital signs, pertinent medical history, home medications and allergies, and documentation regarding the care provided, response to treatment, and any plan for follow-up care of transfer of care to a medical facility. This documentation is important for communication purposes, quality of care, and medical legal reasons. Moreover, this documentation can be aggregated and retrospectively reviewed and analyzed to understand trends in athlete health and event medical care, and to help prepare for future years. Documentation systems may be paper-based, or electronic using computers, tablets, or encrypted applications on smart phones. Technology is constantly evolving with the goal of making documentation increasingly user-friendly, efficient, and effective in capturing key information. The responsibility of documentation should be assigned to either a dedicated scribe or a designated clinical team member in order to ensure that records are kept for each encounter, even in busy clinical settings [18]. Medical records should be accessed only by designated personnel actively involved in the athlete's medical care, and should be stored on encrypted devices. Protected Health Information should be saved in accordance with local and national regulations for that area [8].

Event Modifications, Postponement, and Cancellations

Just as important as planning for the day of the event is planning for the possibility that the event may not be held as planned. Factors such as weather, concurrent public health events, or other safety concerns could possibly impact the ability to hold a large endurance athletic event safely. Well in advance of the event, it is important to outline, in writing, what circumstances would require the event to be postponed, modified, or even cancelled. In the event of adverse weather conditions (e.g., heat, humidity, severe storms) that may impact participant safety, the event medical director may need to initiate and guide the conversation regarding altering the race or even not starting the event with the event organizers and local leaders. Establishing these parameters in advance, communicating with race organizers and subsequently with event sponsors, and with event participants, can help to mitigate potentially negative community response. Posting the parameters publicly, ideally before time of event registration for participants, allows for transparency and informed agreement from participants at the time of registration. Managing expectations allows participants the opportunity to plan their travel and accommodations, not to mention their training plans, in a way that they may be able to adjust if the event is modified, postponed, or cancelled. Failing to provide this information to participants can lead to disappointment, confusion, and liability.

Unified Command, Public Safety, and Disaster Planning

Endurance event medical coverage includes planning for public safety and emergency planning. In most large endurance events, a UCC has been incorporated into the event, and is present either on location at the event or remotely. The UCC includes the event medical director, event executives, and representatives from all key public safety and community agencies including police, fire, and EMS. It also may include representative from key race operations groups including transportation and logistics teams. The UCC is designed to serve as an interface between these entities that can enable rapid response to emergencies and unexpected events [19]. Should an event disruption occur due to weather, traffic interruptions, fire, or flooding on or near the course, or terrorist threat, the UCC would coordinate the response. Each representative remains in direct communication with their respective groups using multiple forms of communication including two-way radio, phone, along with video and data surveillance tools to monitor activity the event course and within the medical facilities. Each representative, in turn, can receive high-level updates directly from other key groups and direct any response necessary.

Even before the day of the event, contingency plans are imperative and should be generated in collaboration with local agencies including police, fire, EMS, hospitals, and public works departments.

Weather-related issues are the most common to impact endurance race events. Heat has impacted several major endurance race events in recent years. The WetBulb Globe Temperature (WBGT) is used by most leading endurance event organizations in safety decision-making; it is a measure of the heat stress in direct sunlight, which takes into account temperature, humidity, sun angle, cloud cover (solar radiation), and wind speed [20]. In recent years, excessive WetBulb Globe temperatures have led to the decision to change start times, to cancel the event before race start, or to end the race during the event itself. In other instances the race has proceeded despite high temperatures and saw greater than normal numbers of medical encounters. Lightning is another weather-related issue that can require sudden disruption to an event and may necessitate participants to shelter in place, in which case predetermined safe areas along the course or at the start/finish areas would be necessary where participants can move to during event stoppage. All of these scenarios require extensive multidisciplinary contingency planning. Efficient and accurate communication is key, and protocols and specific chain of command for these different types of scenarios should be preestablished. The IIRM has endorsed the Event Alert System, created by the American College of Sports Medicine, as an effective communication tool for streamlined advisements regarding weather-related and other situational risks that may occur in the setting of endurance events [21].

Medical Management

In a high-volume endurance event setting, medical encounters need to be handled efficiently and systematically. Triage and treatment protocols can help in this regard. Medical triage is based on assessment of an athlete's ambulatory status, mental status, vital signs (heart rate, respiratory rate, blood pressure, temperature), and their presenting symptoms. Based on these parameters, athletes can be classified and triaged in terms of their level of severity.

Dehydration: Dehydration is defined as 3 percent reduction in body weight, caused by an imbalance of fluid losses (through sweat and insensible losses) with fluid intake. This leads to progressive volume depletion, impairment in performance, and ultimately can lead to collapse along the race route or at the finish line. Dehydration contributes to the risk of hyperthermia by limiting the amount of blood that can be shunted to the skin to evaporate heat loss. A dehydrated athlete commonly presents with hypotension, tachycardia, nausea, dizziness, and weight loss (it is recommended that prerace weights be written on event bibs or other available materials for reference by a medical team). The skin turgor may be decreased, mucus membranes dry. If the temperature is normal, they should be given oral fluids. Most athletes will not need (IV) hydration. IV lines may be considered if fluids cannot be taken orally, however IV fluids should be administered only after electrolytes are tested, in particular to identify sodium levels and rule out hyponatremia. In the absence of hyponatremia, an athlete typically improves with the infusion of one to two liters of replacement fluids (e.g., normal saline, lactated ringers, or plasmalyte) with both vital signs and clinical status normalizing [22].

Exercise Associated Heat Illness: Exercise Associated Heat Illness may occur on a spectrum including: heat cramping, heat exhaustion, heat syncope, and heat stroke/hyperthermia. Environmental conditions (WBGT) and exercise intensity are the two most important factors that influence the rate of rise in core body temperature and put athletes at risk of heat illness. Athlete-specific factors including clothing, equipment, hydration status, and acclimatization status also play a role in exercise heat tolerance.

For heat cramping, athletes present with severe muscle cramps of the lower extremities and trunk, sweating, and typically have normal vital signs. Treatment includes rest, cool environment, muscle therapy, salty fluids and food intake [23]. In heat exhaustion, athletes present with symptoms that may include headache, nausea, feeling dizzy or lightheaded, cramping, chills, and clammy skin. Treatment involves resting in a cool area, fluid intake, and removing excessive clothing. The athlete may be cooled simply with ice

bags or wet towels over the chest area and over the extremities [24]. On the most severe end of the spectrum, heat stroke/hyperthermia is defined as high body temperature (rectal temperature ≥104°F or 40°C), and is a medical emergency. Early signs may include emotional lability, irrational behavior, irritability, undue fatigue. Vomiting, belligerence, and lethargy may develop. An athlete may develop hyperventilation or paradoxical chills, and ultimately may lose consciousness. Athletes are at risk for neurologic compromise including seizures. Rectal temperature monitoring is key for diagnosis and management, with emergent need for cooling in an ice bath. Tympanic temperature checks are not sufficient if hyperthermia is suspected as they may underestimate core temperature. Ice tub water should be stirred vigorously, and the rectal thermometer monitoring should continue for approximately ten minutes after removal from ice bath to monitor for any rebound hyperthermia or excessive cooling causing hypothermia. Cooling is the emergent medical necessity, and should not be delayed for transport to a local emergency department [25]. Once a patient has been cooled to appropriate thresholds, patients with moderate to severe hyperthermia or underlying medial conditions should be transferred to a local hospital for continued monitoring.

Exercise Associated Hyponatremia: Exercise Associated Hyponatremia (EAH) occurs in the setting of excessive hydration during the event or after the race. It can be severe and life-threatening. Presenting symptoms may include malaise, nausea, fatigue, headache in moderate cases, or may progress to seizures, coma, or even death in severe cases. Weight gain during the event, a long racing time, and body mass index (BMI) extremes are associated with hyponatremia, and nonsteroidal anti-inflammatory drug (NSAID) use can increase one's risk. Low sodium levels as well as rate of change of serum sodium both contribute to EAH. Medical management is based on clinical hydration status and sodium levels, along with clinical signs and symptoms. Treatment for mild to moderate cases includes fluid restriction until urine is produced. Severe mental status alteration and sodium levels may warrant administration of 3 percent saline boluses (100 ml every 10 minutes until symptoms improve) followed by a continuous infusion and frequent sodium monitoring. Athletes should be transferred to a hospital thereafter for monitoring [26].

Athletes with Impairments

Athletes with mobility, sensory, and intellectual impairments all have the ability to regularly participate in endurance events. A number of organizations support athletes with impairments in their endurance sport goals. Promoting accommodations and access is paramount in race planning. Access to guides for the visually impaired is also needed. Coordination of start times, allowing for a field clear of obstacles for wheelchair and hand cycle athletes, is necessary given the high rate of speed at which they travel. Unique considerations including risk for high speed traumatic injuries in athletes using wheelchairs or more chronic concerns including skin breakdown, differences in temperature regulation, and autonomic dysreflexia should be considered, and medical teams should be prepared to assess and treat these conditions when they arise.

Athlete Education

Providing education for athletes before an endurance event may help in preventing injuries and avoiding medical emergencies. Educating athletes on topics including appropriate nutrition, training strategies, and apparel planning can be useful. Athletes commonly lack familiarity about proper hydration approaches, putting them at risk for issues including dehydration and hyponatremia, and it is important for athletes to be provided with reliable information about this critical issue. Information can be disseminated electronically before the event, and paper education materials can be included in the athlete's prerace materials distributed before the event.

Information can be provided that includes logistics information such as locations of hydration stations and medical stations. Information on injury prevention and precautions regarding specific medical conditions and risk factors, for example respiratory disease, heart disease, renal issues, and returning to sport after any recent illnesses all can be important in helping athletes prepare safely. Athlete's bibs should include an area to write in key medical information, active medications, allergies, emergency contact information, and prerace weight on the back of the bib, for medical teams to reference if needed. Some events host injury and medical screening clinics which can help reduce risk for morbidity [27]. Another opportunity to promote an environment of preparedness is through hosting CPR training opportunities for athletes and community members in the timeframe leading up to the event [27]. Sport-specific education including water safety for swimming and rowing athletes and education on sport-specific attire selection to optimize thermoregulation and prevent dermatologic issues for various sport needs (i.e., wetsuits during open water swim below a certain temperature, foot/skin care during ultra-endurance races) can be offered to athletes before an event. Event-specific nutrition education can also be informative for athletes and tailored to race distance and expected energy expenditure levels. As always, prevention is the goal, and good communication strategies and community engagement is paramount in helping athletes stay healthy and well so they can safely succeed in their endurance event goals.

Summary

Medical coverage for endurance events is a multifaceted responsibility that requires extensive planning and preparation. Medical plans should be developed in partnership with community organizations and event directors. Treatment protocols help in standardization of quality medical care that is delivered efficiently. As always, prevention of injury and illness is the ideal, and there are many opportunities for prevention through athlete education before the event. The overall goal is safety for event participants, staff, and the surrounding community.

References

1. Lund A., Turris S. A., Bowles R., et al. Mass-Gathering Health Research Foundational Theory: Part 1 – Population Models for Mass Gatherings. *Prehospital and Disaster Medicine*. 2014;29(6):648–654.

2. Schwellnus M., Kipps C., Roberts W. O., et al. Medical Encounters (Including Injury and Illness) at Mass Community-Based Endurance Sports Events: An International Consensus Statement on Definitions and Methods of Data Recording and Reporting. *British Journal of Sports Medicine*. 2019;53(17):1048–1055. doi: 10.1136/bjsports-2018-100092.

3. Asplund C., Miller T. K., Creswell L., et al. NRP10 Triathlon Medical Coverage: A Guide for Medical Directors. *Current Sports Medicine Reports*. 2017;16(4):280–288.

4. Breslow R. G., Giberson-Chen C. C., Roberts W. O. Burden of Injury and Illness in the Road Race Medical Tent: A Narrative Review. *Clinical Journal of Sports*

Medicine. 2021;**31**(6):e499–e505. doi: 10.1097/ JSM.0000000000000829.

5. Roberts W. O. A 12-yr Profile of Medical Injury and Illness for the Twin Cities Marathon. *Medicine and Science in Sports and Exercise*. 2000;**39**:1549–1555.

6. Tang N., Kraus C. K., Brill J. D., et al. Hospital-Based Event Medical Support for the Baltimore Marathon, 2002–2005. *Prehospital and Emergency Care*. 2008;**12**:320–326.

7. Schwabe K., Schwellnus M., Derman W., et al. Medical Complications and Deaths in 21 and 56 km Road Race Runners: A 4-year Prospective Study in 65,865 runners – SAFER study I. *British Journal of Sports Medicine*. 2014;**48**:912–918.

8. Roberts W. O., Nicholson W. G. Youth Marathon Runners and Race Day Medical Risk over 26 Years. *Clinical Journal of Sport Medicine*. 2010;**20**:5.

9. Schwellnus M., Kipps C., Roberts W. O., et al. Medical Encounters (Including Injury and Illness) at Mass Community-Based Endurance Sports Events: An International Consensus Statement on Definitions and Methods of Data Recording and Reporting. *British Journal of Sports Medicine*. 2019;**53**:1048–1055.

10. Riebe D., Franklin B. A., Thompson P. D., et al. Updating ACSM's Recommendations for Exercise Preparticipation Health Screening. *Medicine and Science in Sports and Exercise*. 2015;**47**(11):2473–2479.

11. Thompson P. D., Franklin B. A., Balady G. J., et al. Exercise and Acute Cardiovascular Events Placing the Risks into Perspective: A Scientific Statement from the American Heart Association Council on Nutrition, Physical Activity, and Metabolism and the Council on Clinical Cardiology. *Circulation*. 2007;**115**(17):2358–2368.

12. Harris K. M., Creswell L. L., Haas T. S., et al. Death and Cardiac Arrest in U.S. Triathlon Participants, 1985 to 2016: A Case Series. *Annals of Internal Medicine*. 2017.

13. Turris S., Lund A., Mui J., Wang P., Lewis K., Gutman S. An Organized Medical Response for the Vancouver International Marathon: When the Rubber Hits the Road. *Current Sports Medicine Reports*. 2014;**13**(3):147e154.

14. Ewert G. D. Marathon Race Medical Administration. *Sports Medicine*. 2007;**37**(4–5):428–430. doi: 10.2165/ 00007256-200737040-00040.

15. Ross C., Başdere M., Chan J. L., Mehrotra S., Smilowitz K., Chiampas G. Data Value in Patient Tracking Systems at Racing Events. *Medicine and Science in Sports and Exercise*. 2015;**47**(10):2014–2023. doi: 10.1249/ MSS.0000000000000637.

16. American College of Sports Medicine. Mass Participation Event Management for the Team Physician: A Consensus Statement. *Medicine and Science in Sports and Exercise*. 2004;**36**(11):2004–2008. doi: 10.1249/01. mss.0000145452.18404.f2.

17. Cohen S., Ellis E . Death and Near Death from Cardiac Arrest During the Boston Marathon: Pacing and Clinical Electrophysiology. *PACE*. 2012;**35**:241–244. doi: 10.1111/j.1540– 8159.2011.03248.x.

18. Pickard L., Agar C., Butler L., Bhangu A. Adequacy of Immediate Care Documentation at a Major United Kingdom Endurance Event. *European Journal of Emergency Medicine*. 2010;**17**(3):170–172. doi: 10.1097/MEJ.0b013e3283307b23.

19. Yao K. V., Troyanos C., D'Hemmecourt P., Roberts W. O. Optimizing Marathon Race Safety Using an Incident Command Post Strategy. *Current Sports Medicine Reports*. 2017;**16**(3):144e149.

20. Montain S. J., Ely M. R., Cheuvront S. N. Marathon Performance in Thermally Stressing Conditions. *Sports Medicine*. 2007;**37**(4–5):320–323. doi: 10.2165/ 00007256-200737040-00012.

21. Hanken T., Young S., Smilowitz K., Chiampas G., Waskowski D. Developing a Data Visualization System for the Bank of America Chicago Marathon (Chicago, Illinois USA). *Prehospital and Disaster Medicine*. 2016;**31**(5):572–577. doi: 10.1017/ S1049023X1600073X.

22. Kenefick R. W., Sawka M. N. Heat Exhaustion and Dehydration as Causes of Marathon Collapse. *Sports Medicine*. 2007;**37**(4–5):378–381. doi: 10.2165/ 00007256-200737040-00027.

23. Miles M. P., Clarkson P. M. Exercise-Induced Muscle Pain, Soreness, and Cramps. *Journal of Sports Medicine and Physical Fitness*. 1994;**34**(3):203–216.

24. Gauer R., Meyers B. K. Heat-Related Illnesses. *American Family Physician*. 2019;**99**(8):482–489.

25. Sloan B. K., Kraft E. M., Clark D., Schmeissing S. W., Byrne B. C., Rusyniak D. E. On-Site Treatment of Exertional Heat Stroke. *American Journal of Sports Medicine*. 2015;**43**(4):823–829. doi: 10.1177/ 0363546514566194.

26. Hew-Butler T. Exercise-Associated Hyponatremia. *Frontiers of Hormone Research*. 2019;**52**:178–189. doi: 10.1159/000493247.

27. Schwellnus M., Swanevelder S., Derman W., et al. Prerace Medical Screening and Education Reduce Medical Encounters in Distance Road Races: SAFER VIII study in 153,208 Race Starters. *British Journal of Sports Medicine*. 2018;**0**:1e7.

Mass Gathering Events: Extended Duration Events

Sarah Kleinschmidt and Rebecca G. Breslow

Introduction

On May 22, 2021, at 9:00 am the gun went off to start the Yellow River Stone Forest Ultramarathon in the Gansu Province of China. Racers paced down the trail, among them some of the country's most elite ultra-runners [1]. Less than halfway through the race the weather changed, bringing hail, strong winds, and freezing temperatures to a mountainous section. Over the next day and night over 1,200 volunteers, technical teams, drones, and helicopters participated in an enormous rescue effort to find, treat, and recover runners who were injured, hypothermic, lost, or dead. Of the 172 runners who began that race, 21 died and dozens more were hospitalized. It was the deadliest athletic competition in recent memory.

Though tragic, this event is also instructive to those providing medical support to events that are longer, more remote, and more complex than standard road races. Athletes faced unique stresses from the distance and environment. Support and rescue efforts also faced significant challenges from the same terrain, distance, and conditions, slowing response times and posing physical risk to medical teams. Though the number of participants was small, significant resources were required to manage these unique circumstances. Healthy, well-trained participants encountered increased risk and a catastrophic outcome due to the extreme conditions.

This event led to a ban on all ultramarathons in China while national officials investigated further. All practitioners involved in mass participation event medical planning should consider similar questions. This chapter covers medical support for planned events lasting longer than six hours, including endurance events, multisport and remote races, and multiday festivals. We encourage review of prior chapters for information on overlapping, relevant areas. Although they share many common features, we will not specifically discuss the medical needs of military units, prolonged expeditions, or small groups that live and travel in remote locations.

The highly variable nature of events makes it difficult to draw consistent conclusions regarding medical risks and support. Providers must carefully evaluate the specifics of each event and must tolerate a higher degree of uncertainty than with more traditional race formats, distances, and settings. Complexity is the only constant, as each of the listed factors can impact the logistics of preventing medical incidents, providing tangible support, and evacuating participants. Medical providers must be in close contact with race organizers to manage these challenges, as well as contribute to risk management decisions throughout the planning process.

Event Classification

Extreme mass participation events may be categorized by their size, duration, sport or activity, and location. The unique characteristics of each race contribute variable risks and considerations. Traditionally, mass gathering events include 1,000 or more participants, however, many extreme or prolonged events are significantly smaller. The event duration may include both the duration of components of the event and of the entire event. For example, a multistage or relay race may have operations that extend over multiple days, though each part may consist of shorter athletic efforts [2]. The geographic and political location affects the medical and rescue supports available, as well as legal or operational constraints. The route is also crucially important. This defines access for support or evacuations, and presents specific environmental or terrain hazards.

Individual events present their own challenges. Most ultramarathons take place on remote wilderness trails, but some include significant portions within an urban area or consist entirely of repetitions of a single city block [2–4]. A music or cultural festival may be in a remote area, and though not an athletic competition, may pose similar physiologic stresses of prolonged exertion and exposure. Open water swimming may be a brief but risky segment of a multisport event, or may include a single, multihour or even multiday effort. Orienteering or way-finding competitions may not have a predictable distance or route. Even more extreme, the newer "Last Person Standing" running races define a route which is repeated at a specific interval (usually 4.17 miles each hour), but this cycle continues indefinitely until only one participant is able to continue [5].

Epidemiology

Though highly variable and complicated, there are some patterns to medical encounters at extreme endurance events that can guide preparation. Longer events tend to have a higher rate of encounters per participant, though the vast majority are for minor complaints and do not require evacuation. Serious, life-threatening medical encounters do occur at extreme events. However, providers should also be prepared for more benign but atypical complaints, such as skin injuries, gastrointestinal complaints, and infectious diseases. Multisport and remote events have higher rates of traumatic injuries. Any life-threatening event in a remote setting can become catastrophic due to inevitable delays in response time.

Participation in ultra-endurance events has exponentially increased during recent years both by the number of events and by the number of participants [6, 7]. As a cohort, endurance athletes tend to be somewhat older than other athletic cohorts, with an average age of 42.3 years in one large survey [8]. The same survey found that the majority (68 percent) were men, and that overall participants reported low rates of chronic medical conditions. However, both women and children have also shown increasing participation in endurance events, with unclear implications for medical encounters and needs [6, 9].

Multiple studies have shown an overall higher rate of medical encounters in ultramarathons compared to shorter distance events, although these are mainly heterogeneous case reports so may not be appropriate for direct comparison. One meta-analysis gathering data from 1983 through 2014 estimated that 65.6 percent of ultramarathon runners required medical attention during their event, compared to 7.8 percent

for marathon runners [10]. However, one large ultra-marathon reported only 8.2 percent of participants requiring medical care [11]. Longer events appear to have even higher incidence rates; for example, up to 85 percent of participants required medical care at a seven-day stage ultramarathon [12]. A direct multi-year comparison of participants in 21 kilometer versus 56 kilometer road races showed 12.98 medical complications per 1,000 runners for 56 kilometers, compared to 5.14 per 1,000 for 21 kilometers [13]. The only two deaths occurred in the shorter distance races and there was no significant difference in the incidence of serious medical complications.

Medical encounters at endurance events are largely for non-life-threatening complaints. For instance, although most runners in a seven-day stage race participants required care, 95 percent of these complaints were minor, and included skin pathology (74.3 percent), musculoskeletal injuries (18.2 percent) or other minor medical complaints (7.5 percent) [12]. A smaller but similar stage race reported a medical encounter rate of 56 percent of participants [14]. In this study, the most common complaints were blisters (33.3 percent), chafing (9.1 percent) and lower limb musculoskeletal injuries (22.2 percent). A single day 65 kilometer race reported 37.7 percent of participants suffered fatigue, followed by cramps (26.2 percent), headache and vomiting (both 9.8 percent), dehydration/heat (6.6 percent), and other gastrointestinal complaints (4.9 percent) [15]. A larger event reported that the most common medical illnesses were dehydration or exercise-associated muscle cramping [16].

Race-Level Factors: While endurance running events have the most robust studies, endurance cycling has a similar medical encounter incidence, with a trend toward more severe injuries. A multiday stage race in Turkey reported an overall incidence of 5.83 per 1,000 cycling hours, or 18.6 percent of participants, comprising mostly skin and musculoskeletal complaints. Only one participant was hospitalized; this was for a traumatic pneumothorax [17]. Similarly a review of Tour de France cyclists found that most withdrawals from the race were due to acute trauma, most frequently fractures [18]. Another study of a 315 kilometer cycling race in Sweden found that a total of 0.35 percent of hospitalized starters had fractures, largely to the upper body [19].

Cycling injuries may be highly variable based on terrain and collisions and are influenced by both course and competition characteristics. A study of road cycling events in Flanders showed that over 30 percent of riders sustained a serious injury. The most common cause was collision with another rider [20]. In contrast, recreational cycling tours have a much lower rate of overall injury (3.6 percent and 4.2 percent in two separate studies) [21, 22]. Although there is limited evidence on competitive off-trail cycling endurance events, recreational studies suggest that trail riding may have a higher rate of injury, with fewer head injuries but more thoracic trauma [23].

Triathlons and multisport events have more limited evidence. A survey of triathlons found a low fatality rate for all race distances, with most occurring during the swim portion [24]. Reviews of all medical encounters during shorter races suggest a low overall rate, and the majority were musculoskeletal and skin injuries sustained during running or cycling [25]. A half Ironman triathlon race, comprising a 1.2 mile swim, 56 mile cycle, and 13.1 mile run, reported that most encounters were for traumatic injuries sustained during the run portion, though five fatalities occurred during the cycling portion [26].

Some specific race types and locations may raise risks for illness, injury, or death. A report of a trail race occurring in Nepal at high altitude described an evacuation for high altitude pulmonary edema, though 35 percent of participants used diuretic prophylaxis [27]. A large long-distance ski race had a rate of cardiac arrests of 2.16 per 100,000 participants, and they primarily occurred during the first third of the course. The authors speculated that temperature may have influenced cardiac events in this setting [28]. Obstacle course races report a lower incidence of acute injury (2.4 percent), though this may reflect their generally shorter distances [29].

Music and cultural festivals have wide variation in the number and nature of medical encounters, ranging from 0.13 to 20.8 encounters per 1,000 participants in one review [30]. Most encounters were for minor illness such as headaches or abdominal complaints. A review of Australian gatherings found that the rate of encounters increased if alcohol was present, the crowd was predominantly male, or in adverse weather conditions [31]. A report of the seven-day 2011 Burning Man festival described 2,307 of 53,735 participants who received medical care, most for minor soft tissue injuries, dehydration, eye problems, and urinary infections [32]. There was one death from subarachnoid hemorrhage and one patient who survived a cardiac arrest due to aortic dissection.

Participant-Level Factors: Participant characteristics may also predict medical risks at an event. At multiple distances, less racing experience, slower pace, older age, and female gender have been associated with a variety of complications including gastrointestinal distress and postural hypotension. Cramping and skin problems are also pace-dependent, and are primarily found in faster runners [33]. Female gender, older age, running speed, wind speed, and heat also influence encounter rates during cycling events. Slower speed has been associated with illness complaints and faster speed with traumatic incidents [34, 35].

Medical Concerns

Prolonged exertion leads to a broad and unique set of physiologic stressors, distinct from higher intensity, shorter efforts. Almost all finishers of endurance races have pathology of multiple organ systems, including significant caloric deficits, renal strain, skeletal and cardiac muscle damage, hemolysis, hormonal deficits, transaminitis, acute inflammation, and immune suppression [36]. While we will focus here on problems likely to be either symptomatic or emergent, providers should recognize that most patients will have multiple underlying pathologies. Both trauma and environmental injuries, as well as a patient's cognitive or mental health status may introduce unique pathology and considerations for the treating provider.

Cardiac: Marathon running has been shown to increase the risk of sudden cardiac death, exercise associated collapse, and tropinemia, but these risks appear to be more related to exercise intensity than duration. In fact, there is some evidence that cardiac biomarkers are less deranged following longer events, presumably due to the lower exercise intensity [37, 38]. Faster runners at one ultramarathon showed significantly more cardiac biomarker elevation than finishers near the cut-off time [39]. One of the most dramatic troponin elevations found in sporting activity (mean 900 percent) was found in runners of an uphill only trail marathon [40].

Multiple studies describe only modest and temporary changes to cardiac markers after other prolonged events [36]. In a study of participants in a 63 kilometer ultramarathon, left ventricular ejection fraction (LVEF) and cardiac output were decreased initially postrace, but normalized within twenty-four hours [41]. Both tropinemia and brain natriuretic protein (BNP) also normalize within hours [42]. In participants of one twenty-four-hour race, troponin continued to increase with distance, while BNP elevation peaked at marathon distance and LVEF improved over the course the race [43].

Sudden cardiac death is a rare event. There is no evidence that endurance events pose a specific risk compared to marathon or shorter races [13]. However, multiple cardiac events have been reported during these races. Ultra-endurance athletes tend to be older with a higher proportion of male participants than shorter-distance cohorts [36, 44]. Cold environments like those found in open-water swimming and cross-country skiing may pose a specific risk, possibly due to vasoconstriction [24, 28]. Atraumatic cardiac arrests at music or cultural festivals are largely associated with toxic ingestions or overdoses [45]. Providers should therefore be prepared to provide advanced life support including treatment of causative factors.

Exercise-associated collapse (EAC) has been well documented at endurance events and shorter road races [36]. The rate of asymptomatic postural hypotension after finishing an ultramarathon may be as high as 68 percent, likely related to dehydration and vascular dysregulation [46]. One running ultramarathon found that a full 56 percent of participants who did not finish also experienced EAC. Though EAC is generally a benign condition, medical evaluation and response may be complicated if they occur at locations other than the finish line [2]. Treatment consists of supine or Trendelenburg positioning, oral hydration and cooling, and further evaluation and treatment if the patient does not improve rapidly.

Dermatologic: While skin conditions are rarely severe, providers should be prepared for a high volume of performance-limiting complaints. Chafing can result from friction with moist skin or clothing, and can be treated with lubricating and barrier creams [47]. Abrasions are common in trail or multisport events, as well as nonathletic gatherings. Cycling crashes may result in extensive, contaminated or deep abrasions requiring debridement and bandaging [48]. Lacerations should be thoroughly cleaned and bandaged. If repair is required, the patient should be transported for further evaluation and infection control. Sunburn prevention and treatment is another frequent medical intervention. Soft tissue infection may develop during multiday events, and repeated dressing changes, compresses, antibiotics, and even drainage may be required [12].

Blisters are one of the most common complaints by ultra-endurance athletes, especially in running events. In one stage race, 76 percent of participants had clinically significant blisters, most frequently on their toes [49]. Prior race experience may decrease the risk, though other preventative methods that have been studied (including different socks, antiperspirants and mechanical barriers) are not effective [50]. Paper tape may provide some protection, and various taping techniques are a mainstay of treatment once an area of friction develops [51, 52]. To prevent further friction, many providers advocate for low profile tapes or dressings, contouring dressings to the foot, and using adhesive agents such as tincture of benzoin. Large blisters may benefit from field drainage, especially if ongoing friction is expected, the blister is affecting gait or shoe fit, and it can be appropriately drained in clean conditions [53, 54].

Gastrointestinal and Nutrition: The well-known ultra-endurance athlete Ann Trason called ultramarathons "an eating and drinking competition, with a little bit of running thrown in" [55]. Consequently, ultra-endurance events have a higher incidence of gastrointestinal concerns, and significant ramifications if affected athletes are not able to maintain hydration and nutritional status. Race distance, as well as slower speed, appear to be the strongest predictors for developing significant GI distress [56, 57]. Lower GI symptoms of bloating, diarrhea, and flatulence may be even more prevalent than nausea, especially during running events [58].

Gastrointestinal symptoms reduce caloric, macronutrient and fluid intake [59]. Lower gastrointestinal symptoms may lead to self-restriction of calories, and fluid and electrolyte losses from diarrhea [60]. Even in ideal circumstances, the caloric demands of endurance events almost always outpace intake, leading to measurable caloric deficits of over 4,000 kilocalories and a decrease in body mass, adipose tissue, and muscle [61]. Recent guidelines recommend intake of 150 to 400 kilocalories/hour to "attenuate" caloric deficits [62]. Greater caloric deficits increase the likelihood of not finishing, and also increase the risk of significant medical issues such as renal dysfunction, hypothermia, skeletal and cardiac muscle stress [63]. Gastrointestinal symptoms are among the most common reasons for athletes to withdraw from endurance events [36].

Oral ondansetron is commonly used to treat ultra-marathon-associated nausea, however, a recent randomized controlled trial showed no significant effect [64]. This may be due to the wide range of underlying causes of nausea, including hormonal or electrolyte imbalances, heat stress, altitude, supplements or medications, anxiety or infection, or ill-chosen fasting, food, or beverages [57]. Splanchnic blood flow changes can lead to intestinal ischemia and permeability, while neuroendocrine stress slows motility [36, 65]. Gastrointestinal symptoms may demand supportive care, rest, temperature management, and medication to restore normal functioning. In addition to traditional anti-emetics, simethicone and artichoke and ginger extracts have shown promise for both upper and lower gastrointestinal symptoms [66]. During multiday, wilderness or international events, providers may also consider treating for infectious gastroenteritis, especially with known exposures or symptom clusters.

Musculoskeletal: Musculoskeletal injuries are extremely common during endurance events. Although traumatic injuries may occur (especially during cycling, multisport, or technical mountainous events), endurance athletes are also at significant risk for atraumatic overuse injuries. Common complaints include patellofemoral syndrome, Achilles tendonitis, or lower limb stress fractures, which may present at any point during a training cycle or event [36] [1]. Participant screening may limit this risk [67]. Providers may be asked to assist athletes who frequently continue to compete through their injury. This may not always be detrimental; some MRI studies have demonstrated cartilage regeneration and active adaptation during extended stage races [61].

Rhabdomyolysis deserves special consideration, given the overall high prevalence of renal injury in ultra-endurance athletes [36]. Most ultra-runners experience muscle damage, and have significantly elevated creatinine kinase (CK) enzymes compared to baseline following their event, with values after a 67 kilometer run averaging 2573 U/l and those after a 100 mile race averaging 14,569 U/l [68, 69]. CK levels increase during longer distance races compared to shorter distance races [37]. Additionally, the eccentric stress of downhill running or warm conditions can result in elevations in CK [36]. Individual variation can be significant and may correlate with training load as well as experience [70, 71]. For instance, at the 2012 100-mile Western States Endurance Run two-thirds of runners had significant CK elevation, ranging from 1,500 to 264,300 U/l, and 6 percent of finishers had values above 100,000 U/l [72]. However, other studies (including prior years at the same event) have found only rare CK elevations above 20,000 U/l [36].

Most athletes with elevated CK levels remain asymptomatic and do not require major medical interventions [69]. Follow-up studies show that within days the majority of athletes recover normal muscle function and CK levels [73]. One comparison of highly trained athletes versus amateurs showed that though the former had higher serum markers of muscle damage, they exhibited a higher level of neuromuscular performance [74]. Another study failed to find correlation between CK elevation and reduced postrace physical activity after an 118 kilometer mountain ultramarathon [75].

Although CK elevation and renal injury are both common in ultra-endurance athletes, it is not clear that rhabdomyolysis is a common mechanism for the renal injury. Several small studies have shown that elevated creatinine and urea concentrations precede pathologic CK elevation [76]. There are no studies correlating CK levels with the extent of renal injury, and most CK elevations in the context of endurance racing remain at the low end of the range known to cause rhabdomyolysis [36, 68]. The largest report of acute renal failure after an ultramarathon showed no relationship between this condition and CK concentrations [77]. In fact, multiple studies suggest that rhabdomyolysis is more common with preceding or concurrent hyponatremia [78, 79]. Taken together, these findings suggest that ultra-endurance athletes will rarely present with renal dysfunction purely from rhabdomyolysis. Muscle breakdown may instead be both an effect of and a contributor to combined metabolic derangements.

Neurologic and Psychiatric: Although primary neurologic pathology is uncommon during endurance events, the metabolic demands of endurance racing can impact cognitive function. Multiple imaging studies have documented changes in brain volume following endurance events [80, 81]. Runners are often sleep deprived, and some studies even show that forgoing sleep leads to faster finishing times, likely due to less time spent at rest [82]. Increasing sleep time prior to a race does not compensate for lost sleep from near continuous running for over twenty-four hours. Some studies and many anecdotes describe a range of effects, from decreased response times to hallucinations and delusions [83, 84]. This may severely challenge athletes' functional abilities, including route-finding, navigating technical terrain, and managing physiologic needs.

Endurance exercise does have well-documented benefits for mental health [80, 85, 86]. Many runners report achieving a desirable "flow" state, and racers tend to have high levels of mental toughness, resilience and self-efficacy [87, 88]. However, athlete cohorts also carry a higher prevalence of preexisting mental health diagnoses, and individual athletes may demonstrate maladaptive dependence on exercise as a coping strategy [89, 90]. These combined neuropsychiatric characteristics may lead medical providers into complex decisions around runners who wish to continue racing despite decreasing physiologic and cognitive functioning.

These situations will be smoother if medical staff, race officials, participants, and support teams have a shared ethical and risk management framework [2]. For instance many races now specify that medical staff may force an athlete to withdraw if doing so would pose a risk to themselves or others. Other events may permit participants to continue against medical advice, but the athletes should be reminded of risks to their future training and performance as well as their overall health. They should be applauded for the training and fortitude to reach their physiologic limits. And if they choose to continue, medical staff should make every effort to have close monitoring and support available if their condition deteriorates.

Renal Issues, Fluids and Electrolytes: Most endurance athletes suffer from renal and electrolyte derangements, which presents challenges for the field practitioner. Significant volume depletion is common, although body mass measurements are complicated by concurrent caloric deficits [91]. Multiple studies have shown weight loss of up to 8 percent without symptoms or pathology, and racers who lose more bodyweight can have faster performances [92–95]. Weight loss occurs early in endurances races, after which most participants can self-regulate intake to achieve a steady state. Fluid consumption often decreases at greater distances [96, 97].

Although most athletes can maintain equilibrium without symptoms, some develop impaired renal function. Multiple studies have shown creatinine elevation in the range of 1.3 to 2.0 mg/dL deviations from baseline in a substantial number of athletes [36, 97]. Intra-race measurements of creatinine and

BUN suggest a similar pattern to hydration for these markers, which increase before the first checkpoint and then obtain a steady state until after the race [76]. Multiday stage races appear to have even higher risk. One multiday running event found a cumulative incidence of renal injury of 41 percent, with higher rates on later days, suggesting ongoing stress combined with incomplete recovery between stages [98].

More significant renal injury is less common. In one 100-mile race, 4 percent of finishers more than doubled their serum creatinine over the course of the race, though the majority remained asymptomatic [72]. The same race did report 5 of 400 starters hospitalized with either hyponatremia, renal injury, rhabdomyolysis, or a combination of these disorders. Three participants developed renal failure [77]. Most studies show no clinical effect associated with lab derangements and almost all subjects studied recover normal function within twenty-four hours [76, 97]. Athletes who suffer from acute kidney injury (AKI) are likely to have similar dysfunction after future stresses, but have no specific increased risk [71]. Although long-term effects in endurance athletes are unknown, general population studies suggest repeated AKI episodes are associated with chronic renal disease [99].

Sodium balance can also be deranged, with variable prevalence and with a general trend toward hypernatremia versus hyponatremia [36]. For instance, one study of collapsed runners found that 45 percent had hypernatremia while only 2 percent had hyponatremia, and both groups required additional medical care compared to normonatremic athletes [100]. Similar findings from a multistage race showed that hypernatremia is three times more common than hyponatremia, though the prevalence of both increases during successive days of racing [12]. Other studies have reported rates of hyponatremia as high as 42 percent without symptoms, though most estimates are below 10 percent [36, 101]. Hyponatremia may be due to overconsumption of water and inappropriate maintenance of prerace weight [12, 36]. The prevalence of exercise-associated hyponatremia increases with longer event duration, higher ambient temperatures, female sex, and specific sport disciplines. It occurs more frequently during swimming, triathlon, and running events than cycling events [102].

Prevention of AKI and hyponatremia can be achieved by decreasing the intensity and duration of exercise, though this may not be compatible with training or competing in endurance events. Athletes should be counseled to drink to thirst, avoid over-hydration, and balance fluid intake with appropriate calories and electrolytes. Heat stress should be monitored and mitigated where possible. Sodium supplementation has no significant effect [103]. Many endurance athletes report non-steroidal anti-inflammatory medicine (NSAID) use during prolonged training or racing, which may also carry risk [104, 105]. One placebo-controlled study of ultra-marthoners found that ibuprofen significantly increased the risk of AKI, and the number needed to harm was only 5.5 participants [106]. NSAID use has also been associated with exercise-associated hyponatremia [107]. Athletes should avoid these medications and medical practitioners should educate and counsel against their use prior to or during endurance training or competition [108, 109].

Field management largely rests on symptoms, including empiric provision of oral fluids to the majority of patients with minor symptoms [2, 110]. Patients with clinical suspicion for hyponatremia may be provided hypertonic solutions such as broth, with minimal risk of worsening other derangements. Targeted or intravenous correction is limited by laboratory testing capabilities. Though portable equipment is available, it is expensive and has many logistical barriers to field implementation. Physical examination should be performed, but vital signs, weight, skin turgor and edema may have limited sensitivity and specificity for clinical dehydration in the endurance runner [111]. Urine dipstick proteinuria and hematuria have good sensitivity and specificity for renal injury, though specific gravity may not reflect volume status if regulatory mechanisms are disrupted [112, 113]. Rest is also essential and may lead to spontaneous diuresis of the dysregulated hyponatremic patient: as Grand Canyon medical staff are directed, "when in doubt, sit it out until they pee it out" [114]. A patient with altered mental status or seizures and a high suspicion for hyponatremia may warrant empiric treatment with small hypertonic saline boluses even without plasma values, as the benefit of rapid correction likely outweighs the risks [109]. Any patients with persistent or severe symptoms should cease racing and be referred to a setting with laboratory monitoring to guide correction.

Traumatic: Traumatic injuries are expected at endurance events and can range from minor to catastrophic. Traumatic deaths at music or cultural festivals may involve intentional and penetrating injuries [45]. Cycling, multisport, and mountain athletes are also at higher risk for blunt trauma, including multiple deaths that have occurred from crashes or falls [20, 25]. Participants who experience minor traumatic injuries should be evaluated and treated for skin, soft tissue, and musculoskeletal pathology. Evaluation of more severe injuries should focus on identification of injuries, stabilization, and transport. Interventions may include hemorrhage control, basic life support, immobilization, and rapid transport. Transport may require outside resources or technical rescue. Especially in remote environments, providers should consider selective spinal immobilization using either NEXUS or Canadian C-spine Rules [115]. Head injuries, and particularly those sustained in high speed accidents during cycling events, can be severe. Providers must recognize the need for further imaging and should evaluate thoroughly for concussion. This generally requires removal from competition to prevent secondary injury [116].

Environmental: Both hyper- and hypothermia are serious medical complications of endurance events and can be life-threatening. Even modest heat, generally measured via wet bulb globe temperature (WBGT), increases the risk of renal injury, hyponatremia, intestinal permeability, rhabdomyolysis, cardiac strain and sudden death [39, 102, 117]. In hotter conditions, a significant portion of racers may have elevated core body temperatures and develop exertional heat stroke. This condition is defined as a core body temperature of greater than 40 degrees Celsius and altered mental status, and can be fatal if not promptly treated [118]. High levels of individual fitness and acclimatization may be protective. There are also race-level prevention measures, which include frequent rest stops, fluid stations and cooling modalities. Rarely, in extreme conditions, races may be cancelled [2, 119, 120]. Treatment consists of rest and cooling. In cases of exertional heat stroke, confirmed by rectal core body temperature measurement, rapid cooling via cold water immersion to a temperature of less than 39 degrees Celsius within 30 minutes of presentation is critical to prevent end organ damage and death [118, 121].

Cold stress presents different challenges. While there is some evidence that moderately cold conditions improve endurance performance, cold exposure can also increase caloric needs, auto-diuresis from vasoconstriction and rates of exercise-associated sudden cardiac death [28, 122, 123]. Inhaling cold air can cause bronchospasm even in otherwise healthy individuals [123, 124]. Precipitation and wind increase evaporative and convective losses and may result in life-threatening hypothermia, especially if weather changes are sudden. Even milder conditions may become deadly for racers who become lost, injured, calorie-depleted or otherwise unable to maintain their usually high metabolic output [1]. Event organizers should issue mandatory gear lists to adequately prepare athletes for rapid changes to weather or to their own thermal production. Treatment of hypothermia depends on severity, with mild cases often responding to protection from further heat loss and provision of extra calories as tolerated to encourage metabolic heat production. More severe cases with altered mental status may require a hypothermic wrap, gentle handling, and cardiac monitoring during evacuation to definitive care [125].

High altitude (above 10,000 feet or 3,000 meters) commonly causes acute mountain sickness (AMS) with symptoms of headaches, fatigue, sleep difficulty and nausea [126]. One study reported that one-third of athletes in a high altitude ultramarathon took acetazolamide [27]. Though this medication can prevent altitude-induced symptoms, it is also a diuretic and thus carries the risk of worsening dehydration and renal injury. Severe illness, such as pulmonary or cerebral edema, may also develop during events held at high altitude, and may require more emergent treatment and evacuation. Providers should be familiar with guidelines for both prophylaxis and treatment, which may include oxygen, medications, and repressurization through a Gamow bag [127].

Lightning has killed ultramarathon athletes. Risks include events late in the day, during warm or summer months, local weather patterns, and geographic exposure [109, 128]. Race staff should consider cancelling or rescheduling races with a specific risk of lightning. Given the prolonged and unexpected nature of endurance races, medical directors should also consider educating athletes on preventive measures, and should be familiar with current treatment guidelines [129].

Event Planning

Scope of Care: One of the most important tasks for a medical provider is determining what medical support and precautions are required and reasonable for a particular event. Medical needs and logistical constraints vary widely among extended events due to the diversity of activities, location, terrain, weather, size, and condition of participants. In general, remote endurance races are likely to have increased delays and gaps in support compared to typical road events [2]. On the other hand, a stationary multiday event such as a festival may be able to anticipate and accommodate an increased volume and complexity of medical needs [32].

While medical support should target participant safety, the primary aim is to decrease undue burden on the local medical system, including prehospital or backcountry resources. A survey of endurance athletes found that almost all expect some level of on-site medical support, including simple medications [130]. However, 91.5 percent of surveyed participants felt race organizers should make clear what medical services are available. Organizers should prioritize communication about available services and limitations. They should also communicate early and often with local service providers, especially if they anticipate scenarios requiring additional assistance.

Hoffman et al. recently formulated guidelines for medical standards for ultramarathons, which can be extrapolated to other endurance events [109]. They suggest a tiered system matching medical providers, lay volunteers, and equipment to the size, distance, duration, locale, and environmental conditions of an event. Small or remote events may accept longer access and transport times and a higher burden on local emergency systems due to practical barriers to providing closer support. For very small or remote events, medical support may consist solely of supplies and information for participants, as well as prenotification of responding agencies. Large events with road access and a high anticipated need might provide significantly higher-level care, including multiple shifts of physician staff, basic laboratory tests and imaging, and rapid access to resuscitation and transport. Available local resources may vary widely depending on location, from experienced mountain rescue teams with on board physicians, to areas accessible only by prolonged ground transport with basic life support. In very remote or international locations, there may be no established prehospital system. At a minimum, event staff should notify nearby prehospital and hospital agencies and should gather detailed information, such as the most efficient communication plan and any limitations based on weather, terrain, or nighttime flying. If possible, event and local staff should meet to discuss likely scenarios and preplan a coordinated response, such as by sharing radio communications or staging local units near likely evacuation points.

Preventative Measures: Given the risks to both participants and rescuers, medical directors should coordinate with race leadership on reasonable preventive measures. Medical input may be useful at early stages. This includes planning the length and route of the course, and suggestions on the location and frequency of mandatory rest stops. Medical input on these measures minimizes hazards, maximizes rescuer access, and potentially decreases medical encounters while maintaining the necessary competitive components [109, 120]. The availability of food, fluids, electrolytes, and shelter may be as important as technical medical supplies, and medical directors should advocate for adequate provisions. They may also offer advice on which first aid supplies, clothing or rescue gear participants should carry to decrease the number and severity of medical events. For instance, GPS tracking of participants is highly recommended for remote or large events, while NSAIDs should not be provided due to increased risk of renal injury and hyponatremia [109].

In addition to logistical coordination, medical staff, race directors, and participants should have a shared understanding of ethics, communication, and decision-making prior to the race. Many races emphasize participant autonomy and responsibility for their own safety, relegating medical staff to an advisory and support role. Other races assign medical staff a greater risk management role that may involve mandating participant withdrawal or race cancellation, if indicated. This understanding should be clearly outlined prior to the event so that medical staff, participants, and race directors are aligned with each other, as well as with local laws and cultural practices. Cancelling a race should not be taken lightly, but may be necessary for the safety of participants, volunteers or bystanders due to adverse temperature, lightning, precipitation, air quality, violence, traffic, or myriad other acute risks [109].

Prerace screening to reduce the risk of serious medical encounters should be strongly considered. One longitudinal study found that an online questionnaire followed by automated education of high risk participants led to a significant decrease in all medical encounters (29 percent) and in life-threatening emergencies (64 percent) [67]. Such questionnaires can identify participants who are very high risk due to known cardiovascular disease, high risk due to cardiac risk factors, intermediate risk due to other chronic diseases, injuries or medication risks, or low risk [34, 131]. Specific medical risks include cardiovascular disease or risk factors, seizure disorders, diabetes, asthma, mental health problems, anaphylactic reactions, current pregnancy, and any prior history of exertional hyponatremia, renal injury, rhabdomyolysis, altitude illness, or gastrointestinal bleeding [132].

There are some limits to screening by medical directors, which may be most accurately viewed as a risk management conversation between medical staff, race directors and potential participants [132]. One study showed that over 30 percent of participants met at least one high risk criteria, suggesting that some criteria may be overly broad [131]. Many risk factors are nonmodifiable and possibly discriminatory, such as female sex and increasing age [16]. Risks may be complex and may depend on a participant's medical condition and on the nature of the event. For instance, multiple recommendations advise providers to perform a complete history, exam and counseling for all participants prior to endurance and wilderness activities, which may not be practical for a race medical director [133, 134]. Education can prevent many mishaps, and prerace briefings can be used to prepare participants for common scenarios [135]. Ultimately, providers should recognize risks, educate both participants and race directors, and contribute to any possible risk mitigation decisions including possible removal from the race.

Medical Response

Structure and Staffing: Given the complexity of these events, coordinators should use a formal command structure, such as an incident command system (ICS), if feasible. Within the United States, the ICS is now incorporated into a broader multidisciplinary National Incident Management System, though it was originally developed to manage complex responses to wildfires. Whether or not a formal ICS is established, the principles of delegation of focused tasks, and clear limited lines of communication are crucial for effective management [136]. Contingency planning for both anticipated and catastrophic incidents is essential. While physicians often lead the medical response, it is also reasonable for medical personnel to function as a smaller operational unit within a larger logistical structure.

Most extended distance events require coordination of multiple medical aid sites throughout the course, though many encounters occur at the finish line. In contrast to shorter events, encounters at longer events may not be more frequent during the latter half of the race and should be expected throughout the course [137]. For instance, one large ultramarathon found that 77 percent of encounters occurred on course rather than at the finish line [11]. Specific situations such as swimming, boating, cycling, or technical portions, or sections with anticipated temperature extremes, may require additional medical resources. While cultural or music events have different injury patterns from athletic events, some predictions can still be made based on weather, event schedules, and previous experience [31].

Physicians should lead teams and should be present at all major stations, though other personnel and lay volunteers may provide essential support. Volunteers with basic training may be able to assist with bandaging or may even staff smaller stations. Wilderness medicine training is useful for mobile or transport teams. Language interpretation may be required for international participants or events.

Events over twelve hours duration should provide rest periods for medical staff. Multiple teams may be scheduled in shifts to allow for eating, sleeping, and mental rest at a busy aid station. Smaller races or more remote stations may consider an "on call" model, in which an individual or small team maintains continuous availability for infrequent encounters. These providers must proactively manage physical and mental fatigue to prevent errors in decision-making and may benefit from having well-rested colleagues available for remote consultation. All providers should be briefed, prepared, and trained for their respective roles and shift responsibilities.

Equipment: As described by Hoffman and others, medical equipment should be matched to the size, nature, and location of an event. It should anticipate both the most common and most catastrophic encounters [109]. In remote, rugged, or prolonged environments, supply management may require designated personnel. Supplies should be clearly labeled and stored appropriately for environmental conditions, including waterproofing. Supplies should be prepared

for field response or rescue as well as stationary medical stations. Extremes of temperature must be mitigated for any electronic devices as well as liquid medications. Complex equipment such as electrolyte analyzers, computers, or defibrillators are prone to malfunction in many circumstances, including cold, water, or sand exposure [2]. Many common supplies can be improvised. Medical or wilderness training may be more useful than additional bandages or prefabricated splints. Medical staff should also consider which advanced medical interventions may be futile in remote environments, such as advanced airways in a noncontrolled environment or defibrillation after a prolonged cardiac arrest.

Transport: Access to a severely ill or injured participant in a remote event is often a significant challenge, as is transport to a facility with an appropriate level of medical care. Even a moderately technical trail may require technical rescue for a nonambulatory patient. Participants have gotten lost during races or fallen down significant slopes, requiring a search or a rescue outside the anticipated area [138, 139]. Medical providers should be aware of all possible evacuation routes and resources, including helicopter availability, on-road and off-road vehicles, and local rescue teams. Such evacuations are often prolonged and require outside resources, and medical directors should consider prenotification and prebriefing of any medical, search, or rescue teams [109]. Medical teams can designate "hasty" or "mobile response" teams of individuals who have the fitness, technical skills, and supplies to rapidly find and stabilize patients prior to a larger response, with a goal of reaching victims within thirty to sixty minutes [109].

Communication: Communication may be a significant challenge in remote locations. Cellular phones, satellite phones, internet, and radios are often limited in range, reception, and availability. For instance, cellular and radio service can be affected by sight lines, while satellites may be affected by weather. International borders can alter equipment legality or available radio channels. Therefore, contingency planning should involve backup methods. Each medical station or team should be prepared to function without close online support, or without the support of online medical references.

Communication with racers deserves special consideration, especially in remote or complex event locations. GPS tracking is strongly recommended for endurance or remote events, as it has proven effective in rapidly locating racers who stray from the intended course [109, 138]. Participants may initiate communication with race staff or emergency responders via phone, emergency beacons, or bystanders. Prerace briefing can clarify appropriate and efficient avenues for various racers' concerns. Most importantly, race staff must be notified of any racer who leaves the event to avoid erroneous searches. Similarly, race directors should have predetermined methods for contacting racers in the event of environmental danger or race cancellation.

Legal: Legal considerations depend largely on the location of the event. Some events may cross multiple jurisdictions, or there may be a different country of origin for providers than for participants. Providers should be licensed in the location where they are providing care and should also be familiar with the scope of practice regulations. Medications should be provided in accordance with local prescribing laws. Signed waivers cannot prevent lawsuits or charges for gross negligence. Therefore, liability protection is essential for the event itself and for each licensed clinician [109]. Although so-called "Good Samaritan" laws protect volunteers in many settings, providers in an official volunteer role may not be covered, even if this role is unpaid [140]. Many jurisdictions also have medical privacy laws in place. Providers should share medical information only on a need-to-know basis to best serve their patients.

Follow-Up

Documentation during and after an event supports patient care, preparation for future events, and risk management for any encounters. Any patient who receives more than basic respite or wound care should have documented assessments, usually written in a SOAP (subjective, objective, assessment, and plan) format. Medical staff should follow up with any participant who was transported to a hospital, or who sought hospital care after the event, to provide continuity of care and to collect feedback regarding their race encounter. Even more minor encounters may have a significant impact on supplies and staffing; inventories and provider feedback help improve future planning. Formalized debrief models assist medical and race staff in identifying specific areas of success or potential need for improvement.

Of note, Schwellnus et al. provide a useful classification system for medical encounters [141]. Their comprehensive format recommends collecting information on the severity and timing of a medical event, along with participant demographic information, and details around the medical problem. Information about antecedent illness, overuse injury or acute injuries is also collected. The goal of these recommendations is to standardize data collection at endurance events to facilitate clinical and research collaborations and to improve patient care. Widespread adoption of this system will greatly enhance our knowledge of rates and types of medical encounters at different events and will inform planning and prevention initiatives.

Summary

Extended events encompass a broad range of activities, environments, and logistical challenges to medical care. While each medical team must therefore evaluate specific risks and needs, there are some patterns that can inform planning. Providers should expect to see a higher volume of encounters, including many minor complaints such as wounds or skin pathology, infectious disease, and gastrointestinal symptoms. Providers should be aware of specific risks from endurance exercise and environmental hazards that can contribute significantly to morbidity and mortality.

Life threatening pathology is not necessarily more common but may be much more complicated to manage in remote or extended-care environments. Because of this, it may be impossible to meet usual standards or scope of care, requiring early and clear communication with event staff and participants. In addition, prevention of medical problems becomes much more relevant, through event planning, prescreening of participants, and early recognition of developing pathology.

Ultimately, those who have experienced these events will attest that the rewards greatly outweigh the burden and risks. Extraordinary events may require intentional deviations from standard practices. Prolonged and remote races or festivals may challenge the endurance of volunteers as well as participants. The diversity of events, multiple contingencies and limited evidence base will demand more extensive preplanning as well as tolerance for uncertainty. However, the provider who accepts these logistical and medical challenges will be rewarded with an unforgettable experience.

References

1. Peterson, J. Twenty-One Runners Die in Sudden Cold Weather Exposure During 100 k Ultramarathon in China. *Wilderness Medical Society News*. wms.org/magazine/1108/Breaking-Wilderness-Medicine-News. Accessed June 25, 2021.

2. Hoffman M. D., Pasternak A., Rogers I. R., et al. Medical Services at Ultra-Endurance Foot Races in Remote Environments: Medical Issues and Consensus Guidelines. *Sports Medicine*. 2014;**44**(8):1055–1069.

3. McCarthy P. The Great New York 100 Mile Running Exposition [Internet]. tgny100. [cited November 22, 2021]. www.tgny100.com. Accessed November 22, 2021.

4. Cunningham G. Running Beyond the Marathon: Insights into the Longest Footrace in the World. eText Press Publishing; 2014.

5. Heine P. The Mentally Brutal Big Backyard Ultra Just Keeps Going Until One Person Is Left Standing. *Runner's World*. 2018. www.runnersworld.com/trail-running/a24079861/big-backyard-ultra-winner/. Accessed November 22, 2021.

6. Scheer V. Participation Trends of Ultra Endurance Events. *Sports Medicine and Arthroscopy Review*. 2019;**27**(1):3–7.

7. Stöhr A., Nikolaidis P. T., Villiger E., et al. An Analysis of Participation and Performance of 2067 100-Kilometer Ultra-Marathons Worldwide. *International Journal of Environmental Research and Public Health*. 2021;**18**(2):362–375.

8. Hoffman M. D., Krishnan E. Health and Exercise-Related Medical Issues among 1,212 Ultramarathon Runners: Baseline Findings from the Ultrarunners Longitudinal TRAcking (ULTRA) Study. *PLoS One*. 2014;**9**(1):e83867.

9. Scheer V., Hoffman M. D. Should Children Be Running Ultramarathons? *Current Sports Medicine Reports*. 2018;**17**(9):282–283.

10. Kluitenberg B., van Middelkoop M., Diercks R., van der Worp H. What Are the Differences in Injury Proportions Between Different Populations of Runners? A Systematic Review and Meta-Analysis. *Sports Medicine*. 2015;**45**(8):1143–1161.

11. McGowan V., Hoffman M. D. Characterization of Medical Care at the 161-Kilometer Western States Endurance Run. *Wilderness and Environmental Medicine Journal*. 2015;**26**(1):29–35.

12. Krabak B. J., Waite B., Schiff M. A. Study of Injury and Illness Rates in Multiday Ultramarathon Runners. *Medicine and Science in Sports and Exercise*. 2011;**43**(12):2314–2320.

13. Schwabe K., Schwellnus M., Derman W., Swanevelder S., Jordaan E. Medical Complications and Deaths in 21 and 56 Kilometer Road Race Runners: A 4-Year Prospective Study in 65,865 runners – SAFER study I. *British Journal of Sports Medicine*. 2014;**48**(11):912–918.

14. Scheer B. V., Murray A. Al Andalus Ultra Trail: An Observation of Medical Interventions During a 219-Kilometer, 5-Day Ultramarathon Stage Race. *Clinical Journal of Sports Medicine*. 2011;**21**(5):444–446.

15. Vernillo G., Savoldelli A., Torre A. L., Skafidas S., Bortolan L., Schena F. Injury and Illness Rates During Ultratrail Running. *International Journal of Sports Medicine*. 2016;**37**(7):565–569.

16. Sewry N., Schwellnus M., Boulter J., Seocharan I., Jordaan E. Medical Encounters in a 90-Kilometer Ultramarathon Running Event: A 6-year Study in 103 131 Race Starters – SAFER XVII. *Clinical Journal of Sports Medicine*. 2021.

17. Yanturali S., Canacik O., Karsli E., Suner S. Injury and Illness Among Athletes During a Multi-Day Elite Cycling Road Race. The *Physician and Sportsmedicine*. 2015;**43**(4):348–354.

18. Haeberle H. S., Navarro S. M., Power E. J., Schickendantz M. S., Farrow L. D., Ramkumar P. N. Prevalence and Epidemiology of Injuries Among Elite Cyclists in the Tour de France. *Orthopaedic Journal of Sports Medicine*. 2018;**6**(9):2325967118793392.

19. Sillén K., Wallenius V. Rates and Types of Injuries During the Three Consecutive Years 2016 to 2018 of the Vätternrundan: One of the World's Largest and Longest Bicycle Races. *Traffic Injury Prevention*. 2019;**20**(7):749–752.

20. Decock M., De Wilde L., Vanden Bossche L., Steyaert A., Van Tongel A. Incidence and Aetiology of Acute Injuries During Competitive Road Cycling. *British Journal of Sports Medicine*. 2016;**50**(11):669–672.

21. Pommering T. L., Manos D. C., Singichetti B., Brown C. R., Yang J. Injuries and Illnesses Occurring on a Recreational Bicycle Tour: The Great Ohio Bicycle Adventure. *Wilderness Environ Med*. 2017;**28**(4):299–306.

22. Boeke P. S., House H. R., Graber M. A. Injury Incidence and Predictors on a Multiday Recreational Bicycle Tour: The Register's Annual Great Bike Ride Across Iowa, 2004 to 2008. *Wilderness and Environmental Medicine Journal*. 2010;**21**(3):202–207.

23. Kotlyar S. Cycling Injuries in Southwest Colorado: A Comparison of Road vs Trail Riding Injury Patterns. *Wilderness and Environmental Medicine Journal*. 2016;**27**(2):316–320.

24. Harris K. M., Creswell L. L., Haas T. S., et al. Death and Cardiac Arrest in U.S. Triathlon Participants, 1985 to 2016: A Case Series. *Annals of Internal Medicine.* 2017;**167**(8):529–535.

25. Gosling C. M., Forbes A. B., McGivern J., Gabbe B. J. A Profile of Injuries in Athletes Seeking Treatment During a Triathlon Race Series. *American Journal of Sports Medicine.* 2010;**38**(5):1007–1014.

26. Yang H.-R., Jeong J., Kim I., Kim J. E. Medical Support During an Ironman 70.3 Triathlon Race. *F1000Res.* 2017;**6**:1516.

27. Dawadi S., Basyal B., Subedi Y. Morbidity Among Athletes Presenting for Medical Care During 3 Iterations of an Ultratrail Race in the Himalayas. *Wilderness and Environmental Medicine Journal.* 2020;**31**(4):437–440.

28. Hållmarker U., Michaëlsson K., Arnlöv J., James S. Cardiac Arrest in a Long-Distance Ski Race (Vasaloppet) in Sweden. *J Am Coll Cardiol.* 2012;**60**(15):1431–1432.

29. Rabb H., Coleby J. Hurt on the Hill: A Longitudinal Analysis of Obstacle Course Racing Injuries. *Orthopaedic Journal of Sports Medicine.* 2018;**6**(6):2325967118779854.

30. Alquthami A. H., Pines J. M. A Systematic Review of Noncommunicable Health Issues in Mass Gatherings. *Prehospital and Disaster Medicine.* 2014;**29**(2):167–175.

31. Anikeeva O., Arbon P., Zeitz K., et al. Patient Presentation Trends at 15 Mass-Gathering Events in South Australia. *Prehospital and Disaster Medicine.* 2018;**33**(4):368–374.

32. Bledsoe B., Songer P., Buchanan K., Westin J., Hodnick R., Gorosh L. Burning Man 2011: Mass Gathering Medical Care in an Austere Environment. *Prehospital Emergency Care.* 2012;**16**(4):469–476.

33. Schwabe K., Schwellnus M. P., Derman W., Swanevelder S., Jordaan E. Less Experience and Running Pace Are Potential Risk Factors for Medical Complications during a 56 km Road Running Race: A Prospective Study in 26,354 Race Starters – SAFER study II. *British Journal of Sports Medicine.* 2014;**48**(11):905–911.

34. Sewry N., Schwellnus M., Borjesson M., Swanevelder S., Jordaan E. Pre-Race Screening and Stratification Predicts Adverse Events: A 4-Year Study in 29,585 Ultra-Marathon Entrants, SAFER X. *Scand J Med Sci Sports.* 2020;**30**(7):1205–1211.

35. Killops J., Sewry N. A., Schwellnus M., Swanevelder S., Janse van Rensburg D., Jordaan E. Women, Older Age, Faster Cycling Speed and Increased Wind Speeds Are Independent Risk Factors for Acute Injury-Related Medical Encounters During a 109 km Mass Community-Based Participation Cycling Event: A 3-Year Study in 102,251 Race Starters – SAFER XII. *Injury Prevention.* 2021;**27**(4):338–343.

36. Knechtle B., Nikolaidis P. T. Physiology and Pathophysiology in Ultra-Marathon Running. *Front Physiol.* 2018;**9**:634.

37. Rubio-Arias J. Á., Ávila-Gandía V., López-Román F. J., Soto-Méndez F., Alcaraz P. E., Ramos-Campo D. J. Muscle Damage and Inflammation Biomarkers After Two Ultra-Endurance Mountain Races of Different Distances: 54 km vs 111 km. *Physiol Behav.* 2019;**205**:51–57.

38. Yoon J. H., Park Y., Ahn J., Shin K. A., Kim Y. J. Changes in the Markers of Cardiac Damage in Men Following Long-Distance and Ultra-Long-Distance Running Races. *Journal of Sports Medicine and Physical Fitness.* 2016;**56**(3):295–301.

39. Khodaee M., Spittler J., VanBaak K., Changstrom B. G., Hill J. C. Effects of Running an Ultramarathon on Cardiac, Hematologic, and Metabolic Biomarkers. *International Journal of Sports Medicine.* 2015;**36**(11):867–871.

40. Da Ponte A., Giovanelli N., Antonutto G., et al. Changes in Cardiac and Muscle Biomarkers Following an Uphill-Only Marathon. *Research in Sports Medicine.* 2018;**26**(1):100–111.

41. Christensen D. L., Espino D., Infante-Ramírez R., et al. Transient Cardiac Dysfunction But Elevated Cardiac and Kidney Biomarkers 24 h Following an Ultra-Distance Running Event in Mexican Tarahumara. *Extreme Physiology and Medicine.* 2017;**6**:3.

42. Christensen D. L., Espino D., Infante-Ramírez R., et al. Normalization of Elevated Cardiac, Kidney, and Hemolysis Plasma Markers Within 48 h in Mexican Tarahumara Runners Following a 78 km Race at Moderate Altitude. *American Journal of Human Biology.* 2014;**26**(6):836–843.

43. Żebrowska A., Waśkiewicz Z., Nikolaidis P. T., et al. Acute Responses of Novel Cardiac Biomarkers to a 24-h Ultra-Marathon. *Journal of Clinical Medicine.* 2019;**8**(1):57.

44. Hoffman M. D., Fogard K. Demographic Characteristics of 161-km Ultramarathon Runners. *Research in Sports Medicine.* 2012;**20**(1):59–69.

45. Turris S. A., Jones T., Lund A. Mortality at Music Festivals: An Update for 2016–2017 – Academic and Grey Literature for Case Finding. *Prehospital and Disaster Medicine.* 2017;**32**(1);58–63.

46. Holtzhausen L. M., Noakes T. D. The Prevalence and Significance of Post-Exercise (Postural) Hypotension in Ultramarathon Runners. *Medicine and Science in Sports and Exercise.* 1995;**27**(12):1595–1601.

47. Kercher M. Chafing And Running: How To Prevent It And Deal With It [Internet]. 2021. https://marathon handbook.com/chafing-and-running/. Accessed October 16, 2021.

48. Rooney D., Sarriegui I., Heron N. "As Easy as Riding a Bike": A Systematic Review of Injuries and Illness in Road Cycling. *BMJ Open Sport and Exercise Medicine*. 2020;**6**(1):e000840.

49. Scheer B. V., Reljic D., Murray A., Costa R. J. S. The Enemy of the Feet: Blisters in Ultraendurance Runners. *Journal of the American Podiatric Medical Association*. 2014;**104**(5):473–478.

50. Worthing R. M., Percy R. L., Joslin J. D. Prevention of Friction Blisters in Outdoor Pursuits: A Systematic Review. *Wilderness and Environmental Medicine Journal*. 2017;**28**(2):139–149.

51. Lipman G. S., Sharp L. J., Christensen M., et al. Paper Tape Prevents Foot Blisters: A Randomized Prevention Trial Assessing Paper Tape in Endurance Distances II (Pre-TAPED II). *Clinical Journal of Sports Medicine*. 2016;**26**(5):362–368.

52. Hart R. Blisters. Wilderness Medical Society Magazine. 2015. wms.org/magazine/1140/Blisters-Part-1. Accessed September 20, 2023.

53. Lipman G. S., Krabak B. J. Foot Problems and Care. In: *Auerbach's Wilderness Medicine*. 7th ed. Philadelphia: Elsevier; 2016. pp. 533–549.

54. Blog N. How to Prevent and Treat Blisters [Video] [Internet]. 2015. https://blog.nols.edu/2015/07/21/how-to-prevent-and-treat-blisters-video. Accessed October 16, 2021.

55. Britton R. What to Eat in an Ultra Marathon – Men's Running UK [Internet]. Men's Running. 2017. https://mensrunninguk.co.uk/training/eat-ultra-marathon/. Accessed December 6, 2021.

56. Pillay S., Schwellnus M. P., Grant C., Jansen V. A. N, Rensburg A., Swanevelder S., Jordaan E. Longer Race Distance Predicts Gastrointestinal Illness-Related Medical Encounters in 153,208 Endurance Runner Race Starters – SAFER XVI. Journal of Sports Medicine and Physical Fitness. 2021.

57. Wilson P. B. "I Think I'm Gonna Hurl": A Narrative Review of the Causes of Nausea and Vomiting in Sport. *Sports (Basel)*. 2019;**7**(7):E162.

58. Peters H. P., Bos M., Seebregts L., et al. Gastrointestinal Symptoms in Long-Distance Runners, Cyclists, and Triathletes: Prevalence, Medication, and Etiology. *American Journal of Gastroenterology*. 1999;**94**(6):1570–1581.

59. Costa R. J. S., Snipe R., Camões-Costa V., Scheer V., Murray A. The Impact of Gastrointestinal Symptoms and Dermatological Injuries on Nutritional Intake and Hydration Status During Ultramarathon Events. *Sports Medicine – Open*. 2016;**2**:16.

60. Parnell J. A., Wagner-Jones K., Madden R. F., Erdman K. A. Dietary Restrictions in Endurance Runners to Mitigate Exercise-Induced Gastrointestinal Symptoms. *Journal of the International Society of Sports Nutrition*. 2020;**17**(1):32.

61. Schütz U. H. W., Billich C., König K., et al. Characteristics, Changes and Influence of Body Composition During a 4486 km Transcontinental Ultramarathon: Results from the TransEurope FootRace Mobile Whole Body MRI-Project. *BMC Med*. 2013;**11**:122.

62. Tiller N. B., Roberts J. D., Beasley L., et al. International Society of Sports Nutrition Position Stand: Nutritional Considerations for Single-Stage Ultra-Marathon Training and Racing. *Journal of the International Society of Sports Nutrition*. 2019;**16**(1):50.

63. Mielgo-Ayuso J., Calleja-González J., Refoyo I., León-Guereño P., Cordova A., Del Coso J. Exercise-Induced Muscle Damage and Cardiac Stress During a Marathon Could Be Associated with Dietary Intake During the Week Before the Race. *Nutrients*. 2020;**12**(2):E316.

64. Pasternak A. V., Fiore D., Islas A., Toti S, Hoffman M. D. Treatment with Oral Ondansetron for Ultramarathon-Associated Nausea: The TOO FUN Study. *Sports (Basel)*. 2021;**9**(3):35.

65. Costa R. J. S., Snipe R. M. J., Kitic C. M., Gibson P. R. Systematic Review: Exercise-Induced Gastrointestinal Syndrome: Implications for Health and Intestinal Disease. *Alimentary Pharmacology & Therapeutics*. 2017;**46**(3):246–265.

66. Drobnic F., Fonts S., García-Alday I., et al. A Pilot Study on the Efficacy of a Rational Combination of Artichoke and Ginger Extracts with Simethicone in the Treatment of Gastrointestinal Symptoms in Endurance Athletes. *Minerva Gastroenterol Dietol*. 2022;**68**(1):77–84.

67. Schwellnus M., Swanevelder S., Derman W., Borjesson M., Schwabe K., Jordaan E. Prerace Medical Screening and Education Reduce Medical Encounters in Distance Road Races: SAFER VIII Study in 153,208 Race Starters. *British Journal of Sports Medicine*. 2019;**53**(10):634–639.

68. Hoppel F., Calabria E., Pesta D., Kantner-Rumplmair W., Gnaiger E., Burtscher M. Physiological and Pathophysiological Responses to Ultramarathon Running in Non-elite Runners. *Frontiers in Physiology*. 2019;**10**:1300.

69. Magrini D., Khodaee M., San-Millán I., Hew-Butler T., Provance A. J. Serum Creatine Kinase Elevations

in Ultramarathon Runners at High Altitude. *The Physician and Sportsmedicine.* 2017;**45**(2):129–133.

70. Hoffman M. D., Badowski N., Chin J., Stuempfle K. J., Parise C. A. Determinants of Recovery from a 161-km Ultramarathon. *Journal of Sports Sciences.* 2017;**35**(7):669–677.

71. Hoffman M. D., Weiss R. H. Does Acute Kidney Injury from an Ultramarathon Increase the Risk for Greater Subsequent Injury? *Clinical Journal of Sports Medicine.* 2016;**26**(5):417–422.

72. Hoffman M. D., Stuempfle K. J., Rogers I. R., Weschler L. B., Hew-Butler T. Hyponatremia in the 2009 161-km Western States Endurance Run. *International Journal of Sports Physiology and Performance.* 2012;**7**(1):6–10.

73. Bird S. R., Linden M., Hawley J. A. Acute Changes to Biomarkers as a Consequence of Prolonged Strenuous Running. *Annals of Clinical Biochemistry.* 2014;**51**(Pt 2):137–150.

74. Pradas F., Falcón D., Peñarrubia-Lozano C., Toro-Román V., Carrasco L., Castellar C. Effects of Ultratrail Running on Neuromuscular Function, Muscle Damage and Hydration Status. Differences According to Training Level. *International Journal of Environmental Research and Public Health.* 2021;**18**(10):5119.

75. Martínez-Navarro I, Collado E, Hernando C, Hernando B, Hernando C. Inflammation, Muscle Damage and Post-Race Physical Activity Following a Mountain Ultramarathon. *Journal of Sports Medicine and Physical Fitness.* 2021.

76. Belli T., Macedo D. V., de Araújo G. G., et al. Mountain Ultramarathon Induces Early Increases of Muscle Damage, Inflammation, and Risk for Acute Renal Injury. *Frontiers in Physiology.* 2018;**9**:1368.

77. Bruso J. R., Hoffman M. D., Rogers I. R., Lee L., Towle G., Hew-Butler T. Rhabdomyolysis and Hyponatremia: A Cluster of Five Cases at the 161-km 2009 Western States Endurance Run. *Wilderness and Environmental Medicine Journal.* 2010;**21**(4):303–308.

78. Chlíbková D., Knechtle B., Rosemann T., Žákovská A., Tomášková I. The Prevalence of Exercise-Associated Hyponatremia in 24-Hour Ultra-Mountain Bikers, 24-Hour Ultra-Runners and Multi-Stage Ultra-Mountain Bikers in the Czech Republic. *Journal of the International Society of Sports Nutrition.* 2014;**11**(1):3.

79. Cairns R. S., Hew-Butler T. Proof of Concept: Hypovolemic Hyponatremia May Precede and Augment Creatine Kinase Elevations During an Ultramarathon. *European Journal of Applied Physiology.* 2016;**116**(3):647–655.

80. Wollseiffen P., Schneider S., Martin L. A., Kerhervé H. A., Klein T., Solomon C. The Effect of 6 h of Running on Brain Activity, Mood, and Cognitive Performance. *Experimental Brain Research.* 2016;**234**(7):1829–1836.

81. Freund W., Faust S., Birklein F., et al. Substantial and Reversible Brain Gray Matter Reduction but No Acute Brain Lesions in Ultramarathon Runners: Experience from the Transeurope-Footrace Project. *BMC Med.* 2012;**10**:170.

82. Poussel M., Laroppe J., Hurdiel R., et al. Sleep Management Strategy and Performance in an Extreme Mountain Ultra-Marathon. *Research in Sports Medicine.* 2015;**23**(3):330–336.

83. Hurdiel R., Pezé T., Daugherty J., et al. Combined Effects of Sleep Deprivation and Strenuous Exercise on Cognitive Performances During the North Face® Ultra Trail du Mont Blanc® (UTMB®). *Journal of Sports Sciences.* 2015;**33**(7):670–674.

84. Huang M.-K., Chang K.-S., Kao W.-F., et al. Visual Hallucinations in 246-km Mountain Ultra-Marathoners: An Observational Study. *Chinese Journal of Physiology.* 2021;**64**(5):225–231.

85. Krogh J., Speyer H., Gluud C., Nordentoft M. Exercise for Patients with Major Depression: A Protocol for a Systematic Review with Meta-Analysis and Trial Sequential Analysis. *Systematic Reviews.* 2015;**4**:40.

86. Kvam S., Kleppe C. L., Nordhus I. H., Hovland A. Exercise as a Treatment for Depression: A Meta-Analysis. *Journal of Affective Disorders.* 2016;**202**:67–86.

87. Méndez-Alonso D., Prieto-Saborit J. A., Bahamonde J. R., Jiménez-Arberás E. Influence of Psychological Factors on the Success of the Ultra-Trail Runner. *International Journal of Environmental Research and Public Health.* 2021;**18**(5):2704.

88. Brace A. W., George K., Lovell G. P. Mental Toughness and Self-Efficacy of Elite Ultra-Marathon Runners. *PLoS One.* 2020;**15**(11):e0241284.

89. Buck K., Spittler J., Reed A., Khodaee M. Psychological Attributes of Ultramarathoners. *Wilderness and Environmental Medicine Journal.* 2018;**29**(1):66–71.

90. Hoffman M. D., Krouse R. Ultra-Obligatory Running Among Ultramarathon Runners. *Research in Sports Medicine.* 2018;**26**(2):211–221.

91. Hoffman M. D., Goulet E. D. B., Maughan R. J. Considerations in the Use of Body Mass Change to Estimate Change in Hydration Status During a 161-Kilometer Ultramarathon Running Competition. *Sports Medicine.* 2018;**48**(2):243–250.

92. Knechtle B., Knechtle P., Wirth A., Alexander Rüst C., Rosemann T. A Faster Running Speed Is Associated with a Greater Body Weight Loss in 100-km Ultra-Marathoners. *Journal of Sports Sciences.* 2012;**30**(11):1131–1140.

93. Rüst C. A., Knechtle B., Knechtle P., Wirth A., Rosemann T. Body Mass Change and Ultraendurance Performance: A Decrease in Body Mass Is Associated with an Increased Running Speed in Male 100-km Ultramarathoners. The *Journal of Strength and Conditioning Research.* 2012;**26**(6):1505–1516.

94. Hoffman M. D., Stuempfle K. J. Hydration Strategies, Weight Change and Performance in a 161 Ultramarathon. *Research in Sports Medicine.* 2014;**22**(3):213–225.

95. Landman Z. C., Landman G. O., Fatehi P. Physiologic Alterations and Predictors of Performance in a 160-Ultramarathon. *Clinical Journal of Sports Medicine* 2012;**22**(2):146–151.

96. Martinez S., Aguilo A., Rodas L., Lozano L., Moreno C., Tauler P. Energy, Macronutrient and Water Intake During a Mountain Ultramarathon Event: The Influence of Distance. *Journal of Sports Sciences.* 2018;**36**(3):333–339.

97. Kao W.-F., Hou S.-K., Chiu Y.-H., et al. Effects of 100-Ultramarathon on Acute Kidney Injury. *Clinical Journal of Sports Medicine* 2015;**25**(1):49–54.

98. Lipman G. S., Krabak B. J., Waite B. L., Logan S. B., Menon A., Chan G. K. A Prospective Cohort Study of Acute Kidney Injury in Multi-Stage Ultramarathon Runners: The Biochemistry in Endurance Runner Study (BIERS). *Research in Sports Medicine.* 2014;**22**(2):185–192.

99. Scheer V., Tiller N. B., Doutreleau S., et al. Potential Long-Term Health Problems Associated with Ultra-Endurance Running: A Narrative Review. *Sports Medicine.* 2021;1–16.

100. Hew-Butler T., Sharwood K., Boulter J., et al. Dysnatremia Predicts a Delayed Recovery in Collapsed Ultramarathon Runners. *Clinical Journal of Sports Medicine* 2007;**17**(4):289–296.

101. Costa R. J., Teixeira A., Rama L., et al. Water and Sodium Intake Habits and Status of Ultra-Endurance Runners During a Multi-Stage Ultra-Marathon Conducted in a Hot Ambient Environment: An Observational Field Based Study. *Nutrition Journal.* 2013;**12**:13.

102. Knechtle B., Chlíbková D., Papadopoulou S., Mantzorou M., Rosemann T., Nikolaidis P. T. Exercise-Associated Hyponatremia in Endurance and Ultra-Endurance Performance-Aspects of Sex, Race Location, Ambient Temperature, Sports Discipline, and Length of Performance: A Narrative Review. *Medicina (Kaunas).* 2019;**55**(9):E537.

103. Lipman G. S., Burns P., Phillips C., et al. Effect of Sodium Supplements and Climate on Dysnatremia During Ultramarathon Running. *Clinical Journal of Sports Medicine* 2020.

104. Martínez S., Aguiló A., Moreno C., Lozano L., Tauler P. Use of Non-Steroidal Anti-Inflammatory Drugs among Participants in a Mountain Ultramarathon Event. *Sports (Basel).* 2017;**5**(1):E11.

105. Chlíbková D., Ronzhina M., Nikolaidis P. T., Rosemann T., Knechtle B. Non-Steroidal Anti-Inflammatory Drug Consumption in a Multi-Stage and a 24-h Mountain Bike Competition. *Frontiers in Physiology.* 2018;**9**:1272.

106. Lipman G. S., Shea K., Christensen M., et al. Ibuprofen Versus Placebo Effect on Acute Kidney Injury in Ultramarathons: A Randomised Controlled Trial. *Emergency Medicine Journal.* 2017;**34**(10):637–642.

107. Page A. J., Reid S. A., Speedy D. B., Mulligan G. P., Thompson J. Exercise-Associated Hyponatremia, Renal Function, and Nonsteroidal Antiinflammatory Drug Use in an Ultraendurance Mountain Run. *Clinical Journal of Sports Medicine* 2007;**17**(1):43–48.

108. Rotunno A., Schwellnus M. P., Swanevelder S., Jordaan E., Janse Van Rensburg D. C., Derman W. Novel Factors Associated with Analgesic and Anti-Inflammatory Medication Use in Distance Runners: Pre-Race Screening Among 76 654 Race Entrants-SAFER Study VI. *Clinical Journal of Sports Medicine* 2018;**28**(5):427–434.

109. Hoffman M. D., Khodaee M., Nudell N. G., Pasternak A. Recommendations on the Appropriate Level of Medical Support at Ultramarathons. *Sports Medicine.* 2020;**50**(5):871–884.

110. Bennett B. L., Hew-Butler T., Rosner M. H., Myers T., Lipman G. S. Wilderness Medical Society Clinical Practice Guidelines for the Management of Exercise-Associated Hyponatremia: 2019 Update. *Wilderness & Environmental Medicine.* 2020;**31**(1):50–62.

111. McGarvey J., Thompson J., Hanna C., Noakes T. D., Stewart J., Speedy D. Sensitivity and Specificity of Clinical Signs for Assessment of Dehydration in Endurance Athletes. *British Journal of Sports Medicine.* 2010;**44**(10):716–719.

112. Hoffman M. D., Stuempfle K. J., Fogard K., Hew-Butler T., Winger J., Weiss R. H. Urine Dipstick Analysis for Identification of Runners Susceptible to Acute Kidney Injury Following an Ultramarathon. *Journal of Sports Sciences.* 2013;**31**(1):20–31.

113. Khodaee M., Saeedi A., Irion B., Spittler J., Hoffman M. D. Proteinuria in a High-Altitude

161-km (100-mile) Ultramarathon. The *Physician and Sportsmedicine*. 2021;**49**(1):92–99.

114. Hawkins S. C. *Wilderness EMS*. Philadelphia: Lippincott Williams & Wilkins; 2017.

115. Hawkins S. C., Williams J., Bennett B. L., Islas A., Kayser D. W., Quinn R. Wilderness Medical Society Clinical Practice Guidelines for Spinal Cord Protection. *Wilderness & Environmental Medicine*. 2019;**30**(4):S87–99.

116. Harmon K. G., Clugston J. R., Dec K., et al. American Medical Society for Sports Medicine Position Statement on Concussion in Sport. *British Journal of Sports Medicine*. 2019;**53**(4):213–225.

117. Pires W., Veneroso C. E., Wanner S. P., et al. Association Between Exercise-Induced Hyperthermia and Intestinal Permeability: A Systematic Review. *Sports Medicine*. 2017;**47**(7):1389–1403.

118. Roberts W. O., Armstrong L. E., Sawka M. N., Yeargin S. W., Heled Y., O'Connor F. G. ACSM Expert Consensus Statement on Exertional Heat Illness: Recognition, Management, and Return to Activity. *Current Sports Medicine Reports*. 2021;**20**(9):470–484.

119. Alhadad S. B., Tan P. M. S., Lee J. K. W. Efficacy of Heat Mitigation Strategies on Core Temperature and Endurance Exercise: A Meta-Analysis. *Frontiers in Physiology*. 2019;**10**:71.

120. Joslin J., Mularella J., Bail A., Wojcik S., Cooney D. R. Mandatory Rest Stops Improve Athlete Safety During Event Medical Coverage for Ultramarathons. *Prehospital and Disaster Medicine*. 2016;**31**(1):43–45.

121. Belval L. N., Casa D. J., Adams W. M., et al. Consensus Statement: Prehospital Care of Exertional Heat Stroke. *Prehospital Emergency Care*. 2018;**22**(3):392–397.

122. Gatterer H., Dünnwald T., Turner R., et al. Practicing Sport in Cold Environments: Practical Recommendations to Improve Sport Performance and Reduce Negative Health Outcomes. *International Journal of Environmental Research and Public Health*. 2021;**18**(18):9700.

123. Castellani J. W., Young A. J., Ducharme M. B., et al. American College of Sports Medicine Position Stand: Prevention of Cold Injuries During Exercise. *Medicine and Science in Sports and Exercise*. 2006;**38**(11):2012–2029.

124. Koskela H. O. Cold Air-Provoked Respiratory Symptoms: The Mechanisms and Management. *International Journal of Circumpolar Health*. 2007;**66**(2):91–100.

125. Dow J., Giesbrecht G. G., Danzl D. F., et al. Wilderness Medical Society Clinical Practice Guidelines for the Out-of-Hospital Evaluation and Treatment of Accidental Hypothermia: 2019 Update. *Wilderness & Environmental Medicine*. 2019;**30**(4):S47–69.

126. Roach R. C., Hackett P. H., Oelz O., et al. The 2018 Lake Louise Acute Mountain Sickness Score. *High Altitude Medicine and Biology*. 2018;**19**(1):4–6.

127. Luks A. M., Auerbach P. S., Freer L., et al. Wilderness Medical Society Clinical Practice Guidelines for the Prevention and Treatment of Acute Altitude Illness: 2019 Update. *Wilderness and Environmental Medicine Journal*. 2019;**30**(4S):S3–18.

128. Boren C. Ultramarathoner Killed by Lightning Strike During Italian Race. *Washington Post*. www.washingtonpost.com/sports/2019/07/30/an-ultramarathoner-caught-between-aid-stations-is-killed-by-lightning-italy/. Accessed December 10, 2021.

129. Davis C., Engeln A., Johnson E. L., et al. Wilderness Medical Society Practice Guidelines for the Prevention and Treatment of Lightning Injuries: 2014 Update. *Wilderness & Environmental Medicine*. 2014;**25**(4):S86–95.

130. Hoffman M. D. Participant Opinions and Expectations about Medical Services at Ultramarathons: Findings from the Ultrarunners Longitudinal TRAcking (ULTRA) Study. *Cureus*. 2019;**11**(9):e5800.

131. Schwabe K., Schwellnus M., Swanevelder S., Jordaan E., Derman W., Bosch A. Leisure Athletes at Risk of Medical Complications: Outcomes of Pre-Participation Screening Among 15,778 Endurance Runners – SAFER VII. *The Physician and Sportsmedicine*. 2018;**46**(4):405–413.

132. Joslin J., Hoffman M. D., Rogers I., Worthing R. M., Ladbrook M., Mularella J. Special Considerations in Medical Screening for Participants in Remote Endurance Events. *Sports Medicine*. 2015;**45**(8):1121–1131.

133. Sedgwick P. E., Wortley G. C., Wright J. M., Asplund C., William O. R., Usman S. Medical Clearance for Desert and Land Sports, Adventure, and Endurance Events. *Wilderness & Environmental Medicine*. 2015;**26**(4):47–54.

134. Joy E., Baak K. V., Dec K. L., et al. Wilderness Preparticipation Evaluation and Considerations for Special Populations. *Wilderness & Environmental Medicine*. 2015;**26**(4):76–91.

135. Larson H. H., Khalili-Borna D., Uzosike E., Sugiyama D. Medical Coverage of Ultramarathons and Its Unique Challenges. *Current Sports Medicine Reports*. 2016;**15**(3):154–160.

136. Yao K. V., Troyanos C., D'Hemecourt P., Roberts W. O. Optimizing Marathon Race Safety Using an Incident Command Post Strategy. *Current Sports Medicine Reports.* 2017;**16**(3):144–149.

137. Nash C. J., Richards C. T., Schwieger G., Malik S., Chiampas G. T. Medical Care at a Large Vertical Running Event. *Prehosp Emerg Care.* 2018;**22**(1):22–27.

138. Hoffman M. D., Longobardi C., Burt C., Nardi T. GPS Tracker-Enabled Rescue of a Lost Runner During a Wilderness Ultramarathon: A Case Report. *Current Sports Medicine Reports.* 2018;**17**(10):332–334.

139. Metzler, B. Czech Runner Dies from Falling During UTMB's TDS Race in Chamonix. *Trail Runner Magazine.* 2021. www.trailrunnermag.com/people/news-people/czech-runner-dies-from-falling-during-utmbs-tds-race-in-chamonix. Accessed December 7, 2021.

140. Ross D. S., Ferguson A., Herbert D. L. Action in the Event Tent! Medical-Legal Issues Facing the Volunteer Event Physician. *Sports Health.* 2013;**5**(4):340–345.

141. Schwellnus M., Kipps C., Roberts W. O., et al. Medical Encounters (Including Injury and Illness) at Mass Community-Based Endurance Sports Events: An International Consensus Statement on Definitions and Methods of Data Recording and Reporting. *British Journal of Sports Medicine.* 2019;**53**(17):1048–1055.

At-Risk Populations within Mass Gathering Events

Megan C. Marino, Andrew L. Garrett[*], Aileen M. Marty, and Paul E. Pepe

Introduction

At most mass gathering events, there will be individuals and groups who are at a higher risk for requiring specialized healthcare services. Persons at extremes of age, those displaced from their homes, and people with medical or behavioral health conditions can be expected to possibly require specialized medical treatment, even during the event. It should be anticipated that vulnerable populations can be in attendance at any type of mass gathering, but events of heightened concern might include a scheduled international assembly of people attending a large religious gathering, a large public festival, or a major cultural celebration. Another concern is the sudden and unplanned gathering of displaced persons who collect together in the aftermath of a major natural disaster, humanitarian crisis, political conflict or war. Accordingly, religious events like the annual Hajj pilgrimage or a long-anticipated Papal visit, or the diaspora resulting from the 2005 Hurricane Katrina aftermath, the 2011 Fukushima incident, or the 2022 Ukraine–Russian war, all exemplify the various types of situations in which certain at-risk individuals may be placed at an escalated and disproportionate disadvantage in terms of encountering circumstances that negatively impact their well-being. What comprises the "whole community" in modern society is changing significantly. For example, in the United States alone, the number of living persons aged sixty-five and older had increased by nearly fifteen million in 2019 compared to a decade earlier. This older population is now projected to reach 80.8 million by 2040 and 94.7 million by 2060. All but a very small percentage of these elders live in noninstitutional settings.

Currently, there are more than sixty-one million people with disabilities in the US, but modern medical science and ever-increasing options for pharmacotherapy and assistive devices has improved the ability of these persons, not only to manage their complex medical conditions outside of medical facilities, but also routinely participate in independent recreational and work opportunities outside the home. In addition, according to recent census reports, about 9 percent of the US population under sixty-five years of age self-identifies themselves as having a disability in one or more of the four basic areas of functioning, namely hearing, vision, cognition, and ambulation [1]. Similarly, minors comprise about 22 percent of the population and about half of them are dependents under the age of ten. Approximately 19 percent (fourteen million minor children) self-identify as having a special health care need and about 25 percent of homes report having a one or more children residing with special health care needs [1]. All of these evolving statistics highlight the need for event planners and emergency managers to be able to accommodate escalating populations who may now need to rely more upon others for their health and safety. Again, all of these at-risk populations are growing, with older Americans being one of the fastest-growing demographics in the US and other nations [1].

One readily observable example of this shift in the public domain has been the growing need for commercial airlines to further adapt to larger numbers of persons whom they need to "preboard" with wheelchairs, canes and service animals on each flight. It is anticipated that this evolving pattern will continue to grow even more over the next decade. As such, these types of population changes will also become a major factor in planning for mass gatherings and the related medical planning, whether they involve planned or even unscheduled events. Of further relevance in this discussion about mass gatherings is that, in general,

---

[*] The views expressed do not necessarily represent the views of the U.S. Department of Health and Human Services or the United States.

the prevalence of people with some form of a higher risk condition is about 25 percent [1].

As indicated in the airline boarding analogy, the anticipated growing accommodations for these special populations will also affect the broader population as well. As will be indicated in this ensuing discussion, anticipating and meeting the medical and supportive needs of all individuals attending mass gatherings can represent an extreme challenge, even under the best of circumstances. However, with at-risk populations already constituting a large portion of many mass gathering situations, those challenges will be amplified even further in the future.

Most medical personnel typically think of mass gatherings in terms of major professional sporting events, popular rock music concerts or festivals. However, civil unrest, warring nations, public health threats, or sequelae of climate change can also lead to mass migrations with resulting mass sheltering scenarios. Many of these situations are more likely to involve underserved populations and individuals most likely to be from at-risk communities and vulnerable populations who may now congregate together in potentially vast numbers and in close quarters to each other at distant harboring locations. In the case of mass gatherings that result from such crises, the challenge of meeting the needs of the public are exacerbated by loss of the comforts, sense of security, and the day-to-day routines of their former homes, including frequent separation from caregivers, medical professionals, therapists, and pharmacies. The additional lack of proper sleep, the toll of long journeys, and the extraordinary psychological stressors of their situation all place these evacuees at greater states of immunocompromise and worsening of underlying medical conditions. Compounding these consequences will be the possibility that many in attendance may not have had enough time to bring everything they needed to maximize their independence, such as mobility aids, medical records, and medications let alone sufficient clothing, change of clothes and the ability to launder them.

Following the Fukushima Daiichi tsunami and nuclear disaster in Japan in 2011, the major health threat became the sudden displacement of tens and tens of thousands of at-risk individuals. That problem turned out to be more of a threat than the radiation contamination in the region. Likewise, in the US, after Hurricane Katrina, the displacement of at-risk individuals became one of the most catastrophic consequences of the disaster with the resulting formation of several distant mass gathering shelters with each harboring tens of thousands of disadvantaged evacuees over several weeks. Most of these displaced persons had been transported hundreds of miles under austere conditions before arriving at destinations like Dallas (814 kilometers), Houston (558 kilometers), and many other far-reaching sites of shelter including Hawaii.

With these perspectives in mind, there is both an ethical and a legal mandate to ensure that mass gatherings are well-positioned to respond to the "whole community" appropriately. This goal also requires that event organizers and emergency managers become familiar with the many regulations that could apply across the community hosting a mass gathering. These regulations and policies may include federal, state, county, and local laws and ordinances. While many of these requirements will become apparent in the permitting process for a scheduled mass gathering, during an unscheduled event such as the opening of a disaster shelter, the onus may be on the site coordinators to ensure that they are in compliance.

In the US for example, the 2019 Pandemic and All-Hazards Preparedness Act now requires planning for those in at-risk communities to ensure that they receive adequate resources during a public health emergency. Likewise, the US Americans with Disabilities Act (ADA) 42 U.S.C. § 12101, a federal civil rights law established in 1990, broadly prohibits discriminating against those with disabilities and their service animals. It has several subtitles that include: (1) employment equity, (2) discrimination by public entities including transportation systems and housing, and (3) public and commercial accommodation for those with disabilities [2]. Similar counterpart statutes and regulations are enacted in many other nations as well and, accordingly, all of these regulatory issues are germane to those who organize and plan mass gathering events or who called in to manage sudden and unexpected mass gatherings. More specifically, the US ADA does require that disaster and emergency preparedness activities encompass the domains of alerting, sheltering, lodging, social services, relocation, recovery, and enabled access as part of planning and preparation for disasters in order to ensure the availability of ample resources and proper accommodations for those individuals with disabilities. Given this information, it is no surprise that many large event planners and emergency managers have ready access to legal counsel and other special advisors to ensure that they are in compliance with the many rules that exist for these situations. Regardless of such disaster scenarios or if they are planned celebrations, concerts, religious or political events, mass gatherings need to address the special medical and logistical needs of disabled and vulnerable populations such as children, the elderly and other populations at higher risk for illness or injury.

Special Planning for Children

Children's healthcare needs differ from those of adults, and mass gathering planners or organizers need to anticipate those special needs. Children cannot speak for themselves, nor can they properly understand and act on risks to their health and safety. There are also challenges in their ability to follow verbal or written directions.

In displacement situations, children are especially vulnerable if they are separated from parents or caregivers, either intentionally, inadvertently or because of criminal abduction. Very young children, especially the unvaccinated, are at higher risk of dying from disease. Depending on the nation of origin or region, even older children may not have adequate vaccinations. In addition, infants and children have special dietary needs. Breastfeeding mothers need a safe and private place to feed their children. Mothers of formula-fed infants need access to clean water and safe ways to mix formula, assuming it is even available under certain circumstances. Improperly mixing of formula can lead to life-threatening electrolyte abnormalities in infants. Likewise, sanitation and clean water are critical for young children since they are at higher risk of dehydration and even death from diarrheal illnesses. It is developmentally appropriate for toddlers to crawl on the floor and they also will have direct contact with various other contaminated surfaces and possibly infectious persons. It is also typical for them to quickly put various items, usually now contaminated, in their mouths. These behaviors put toddlers at an increased risk of exposure to physical, infectious, and chemical hazards. Creating a safe space for children to play safely and providing them with adequate access to diapers, bathrooms, laundry, hand-washing, and sanitizers are all essential considerations in caring for children. At the same time, bringing children together in a safe place may also increase certain contagious risks as well. Children can rapidly spread disease to each other, they can also place healthy adults at risk, particularly the elderly, pregnant women, and those otherwise compromised by the circumstances.

Even in a single one-day mass gathering event such as a music festival or protest rally, the risk for physical injury can be elevated depending on the degree of alcohol consumption, environmental heat, humidity, or the stability of the crowd and its movements. Many times, bringing a young child to a mass gathering event may be a care-taking necessity or simply a special wish of the parent, but the ambient noise, crowds and unfamiliar faces can also create additional stressors that parents may not have anticipated. Having first aid support, and consideration of special mechanisms for hearing protection and sun protection, go hand in hand with hydration techniques and places to be cooled. Like adults, children occasionally may become relatively dehydrated at many mass gathering or have an unexpected seizure, allergic reaction or asthma attack. Therefore, proper modes of therapy, including medications and delivery methods, should be stocked and readily available in case of such an event. In addition, medical organizers should have a definitive plan for transport as indicated to a dedicated children's hospital and, if different, the optimal trauma center for children.

Special Planning for Women

In terms of mass gatherings, women do have distinct needs, but especially in evacuee encampment settings where nutrition and healthcare needs of women do differ from the needs of men. Likewise, clinical presentations often differ for women and serious illness may be underappreciated or lost in the shuffle of mass gatherings. For example, the only present signs of life-threatening coronary artery syndromes or other types of cardiac events may be abdominal pain or nausea which may get attributed to other common illnesses that are less life-threatening. While both men and women may possess various elements of stoicism, in some cultures, many women may have clear reticence to reach out to others. Beyond medical presentations, women also are at higher risk of becoming victims of rape, violence, and human trafficking, particularly in the circumstances of poorly secured mass gatherings, and often in the case of unplanned emergencies. Even in the one-day and more routine mass gathering event, pregnant women may have problems with mobility and may not be able to walk as far or as quickly as others which may put them at higher risk of injury in large crowds. Late-stage pregnant women in particular will routinely need places to sit or even recline depending on the ambient circumstances, air quality and their state of hydration and nutrition. Pregnant women are at higher risk of becoming dehydrated and they are at also higher risk of complications from various illnesses.

In displacement situations where nutrients are scarce, malnutrition and starvation can cause irreparable damage to a developing fetus. Exacerbating this concern is the overriding concept that prenatal care varies significantly among people from different backgrounds, nations, cultures and regions. Cultural and language barriers can make it much more difficult to fully assess the prenatal care that a mother has received or to ascertain any prenatal diagnoses that a baby may have, let alone the mother. Also, planning for a woman in labor will differ based on cultural and societal values. For some women, being alone with a man or even shaking hands with one is considered improper. In some cultures, for example, it is imperative that a woman in labor only has female healthcare providers or that other family members are present if a male healthcare professional examines the expectant mother. Some women, especially those with chronic illness, including drug addiction, are at higher risk of having a premature baby or having a baby requiring a higher level of care. Likewise, even for a single day or short duration mass gathering event, knowledge of the proper receiving facility for women is essential, particularly those visitors to the community who are pregnant or even in labor. Beyond trauma, stroke, and cardiac care centers, an important part of mass gathering planning and preparation, is knowing where to bring pregnant women for optimal care.

Planning for the Elderly, Chronically Ill, and Disabled

Elderly, chronically ill, and disabled persons are at risk of being neglected, abused, or even being left behind in a disaster, especially those living alone or those with limited mobility. Some older adults may also become confused or disoriented and get separated from their family members even in a more routine circumstance, let alone a mass gathering event. Beyond these general concerns, the elderly, chronically ill, and disabled also have distinct needs during a mass gathering be it a disaster-related gathering a routine scheduled mass gathering sporting or entertainment event. As such, it is critical that the medical evaluation and triage plan and the allotted resources include considerations for

the managing the medical and sociological welfare of these vulnerable groups.

Many of the risks for the elderly stem from underlying medical conditions that are uncontrolled or exacerbated during the event, including previously undiagnosed conditions. They may be unable to accurately remember or disclose what conditions they have or all of the medications that they are taking, let alone dosing. Some chronically and disabled persons depend on electrical power for life-sustaining devices and this concern was emphasized by the massive, unexpected power failure created during the week-long deep freeze catastrophe in the US state of Texas in February 2021. Power-dependent devices at risk included ventilators, suction apparatus, nebulizer machines, oxygen concentrators, continuous positive airway pressure (CPAP) machines, left ventricular assist devices (LVAD), and dialysis machines. While access to some of these devices and electrical power may only be of critical concern for the situation of displaced elders requiring mass gathering shelters, some patients may still require frequent supplemental oxygen replenishment or refrigeration for their medications and someone to access and distribute these medical needs. All attempts should be made to accommodate the at-risk populations accordingly.

A Framework for Meeting the Needs of the Whole

Given the significant numbers and varieties of individuals who could fall into one of many "at-risk" categories when attending mass gatherings, it is difficult to accurately identify and meaningfully plan for every person's specific needs, be it for a transient one day activity or a protracted mass gathering. However, many emergency managers and event planners have adopted the *Communication, Maintaining Health, Independence, Support/Safety and Transportation* (CMIST) Framework (Figure 18.1) to help facilitate a more methodical and comprehensive approach toward tailoring their planning processes. In the simplest of descriptions, the CMIST Framework is a strategy to help organizers, including medical care providers, better consider and plan for accommodating the general *access and functional needs* (AFN) common to many at-risk individuals, particularly conditions and situations that may interfere with their ability to remain safe and receive appropriate care during any type of mass gathering.

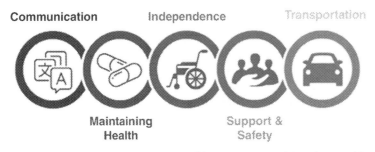

Communication **Independence** Transportation

Maintaining Health Support & Safety

Figure 18.1 Depiction of the components of the CMIST Framework from the United States Department of Health and Human Services, Office of the Assistant Secretary for Preparedness and Response. www.phe.gov/emergency/events/COVID19/atrisk/discharge-planning/Pages/CMIST-framework.aspx

The framework approach does not eliminate the requirement to undertake specific planning efforts for certain at-risk persons, but it does provide a pathway for finding meaningful solutions in many uncharted situations. The framework is designed to help achieve improved equity in terms of health and safety for all individuals attending a mass gathering. In some respects, this overview and conceptual paradigm is akin to a unified "all hazards" approach to disaster preparedness and the respective related planning for most disasters to achieve efficient and successful resource utilization as problems arise.

Each category within the CMIST Framework is intentionally broad, requiring planners and organizers to at least consider the types of individuals that might expected at their site. Nevertheless, the CMIST framework is also useful for specifically anticipating the range of special needs that fit into each subcategory. Throughout the subsequent discussion, examples will be provided as to how the CMIST framework can work within the context of various types of mass gathering situations. As expected, there is significant overlap across the various scenarios, but there are also specific nuances to consider within each of the given examples.

Overall, when exploring the various elements of the framework, the *Communication* category includes assurances that there is signage and emergency notification capability for those who are sensory impaired and those who may not be able to see, speak, or hear. It includes mechanisms to address the challenges some individuals will have in verbalizing their concerns or their ability to understand both routine and emergency messaging. This subcategory of CMIST includes those with limited language proficiency, particularly for those struggling with the regional language used in the locality of the mass gathering.

Maintaining health includes plans for meeting the goal of preventing illness and injury, meeting ongoing health maintenance needs of individuals (such as food, water, medications, breastfeeding, or sheltering), mitigating preventable medical conditions, and assuring the ability to provide routine and emergent medical care as needed. It also includes establishing special medical facilities and even pharmacies and certain specialists on-site for the more protracted events.

Independence involves mechanisms to optimize access and functional needs (AFN) requirements such as assistive technology, mobility aids, and service animals to help individuals maintain their self-reliance. As a general rule, it is critical to avoid the separating individuals from their assistive technology, devices, service animals, professional aides, or supportive family members whenever possible. Plans and training for mass gathering medicine tasks should include mechanisms to facilitate that goal.

The *Support and safety* category focuses on meeting the safety and support needs of individuals such as those who may become separated from their caregivers or children with cognitive or behavioral health needs. These categories of vulnerable populations may have an extremely difficult time coping during a disaster-related assembly or any other mass gathering situation. The component of CMIST also identifies mechanisms to provide security for vulnerable populations at great risk for criminal exploitation or intentional injury during certain mass gatherings.

Transportation involves assurances that individuals, regardless of their abilities, are provided mobility within and during the event and access leading into and exiting the event. This concept of ensuring mobility should also include mechanisms to provide appropriate and safe transportation to receive medical care and access to emergency medical services, either on-site or at receiving facilities. In addition, there should be built-in assurances that any on-site transportation options, such as shuttles or city buses, are accessible to all without requiring that individuals be separated from any of their adaptive technology or devices. It also involves anticipation of many more additional disability placard parking spaces for certain events.

Applying the CMIST Framework Across Various Scenarios

This textbook describes a myriad of scenarios in which people may congregate in large numbers. The types of mass gatherings are as varied as the people who attend them. To describe the utility of the CMIST Framework, four representative types of mass gatherings with higher risk for vulnerable populations will be discussed in the ensuing text: (1) large religious events; (2) political rallies; (3) large public celebrations/festivals; and (4) disaster sheltering circumstances.

Religious Gatherings

Gatherings rooted in religious tradition have historic-ally generated some of the largest mass gatherings ever observed worldwide. The Kumbh Mela, occurring every twelfth year in India, is a Hindu pilgrimage and festival that reportedly attracts thirty to fifty million devoted pilgrims across only a few weeks' time. The Shia Muslim annual event, called the Arba'een Pilgrimage, routinely entails tens of millions of participants. The Hajj pilgrimage to the House of God in Mecca carries notoriety, not only for the sheer volume of international attendees, numbering in the millions, but also the history of unfortunate events that periodically have led to the loss of hundreds of lives due to the unpredictability of crowd dynamics, fires, and protests. In 1990, due to a tunnel stampede, nearly 1,500 persons were killed during the Hajj pilgrimage and many more were injured. Despite governmental attempts to curtail such situations over the years, a similar stampede ("the Mina Stampede") occurring on September 24, 2015, was associated with nearly 2,500 deaths according to press reports. Other threats, including infectious disease outbreaks have also complicated these events.

As in the Hindu and Muslim religious communities, many Roman Catholics from around the world will also attend extraordinarily large mass gatherings when the Pope travels outside of the Vatican. Visits from the sitting Pope frequently draw very large crowds reaching into the millions with the attendees traveling from many global destinations to garner a glimpse of the Holy Father. Again, depending on the venue, accessibility and climate, these events can be extraordinarily challenging and the involvement of such a celebrated figure also raises the threats of assassination, terrorism and other types of malfeasance and exploitation.

Given the lifelong devotion many pilgrims will possess, it is not surprising that these religious events often attract a disproportionately higher number of at-risk individuals compared to other mass gatherings. These vulnerable populations may include attendees at the extremes of age, those with chronic or fragile medical conditions seeking possible healing, and those who may overextend themselves physically and mentally to attend the event, even to the point of injury or incapacitation.

Events of this scale also escalate the complexity and need to mitigate a higher risk of serious safety threats that can range from the augmented interactions that can occur between vehicular traffic and the disabled or slower-reacting pedestrians to the impact of extremes in weather such as heat, precipitation, and lightning. Many have traveled long distances that must be traversed to access the event. Beyond language and impairment barriers, organizers must further ensure reliable access to water and food, specialized viewing areas and toilets, and unique precautions in terms of crowd dynamics and the more subtle environmental threats such as mosquitos and other local zoological threats. These threats are described extensively in other sections of this textbook, but, in the special case of the more vulnerable populations, using the CMIST framework, organizers and medical teams may be able to better analyze the event and anticipate the needs of at-risk attendees, framework, organizers and medical teams may be able to better analyze the event and anticipate the needs of various at-risk attendees.

For example, in terms of *Communication*, planning must consider those with sensory impairments such as vision or hearing issues. Sensory impairment issues introduce the need to consider having multiple redundant messaging capabilities for routine and emergency operations at the gathering and to advise the use of accompanying "buddy systems" (younger, healthier companions) for such individuals. Wireless communications can become tremendously unreliable at very high-density events, and the ability to utilize text messaging and wireless alerts could also be degraded severely.

Many events utilize loudspeaker announcements but this may be ineffective for those with hearing impairment who constitute approximately 5 percent of the general population, and likely larger proportions under these special circumstances. Large visual messaging boards and Megatron-type displays provide additional options for messaging. On a case-by-case basis, event planners need to ensure that routine and emergency messaging is conducted, not just in the local language, but also in numerous languages based on the likely community in attendance. In recent years, English has become a very useful and a common global language, especially for younger generations, but it still may not be as useful for many of the elderly in attendance or children.

Papal Visit to Philadelphia (2015)

Planning estimates were that over half of the anticipated two million attendees for Sunday mass would be senior citizens. To attend, most of these elderly would be required to undertake a long trek during warm and humid conditions, from a site in New Jersey, the closest point for vehicle and mass transit access. This trip included a 1.5 mile walk over the Benjamin Franklin Bridge with its 135 feet of steep incline. It is also likely that the return trip would occur in the dark. This set of circumstances immediately exemplifies the importance of using a framework such as CMIST to identify and mitigate the vulnerabilities of at-risk individuals who were expecting to attend this mass gathering in a well-resourced environment.

In fact, one of the specific US ADA requirements regarding large public events is the directive to provide "auxiliary aids and services" to accommodate those with hearing, vision, or speech disabilities. This stipulation could include requirements for adaptive technology such as sign-language interpretation, closed-captioning on video screens, or assistive listening systems. Especially for event planning purposes, as of 2018, the US Department of Justice has determined that websites are now sites of public accommodation and that specific requirements must be in place so that adaptive reader technology can access the electronic information on a website.

Maintaining Health: Since persons in the extremes of age and those with serious chronic medical conditions often attend religious gatherings in larger numbers, it is imperative to have a well-designed and well-researched medical plan that accommodates their special needs. Religious mass gatherings can potentially involve individuals from a large cross-section of demographics, largely based on religious customs and locale, but data from previous similar events can provide pivotal information in terms of planning.

One priority in terms of the maintaining health component is to create strategies that would prevent individuals from ever developing a medical emergency at the event. This contingency work requires a layered strategy addressing numerous areas of often under-recognized concerns. For example, for some types of events, it is essential (yet very often overlooked) to have supplies that support the hydration and nutrition of infants and children if their presence is anticipated at the religious mass gathering (or any other event). Beyond an abundance of water supplies, provisions of infant feeding formulas, disposable feeding supplies, and areas for breastfeeding should be incorporated into planning. Ensuring access to disposable diapers and appropriate disposal mechanisms also mitigates serious sanitation issues that can quickly develop when hundreds, if not thousands, of babies populate the event. Having adequate, well-maintained toilets and trash disposal systems on-site are also essential components as well as readily accessible and omnipresent options for hand-sanitizing hygiene, and their continuous replenishment as indicated. These supplies have all been found to be essential for preventing illness especially in child care areas or under the sheltering circumstances for disaster evacuees.

For all populations, let alone those at risk, comprehensive food safety plans must be in place to ensure that items for purchase at the event are not only safe and hygienic, but that they also meet the nutritional needs for people of all ages. Prolonged ambient heat exposure, poorly stored food or liquids, and under-refrigerated items brought into the site(s) can be a significant threat. Also, for the very young and elderly, having access to cooling facilities or ventilated shade can help to prevent serious environmental emergencies. Sunscreen, insect repellent and similar precautions should become part of the supply stocking portfolio. For those with applicable disabilities, viewing areas in singular events such as a papal visit or concert should also prioritize those protections.

When a medical emergency does occur, it is essential that the health and safety plan involves the ability to rapidly assess, treat, and safely transport persons of any age or size experiencing a behavioral or physical emergency. Crowds and heat often exacerbate those with bariatric challenges. Very large and heavy persons constitute a growing portion of the population and they can require additional care and resources when they become ill or injured. Common issues such as heat emergencies, dehydration, vomiting, and physical injuries can disproportionately impact the very young, the elderly, and those with chronic medical conditions, especially if they are not identified and managed quickly. As indicated in prior chapters, well-researched *medical threat assessment* will ensure that care stations and personnel are adequate in number and properly equipped for the type and volume of care that they can be expected to deliver. Marked medical aid stations and roving medical patrols in the crowd are some of the best practices that better ensure that these needs are met and accessible to all.

Independence: Extremely crowded conditions and variable terrain can challenge the independence of those who routinely require and use mobility adjuncts or other assistance, including service animals. These challenges are exacerbated when there are long and exposed distances to traverse to gain entrance into the event site. Chokepoints in the flow of the crowd such as tunnels, stairs, ramps, or sharp corners and turns can enhance the threats where a trip and fall can occur. If not at the time of injury, particularly for those taking anti-coagulants, such traumatic events can lead to a life-threatening injury such as the eventual sequelae of a hip fracture in someone over seventy years of age. Resulting crowd crush situations also impose higher risk for pregnant woman and those elderly or impaired with less compliant skeletal tissues. While barricades and other strategies can prevent such tragedies, stampedes are still a problem as has been the case with the Hajj, recent music festivals in the US, or past football matches in Europe. As a result, for risk management purposes, planners should ensure that the event can and will meet the requirements of the ADA in the US and similar regulations in other nations. Following ADA rules is particularly important for ensuring regulatory-required

equitable access to viewing areas and all necessary resources, including medical care during normal and contingency operations at the site.

Support and Safety: Having a system in place to facilitate the reunification of lost individuals, including, but not limited to children or those with cognitive impairment, is an essential element at any type of gathering. Given the numbers of persons attending, the likelihood of wireless communication shortfalls will be augmented. It is also important to ensure that this reunification system incorporates the medical and law enforcement officials at the site. Unaccompanied individuals or their separated caregivers often appear at a first aid or medical station as their first stop. Chapter 4 discusses, in detail, some evolving systems for attendee tracking.

Large gatherings may be extremely stressful for certain individuals with behavioral health conditions. The emotions involved with attending a mass religious event can exacerbate a crisis in some. A preestablished system for managing behavioral health emergencies that works closely in conjunction with the on-site medical and security staff is a best practice that can help deescalate these types of crises before they become unfortunate law enforcement situations or result in injury to those persons or others.

Transportation: Travel-limiting disabilities are very common in most nations hosting religious events, with some more impacted than others. In the US, the prevalence of travel-limiting disabilities increases steadily with age (Figure 18.2), reaching a peak of well over 30 percent after eighty years of age [5].

This type of information is an elemental consideration in a religious mass gathering. Religious events have greater numbers of persons with disability-related parking placards on their personal vehicles compared to most athletic or musical events. Many attendees may also arrive with mobility assistance devices ranging from canes and walkers to personal scooters. Event planners should therefore anticipate the need for supplementing additional areas to provide adequate accessible parking spaces. They should also emphasize planning for more accessible, shorter, and easier routes leading into the venue and within the venue. Alternative mechanisms or procedures to accommodate and bypass the usual turnstiles at security checkpoint barriers should be planned. When transportation vehicles are part of the event plan,

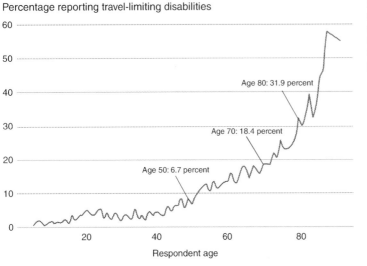

Percentage reporting travel-limiting disabilities

Age 80: 31.9 percent

Age 70: 18.4 percent

Age 50: 6.7 percent

Respondent age

Figure 18.2 The percentage of persons now reporting that they have travel-limiting disabilities stratified by age indicate significant escalating numbers for those over fifty years of age and sharper rises in percentage numbers after the age of eighty years

such as a shuttle service, they must accommodate those with disabilities and their assistive equipment and be present in numbers that are adequate and efficient support for the number of attendees that may require such accommodations. When an event provides emergency medical transportation on-site or off-site, it must include the capacity for safe transport of infants and children in appropriate car seats or other appropriate restraint systems. While these considerations appear more in the wheelhouse of organizers, medical leaders should also become stakeholders that ensure that their implementation. Not only will these interventions help in the prevention of medical illness and injury for vulnerable populations, they will also help to decrease subsequent overall workload for medical professionals serving the event.

Political Mass Gatherings

Large gatherings to support, protest, or even commemorate political activities are a time-honored tradition worldwide. However, as in the case of religious events, they can pose important challenges for vulnerable populations. An example is the January 2009 presidential inauguration of US President, Barack Obama, at which over two million attended. That mass gathering event, which lasted for hours, involved spectators huddling at National Mall in extremely frigid weather. A large percentage of those attendees

were elderly and disabled spectators. It is not uncommon for millions of others to attend other political mass gatherings that pose similar environmental risks such as state funerals, political rallies, and even birthday or coronation celebrations for world leaders.

While political mass gatherings face many of the same challenges seen for religious events, there are also some distinctive aspects. Politically motivated mass gatherings have some unique threats relative to those individuals who have special access and functional needs. Unfortunately, those events also bring a higher likelihood of violence and other sudden threats, thus creating greater risk for the more fragile and lesser mobile persons attending the event.

Often, political events can be unexpectedly scheduled with relatively short notice requiring an extremely accelerated planning schedule and sometimes no time whatsoever. Such suddenness can compromise the more preferable and typical comprehensive planning phase using the CMIST framework. Additionally, political events often hold the potential for demonstrations or civil disobedience which have the potential to escalate unexpectedly. As seen during the "Black Lives Matter" rallies and protests during the summer of 2020 in the US, or the 2018 antigovernment rallies in Paris, or January 6, 2021 riot at the US Capitol, violence can sudden erupt. Often instigated by extremist factions who imbed themselves into such events, this additional factor can lead to the use of law enforcement interventions such as chemical agents and a large police presence using force with resulting physical injuries. As previously indicated, these factors can pose a greater impact on the more vulnerable populations under discussion.

For at-risk individuals, these combinations of factors increase the possibility that the vulnerable populations in attendance could be put into a disproportionately dangerous situation when organizers are likely to be inadequately prepared to extricate them from such circumstances safely or if the at-risk attendees are not positioned to do so because of unforeseen logistical reasons or imposed law enforcement and security factors. Nonetheless, the CMIST strategy along with "just-in-time" training may still provide some degree of improved preparation to mitigate tragic outcomes.

Communication: In addition to the various regulatory and best practices requirements described previously with religious events, it is critical to think about how to provide emergency messages if an unforeseen or unexpected problem occurs during a political event. One good example would be the individual with hearing or vision impairment who needs to have access to information about sheltering in place or evacuating the venue when an explosion or fire occurs. In addition to having the ability to deliver emergency messages by mobile phone, which may be limited or not applicable to some individuals, it is important to consider the use of instructions that

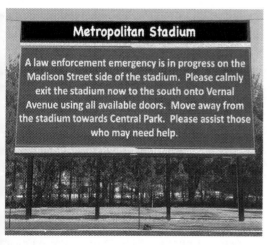

Figure 18.3 Demonstration of the use of a visual messaging board for emergency situations occurring during mass gatherings

Photograph taken and provided with the permission of Dr. Andrew Garrett

a public address system could broadcast, and also via digital emergency messaging delivered via large screen technology or scoreboards (Figure 18.3). In the past, such emergency messaging has not always been posted or broadcast as rapidly as possible while the message content was reviewed and approved by supervisors. Event planners may now mitigate this delay by drafting a series of preapproved messages with each being applicable to a given potential crisis. This approach can be fine-tuned by practicing emergency message dissemination during drills and exercises and by delivering "routine" safety messages during the actual event itself to familiarize attendees with such processes and notifications. Similar to the safety demonstrations that are delivered before departures on commercial aircraft, attendees can be alerted to emergency evacuation and assembly areas "in case of an emergency." Lastly, organizers and medical personnel should ensure that all event messaging uses proper terminology whenever referring to at-risk individuals in a manner that further minimizes the risk that someone would be offended by the messaging. This would appropriately include the use of "people first" language.

Beyond stadia, hotels, and arenas being used as a political rally sites, many political mass gatherings are held in outdoor areas without such large-scale messaging apparatus except perhaps the speaker's microphone and social media, such as that utilized at the beginning of the well-publicized January 6, 2021 incumbent president's rally in Washington, DC. Likewise, protest rallies are often parade-like as are celebratory motorcade routes for heads of state or royalty. The June 2, 2022, carriage procession during the Platinum Anniversary celebration of the coronation of Queen Elizabeth II had compacted crowds lining the route of travel. This type of event not only needs longitudinal planning, but also prior education of the public about using companion "buddy systems" with each person watching out for the other and purposely knowing where the closest public safety officer is posted. Even so, for all the reasons previously discussed, the risks remain higher for those vulnerable populations under consideration here.

Maintaining Health: Similar to most mass gatherings, political events often include the full spectrum of at-risk individuals with special access and functional needs attending the event. These attendees range across extremes of age, those with sensory, mobility, and cognitive challenges, and across those with preexisting medical conditions of all kinds. Dense crowding, extremes in temperature, loud noises, and long periods of time elapsing without adequate rest, food, and hydration, all can exacerbate the potential for any attendee, particularly at-risk individuals to experience a true emergency or worrisome sign or symptom. Organizers should anticipate the healthcare maintenance needs for the whole community to ensure the best outcome for the event itself. A goal of planning should have the goal that all attendees will have equal access to high-quality, age and gender-appropriate emergency medical services at all locations along the route or within any "brick and mortar" structure, and that they receive on-site medical treatment from well-qualified clinical teams familiar with managing the very young, the very old, and those with other disadvantageous physically and cognitively.

Independence: Impromptu rallies and protests can often occur very soon after a tragedy such as a police-involved shooting or news of the pending passage of unpopular legislation. As such, these mass gatherings may not allow for adequate planning to accommodate the needs of all at-risk individuals. In addition, the at-risk persons may also be caught up in such events without active participation and, instead, simply become involved by proximity at the time of the event. As attendance grows, so does the possibility that a dangerous situation could evolve in which it may not be possible for a mobility-impaired person to continue to move independently either within or near the crowd. Again, such scenarios can lead to a fall, trampling, or crush situation, let alone the physiological stress emanating from fear of the situation. Likewise, if truly involved in the rally or protest, access to on-site resources such as food, water, and shady sites should be equitable for at-risk attendees and hopefully without needing third-party assistance. In some situations, some third-party entities such as the Red Cross may indeed be able to assist on short notice, as they often do locally on short notice with major displacement disasters such as a very large residential complex fire. Nonetheless, such a response should only occur in close cooperation and guidance from public safety officials responsible for dealing with the incident.

As for any other mass gathering, access for service animals is also an important consideration here. They are a critical tool to maintain the independence of some at-risk individuals, and their presence, for example, is protected under regulations in many jurisdictions such as the US, where the ADA stipulates that there must be accommodation and protection for the animals. While the animals may sometimes be a protective deterrent during marches and rallies, they may also become a target in certain circumstances. They will also need areas and accommodations (such as small plastic bags) for bowel movements and urination needs as well as access to water. In addition, it is important to note that, in contrast to service animals, emotional support animals (ESA) are not covered by the ADA and other nations' protective regulations as they are not specifically considered "service animals" such as the traditional "seeing-eye" dogs. A service animal, by definition, is trained to provide a specific action to protect the owner whereas an ESA, as defined by the US Department of Justice, is "an animal that provides comfort by its presence."

Support and Safety: Similar to the comments provided regarding religious mass gatherings, adequate planning and resource allotments need to be in place at political mass gatherings to ensure a system for the reunification of separated individuals, including children and those with cognitive impairment. It is often suggested that certain qualified individuals become part of an on-site coordinated response plan for attendees who may experience a behavioral health emergency such as an anxiety attack, the development of altered mental status or even a sudden episode of combativeness. Likewise, as discussed in subsequent text, planning for deteriorating security on a mass scale is also warranted.

As noted previously, on January 6, 2021, the world did witness firsthand the devolution of a scheduled political mass gathering. In short, the political rally rapidly became a disorganized riot that endangered public safety and the function of the national governmental. In that incident, a permitted, relatively small political rally involving the sitting U.S. President on the National Mall in Washington, DC, rapidly transitioned into a political insurrection with an assault on the US Capitol building where lawmakers were in session. The widespread violence that ensued even included the use of various standard and improvised weapons and chemical agents which all led to many injuries, some severe, and even fatalities. While few persons in the rioting crowds were elders or disabled, many of the persons within the capitol building were such vulnerable persons. In that respect, therefore, planning for a large political event should also take into account a contingency for a spontaneous eruption of civil unrest and mayhem for the vulnerable populations being discussed here. That aspect of planning should consider options for safe means of egress from the venue for all attendees regardless of their access and functional needs.

Transportation: More often than not, political mass gathering events will, fortunately, be held in "improved" public or commercial areas such as arenas, auditoriums, or public spaces that have appropriate existing infrastructure for at-risk groups such as public transportation, parking lots, and sidewalks adapted for those groups. In turn, this also increases the likelihood that the venue and surroundings will already meet accessible access and movement regulations for those with mobility challenges. However, as described previously, event planners also need to consider the special needs of sensory or mobility-impaired attendees while at the venue.

In essence, the planning evaluation should cover the special populations' experience from start to finish, including their means for arriving at the event and the distance to travel, be it on foot or with a mobility aid device. Best practices would consider the question, "if this were your family member, what do we need to do (for him or her)?"

These considerations are most appropriate when addressing the need for public transportation or easy, well-marked access for disable placard parking. It would also consider transit or shuttles to and from the event and mobility strategies within the venue while attending the event. Again, the plan should include all potential opportunities and mechanisms to help the vulnerable populations safely evacuate away from any hazards in the event of a life-threatening emergency. As for events away from such established infrastructure, there is still a need to address instant adaptations, which often pose a challenge. With more elders participating in such events, it is important to expect that there will be more and more vulnerable populations present at mass gatherings, including political rallies outside the mainstream of typical crowd medicine scenarios.

Celebrations

Large celebrations that bring millions of people together to the same location to participate in a shared experience are not only held across many nations, but they are becoming more and more popular. As discussed previously, bringing large numbers of people together has many inherent dangers regardless of the type of event, but those dangers can be further compounded by some perilous activities that are often associated with large public celebrations.

Many consider the pre-Lenten Carnival in Rio de Janeiro, Brazil, to be the largest party in the world, during which over five million people gather to celebrate publicly over five days. The streets are filled with many inebriated, dancing people celebrating cheek to cheek and watching parades and other events. On many of the forty-foot floats that travel many distances along city streets in the heat and humidity, one can typically see the float crews and guest riders aboard them dancing and singing as they pass along. Likewise, Carnival in Venice, Italy, attracts three million visitors a year, but there the jammed waterways can create a different set of hazards and risks. In New Orleans, Louisiana, Mardi Gras activities are held annually with a much smaller celebration, but one that still encounters one million people from many parts of the world crowded into a much smaller area of festivities during a similar five-day period. As is the case in Rio, the Mardi Gras floats themselves create well-known risks, not only for those on the floats, but also for those on the streets. That, however, is just one of many other special hazards routinely encountered at these events.

Despite their festive intent, all three of the mentioned events are regularly marred by the effects of protracted overuse of alcohol, float mishaps, and the usual challenges to public safety and risks for vulnerable populations. Nonetheless, they remain an annual staple for those locales despite incumbent tragedies. Moreover, during the Pamplona Encierro, also known as the "Running of the Bulls" in Pamplona, Spain, one million people also gather together and, every year, it is expected that people will be severely injured at this event. Those injuries are even considered by many to be part of the routine festivities. Accordingly, preparations must include retrieval plans to work around this very unusual "hazard" and it also incumbent upon local governmental officials and event planners to consider the special needs of at-risk populations when preparing to host these city-wide, extremely populous and often aimlessly migrating parties. Beyond the enhanced risks for all others in general, those with vulnerabilities face additional threat of harm as these individuals often lack the agility to avoid injuries or other threatening exposures.

New Orleans

New Orleans is best known for two types of experiences: parties and disasters, both of which result in mass gatherings. The misery inflicted by the combination of living at or below sea level, and the never-ending supply of natural and technological hazards, has led to a culture where celebration is consequently embraced. New Orleans has a festival for everything: tomatoes, satsumas, oysters, cocktails, po-boy sandwiches, beignets, and crawfish, just to name a few culinary celebrations. In turn, New Orleanians love food which is why, not surprisingly, the region perennially ranks at the top – for rates of obesity, diabetes, and heart disease. Over half of the people living in New Orleans report at least one chronic medical condition [1]. This medical matter is compounded by high rates of poverty and pervasive health care inequities. Therefore, planning for mass gatherings in New Orleans, be it a Mardi Gras or hurricane evacuation gathering, includes a close evaluation of the needs of those at high risk for medical complications. As a result, the New Orleans Special Needs Registry is updated regularly and includes a reasonably current list of those people who will likely need additional support during an emergency. Of note, this registry includes the specific needs of each individual.

Communication: Experience has shown that mobile phone towers quickly become overwhelmed when large numbers of people descend upon a small area, making phone communications difficult. But cheering shouting crowds, event music, and other sources of loud noises prevent reasonable conversations in either direction, calling in or out. Similarly, loudspeaker announcements may not be heard over the din of the crowds, the loud rock music, or marching bands. Elderly people, those with hearing impairment, and international visitors who do not speak the native language, will clearly have trouble hearing loudspeaker announcements as presbycusis and other hearing deficits often prohibit accurate delineation of those sounds. Even on well-lit billboards, written communication may be overlooked amid the reveling. The elderly and younger children are more likely to get separated from their families in large crowds, especially when caretakers are understandably turning their attention toward a passing parade float and being distracted by antics on those floats or among the partying attendees. Especially with migrating crowds, children, pregnant women, the elderly and those with chronic diseases are more likely to have trouble keeping up with the pressing crowd and rate of migration. As a result, they are more likely to be separated from their loved ones, a frequent problem in these events. Similar situations in rapid exiting, and particularly with rapid evacuations away from a hazard such as a fire, explosion, active shooter, or police incursion.

Maintaining Health: Float mishaps are common, often resulting in serious injuries and even death. In 2020 in New Orleans, two people were killed – in two separate incidents at different locations. In both cases, floats ran over them. Balconies of old buildings have collapsed under the weight of unusually large groups of people pressing into them for a closer view of events below. As with a pressing crowd, children and the elderly are at higher risk of being injured or crushed by such collapses or by being pushed and crushed by a resulting stampeded crowd. Anxious to still celebrate, those with chronic medical conditions may not find themselves tolerating the conditions of being outdoors or standing on their feet all day. As an expected and traditional part of the festivities, even those at risk may be consuming alcoholic beverages all day and often without eating their regular or appropriate meals. In such situations, many persons, including the young and healthy, can collapse from exhaustion after dancing throughout heat of day and continuing to experience the usual combination of alcohol and dehydration.

Therefore, it is important to have many easily accessible medical triage and first aid stations assembled and ready to triage, assess, and transport as indicated. Roving paramedics, on foot with backpacks, should also be considered for a first-in response as vehicles, even small carts, may be delayed. A prospective plan including resources for providing treatment in place or treat and release decisions can be particularly helpful. Transporting patients out of the city-wide crowded environments can be very difficult and, typically, hospitals are already being overcrowded with routine problems largely due to additional large populations of visitors coming into the community and also walk-ins not seen at the site. As in the case of music festivals, indeterminate drug use can become rampant and create both behavioral threats and sudden medical emergencies across many attendees. Such mini-epidemics can therefore compromise and compete with the prioritization of care for the more vulnerable, not only on-site, but also across the community. Having a plethora of resources available on site for the majority of party goers who will only require hydration, monitoring, some sobering and some period of observation, is a more prudent tactic than just steadily evacuating persons who, in most cases, can readily be treated and released on site. This also preserves some transport priority for the more vulnerable populations.

Independence: Intuitively, independence for those with limited mobility is particularly difficult in large gatherings, but creating clearly barricaded lanes and a clear pathway for wheelchairs and mobility devices, can help to overcome those concerns, especially when considering what a sudden evacuation would entail for them. Those who depend on wheelchairs and mobility devices can get trapped in a crowd, and those less than agile persons may be unable to extricate themselves, especially if they pushed over in a wheelchair and tossed onto the ground.

Having a designated viewing area for those with limited mobility or those requiring mobility devices is also important, but if the event is in a building with multiple floors, a plan should be in place that addresses how to safely evacuate those who cannot rely on evacuating themselves via a stairwell. This concern includes children and those with impaired mobility who depend on mobility devices. In addition to ensuring that the toilets have support bars and are of appropriate height, it is also important to ensure that the toilets are accessible via ramps for those in a wheelchair. Likewise, the sink and soap sources should be accessible as well. Avoiding mishaps is the most logical task.

Support and Safety: In such public celebrations, certain persons misuse the large crowds as a cover or distraction for their own violent or predatory behavior. Many criminals operate under the assumption that their crimes will likely go unnoticed amid a massive crowd and the allure of the events. Compounding this concern, experience reveals that women and children are at a higher risk of being separated from their friends and families in such crowds and that they have sometimes been abducted and even forced into human trafficking during large festivals [9]. Other perpetrators have specifically used the crowd setting for executing gang assassination plots when firing gunshots or automatic weapons into the crowd (and not just at their intended target) and then, in turn, disappearing among the other mass gatherers.

These instances involving firearms are particularly dangerous for the disabled because an additional risk for injuries can result from the stampeding that follows. The startle reflex from the loud gunshots and the witnesses seeing the wounded collapsing can create chaos and indiscriminate scrambling. Also bullets hitting hard pavement in inner city locales can ricochet and thus cause additional injuries and drive more persons onto the ground, further impeding avenues of escape or access. At-risk populations are disadvantaged during these crises because they may have even more difficulty protecting themselves from a stampede and may be unable to run away. Several active shooter events have demonstrated that the elderly and the less mobile were the primary victims for that reason such as that observed during the shooting incident at the Fort Lauderdale airport baggage claim area on January 6, 2017.

Also, if in a wheelchair and therefore closer to ground level, the risk of ricocheting bullets hitting a vital organ can be enhanced. Creating protected viewing areas for at-risk individuals and their families can provide more of a buffered space that offers additional protection from the crowds and such criminal malfeasance.

Creating safe and guarded spaces for breast-feeding mothers, along with family-friendly bathrooms, and places for diaper changes can also help deter predatory crimes against at-risk people at any mass gathering. Assigning event staff or security personnel to closely monitor this special location designed for these vulnerable populations is highly recommended and should be supported by medical planners as part of a holistic and prevention strategy for medical staff.

Transportation: As previously described, large celebrations usually require the participants to walk significant distances without many areas for resting or even sitting. Therefore, specially identified and reserved benches should be strategically staged throughout the event to allow the elderly, chronically ill, injured, and pregnant persons to rest when walking from one part of the event to the other. Transportation options during large celebrations often do not meet the needs of at-risk populations especially those who are mobility-impaired. However, transportation plans for a large celebration should include wheelchair-compatible buses and shuttles which are allowed to use specialized traffic lanes. Those lanes should be established and well-marked to allow drop-off access as close to the event as possible. Again, these logistical issues have overlap with medical practitioners' interest in terms of injury and illness prevention.

Disasters

Unlike most other mass gathering events, those that have evolved as a result of some major catastrophe can pose some of the most unpredictable challenges. Even with the best governmental planning and preparation, disasters can be sudden and insidious. It must recognized that no two disasters are truly alike, and it is impossible to create a perfect plan for each. When a sudden flood, wildfire, typhoon, earthquake, or military conflict force human beings to leave their homes and find shelter, poorly defined and demographically unpredictable mass gatherings can result, very often without any preplanning whatsoever for the communities tasked with creating safe harbors.

People living in poverty are disproportionately affected by disasters. They are also more apt to have underlying medical conditions that put them at higher risk of acute medical illness and less resilience to withstand environmental exposures and infectious contagion. Those at the highest risk of seeking shelters are more likely to live on a fixed income and those who do not have adequate savings or financial resources to evacuate themselves to a desirable location, let alone prepare for the disaster. Some disasters, like hurricanes and wildfires, may provide a few days' notice, but others, like military bombings, earthquakes, tornadoes, and Tsunamis, may give no notice whatsoever, thus forcing the victims to leave quite rapidly from their often-collapsed homes and as well as their daily routines across a now destroyed community. The rapid onset of wildfire events that were fueled by high winds on Maui, Hawaii, in August 2023, exemplified how killer catastrophes can be very unpredictable, arise out of seemingly nowhere and also disproportionately affect the elderly and other vulnerable populations.

Injured or not, those surviving these terrible disasters will need to immediately leave their homes, destroyed or not, without being able to locate their medications, hearing aids, canes, wheelchairs or eye glasses. In many cases, without having any other resources, these vulnerable and special needs populations will often find themselves in rapidly designated shelters such as arenas, convention centers and other sites far and away from their homes. They will also find themselves in close and privacy-lacking contact with others of similar disadvantage seeking shelter.

Therefore, being prepared for the needs of at-risk individuals during these unpredictable circumstances is a challenge, but also a critical task to best ensure the health and safety of those affected by the disaster.

A special needs registry, stored electronically, can be one potential aspect of disaster planning as it may help identify those at-risk individuals and their specific needs. Such a registry has now worked well in the City of New Orleans where their share of disasters has been abundant.

It is important to preemptively organize plans with pharmacies that have databases which can help to identify current medications for each patient, even when the hometown pharmacy is destroyed. Prospective public education, media service announcements and prompts from primary care professionals can emphasize that each person should maintain a list of medical conditions, medications, and allergies in a protected manner, perhaps within their mobile phones, a universal denominator for most, even the elderly and disabled. This latter recommendation has been suggested with the understanding that most persons or their loved ones will have such a device and know how to manage the security of the information.

Hurricane Ida (2021)

On Monday, August 30, 2021, in the wake of Hurricane Ida, the public 911 emergency call center operations in New Orleans were disabled for thirteen hours making it almost impossible for its citizens and visitors to reach out for help. The Orleans Parish Communications Dispatch (OPCD) ran social media posts that asked emergency callers to walk to their local fire house to ask for help. Local radio stations started receiving calls from stranded people who gave their name, address and emergency details asking for help. Text-to-911 was operational during this time which was only available to those who had working mobile phones. Many people also turned to the Twitter and Facebook social media sites to ask for help from first responders and the Cajun Navy, a group of volunteers with boats who help those in need during floods. This incident occurred sixteen years to the day after the levees broke following Hurricane Katrina, another event during which the city lost 911 services for an extended period of time. Anticipating such loss of services, all persons and their family members should have an updated preparedness plan must that must go beyond calling 911 for help including rendezvous points, what hospital to go to, packed suitcases or back packs prepared with clothing, medications, glasses and other essentials needed to leave the city as indicated as well as back-up plan for other persons to call.

Communication: During a disaster, the usual avenues of communication may not be operational. Relying on emergency messaging methods, including television, radio, and mass text messaging may not reach at-risk groups, especially those who are elderly, blind, hard of hearing, or living in poverty. Social media are usually not used by several of these groups, and any messaging may need to be in multiple languages based on the languages that are commonly used in the community being managed.

If possible, and when a disaster (e.g., a hurricane) can be somewhat anticipated, individuals on a special needs registry should be called in the days leading up to the disaster. There should be a plan for them to evacuate or go to a shelter and to ensure that they have their medications, eyewear, mobility devices, hearing aids, food, and water. Going door to door can be an effective, though also a slow method of getting the information to the community and ascertaining transportation needs. If a special needs registry has already been created, officials can reach out to those who have already been identified as requiring extra assistance and facilitate those needs. Going door to door after the acute event (e.g., after the tornado or cyclone or earthquake has passed), to those previously identified addresses, can still help to reach those individuals who will need additional assistance or be evacuated. It also helps to prepare for a potential mass gathering either locally or at some distant site.

Maintaining Health: In the aftermath of a disaster, people at risk are more likely to require support than others who have their own resources and are more apt to be evacuated to a shelter with attendant mass gathering circumstances. Setting up medical triage stations can be useful, not only in caring for those with special needs, but all evacuees. Prior studies have revealed that makeshift clinics at the receiving sites will protect local emergency departments from becoming overwhelmed with poorly nourished, poorly hydrated, and at-risk groups who are not faring so well after being transported over long distances and often arriving with newly acquired or exacerbated illnesses and injuries that compounded their underlying conditions [10]. During the disaster, people may have evacuated without their medications, and their chronic medical conditions exacerbated by the stress of the disaster and evacuation processes. Local pharmacies and stores may be closed during the mass gathering incident making it difficult to get medications for those in need. Many medications require

refrigeration or need to avoid ambient temperatures, let alone hot temperatures. Again, preemptive relationships with pharmacies and other supply chains are critical and have been used to create high-efficiency, on-site, and well-stocked pharmacies with top-notch pharmacists assigned to the shelter. This was exemplified by the experience of the City of Dallas at its convention center in 2005.

In the early days of September 2005, following landfall of Hurricane Katrina, thousands of evacuees were transported the City of Dallas from Louisiana for shelter. Evacuees were to be brought to the city's massive convention center where sleeping cots and other basic shelter needs were being set-up. A priority was setting up a on-site pharmacy with imbedded pharmacists on shift and attendant clinics for various ailments and needs. Though it was a first time effort for organizers, the medical response was exemplary and the collaborative medical component was also fully operational by the time some 40,000 evacuees, largely elderly and vulnerable populations arrived from Louisiana hundreds of miles away. With only 1-2 days' notice, the medical community also created prospective relations with local hospitals, medical societies, and public health practitioners who pulled together many volunteer healthcare providers. On the first day of the evacuees' arrival, the volunteer physicians, nurses, paramedics, and other support staff managed over a thousand patients on-site who might have otherwise overwhelmed the local EMS and emergency departments that first evening [10]. The teams treated several thousand more who would have gone to emergency departments over the ensuing weeks.

To facilitate this exceptional mass gathering medicine feat, mechanisms for rapid electronic credentialing and time-keeping for service hours also helped with subsequent disaster funding and remuneration for resources utilized. Because of this successful experience, and despite less time to act, preparations were ready to go during subsequent hurricanes. Subsequent iterations of these post-landfall mass shelters were arranged for other storms such as Hurricane Ike which made Texas landfall on September 13, 2008. This time, the clinics, pharmacies, and staffing were set-up within a matter of hours.

Before distant travel to designated shelters in another country or region of the same nation, persons with disabilities and other at-risk conditions may be staged in temporary mass gatherings such as the experience at the New Orleans Louis Armstrong international airport (MSY) several days after the initial landfall of Hurricane Katrina, on August 30, 2005. Due to a major breech of levee systems with widespread impassable flooding, many elderly and vulnerable persons became trapped or attempted to evacuate.

With the original intent of transporting evacuees by air to distant locations around the US, it became nearly impossible to effectively evacuate and transport the tens of thousands of evacuees steadily arriving at the MSY airport from all over the greater New Orleans. At the rate they were arriving, difficulties rapidly evolved and became overwhelming with tens of thousands suddenly and unintendedly gathering, including a disproportionate number of the poor, those transferred from skilled nursing facilities and those with disabilities, mobility needs, and a multitude of serious healthcare issues. Even though the airport was being staffed with several specially trained federal disaster medical assistance teams (DMATs) and military medical responders, the personnel on site were rapidly overwhelmed due to the sheer volumes of vulnerable individuals arriving each hour and the lack of supportive infrastructure and staff. Not only was there limited ability to transport patients by air to distant definitive care for several days, but it was relatively hard to see through all of the thousands of evacuees and ascertain who needed medical help.

This experience prompted a movement to reconsider several issues in terms of dealing with such disasters including: (1) how to perform patient triage under such exceptional circumstances; and (2) how to also reconsider other alternatives beyond a single-strategy evacuation plan [11].

Boots-on-the-ground disaster medical leaders who understood the need to adapt under such mass gatherings were able to rapidly adjust the original preplan and rapidly find alternative shelter destinations [12]. This real-time medical decision-making during a challenging mass gathering circumstance provided a remedy and solution for government officials. The medically driven change in strategies resulted in the salvage and survival of dozens of persons who, at first, had been declared "expectant" in prior days and left to die [11]. In addition, many evacuees were transported on austere military transport planes compounding their conditions upon arrival at distant shelters.

Congregate sheltering is a less desirable alternative to providing individual housing during disasters and especially during contagious outbreaks such as the COVID-19 pandemic. However, mass gathering sheltering is often is the only option for many evacuees. In such settings, organizers should ensure that there is adequate air flow and ventilation and a large enough space to separate the individuals as much as possible for both privacy and prevention of illness transmission. The provision of masks and social distancing can help mitigate the risk of transmission of respiratory pathogens. Requiring frequent hand-sanitizing and simple gloving at food stations with protected, properly gloved attendants using the ladles to prevent person-to-person handling is also strongly recommended.

Hurricane Ida (Landfall August 30, 2021)

Before landfall of Hurricane Ida, over 840 nursing home residents from seven different facilities were evacuated to a single warehouse in the path of the storm. The nursing home residents were given mattresses on the floor but were left without access to food, water, or medications. There was no electricity. Seven residents soon died of "storm related" injuries including heat exhaustion. Many of them called the public emergency answering point (911) from their mobile phones but emergency medical technicians (EMTs) were turned away at the door by nursing home staff for unexplained reasons. The evacuees eventually were rescued after multiple calls to 911 and visits by the local mayor and state health department officials. The health inspectors found elderly people lying on mattresses on the floor, some wearing only dirty diapers. Some were crying out that they were having trouble breathing. Ultimately rescued from this evacuation location on September 2, the residents were relocated to sites where they received a medical evaluation including COVID testing. Six of these evacuees required hospitalization. This experienced underscored the importance, even in this modern age, of purposeful, functional, and integrated disaster plans that address the sociological, psychological, physical, and medical support needs of the elderly and chronically ill and particularly those in assisted living facilities.

If possible, providing separate accommodations, such as a hotel room for each family, is preferred to decrease the risk of disease transmission and to decrease the stress of loss of privacy. It also allows for showers, laundry, and other accessories that effect better hygiene. If this approach is not available for all evacuees, prioritization should go to vulnerable populations such as the elderly, those with chronic diseases, pregnant women, and the very young (and parents), as they are more likely to develop complications from transmitted diseases.

Vaccinations are key aspects of mitigating the risk of spreading transmissible diseases in the aftermath of a disaster, particularly when the evacuees are coming from nations or regions where vaccinations are not required, substandard or simply unavailable. The elderly, chronically ill, pregnant women, and young children are at the greatest risk of developing complications from communicable diseases and they should be screened and prioritized if so indicated and feasible. In addition to having public health campaigns that encourage vaccination before any disaster, post-disaster immunization efforts in shelters can help stem the spread or development of disease. More recently, this recommendation has included the provision of COVID-19 and influenza vaccines. In areas with a large number of unvaccinated children, such sheltering medical clinics should preferably include immunizations for measles, chicken pox, pertussis, and other childhood diseases. In addition, vaccination for tetanus, hepatitis, COVID-19, respiratory syncytial virus and possible pneumococcus immunizations should be provided for the vulnerable populations. Consultations with both public health and infectious disease specialists would be most helpful in staging these vaccinations as well.

Hospitals may be destroyed during a disaster or may be overwhelmed by patients. Creating an ongoing post-disaster medical triage and treatment program is recommended as evacuees will have none of their usual medical resources. Having a plan in place before the disaster to meet the needs of at-risk people until a post-disaster medical triage and treatment program is operational, is key to protecting the health and well-being of at-risk groups during a disaster. In addition, preparing for premature deliveries and planning to transport women in labor to the hospital or deliver a baby in place is an important part of preparing for a hurricane. Plans should anticipate persons who may need dialysis, dental emergency

support, and mental health assistance. With limited access to electricity, it is important to have a plan to distribute and refill oxygen tanks as well as find procedural centers such as dialysis units for indicated patients.

In terms of mental health, not only are there profound psychological sequelae from being torn from one's home and country and now being placed in a strange distant environment among strangers, many persons may have recently lost their loved ones to the disaster, the war or the endemic illnesses or political problems that led to the evacuation. Loss of pets can be even more devastating for some. Beyond that, mental health problems are pervasive in most societies and maintenance of care for the schizophrenic, the depressed, bipolar, and other mental health patients should be a priority. Practitioners with extraordinary experience in disaster care have provided excellent outlines for such preparations [13].

Independence: In considering evacuation and sheltering options for nursing home residents specifically, it is even more intuitive to consider the needs of the elderly and the chronically ill. The checklist includes:

- Mobility Issues – Can the persons being evacuated move around on their own, or do they need assistive devices? Are there clear pathways for wheelchairs? Do they need elevated cots for sleeping?
- Nutritional Issues – Can the evacuated people eat prepackaged Meals-Ready-to-Eat (MREs)? Do they need soft diets or other special nutritional supplements?
- Sanitary Issues – Can they use a bathroom/toilet unassisted or do they need help? Do they usually wear diapers?

Support and Safety: As previously indicated, women, children, and those individuals with intellectual disabilities are at higher risk of becoming victims of violence and human trafficking during a disaster. Some traffickers and other criminals use disasters as a cover for violent or predatory behavior believing that law enforcement will likely be preoccupied with other disaster-related responses. Families are often separated during disasters posing further danger and disadvantages for the elderly and chronically ill. Family reunification plans should be part of every mass gathering event, especially those arising from disasters. Creating separate living areas for at-risk individuals and families in shelters can help create a buffered space that can offer additional

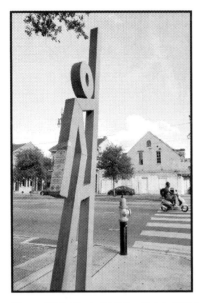

Figure 18.4 City Assist Pickup Points (CAPP). After Hurricane Katrina, the City of New Orleans created the CAPPs which are marked by large sculptures that can be seen from far away

Photograph (November 14, 2021) taken and provided with the permission of Dr. Megan C. Marino

protection, particularly from predators. Having safe, family-friendly places of refuge with security can also help deter predatory crimes against at-risk people.

Transportation: A pre- and post-disaster transportation plan is critical for caring for at-risk groups during a disaster. Many elderly and chronically ill people cannot drive themselves or have access to other modes of transportation. Pregnant women and young children are more likely to live in poverty and not have access to funds or resources to evacuate independently. Creating meeting places for those needing evacuation is a critical step. During some disasters, like a flood or a fire, the agreed meeting locations may look very different during the disaster. Large, easily identifiable landmarks can help the needy to know where to go during a disaster, even if there are language or literacy barriers (Figure 18.4). Ensuring that the mass transportation before and after a disaster includes options for those who have limited mobility is important and this includes wheelchair-accessible busses and trains. However, mass transportation for at-risk people presented new challenges during infectious disease outbreaks such as the COVID-19 pandemic since the pregnant, elderly, and chronically ill populations are at higher risk of serious complications or even death from COVID-19 and similar infectious disease threats.

Nonetheless, these relative risks must be weighed against the risk of remaining in a disaster zone when no other options are available. Providing proper (N-95, KN-95) masking and other protective shields can help to mitigate the threat and sequester those with likely disease because of a persistent cough, fever, or other signs of a contagious disease.

Summary

It is important to consider the special needs of women, children, the elderly, chronically ill, immune-compromised, and disabled when planning for mass gathering events or when anticipating the mass gatherings that occur after a disaster. Using the framework of CMIST (Communication, Maintaining Health, Independence, Support and Safety, and Transportation) to anticipate the various types of needs of these at-risk populations will help leaders and organizers to improve the design of plans for mass gatherings that better serve the needs of each individual involved.

References

1. US Census Bureau, 2020 Census data: www.census.gov/topics/health/disability.html. Accessed September 21, 2023.

2. Americans with Disabilities Act Regulations for Special Events: https://onsiteco.com/ada-regulations-for-special-events/. Accessed September 21, 2023.

3. www.ennonline.net/attachments/1321/module-17-infant-and-young-child-feeding-full.pdf. Accessed September 21, 2023.

4. www.phe.gov/Preparedness/planning/abc/Pages/at-risk.aspx. Accessed September 21, 2023.

5. www.ada.gov/effective-comm.htm. Accessed September 21, 2023.

6. Bureau of Transportation Statistics: www.bts.gov/travel-patterns-with-disabilities. Accessed September 21, 2023.

7. https://nasemso.org/wp-content/uploads/Safe-Transport-of-Children-by-EMS-InterimGuidance-08Mar2017-FINAL.pdf. Accessed September 21, 2023.

8. Americans with Disabilities Act Regulations for Service-Animals: www.ada.gov/regs2010/service_animal_qa.html. Accessed September 21, 2023.

9. Banford A., Froude C. K. Ecofeminism and Natural Disasters: Sri Lankan Women Post-Tsunami. *Journal of International* Women's Studies 2015;**16**:170–187. https://vc.bridgew.edu/jiws/vol16/iss2/11. Accessed September 21, 2023.

10. Eastman A. L., Rinnert K. J., Nemeth I. R., Fowler R. L., Minei J. P. Alternate Site Surge Capacity in Times of Public Health Disaster Maintains Trauma Center and Emergency Department Integrity. *Journal of Trauma.* 2007;**63**:253–257. doi: 10.1097/TA.0b013e3180d0a70e

11. Klein K. R., Pepe P. E., Burkle F. M., Nagle N. E., Swienton R. E. Evolving Need for Alternative Triage Management in Public Health Emergencies. *Disaster Medicine and Public Health Preparedness.* 2008;**2** (Suppl 1):S40–S44.

12. King R. V., North C. S., Larkin G. L., et al. Attributes of Effective Disaster Responders: Focus Group Discussions with Key Emergency Response Leaders. *Disaster Medicine and Public Health Preparedness.* 2010:**4**:332–338.

13. North C. S., King R. V., Fowler R. L., Kucmierz R., Wade J., Hogan D., Carlo J. Planning for Mental Health Care in Disaster Shelters. https://hazards.colorado.edu/news/research-counts/mental-health-needs-in-a-large-scale-shelters-lessons-from-dallas. Accessed September 21, 2023.

Chapter 19

Crowd-Related Considerations at Mass Gathering Events: Management, Safety, and Dynamics

Katie Klatt, Richard Serino, Edward Davis, and Jennifer O. Grimes

Crowd Management

Providing medical care during a mass event requires important situational awareness and preparation, in addition to standard medical training. Concerts, marathons, political events, and other large-scale celebrations can draw crowds of 100,000–500,000 people – roughly the equivalent of a city. Among a population of that size, medical issues would be expected in some individuals as a statistical probability: every area has daily medical requirements. However, distinctive demands imposed by properties of the event itself and crowd dynamics further complicate the demand profiles and requires special planning for such contingencies. The goal of this chapter is to provide a foundational understanding of these unique considerations from which any member of the medical team can make decisions in real-time. As crowd management layers on additional considerations in the planning, response, and after-action phases, relationship building and communications are vital.

Preparedness: The Planning Phase

Any event that draws a crowd will naturally consist of elements of predictable and unpredictable nature, to which the on-site medical team must have the ability to respond. To ensure that crowd safety remains prioritized, preparedness efforts must begin well in advance. Importantly, these preparation efforts include the establishment and maintenance of community relationships and dedicated advanced planning efforts.

Relationships: Forming Partnerships

Leveraging inter-agency partnerships is one of the most vital activities to ensure successful crowd management [1]. Working across jurisdictions, even within just the medical field, can be challenging – but a lack of familiarity with the functionality and personalities of other jurisdictions can hamper any response [1]. As seen time and time again, large events cannot be handled by a single agency – cooperation and communication among agencies is essential [2]. For example, in the fatal crowd catastrophe at the Astroworld Festival in Houston in 2021, improved communication between the emergency responders on the ground and the event producers could have facilitated a response that stopped the performance before the crowd surge occurred.

These partnerships might include public-private partnerships [1], especially if events are organized by private entities, or if crowds might gather on private property. It should also include local leaders, event and venue managers, public transportation, public utilities, public works, local hospitals, and EMS, police, and fire departments [2]. In particular, EMS and law enforcement partnerships are integral in responding to large-scale events. Even some of the less obvious partners should be considered in collaboration regarding event processes, as they likely have experience with similar events [2]. It is even suggested to attend similar events prior to the scheduled one, in conjunction with one of these organizations, to observe their operations in real time [2]. Bringing these groups together in advance of the event establishes these relationships to ensure the medical team's familiarity with procedures, and also to facilitate more inclusive logistics planning, with sharing of key insights into how the crowd will be moved, how an evacuation might be carried out, or where bottlenecks might occur. It can even open the door for partnering a medical responder with a law enforcement officer during an event, so medical services can be delivered quickly and safely [3]. The ability to do this requires preestablished relationships so everyone knows what to expect and agencies can work in tandem in a coordinated manner.

Preestablished relationships are also crucial in gaining an awareness of the political undercurrents that could play a role in an event. Often, political undertones can influence decision-making, and may happen behind closed doors, outside of the medical team's influence. Historical rivalries, for example, can counteract good intentions or operations [1]. Even a particular desire for publicity can counteract operations. Understanding these political currents allows for the avoidance of ego or competitiveness among agencies [1].

Learnings from the Boston Marathon Bombings: In the event of a disaster at a mass gathering, preestablished partnerships can be vital in ensuring the least harmful outcome. In the Boston Marathon bombing response, local leaders had been building and maintaining cross-sector relationships for over a decade before the bombings occurred [1]. The identification of key stakeholders in the planning stage meant, as one example, involving emergency room personnel in training exercises with police and EMS. In addition, having these separate entities together at the table prior to the event allowed for a discussion (and negotiation) about goals and resources. After these discussions and training exercises, it opened the door for police to respond to emergency rooms to secure victims and identify potential terrorists.

While not every crowd scenario will see a medical crisis such as this, it demonstrates the importance of developing relationships before events. Understanding the roles and resources of stakeholders and cultivating cooperative inter-agency interactivity before the event fosters flexibility. In this example, the response was able to shift swiftly from operations expected of a marathon to meet the unexpected demands of a bombing mass casualty incident. A history of productive relationships helps an event run smoothly and establishes expectations beforehand of how crowd management will be approached by each organization, and it also makes the system more adaptable.

Planning

The planning phase should begin in the months leading up to a planned event, and is the most important part of the run up to the event. Experienced personnel, including high-level decision-makers [4] from among the various stakeholders, should gather to work out the details. Research on past incidents is vital, and it is beneficial to plan for more standby than expected even based on previous events [3]. Scenarios can be proposed and problem-solving should be employed to identify and preemptively eliminate issues. Tabletop exercises are extremely valuable for a planned event. Identifying issues in communication, training, and command and working those issues out can make the difference between success and failure. Command is often prescribed by local and state laws as well as the National Incident Management System (NIMS), and often requires notifying local response offices (consider any agency that may be involved in crowd management) for approval and filing permits. Many large events may require logistics around staffing, deployment, supplies, housing, fuel, provisions, and downtime, and contractors are vital at this stage. The list of contingencies is extensive and changes with the assignment.

The planning stage is meant to establish a common vision, or unity of mission [1], to ensure all stakeholders are on the same page serving the same overarching goal. Without unity of mission, management plans are often hindered [1]. Previously established relationships come in handy at this stage, when the creation of formal coordination protocols within and among agencies becomes necessary [5]. This formal planning takes time; account for the amount of time it may take to develop plans and carry out training exercises [3]. Planning can be folded into other typical activities [4], like training or supply management, as a way to time-manage.

Components of emergency management to include during the planning phase are risk assessment, surveillance, and response [6]. Consider the existing health risks, plus possible scenarios of what could happen and their likelihood, in order to create an initial planning framework [6]. Then reflect on how the team will become aware that any of these scenarios has occurred, and what to do in response [6]. Not every occurrence can be accounted for, as there will likely be spontaneous aspects to the planned event. It is important to include worst-case scenario planning, as well as mid-course corrections [2], recognizing that there will always be unpredictable pieces to any event that gathers a crowd. Having a baseline allows responders to resort to an appropriate level of training when the unexpected occurs, requiring adaptability [3]. While maintaining flexibility, it is also important to remember that life goes on outside of the crowd; plan for continuity, and ensure there are medical responders available for incidents outside of the event [2].

Do not accept all assumptions that subsist on the status quo [2]. Remember that whatever plans are established, or have previously been established, should be updated on a regular basis [3]. For example, medical crowd management plans required extensive updates for the COVID-19 pandemic. When crowds gathered for racial justice demonstrations during the pandemic, medical professionals needed to be prepared to add the layer of COVID-19 precautions into their crowd management and patient care. Local health providers also had to consider adequate laboratory and testing capacity in the aftermath [6].

Training

Training becomes an inherent part of the planning process. Researching past incidents at the specific location, as well as other locations, will dictate what type of training is necessary. Team members will respond to a crisis in the way they are trained; there is no such thing as too much training. It is absolutely necessary for successful outcomes in the stressful and high-intensity situations that often exist within crowd management. This can help team members to understand and manage nuances of how responder actions impact crowd dynamics, such as appropriate deployment of equipment: Premature use of crowd control equipment such as helmets or shields, for example, may incite the crowd, while holding off on their use until they are truly necessary is more likely to reduce stress within the crowd. Joint exercises should be conducted [2] to bring awareness to what other agencies will be doing in tandem [7]. These can take the format of lectures, simulations, or field exercises, and should occur with the specific event team when possible [2]. Training can also be used as an opportunity to practice under Incident Command System (ICS) structures [7], as other agencies will likely also be operating under these protocols.

Communications

The planning phase should include the establishment of ways to communicate within the team, as well as with the public. Ensure that any form of communications infrastructure and technology will function properly in a crowd, where bandwidth might be impacted by the density of the crowd [5]. Dedicated radio channels are vital [7]: channels that exist solely for medical communications, as well as established channels for inter-agency communication between production staff, performers, and responders. Radio channels contribute one aspect of the more fundamental task of planning how to strategically disperse information from leaders to team members in the field, and how they can communicate back [3], as well as how leadership plans to communicate with each other. Mechanisms to filter the unnecessary "noise" must be established so the right people get the important information, and superfluous details do not impede [5]. Additionally, backup methods of communication should be established in case radio communication fails. Ensure emergency communication is clearly outlined, with separate protocols from standard operations.

Plans to communicate with the public encompass several aspects. Social media, which is addressed later in this chapter, is just one of them. Mechanisms need to be established to communicate with family/group members of injured crowd members (perhaps a call center or responsive social media account), as well as ways for crowd members to find locations to be treated [5]. Clear role indicators like vests serve as physical communication that identify medical team members in a crowd.

Event Type

It is vital to take the type of event into consideration in the planning stage. The demographics of attendees as well as their emotional and behavioral states will vary by event; consider a typical participant and adjust medical expectations accordingly. For example, sporting events tend to provoke certain hazards that are more probable to occur. "Regardless of whether their team wins or loses, historically there is something that has attracted fans to get rowdy and light stuff on fire after championship games" [8]. Anticipate the emotions that come with certain events, and prepare to be adequately staffed and supplied. Anticipate whether medical translators might be needed.

Size of Event

Using ticket sales and social media surveillance, rough estimates can be made of expected crowd size. Generally, 1–2 percent of any crowd will require some sort of medical treatment [6]. Of those that require treatment, about 10 percent will need ongoing care and about 1 percent will need to be transported to the hospital [6]. These estimates increase with a more high-risk crowd [6]; see the "Injuries and Illnesses to Expect in a Crowd" section for more information of the types of injuries that are associated with certain crowd demographics. In raw numbers, research has shown 0.5 to 2.6 patient presentations per 1,000 crowd members [9].

To address this need, medical staff should be appropriately deployed on-site. Research suggests that two medical response teams (consisting of two paramedics/nurses or a paramedic paired with an EMT) per 10,000 people should be adequate, if spaced appropriately around the site [10] (and accounting for the possible necessity of additional teams for rowdier crowds). It is recommended to have physicians present, approximately two per 50,000 people [10]. Having physician care at events reduces the number of patient transports to hospitals, which eases the burden on local EMS and the community health systems [11]. While these measures are likely to minimize the impact of the event on local health services, it is still important to ensure that the community is prepared for increased demand at medical centers, including having transfer arrangements with local hospitals and communication pathways sharing bed availability [12].

Location

Staging of the venue or site ahead of time allows for the creation of hard and soft staging zones and the inclusion of other relevant ancillary locations. The identification of treatment stations, secure facilities where team members can meet in an emergency [5], locations to prestage supplies [3], and paths to direct crowd members are all necessary components of location scouting. Planning for each main venue and even those that are ancillary could become important [4]. Medical treatment areas will require tents or other forms of shelter, electricity, potable water, and waste disposal [6], and they may need to be differentiated and specialized by first aid stations and field hospitals [12]. When planning treatment areas, consider access and clear indication to the public [6]. Also consider who will be treated; the type of event may necessitate separate facilities for performers, officials, and audience, for example [6].

A vital component of location planning is determination of transportation logistics. It is necessary to have a system for how to access anyone within the crowd, as well as egress routes out to the medical stations and from the medical stations to the receiving hospitals. These ingress and egress routes need to be established for emergency vehicles, participants, medical aid stations, staff rest and rehabilitation stations, and out-of-sight spare and emergency equipment. Ensure emergency vehicles will be parked in ways that prevent obstruction [5] and allow for the most expeditious route to get to hospitals. Establishment of at least one alternative route of access and egress is always advised. In the event of an emergency, personnel must be prepared to evaluate whether evacuation or sheltering in place is a more appropriate option for injured individuals. Under some circumstances, moving patients may be more dangerous. Similarly, such decisions become important in active shooter situations. Robust planning should underpin these decisions should they present at the event.

Managing crowd distribution can improve access, as well. Depending on the venue setup and the local terrain, it may be helpful to build lanes in the crowds. Inclusion of various types of vehicles improves the ability to maneuver in a crowd [7] for security access, patient transportation, and medical access. These include bicycles, golf carts, foot teams, boats, and other modes of transportation. Utilizing these alternative methods also requires proper training on use, docking/parking when caring for a patient, and possible requirements for personal protective equipment (PPE) such as helmets, protective gear, turnout gear, and bullet proof vests.

One of the most challenging aspects of medical care in mass gatherings is finding patients within a crowd. There are generally two types of patients in crowded settings; those who can seek care themselves, and those who require assistance or outreach [13]. Those who can seek out care stations or medical professionals often have minor injuries or illnesses [13]. However, those who cannot need to be spotted in a crowd and identified as needing assistance [13]. In some instances, medical professionals who patrol for patients [13], "roving medical spotters," can radio and flag to signal their location while in the meantime providing immediate care [14]. If there are not enough medical personnel to assist with finding patients or patient transport out of the crowd, established relationships with ushers, police, security, or other event personnel could contribute to this team effort [14]. Also, the use of drones, portable cameras, and other such devices, usually by law enforcement but also with medical staff located at the command post, will help in locating patients in a crowd.

Team and Team Dynamics

Once the event dynamics have been established, a medical response team can be assembled that best fits the anticipated needs. Within the larger medical team, assigned roles and defined authority need to be established [1]. Those assigned to leadership positions must remain focused on the broader picture without succumbing to a natural tendency to focus more operationally on their accustomed role in clinical care; leaders must maintain perspective and avoid distractions [1, 15]. Within the medical team, clear structure and command includes establishment of who is in charge, and what the chain of command is [2]. Once these leadership and response roles have been established, their associated expectations and goals must be communicated ahead of time [7]. Ensure that everyone involved knows who is in charge of what (within the medical team and among agencies), and who reports to whom (to whom within the medical team to report, and to whom the medical leader should report out) [3].

In a dynamic crowd situation, the medical team itself will likely need to split for greater crowd coverage; consider specialized units, or area coverage [2]. If splitting the team, always work in a minimum of pairs or larger groups; team members should never operate alone. Having a response hierarchy will help control "self-deployment" [5], allowing for an organized response to any incident that does not incapacitate the ability to respond to other incidents. Consider the use of technology like GPS to increase awareness [6] of team position in relation to the crowd [16].

When creating the medical team, ensure depth to allow for rest, rotations, meals, breaks [5], and shift overlap [10]. If the personnel is available, it is advisable to plan for higher numbers than expected. As an example, compare the responses to the riots that broke out after the Stanley Cup final in 2011. While the Chief of Police in Vancouver deployed 600 officers and lost the city to riots, the Boston Chief deployed 2,000 officers, teamed up with Boston EMS personnel, and stopped the rioting [17]. While this is specifically a police force example, it still gets to the heart of how

adequate preparation and response with sufficient personnel can prevent overwhelming events. If riots were to occur in any crowd, medical needs would be tremendous, and worsening of injuries would be preventable by having adequate staff.

If the upcoming event is unusual and outside of the comfort zone for many team members, traditional structures can be adapted to meet these unique needs. Consider the following strategy from the Boston Marathon bombing response. The director of a trauma center created "micro-sites," or areas within the emergency room where the treatment teams could focus on just their patient, rather than be overwhelmed by the many patients inundating their unit [5]. This director helped create a more routine environment, fashioned to be as close to their typical working conditions as possible, distracting from the fact that they were working in the middle of a mass casualty event [5]. Designing settings within an unexpected event in which responders could function under routine conditions allowed for successful hospital management. This can be an effective strategy in medicine, in which the focal point is treating patients, by applying appropriate environmental design elements to influence the management of a chaotic and stressful crowd environment.

Special Considerations

While much focus has centered on gatherings and crowd movements within a specific venue, many of these principles can be extended to moving crowds, as occur during parades, rolling rallies, and marches. Thus, such events also require working with other public safety partners to maintain order, and an emergency operations center (EOC) or unified command provides a vital common point for convergence of public safety and event organizers. Some management aspects require adaptation to cover the mobility and projected course of the crowd. Medical access and treatment areas can be set up at a central location, endpoints, and/or at strategic locations along the route of the event. Predetermined access routes running parallel to the crowd can be maneuvered by medical personnel using bicycles and other small vehicles. Resources can be leapfrogged along the course to keep up with greatest need. While television station and other camera feeds using public and private sources are helpful to track crowd occurrences including medical emergencies and asset movement, social media is a critically important tool and should be closely monitored.

Spontaneous events also capitalize on the teachings of planned events, as they benefit from advanced planning and training. Key training elements to address this include: situation evaluation, in-the-moment decisions, documentation, communications, and supply utilization [2], along with accounting for unexpected twists, fluctuating crowd sizes, and weather changes.

The occurrence of spontaneous events is often predictable by monitoring sociopolitical developments that are conducive to the formation of a gathering in reaction. Marches are a unique entity that are moving and may be spontaneous, without formally established advance notice of crowd magnitude or projected course, but many marches and rallies require similar management tools as large parades. Social media can yield information about projected crowd size, how quickly the gathering will form, and what resources should be allocated to meet its needs. Plans should allow flexibility to react to evolving circumstances and for rapid movement of resources as demands change. Plans should cover how to expand if event requirements overwhelm capabilities on scene and should yield the ability to institute mass casualty protocols. Arrange for backups and agreements with partners that can help scale up as needed. Ensure that the correct personal protective equipment is available, including helmets and ballistic vests. Be aware of counter-protests, volatility, and counter-demonstrations. A unified command or EOC promotes good communication among entities to respond to such emergent threats within a crowd. US Department of Homeland Security resources are also available to support local efforts for special security events (for more information, please consult www.dni.gov/index.php/nctc-how-we-work/joint-ct-assessment-team/first-responder-toolbox and www.dhs.gov/major-event-security-cases).

Components of an Operations Plan

Utilizing all of the aspects detailed above, an internal operations plan should be published with enough time leading up to the event for all involved to become familiar with the operations, at least a week before the event. The details of the plan itself can be customized to the particular event and organization but listed below are crucial sections and components to include in each. This section can be utilized as a template [18], in which

Checklist: Operational Plan Components
- ☐ General operations
  - ☐ Event specifics, including size, location, weather, and demographics
- ☐ Goal of operations
  - ☐ Unity of mission[1]
- ☐ Medical operations
- ☐ Continuity of medical operations
- ☐ Medical direction and leadership
- ☐ Incident management
- ☐ Security and safety plan
- ☐ Crisis management
  - ☐ Emergency plans
- ☐ Tables, infographics, and maps

Figure 19.1 Overview of necessary components of an event operational plan

to fill in components relevant to any event or operation. See Figure 19.1.

General Operations

Any plan needs to offer event specifics, such as location, weather forecast, uniform, and timing and nature of event [19]. It is important to include estimated participant numbers [19], as well as the preevent briefing time and location [19]. This sets the stage for all other plans put forth in the document.

Goal of Operations

The objective of medical operations should be clearly stated. They should include the assurance that an event does not compromise the ability to provide standard medical and emergency care to the community, and that plans include measures that can mitigate any consequences to the community's health care facilities [20]. Examples from the Boston Emergency Medical Services 2019 Operations Plan for the 4 July Esplanade Event include:

(1) "Boston EMS' primary objective is to ensure this event does not compromise the provision of emergency medical care to Boston's residents and neighborhoods. Moreover, Boston EMS will

institute an operational plan that is designed to mitigate the medical consequences and potential surge impact to Boston's healthcare facilities" [20].

(2) "Our presence on the esplanade is to serve as the medical consequence lead, which includes providing on scene medical care, rapid transport resources, and a forward leaning posture should a larger emergency arise" [21].

Medical Operations

This section should contain the bulk of the medical direction in relation to the event and crowd dynamics. Often, the provision of first-aid care will cover the majority of injuries, and can reduce the necessity of transporting patients to hospital. On-site medical coverage should include the establishment of field stations to provide such care [20]. Prehospital treatment for likely illnesses and injuries needs to be spelled out; any additional care that can be made accessible is also worth considering, such as bicycle units [21], intravenous (IV) hydration stations, or blood testing stations. Include in any medical outlines the necessary documentation that should be completed for each patient encounter [20], as well as a list of medical assets such as supplies and staff [19]. Specifically spell out basic life support (BLS) and advanced life support (ALS) requirements [19], and establish a triage strategy [12] and a strategy for patient stabilization [13].

This section should also include patient access and transportation requirements. Locating and accessing patients will hinge on the availability of different mobile units and the modes of transportation available, all of which should be discussed here. Including a decision tree could be helpful for guiding decisions around whether to transport patients from field sites to hospitals.

Medical Direction

Leadership structure should be established by directly stating the medical lead and hierarchy, along with contact details of all in charge [19]. If zones will be utilized during the event, supervisors per zone are necessary. Having a clearly defined order of reports and decision-making ensures continuity of operations during the event.

Communications

The communications section will cover a broad range of topics. The infrastructure for communications and specifics such as radio channels should be discussed here. Additionally, this should include a discussion of media request protocols, such as to whom requests should be directed and what media contact is allowed [21].

Incident Management

ICS is often the functioning structure of municipal operations (refer to Chapter 7 on this topic). Any ICS structure that will exist during the event should be spelled out in this plan section. Medical responders participating in an event will likely be pulled into this command structure, so it is essential to have a basic grasp and a willingness to collaborate and work dynamically within the structure [1]. ICS and NIMS provide a consistent framework, so even teams with different expertise will understand how others are operating [5]. Many EMS services operate under ICS structure [22], and medical command can often tailor these structures to fit operations. It can be expected that the medical team leader will report to the Unified Command Center [7], so find out and communicate in the plan where this will be and who should report there.

Security and Safety Plan

Contingencies for the safety and security of both the crowd members and public safety officers should be addressed in this section; consider all possibilities of crowd density in doing so [20]. It can be helpful to staff a medical liaison in different operational areas, such as with law enforcement or at EOCs [20] to establish direct lines of communication among event partners. Public safety officers should be prioritized for treatment [20] to allow them to enter back into the team if possible.

Crisis Management

In case of disruption within the crowd, flexibility and autonomous decision-making within defined boundaries are important to establish here [23]. Identifying casualty collection points, on-call staff in case the crowd grows or gets out of hand, and plans for what to do if a unit becomes compromised are all valid contingencies that should be included in this section's plans [20].

Tables/Infographics

Providing visuals or easy-to-read tables communicates important information clearly. Include a map of treatment zones and unit locations, unit assignments, an event timeline, moving crowd locations [20], fluctuating transport routes, and road closure information. Some providers, including emergency medical services (EMS), physicians, nurses, law enforcement officers, and others, may be from out of the area and thus unfamiliar with the local geography, both of the venue and the host city. Therefore, it may prove helpful to provide printed maps (e.g., on Tyvek material) of the area presented in a grid format marked with specific locations. These maps should also be made available electronically for easy access via phones or tablets.

Allowing for Flexibility

Changing community or even global situations may indicate the need to redesign any previously created templates or plans, even last minute. For example, in 2020, Boston EMS plans were rewritten to include considerations for COVID-19 and racial justice marches [24]. The plans were reworked to include language on standard PPE and PPE needed for suspected COVID-19 cases [24]. They also included encouragement of physical distancing, recommending crowd engagement only when treating patients, and extracting personnel from congregation areas when not providing care [24]. The Medical Operations section additionally provides clinical care instructions and personal protection strategies specific to the use of riot control agents [24].

Following a process of discussion, creation, revision, and finalization, the plan should be ready to be distributed to the response team with adequate time to prepare for the mass gathering.

Response: The Event Itself

When the day of the event arrives, the plan should have already been distributed and understood by each team member. Preparation for the event starts early. Medical responders and all other event management agencies will arrive well ahead of time. There should be a preevent briefing [2] on the plan, including anticipated problems that may emerge. Also important to include in the briefing are [6]:

(1) Command structure

(2) Location of medical treatment stations, and expertise and supplies at each
(3) Communications plan
(4) Updated event details
(5) What to do in an emergency

In some cases, with very specific medical engagement plans, cards can be distributed to each team member to remind them of exact rules and guidelines. Teams are deployed to zones or sites and are ready to respond as the crowd slowly trickles in.

Swarm Intelligence

In an ideal event, once relationships have been established and the preplanning has been completed, the foundation has been laid for a successful event. Elements of swarm intelligence that manifest in leadership patterns throughout the response structure [1, 23] should emerge during any incident in the crowd, whether disaster or a minor medical issue. This concept of "swarm leadership" was developed by the National Preparedness Leadership Initiative (NPLI) at Harvard University and encompasses several key elements of effective teamwork and leadership. The following principles of swarm leadership are meant to be embraced and acted upon at all levels of medical management [1, 23]:

(1) Unity of mission
(2) Generosity
(3) Respect for the roles and authority of others
(4) "No ego, no blame"
(5) Trust

Medical responders who utilize these principles to develop situational awareness and accept flexible task allocation will contribute to a more successful response to any medical emergency that occurs, big or small.

Communications

As discussed in the previous section, adequate communications planning can make or break an event response. When a crowd gets rowdy, or the unexpected starts to happen, communications are generally the first thing to suffer [7]. Therefore, it is important to not only have a robust communications plan in place beforehand, but to commit to maintaining those guidelines during any scenario that may play out. Ensure there is awareness of where team members may have deployed in the crowd [2], and track the use and whereabouts of resources [7].

Communications encompass those within the team, as well as with other event managers. It should also encompass avenues of communication with area hospitals (for variables like awareness of surge capacity, decontamination at the hospital, and reciprocal awareness for the hospitals of what is going on at the event), public health authorities, and other stakeholders perhaps not directly involved in the event but of relevance. Be proactive in seeking these channels out [3]. Communication must be influenced by current intelligence and adapted to the situation at hand, while remaining context-appropriate [6].

The Media and Social Media

In the modern crowd, the media (here meant to encompass both news sources and social media unless otherwise specified) has evolved to be everywhere, all the time. The ubiquity of the media and the impressive extent and immediacy of its influence, coupled with its potential to spread both helpful information and dangerous misinformation, render it an important tool that must be actively monitored with prompt response. While a designated public relations expert should be consulted to fulfill this role, media interactions may spontaneously arise and be addressed to other parties. As such, any medical responder should be prepared for how to handle media requests, involuntary media involvement, and any other media scenarios.

Transparency is key and can lead to credibility and trust [1]. However, confidentiality of attendees who require medical care must be protected. Therefore, both the content and presentation of the information should be carefully considered. Having a planned message that can be adapted to the crowd and situation at hand prepared by a predetermined spokesperson makes it easy to direct media attention to certain focal points. One medical point of contact, determined ahead of time and shared with the media outlets, helps them know who to contact rather than distract other medical responders.

An event can be used to the advantage of the medical team to spread relevant health information and encourage community resilience, arming the crowd with knowledge. If event officials say nothing, social media will try to fill the silence with something, which could be speculative, untrue, or misleading [5]. Early, open, and simple communications with the media is a way to thwart misinformation.

A public relations and media plan is a vital part of the overall plan and should involve professional expertise. Public relations experts should be consulted to develop a specific plan for media engagement and a specific social media plan to push information out to the public. This plan allows for medical responders to educate and reassure the crowd about various contingencies, should they arise [2]. If something goes wrong, key elements of any communication are reassurance, simplicity, brevity, how to find help, and how to contact someone for details on an ill or injured loved one [2]. Engaging the community [7] through direct communication of plans of action increases the likelihood of improved crowd compliance. Additionally, active medical team monitoring of social media coming from fans at the event can produce a more proactive response to any unfolding circumstances.

Injuries and Illnesses to Expect in a Crowd

Events that draw a crowd can raise issues particular to congested scenarios. Surveillance of the crowd needs to be sensitive to quickly catch warning signs indicating individual or larger issues [6]. When patterns are noticed, established reporting protocols for certain symptoms should be followed [6]. Medical professionals can gather real-time data through triage, improving the ability to find vulnerabilities and hazards [12]. This can expand the ability to risk-assess for individual patients and the crowd as a whole, identify those at highest risk for any health hazard, and be prepared to intervene early [13]. Risk mitigation allows preventative care in crowds.

The most common care requirement is basic level care [25]. Treatment of minor injuries and illnesses in the field prevent burdening local hospitals and ensure adequate resources for more urgent patients, with the ability to scale as needed [6]. In the most urgent cases, field care should focus on maintaining the "chain of survival," or actions that reduce mortality from cardiac arrest [6].

Medical care, rather than bodily injury, tends to be the most common need, although events with precipitation and rock concerts are the most likely to see bodily injuries [25]. Event type and event temperature are the best predictors of medical usage rates [25]; research has found a higher frequency of patient visits at papal masses, rock concerts, and in hot weather

[26]. Papal masses and sporting events tend to see the most cardiac arrests [26].

While this list is nowhere near exhaustive, it is a good idea for all medical responders to have a familiarity with caring for the following [6, 12, 13]:

(1) Respiratory illnesses
(2) Minor injuries, falls
(3) Headaches
(4) Hypoglycemia
(5) Abrasions, blisters, sunburn
(6) Altered mental status
(7) Chest pain
(8) Airway obstruction
(9) Allergic reaction
(10) Cardiac arrest
(11) Panic attacks, claustrophobia
(12) Drug overdoses, including with underage users
(13) Alcohol intoxication, including with underage users
(14) Heat exhaustion, heat stroke
(15) Dehydration
(16) Freezing injuries, frostbite
(17) Transmissible diseases
(18) Active shooter situations
(19) Active terrorist activities
(20) Mass casualty situations, accidents
(21) Trampling, crush injuries
(22) Medical screening or treatment of prisoners
(23) Public health surveillance
(23) Chemical, biological, or radiological monitoring at a high-profile event

Consider the nature and timing of the event in assessment and treatment. As previously noted, it is wise to analyze collected health data on an ongoing basis for trends in injuries and illnesses; the initial patients could indicate worrisome patterns [4].

Environmental health measures that exist outside of typical controlled medical settings could include anything from the availability of potable drinking water to sanitation stations and shade [6]. Necessary infrastructural and access needs could vary wildly among crowd members over the course of a single event [27]. These demands include wheelchair access or other accommodations, but needs may change over time, as occurs during multiday events. For example, attendees of events such as Burning Man, Coachella, and the Democratic National Convention may stay overnight at the venue, requiring safe accommodations.

It is also important to monitor the health and safety of medical responders on duty. Fatigue from a long event or handling a large crowd has been shown to impact decision-making [7]. Watch for signs of fatigue, hunger, thirst, and impaired decision-making in all members of the medical team, and allow breaks and care for team members. These considerations are especially important as staff work in extreme weather, including heat and cold, but also with rain and other complicating meteorological conditions.

Psychosocial Considerations

Psychosocial factors are often neglected in crowd dynamics, but can contribute to crowd behavior [6]. The audience may respond in certain ways depending on the mood or "emotional excitement" [16] of the crowd, the political and cultural climate, and the environment [6]. Harm minimization and situational awareness are key, and surveillance activities should include noting the nature of the event, the demographics of the crowd, and crowd behavior [6]. Encouraged audience participation activities, such as mosh pits, also contribute to the psychosocial factors at play [12].

Crowd Management

As opposed to typical individual treatment of patients, a crowd adds dynamic complexity to all medical decision-making where the downstream effects of a decision for one individual could have impacts on the larger group. It involves situational awareness of the crowd, other event managers, and the medical team as a whole. Be aware of the onlookers; if they become immersed in the crowd, they may come under the medical jurisdiction as well [7]. A crowd could even be the result of a small event that takes place during a commute, where the event and rush hour human traffic combine to become a larger crowd [28].

Medical teams should follow formations that law enforcement enact to manage the crowd – do not impede the flow of the crowd while providing care unless absolutely necessary. Officers may try to split crowds into smaller, more manageable segments [2]. If this occurs, be aware of team members' locations in various segments of the crowd. If law enforcement are encircling the crowd, make sure to take a moment to become aware of escape routes, both for the medical team and for the safe removal of injured crowd members [7]. Crowds may move in relation to event programming (such as during a break, changing sets, or at the end) and alter patterns [12]. If the crowd is trying to disperse and can't figure out where to go, there may be trampling; medical providers need to ensure they are not attending a patient on the ground if this were to occur. If a crowd becomes unruly, be prepared for use-of-force or riot control agents to come into play. Medical providers should remove themselves and the patient to the most private location to be found, ensuring the surrounding safety first before focusing on patient care. Additionally, plan to have medical personnel at the holding center site for mass arrests, as there will likely be injuries in those arrested needing treatment. In all instances described, direct consultation with the police on crowd management strategy is recommended [12]. Generally, the overall crowd management goal is to maintain order, control admissions, manage expectations, minimize overcrowding, and promote smooth people flow [12]. As the Australian Institute for Disaster Resilience puts it; "crowd control is a constant reestablishing of public order" [12].

Human Stampede and Crowd Crush

As the population increases and extensive international travel facilitates movement to venues for gatherings, mass gatherings attract increasing numbers of attendees [29]. However, crowd crush injuries are increasing in frequency, as well [29, 30]. While significant media attention to crowd-related injuries has focused on Hajj [31], such incidents occur at music concerts or festivals, sporting events, political events, and other religious gatherings as well as "door-buster" sales events [31, 32].

In spite of the long history of crowd crush disasters [33] and assertions that such casualties are "almost entirely preventable with even minimal preparation" [32], the occurrence of these events is not completely understood. A lack of epidemiological data [31], the complexity of contributing factors [34], and an imbalance of data that under-examines the phenomena in low-income countries where more

fatalities occur, yield an incomplete evidence base from which to develop preventative and mitigative strategies [29]. Older research examining a number of events during the 1970s and 1980s attributed crowd accidents to poor communication, delays in getting people to exits in cases of fire, lack of information-sharing about crowd density, and infrastructural challenges [35]. A delayed warning system can increase the urgency of egress, but addressing communication delays is necessary but insufficient. Creating choke points and bottlenecks, blocking exits, merging flows, flow intersections, and narrow lanes are also contributory [29].

While reports have often shifted the blame for crowd crush disasters onto psychosocial aspects of the crowd by attribution of unruly behavior [32] or panic [34], these explanations do not capture the mechanism of the phenomena and are not applicable to many crowd disasters. Large crowds may have pockets of high density. In these local high-density areas, movements among the people exert forces on adjacent bodies, and the collection of these forces creates a summation of energy that propels people in movements that individuals cannot stop [34]. When crowds of people move with laminar or smooth flow, risk of crowd disasters is low, but these turbulent patterns of crowd movement create favorable conditions for crowd disasters [30]. Thus, the number of attendees less directly predicts risk than the density of groups of attendees and their movement [29]. With sufficient density to change crowd movement dynamics, triggers for stampedes can include rumors of threats, unexpected loud noises, or sudden notice of something important [29].

Crowd crush is often fatal, but medical teams should look for symptoms in survivors with this mechanism of injury. Due to high external pressure, victims suffer acute venous hypertension with impeded venous return, traumatic asphyxia from prevention of respiratory expansion, and crush injuries to the torso [31, 33]. Typical findings include purplish coloration from venous congestion of the head and neck, petechial hemorrhages in the face, conjunctivae, neck, and upper chest, and possible neurological abnormalities ranging from visual deficits to loss of consciousness [33].

Plans to prevent crowd crush should include both infrastructural accommodations and careful management of crowd flow. Limiting crowd densities and preventing congestion is key. At Mecca, changes

BEFORE THE EVENT

Establish Relationships

Public/Private/Non-profit

Local leaders, EMS, Police, Fire, Hospitals, Event and venue managers, Public transit, Public utilities, Red Cross, Other stakeholders

Planning

With decision-makers representing the stakeholders

Establish unity of mission, Risk assessment, Surveillance, Event requirements, Obtain ordinances/permits, Amount of tickets sold *and* requested

Training

Research, Drills/exercises

Communications

Reliability, Radio and channel use, Inter-agency fluency (plain language) including event organizers/producers, Backup methods (e.g., WhatsApp), Public communications, Infographics, Media request protocols

Predictions and Event-Specific Provisions

Event type, Crowd size, Location, Transportation logistics, Medical staffing, Crowd flow dynamics, Safety & security, History of similar type of events

Establish Roles in Teams

ICS use, Hierarchy and contact info within team, Supervisors/zone, Team allocation for optimal coverage, Team assignment, Shifts

Set Operations Objective and Goals

Determine necessary equipment and staffing, Patient access/egress and transportation plans

DURING THE EVENT

Preparation

Before event start time

Briefing with special considerations, command structure, location of medical stations and supplies, communications plans, updates, emergency plans. Test comms with *all* Deployment

Ongoing communication

Within team, to other teams, to attendees

Social media outreach and monitoring

Surveillance

Injuries and illnesses and their patterns, Situational awareness, Psychosocial climate, Crowd movements, Important changes during event

Maintain order

Control admissions and crowd flows to prevent overcrowding

Ongoing pattern-recognition and problem-solving

END OF EVENT

Continue until end of duty

After crowd has departed

Fulfill set roles and responsibilities for concluding event

Leadership assesses and announces end of event

Direct egress

Clear direction of crowd to exits, Fully functional transit leaving venue

Communications

Monitor crowd dispersal and continuing activities in the field

AFTER THE EVENT

After action reports

Lessons learned

Recognition of successes

Public and staff outreach

As appropriate

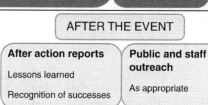

Figure 19.2 Wise counsel for event staff, medical and otherwise

include redesign of the Jamarat Bridge; rerouting of traffic and predicting and monitoring traffic flow were undertaken to assure pilgrim safety. One-way routes are marked, and groups are scheduled to pass through certain areas at certain times to control flow. Interagency communication, public announcements, and continuous supervision are also important [31]. Limiting the absolute number of attendees can also stem the threat of crowd disasters, as can elimination of festival seating [29]. Some researchers assert that congestion is more likely with more than four to five people per square meter [34] and that greater than five people per square meter is high risk for crowd disasters [29, 32], but variance in recommended densities indicates that crowd pressure, which relates to both density and variance of density, is more predictive [29, 36]. Ultimately, careful planning, regulation, and monitoring of crowd movements within the event to ensure smooth flow of traffic, decongestion, and provision of sufficient ingress and egress routes can help mitigate risk.

Crowd Characteristics

The general attributes of a crowd of which one must always be aware are size, composition, intention, and behavior [2]. The crowd could consist of a unified group, or it could be a combined group of different interests that spontaneously came together – there are endless possibilities. The likelihood of violence and injuries may vary depending upon the anticipated proclivities of the population that constitutes the crowd (to determine the possibility that such factors may contribute, it would be wise to utilize intelligence reports from law enforcement prior to the event). On certain occasions, there may be many locations with crowds gathering, of differing sizes, or spontaneous in nature. Situational awareness of crowd characteristics and their possible fluctuating nature is key.

Certain crowd characteristics similarly change the likelihood of necessity of medical care; this can include duration of the gathering, if it is seated or mobile, if the event is contained by a fence and how densely participants are compacted, the geography of the event and environment of the crowd, the mood and average age of attendees, and availability of alcohol or drugs [6]. For example, religious or spiritual events may attract ill or infirm people searching for healing; these types of crowds may need special accommodations or have different health needs [12].

Problem-Solving

In the midst of a chaotic crowded environment, searching for and identifying patterns is a useful skill that can turn chaos into coordination [1, 37]. The thought process of "where am I now, where do I need to be" and "where are they now, where do they need to be" can be a helpful progression to consider [1]. The patterns identified can be used to predict where a medical team member and where a group of the crowd should be directed [1]. Recognize that a nondecision is, by default, a decision to do nothing [1]. As such, avoiding "analysis paralysis" may mean having to make a decision even before being one hundred percent confident [1]. Studying video as well as reports of incidents that have occurred in prior events discloses important information that can aid the problem-solving process. This foundation helps guide intuition, and utilizing real-time intelligence gathered through those previously established relationships will support a robust problem-solving effort.

Using an organized stepwise approach to encourage progression from acquisition of situational awareness through decision-making and action can be helpful to prompt continuous activity and continuous evolution of situational awareness. One such approach, the POP-DOC loop [37], organizes thinking and action into six sequential steps for which the model is named: (1) Perceive, which refers to intentionally acquiring information with a broad perspective; (2) Orient is the discovery of patterns that emerge within the data; (3) Predict refers to anticipation of how these patterns will extend into the future with consideration of options for addressing these projected contingencies; (4) Decide is commitment to a course of action; (5) Operationalize is moving the decision into implementation; (6) Communicate is multidirectional, requiring input from sources to begin to Perceive again for iterative response, and also requiring outgoing information to stakeholders to keep them apprised. Importantly, leaders must progress through these decision-making steps with the understanding that the evolution of an event will require evolution of response, and situational awareness will continue to progress.

Problem-Solving in Action Boston Baseball Championships

Planning for a medical response to unexpected crowd events can utilize the learnings from other expert responders. In Boston, law enforcement observed a number of fights, resulting in arrests, that broke out immediately outside of liquor establishments in the final innings of championship baseball games. Police officers were able to determine that the individuals who flocked to Fenway or to the Kenmore Square area were monitoring the game by looking in the windows of these liquor establishments, watching the game on the easily seen televisions. They could be on site of the celebrations, while simultaneously watching the last minutes of the final. Upon connecting this observation to the outcomes of fights and arrests, in an effort to curb the violence, the police department worked with business owners in the area and managed to cover windows so the game could not be seen from the outside. No crowds gathered and no violence occurred in those areas after the intervention. To improve situational awareness and expand the ability to observe these developments, video cameras placed throughout the city and its colleges can monitor crowd movement and activity before, during, and after an event.

Finding Ways to Improve

After a number of incidents in which people lost their lives, in consultation with the mayor's office, it was determined that an independent observer should be part of all law enforcement responses. Attorneys with experience in government operations were invited to participate. These individuals were then brought to each component of the process: They were present in the command post, even accompanied officers on the street. If anything went wrong, they were independent entities that could certify what was successful, as well as make suggestions for improving the process for future situations.

End of Event

The end of an event is just as important to plan and execute as the event itself. For responders, the event does not "end" at the allotted time, and the crowd does not disperse on a dime. A protocol for standing down must be established to provide a clear indication of roles, responsibilities, and end of duty [2]. This is important to ensure the end of the event is not prematurely announced to responders, and medical team members are no longer available or active when still needed. It is extremely dangerous to close a command post before the event is over. Solid input from the field is necessary before any decision on wrapping up can be made. Incidents that occur in the waning hours of the event can sometimes be more important than the event itself. Phased closures of medical posts and personnel departures are one avenue of ensuring proper closing [6]; those who are the last to leave any medical post should be those in charge of disposal of medical waste.

Significant input and thought from all leadership, within medical and other command, must be obtained before the end is announced, and the crowd should be dispersed from all sites: Those in command posts must ensure that the venue is empty, medical stations are not overwhelmed, the streets in the area are clear, public transportation is operating and moving freely, and traffic is flowing. The safety of personnel and of the community lies in the balance of this decision.

The efforts do not end when event completion is confirmed. After action reports are extremely valuable. If something went wrong, any incidents can be reviewed and publicized as part of the process of establishing transparency and credibility. All aspects of the event that ran smoothly should also be analyzed in an after action report; the lessons learned are extremely valuable from what worked well.

Having a documented record of events will help in preparation for the next event. Many routine after action reports are done internally, but independent reviews are helpful in exposing gaps. After action reports serve as a record of an organization's success and can point out problems to address in the next round of planning. Transparency and lessons learned are key to this process.

In the unlikely and unfortunate event that major injuries, or even deaths, occur as a result of crowd activities, victim outreach is necessary as well. Public servants have a unique responsibility to show compassion and to reach out to those tragically affected. This process should be a fundamental part of any plan and should include individuals who are trained to work with victims and their families. Actions such as visiting families who are mourning, attending funerals, and providing for financial assistance can go a long way to lessening the impact on the community. Such efforts and considerations should also be extended to response personnel. First responders may require support for their own physical or psychological burdens resulting from the emergency.

As for the successes of the event, it's important to acknowledge the good work and dedication of the individuals engaged in the operations; this is an opportunity for the organization to show their appreciation. A review of the actions of the individuals involved should include identification of outstanding conduct and service to the community. Letters of recommendation, letters of commendation, letters of acknowledgment, and even service medals can be appropriate in these situations. This process directly affects morale, encourages an understanding of the organization, and shows the organization's appreciation of their people.

Conclusion

While mass gatherings introduce many unique challenges involving the safety of large groups of people, elements of crowd management reveal many opportunities to meet these challenges through multiagency collaboration. Many factors can impact event demands and outcomes, including known variables such as event type and unknown variables that present unforeseen problems, including emergencies. Medical, law enforcement, and general logistical issues require careful anticipation and planning and yet also adaptability. Communication and relationship-building facilitates execution of plans with flexibility and improved response to issues as they arise. Creative solutions realized through cooperative partnerships can optimize the safety of a variety of mass events.

References

1. Marcus L., McNulty E., Dorn B., et al. Crisis Meta-Leadership Lessons from the Boston Marathon Bombings Response: The Ingenuity of Swarm Intelligence. National Preparedness Leadership Initiative. The President and Fellows of Harvard College, 2014. https://cdn1.sph.harvard.edu/wp-content/uploads/sites/2443/2016/09/Marathon-Bombing-Leadership-Response-Report.pdf. Accessed August 2021.

2. Narr T., Toliver J., Murphy J., et al. Police Management of Mass Demonstrations: Identifying Issues and Successful Approaches. Police Executive Research Forum, 2006.

3. Police Executive Research Forum. Managing Major Events: Best Practices from the Field. Critical Issues in Policing Series, 2011.

4. Committee on Homeland Security. Public Health, Safety, and Security for Mass Gatherings, 2008. www.hsdl.org/?view&did=485911. Accessed October 2021.

5. Leonard H., Cole C., Howitt A., et al. Why Was Boston Strong: Lessons from the Boston Marathon Bombings. Harvard Kennedy School. The President and Fellows of Harvard College, 2014. www.hks.harvard.edu/sites/default/files/centers/research-initiatives/crisisleadership/files/WhyWasBostonStrong.pdf. Accessed August 2021.

6. Endericks T., McCloskey B., Barbeschi M., et al. (eds.). *Public Health for Mass Gatherings: Key Considerations.* Geneva: World Health Organization; 2015. https://apps.who.int/iris/bitstream/handle/10665/162109/WHO_HSE_GCR_2015.5_eng.pdf;jsessionid=12DCF8A421F3C35DDC7BA4ACCFA594F8?sequence=1. Accessed October 2021.

7. Police Executive Research Forum. The Police Response to Mass Demonstrations: Promising Practices and Lessons Learned, 2018. Office of Community Oriented Policing Services.

8. Fernandez E. 5 Cities That Rioted After Championship Games. *Mic.* October 2014. www.mic.com/articles/102836/5-other-cities-that-rioted-after-championship-games. Accessed September 2021.

9. Arbon P. The Development of Conceptual Models for Mass-Gathering Health. *Prehospital and Disaster Medicine.* 2004;**19**(3):208–212. http://pdm.medicine.wisc.edu. Accessed October 2021.

10. Sanders A., Criss E., Steckl P., et al. An Analysis of Medical Care at Mass Gatherings. *Annals of Emergency Medicine.* 1986;**15**:515–519.

11. Grange J., Baumann G., Vaezazizi R. On-site Physicians Reduce Ambulance Transports at Mass Gatherings. *Prehospital and Emergency Care.* 2003;**7**(3): 322–326. doi: 10.1080/10903120390936518

12. Australian Institute for Disaster Resilience. Safe and Healthy Crowded Places. Commonwealth of Australia, 2018. https://knowledge.aidr.org.au/media/5914/crowded-places-handbook.pdf. Accessed October 2021.

13. Kollek D. An Introduction to Mass Gatherings. The Centre for Excellence in Emergency Preparedness, 2014. https://pdf4pro.com/fullscreen/an-introduction-to-mass-gatherings-192dd.html. Accessed October 2021.

14. Calabro J., Krohmer J., Rivera-Rivera E., et al. Provision of Emergency Medical Care for Crowds. Emergency Medical Services Committee of the American College of Emergency Physicians, 1996. www.acep.org/globalassets/uploads/uploaded-files/acep/clinical-and-practice-management/ems-and-disaster-preparedness/ems-resources/emscrowd.pdf. Accessed October 2021.

15. Marcus L. J., McNulty E. J., Henderson J. M., et al. *You're It: Crisis, Change, and How to Lead When It Matters Most.* New York: Public Affairs; 2019.

16. Harvey M., Lamana J., Russell M., et al. Healthcare Coalition Involvement in Mass Gatherings. Assistant Secretary for Preparedness and Response, 2016. https://files.asprtracie.hhs.gov/documents/aspr-tracie-hcc-webinar-2-mass-gatherings.pdf. Accessed October 2021.

17. Duncan J. Canucks Fans Apologize to Boston for Post-Game Rioting. *Boston Globe*. June 16, 2011.

18. City of Boston Emergency Medical Services. 2018 Boston Marathon: Operations Plan. 2018.

19. District of Columbia Department of Health, Health Emergency Preparedness and Response Administration. Special Events Health, Medical and Safety Planning Guide. 2014. https://doh.dc.gov/sites/default/files/dc/sites/doh/page_content/attachments/2014-0026%20Special%20Event%20Health%20%20Safety%20Plan%20Guide.pdf. Accessed October 2021.

20. City of Boston Emergency Medical Services. 2020 First Night Celebration and Festivities: Operations Plan. 2019.

21. City of Boston Emergency Medical Services. 2019 Boston's 4th of July Esplanade Event: Operations Plan. 2019.

22. Federal Emergency Management Agency. ICS Review Document. Extracted from E/L/G 0300 Intermediate Incident Command System for Expanding Incidents, *ICS 300*, 2018. https://training.fema.gov/emiweb/is/icsresource/assets/ics%20review%20document.pdf. Accessed July 2021.

23. McNulty E. J., Dorn B. C., Goralnick E., et al. (2018). Swarm Intelligence: Establishing Behavioral Norms for the Emergence of Collective Leadership. *Journal of Leadership Education*. 2018;**17**:19–41.

24. City of Boston Emergency Medical Services. 2020 May 31 Rallies and Marches: Operations Plan. 2020.

25. Milsten A., Seaman K., Liu P., et al. Variables Influencing Medical Usage Rates, Injury Patterns, and Levels of Care for Mass Gatherings. *Prehospital and Disaster Medicine*. 2003;**18**(4):334–346. doi: 10.1017/s1049023x00001291

26. Michael J., Barbera J. Mass Gathering Medical Care: A Twenty Five Year Review. *Prehospital and Disaster Medicine*. 1997;**12**(4);72–79. doi: 10.1017/S1049023X00037857

27. South Australian Environmental Health Service, Department of Health. Guidelines for the Management of Public Health and Safety at Public Events. The National Library of Australia Cataloguing, 2006. www.sahealth.sa.gov.au/wps/wcm/connect/b650500045c7337a9262fbac725693cd/publicevents-phcc-100531.pdf?MOD=AJPERES&CACHEID=b650500045c7337a9262fbac725693cd&CACHE=NONE. Accessed October 2021.

28. Johansson A., Batty M., Hayashi K., et al. Crowd and Environmental Management During Mass Gatherings. *Lancet Infectious Diseases*. 2012;**12**:150–156. doi: 10.1016/S1473-3099(11)70287-0

29. Mointinho de Almeida M., von Schreeb J. Human Stampedes: An Updated Review of Current Literature. *Prehospital and Disaster Medicine*. 2019;**34**(1):82–88.

30. Haase K., Kasper M., Koch M., et al. A Pilgrim Scheduling Approach to Increase Safety During the Hajj. *Operations Research*. 2019;**67**(2):376–406.

31. Ahmed Q. A., Memish Z. A. From the "Madding Crowd" to Mass Gatherings: Religion, Sport, Culture and Public Health. *Travel Medicine and Infectious Disease*. 2019; **28**:91–97.

32. Pearl T. H. Far from the Madding Crowd: A Statutory Solution to Crowd Crush. *Hastings Law Journal*. 2016;**68**(1):159–202.

33. Byard R. W., Wick R., Simpson E., et al. The Pathological Features and Circumstances of Death of Lethal Crush/Traumatic Asphyxia in Adults: A 25-Year Study. *Forensic Science International*. 2006;**159**(2):200–205.

34. Helbing D., Mukerji P. Crowd Disasters as Systemic Failures: Analysis of the Love Parade Disaster. *EPJ Data Science*. 2012;**1**(1):1–40.

35. Sime J. D. Crowd Facilities, Management and Communications in Disasters. *Facilities*. 1999;**17**(9/10):313–324.

36. Zhao G., Li C., Xu G., et al. A High-Density Crowd State Judgment Model Based on Entropy Theory. *PloS One*. 2021;**16**(9):e0255468–e0255468. doi: 10.1371/journal.pone.0255468

37. Marcus L. J., McNulty E. J., Flynn L. B., et al. The POP-DOC Loop: A Continuous Process for Situational Awareness and Situational Action. *Industrial Marketing Management*. 2020;**88**:272–277.

Civil Unrest and Terrorism Involving Mass Gathering Events

Pierre A. Carli, Debra G. Perina, and Paul E. Pepe

Introduction

Civil unrest and terrorism, whether they precipitate or complicate a mass gathering event, are both high-risk situations that can clearly potentiate the generic difficulties associated with any large congregation and concentration of people, especially in terms of a compromised emergency response and the sheer volume of potential victims that may require medical care.

However, the eruption of a violent phenomenon targeting the crowd or inciting a violent reaction within the crowd is also a very dangerous circumstance in terms of very real threats to the rescuers as well. Oftentimes, the medical responders and associated receiving hospitals can also be targets [1]. These high-risk environments will not only involve potential direct physical harm to responders, but concomitant law enforcement actions can change the entire landscape of events.

In that respect, as part of the public safety response, the rescue actions and treatment rendered by medical responders will likely be closely scrutinized, formally evaluated, and characterized by the media and official after-action investigators, especially when many innocents are harmed [1–8]. In that respect, such scrutiny can have serious public relations, political, and even judicial consequences. At the very least, they can result in testimonial involvement for medical responders. Particularly when deaths occur, preventability and any relation to the medical response efforts will likely be dissected, analyzed, and either praised or damned, often with very little moderation in tone.

Beyond medical interventions, such review and analysis can include ethical decision-making and triage decision-making. The background and reasons prompting civil unrest, protests, or political rallies already carry an emotionally charged element.

In turn, blame and accountability, be it in the social media, mass media or courts, can have a profound long-term impact on medical responders and their teams, either directly or indirectly [1, 5, 6, 8, 9].

More importantly, these events can result in significant psychological impact on rescuers, not only in terms of physically observing the slaughter of vulnerable innocents, but also in terms of second-guessing one's actions or feeling a sense of guilt for (conceptually) abandoning their life-saving duties when they were held back and staged outside "hot zones" of potential ongoing violence as the scene is being secured by law enforcement. For a number of reasons, protracted events amplify this mental health concern [1].

Compounding these complex associated psychological, logistical, and sociological issues is the reality that exact prediction of the timing and nature of such an event is often quite difficult, especially in the case of a sudden terrorist attack on a "soft" target. For example, many mass gathering shooting events in the United States such as that transpiring at a hometown suburban Independence Day celebration parade (Highland Park, Illinois, July 4, 2022) are typically unexpected and they often occur in otherwise peaceful communities unaccustomed to any type of shootings incidents altogether. Moreover, emergency medical services (EMS) teams standing by at such festive local events can often become victims themselves by being positioned in purposefully visible sites among the crowds [1, 2]. Therefore, if such an event is not anticipated, the medical care providers or police officers can themselves become injured because of a stampeding crowd or as the result of an intended direct hit or ricocheting bullets while attempting to help others [1, 3]. As such, even local events like this should be considered and anticipated as a potential target for a violent "terrorist" incident.

Therefore, while political rallies, civil unrest demonstrations, and overt terrorist attacks are clearly higher risk for violence, any mass gathering involving large congregations of persons lining sidewalks for a small town parade, strolling through a crowded state fairgrounds, singing at a massive church festival, or those gathered for a municipal fireworks celebration, should all be considered at risk for malicious and intended viciousness. As a result, medical crews supporting any mass gathering event should consider plans that keep medical rescuers out of the immediate "kill zone." They should also consider known terrorist tactics such as detonating a smaller ("come hither") bomb and then detonating a larger one once rescuers arrive [2]. Granted, the odds of such incidents occurring in any one small community may be extremely rare, but the escalating number of occurrences of such events demand more attention today and risk planning for any professional involved in mass gathering medicine activities on any scale.

Risk assessments for any mass gathering are neither simple nor always exact. A high-level of mitigation is always the more realistic strategy and it must be carried out according to the type of gathering and the context in which the mass gathering is occurring. Beyond soft targets such as the holiday parade or festival crowd attacked by a single lone gunman, the relatively unplanned political rally or any unscheduled mass gathering does, of course, create greater concern and a broader array of risks including physical harm, obstructed medical and security response and even political and psychological fallout for medical responders [1, 2, 4, 5, 9].

Experience has shown that most well-intended organizers of protests or rallies do not anticipate the possibility of an outbreak of violence during their mass gathering event. Even if has been anticipated as a potential concern, medical response planning is often undersized in retrospect, especially at lower risk events.

Presumed low-risk mass gathering events such as the well-attended country music festival (e.g., Clark County, Nevada, USA, October 1, 2017) or a historically benign and peaceful Black Lives Matter rally (e.g., Dallas, Texas, USA, July 7, 2016) can suddenly erupt into utter mayhem, even when just a single gunman, acting alone, can shoot hundreds of persons within a matter of minutes, or when the gunman specifically targets and assassinates several police officers standing-by at the conclusion of a peaceful march (and do so in a matter of seconds) [1, 3].

In other cases, such as a political rally anticipated to be comprised of vocal but respectful attendees overall, planners should know that these events can suddenly evolve and be ignited into a full-scale show of civil disobedience, and often because of certain malicious persons inserting themselves into the event [4, 5]. What would usually be a peaceful demonstration can quickly erupt into significant violence with resulting injury and deaths, most often when a perpetrating subgroup of protesters or fringe extremists infiltrate the event and purposefully confront the law enforcement officers [5, 6]. These eruptions can be amplified when the police are trying to protect possible targets of the rioters' violent attack (e.g., US Capitol attack, Washington, DC, USA, January 6, 2021) [6].

In other cases, the violent attack can entail a straightforward suicide bombing at a popular rock concert (Manchester, England, UK, May 22, 2017) or perhaps one part of a coordinated multisite terrorist attack simultaneously resulting in numerous deaths at a popular nightclub with a potential for many more injuries across other parts of the city (e.g., Paris, France, November 13–14, 2015) [7, 8]. In essence, these terrible incidents can be very hard to predict, often occurring at the time of the conclusion of the event itself, especially when all appears has been going well (e.g., Boston Marathon bombing, April 15, 2013, the previously mentioned Manchester Arena, 2017 bombing and the 2016 Dallas police ambush) [1, 4, 7]. Also, coordinated multi-site incidents can vary widely in terms of the nature of the weapons and the timing of the attacks (bombs in one place, gunshots in another, chemical attacks elsewhere) [1, 2, 7–9].

Moreover, as previously described, the eventual psychological toll on rescuers and survivors can be quite significant and has become a true burden for many [1]. The spectrum of posttraumatic psychological sequelae can be carried for many months and even years (if not a lifetime). Beyond the frustration of purposely being held back from entering the hot zones where seriously injured patients may laying while the perpetrator is being "neutralized" or secured, subsequent imprinted visions of massacred and macerated bodies (e.g., Uvalde, Texas, elementary school shootings, May 24, 2022; Parkland Florida, high school shooting, February 14, 2018) are difficult to erase. Many such incidents do involve innocent, vulnerable populations such as children, the elderly, or other undeserving and defenseless victims of hate. Moreover, witnessing the deaths of fellow public safety partners or friends can compound this issue [1].

In order to better assist and prepare prospective medical care professionals responding to (or standing-by) such events, this chapter is intended to convey the international experiences of numerous clinicians directly involved in such incidents. Use of these historical examples can help to highlight some of the potential factors and elements to anticipate, recognize, and consider when preparing for the very complex response to such unpredictable and challenging incidents. In addition, the overall plan for this discussion is to attempt to delineate concepts that could be applicable to almost any medical care system in which the civil unrest or terroristic violence will occur. It is also written with the hopeful intent to optimize outcomes and mitigate the fallout from these kinds of brutal tragedies.

Case Examples of Various Terrorist Attacks at Mass Gatherings

The 2015 Bomb Attack at the Stade de France and Concomitant Paris Attacks

A bombing occurred as a part of a multimodal and multisite Daesh terrorist attack on November 13, 2015 which killed over 200 civilians and injured more than 450 others across the city of Paris [8, 9]. Known by its Arabic acronym, Daesh is a militant Islamist group that follows the Salafi jihadist branch of Sunni Islam. Ironically, most of the victims were unlikely to even know of these terrorists existence, let alone their potential threat to do so much harm to so many unsuspecting souls as they started out to enjoy a typical Friday evening in Paris.

An eye-opening aspect of this cross-city incident is that one component did occur within a very high-risk context and the others did not. That higher-risk component was an attack that targeted the spectacular Stade de France, a large, frequently occupied stadium with 80,000 seats for attendees [8]. However, in attendance that evening were several national and international political authorities, including the sitting French President who was there to attend a football match between France and Germany [8].

One of the lessons provided here was that, in accordance with the routine French organization for large-scale sporting events, pivotal security and emergency measures were already predeployed within the stadium and throughout the nearby perimeter

[8, 9]. As later revealed, the planned attack consisted of the intent to detonate suicide bombs inside the stadium just at the beginning of the match, not only with the intent to inflict mass casualties, but also to cause panic in a particular area of the stadium where many major media would be providing both live and recorded audio-visual coverage of the match [8].

Fortunately, several standardized security measures and operational decisions thwarted this plan of attack. The would-be perpetrators were turned back by the security guards in the perimeter and, as a result, the first suicide bomb did explode at the beginning of the match, but it did so outside of the main security perimeter [8]. Consequently, the number of victims was limited. Nonetheless, it must be kept in mind that the extremely large stadium's mass gathering was one of the sources of attraction for this terrorist group and that, despite its mitigation, there were still many resulting casualties [8].

Of particular note in this case, even after the explosion of the first bomb outside of the stadium, the police and national security officials made a purposeful decision not to interrupt the match and not to evacuate the stadium [8, 9]. Instead, the immediate reactive plan was to protect all accesses and also prohibit any entry or exit of the stadium. As a result, the bulk of the crowd did not come within reach of the other suicide bombers outside of the stadium, an important observation and recurrent theme in this discussion.

This decision did seem contrary to the usual immediate evacuation of the public in many typical threat plans. Audience evacuation is usually the first action considered in the event of a major threat event, be it a fire, explosion, active shooter attack, or other uncontrollable violence. In this particular case, however, a decision to evacuate might have caused many more casualties or injuries.

This important observation came from experience. Lone or multiple assailants may purposely attempt to create stampeding evacuations or attempt to "usher" and rush panicked persons within mass gatherings into more vulnerable positions where they can be more easily cornered and directly attacked. Therefore, this example of "adaptability of plans" and real-time risk management is a key element of managing such surprise catastrophes.

Overall, this attack was considered a relative failure for both the terrorists and the French officials. Simultaneous attacks were occurring at other sites. These scattered attacks, meant to be distractors from the main terrorist attack at the stadium, did claim many other victims [1, 8, 9]. These separate but simultaneous attacks involved victims being sprayed with bullets while sitting among the café terraces along a lengthy Parisian boulevard. Another attack was made on those enjoying an evening of music with friends at the popular Bataclan theater where, ironically, the audience was being entertained by a rock group called Eagles of Death Metal.

This 2015 Parisian experience serves to remind counter-terrorism responders and incident commanders that one event may be used to distract rescuers from another attack site. The 2001 (9/11) World Trade Center incident in New York City was compounded by a second aircraft attack, but also it may have served as a distractor for other attacks, namely those targeting Washington, DC, which fortunately was partially thwarted [1]. Accordingly, redundant resources should always be placed on standby and staged at some distance. In other words, resources and response should not be focused on just one site.

Lone Attackers Causing Significant Carnage with Various Tools of Terror

Other surprise terrorist attacks involving mass gatherings can involve a single person with ordinary vehicles in traffic suddenly becoming the threat. One such incident was the violent attack in Nice, France, on July 14, 2016 when a nineteen-ton cargo truck, driven by a single person, was deliberately driven into crowds of people celebrating Bastille Day and gathering for the fireworks on the Promenade des Anglais [9]. This attack resulted in the deaths of 85 people, including 10 children and adolescents and injury to 458 others with 303 taken to hospital [9]. On December 19, that same year, another single-driver truck was deliberately driven into the Christmas market adjacent to the Kaiser Wilhelm Memorial Church at the Breitscheidplatz in Berlin (Germany) [10]. The incident left twelve people dead and fifty-six others injured [10]. Of note, one of the twelve victims was the truck's original driver who was later found shot dead in the passenger seat, presumptively killed by the perpetrator.

That following year, on October 31, 2017, a similar truck attack occurred in New York City when the single driver/attacker drove a rented pick-up truck into cyclists and runners along one mile of the bike path traversing Hudson River Park on the lower east

of the city. Eight persons were killed, including five Argentinian tourists, and eleven others sustained significant injuries. While this specific event and the other cited truck-facilitated attacks in Europe were not classic mass gathering events, they again emphasize that this mode of terrorism is commonly used in many countries for murdering large numbers of persons unexpectedly. It helps to reinforce the need to create true barriers to any type of random traffic access to areas where large numbers of persons may gather or traverse.

This mode of attack is further emphasized by the common use of trucks and lorries for detonating bombs such as the tragic bomb attack in Oklahoma City on the federal government building in the US state of Oklahoma on April 19, 1995, an incident that resulted in 168 deaths and nearly 700 others injured. It was the deadliest "home-grown" terrorist attack in the US. While not a classical portrait of a mass gathering "event," the bomb was still detonated at a large, highly populated governmental structure with many inhabitants. Such events do reinforce the notion that the access of a truck or lorry to a highly populated venue with many people needs to be closely scrutinized and cleared – or curtailed altogether. This scrutiny includes those large trailers that haul large entertainment stage components and other equipment for loading into a large stadium or arena.

Obscured Lone Terrorist Attacks Using Bombs, Guns, or Other Weapons

A key element of understanding terrorist strategies is the consideration of timing of the attack. In contrast to the Paris stadium bombing specifically intended to be triggered at the beginning of the match (to gain more media attention, perhaps assassinate the head of state, and undermine a major international match), other terrorists have chosen to detonate their devices or use their trucks just as crowds were leaving an event [1, 4, 7]. At that later point during a show or match, many persons are still enraptured from the afternoon or evening's wonderful entertainment, especially if also imbibing during the event. At this point, they would not likely be thinking about keeping vigilance or the likelihood of calamity. Even security officials may be more apt to let down their guard as their main principals (i.e., entertainers, athletes, political officials) are already departed and the audience is peacefully evacuating [1, 4, 7].

As previously mentioned, on May 22, 2017, a lone suicide bomber discretely entered the foyer of a large arena in Manchester, UK, when doors were opened wide for the very large exiting audience following a pop music concert with many young adolescents in attendance [7]. Surrounded by that dense exiting crowd, the perpetrator detonated a shrapnel-laden homemade device that killed 23 but also injured 1,017 others as they rapidly exited that concert arena. The subsequent August 12, 2017, vehicle attack in Charlottesville reinforces this same important "take-away' lesson that the major attack may occur just when it appears that the event is over (as was also the case for the 2016 Dallas police ambush previously mentioned) [1, 4, 7].

This Manchester Arena concert, which featured the American singer, Ariana Grande, attracted a majority of attendees who were preteens and young adolescents. Beyond victimization of another vulnerable, innocent population, the resulting impact on the national ambulance service and the additional challenges for both pediatric and trauma surgery resources were all suddenly overwhelming in this off-hours period [7]. Therefore, two key lessons (of many) distilled from this tragedy was that, when crowds are still present, security and medical teams need to remain vigilant for such threats even when the main event has ended [1, 4, 7]. It also meant that, considering the demographics for that given event, preparations in the realm of trauma receiving facilities, including trauma services for children, need to be amply anticipated and resourced with solid back-up plans for additional surgeons, including plastic surgeons, orthopedists and gynecologists, when pediatric trauma surgeons have become overwhelmed as they did in this unanticipated catastrophe [7, 11].

Weapons and Tactics That Are Now Changing the Injury Preparation Calculus

Later that same year (October 1, 2017), a lone sniper marred the festivities at the Route 91 Harvest Festival being held adjacent to Las Vegas Boulevard in Clark County, Nevada. This festive mass gathering became a mass shooting attack when a lone sixty-four-year-old gunman, using a rapid-fire automatic military-style weapon, pummeled the music festival spectators with hundreds and hundreds of destructive bullets [3]. As he was shooting from a distant upper floor

hotel room, it was very hard for anyone to quickly ascertain the source or direction of the attack. This scenario compromised the immediate control of the attack and the audience had no obvious indicators regarding the best direction to head to escape injury. The attack was therefore launched on thousands of "sitting duck" attendees simply having an enjoyable experience at this perennially popular mass gathering music festival. In the end, there were 61 deaths (including the perpetrator) and over 867 were injured, including 411 from the gunfire itself. Many others were hurt in trying to escape or being trampled while doing so. Of note, most attendees were standing or crawling on a hard surface pavement and many bullets ricocheted and caused additional injuries that otherwise would have been avoided if it had been a typical music festival with a grassy field scenario [3].

In most traditional multiple casualty incidents (MCIs), only about 5–10 percent of patients may need immediate advanced life support and urgent attention. Most people will either be killed outright or sustain less immediate life-threatening injuries [2]. However, due to the nature and setting of this particular attack, close to 40 percent of transported patients were (appropriately) classified as critical cases and the absolute numbers of those needing to be resuscitated and go to surgery was clearly extraordinary. As a result, similar to the Manchester bombing, hospital trauma resources and surgeons were overwhelmed early on and secondary triage sites needed to be established outside the hospitals [3, 7].

The event was further complicated by the inability to methodically triage and stage evacuees due to the logistics, geographical-expanse and magnitude of the event as well as the sudden need for many incoming ambulances being unable to access the site when so many thousands were trying to escape the site by any means possible. Compounding these obstacles was a understandable but confounding lack of methodical patient tracking and triage. Many persons were randomly taken from the scene by rideshare vehicles (Uber, Lyft), police units or other private vehicles. The global positioning applications of rideshare vehicles actually helped to pinpoint better evacuation points due to access limitations. Hospitals rapidly became further overwhelmed by these untracked and unanticipated patients.

While having tracking, demographic, and clinical information integrated into a comprehensive electronic medical record is an idealistic concept for a mass gatherings, this experience emphasized that those idealistic concepts may not be practical for many events. Neither was the use of triage tags [2, 3].

As a result of all of these concerns, it was reemphasized that designated public safety personnel, likely someone in the incident command center, should have clear communication capabilities with hospitals. Persons designated to this task should constantly be surveying receiving facilities for their relative capacities, a condition that may be changing rapidly in a dynamic manner. For example, some hospitals may be overwhelmed at one point in time, but they then rapidly regain capacity within ensuing minutes depending on subsequent influxes of persons and types of injuries arriving by various modes of transport. This preparedness concept is further emphasized by the preparations made for the Charlottesville political rally on August 12, 2017, discussed in more detail in following sections of this chapter [4].

One other issue of note from this Clark County incident (and other similar tragedies) is the issue that shooters are now more often taking a high ground position. This same terrorist strategy does date back well over a century (e.g., Centralia, Washington USA, at the 2019 Armistice Day veterans parade massacre) and most famously a half-century later with the assassination of US President John Kennedy. However, attacks from above are becoming more prevalent today such as that observed in this Harvest 91 festival tragedy and the 2016 Dallas police ambush, and the 2022 Highland Park, Illinois, Independence Day parade. The perpetrator in the 2018 Parkland Florida (USA) Marjorie Stoneman Douglas High School rampage had intended to do the same. In that later scenario, the lone shooter had planned to create an panic evacuation of all students and then shoot down at them from a third floor window. Fortunately, this window was hurricane-proofed and resisted breakage avoiding the sitting duck scenario that was planned. This concern should be emphasized in any mass gathering planning recognizing that a trigger event (bomb, fire, shooting) can lead to panic stampedes and/or persons being ambushed from above by high-nested shooters who now have a broader area of direct bullet hits without body-to-body shielding or a risk of being immediately apprehended.

Cases of Civil Unrest or Political Mass Gatherings Gone Awry

The Yellow Vests Demonstrations

From November 2018 to June 2019, a recurrent series of protest events convened in France called the *espect des gilets jaunes* (or "yellow vests" protests / demonstrations) [5, 12]. The origins of these protests emanated largely from multiple grievances linked to an evolving and profound loss of purchasing power among retirees and people with fixed and lower incomes. One of the main drivers was related to increases in fuel prices, but other escalating expenses further exacerbated the social unrest blossoming during this pre-COVID era.

Of interest, despite the core involvement of low income persons and seniors, the movement actually started on the internet with social media instigation. The protests took on two main forms: (1) traditional mass gathering protests in large cities; and (2) the blocking of highway junctions in medium-sized cities [12]. Many demonstrations were organized to take place on weekends and they involved several hundred-thousand participants on any given day of protests.

While these demonstrations were not authorized by the local governments or law enforcement agencies, these rallies were initially nonviolent and only minimally confrontational with respect to police and local authorities. Thus, they were allowed to continue for a while unimpeded. However, significant violence did begin to evolve within a very short period of time. The violence took on two major forms: (1) certain groups of protesters vandalizing luxury shops and bank branches; and (2) international extremist elements, called the Black Bloc, began to infiltrate the protester processions and eventually attacked the police directly [5, 12].

In response, during this phase, security forces set up roadblocks that prevented protesters from approaching official buildings and they also began to make numerous arrests. To do so, they began to deploy and use nonlethal riot weapons such as flash balls and tear gas. In the capital city of Paris, these demonstrations led to a massive police deployment that prohibited protesters from gaining access to certain areas of the city and it also led to the initiation of preventive arrests of certain dangerous demonstrators. It also included substantial deployments of mobile police forces to also protect and supervise the processions recognizing that the majority of marchers were peaceful and that they often included vulnerable persons such as the elderly (see Chapter 18).

Not only did the police confrontations lead to physical injuries, tear gas and flash ball complications, but they also limited rapid access into the injured crowd as well as expeditious evacuations to appropriate hospitals. Beyond the police security forces, firefighter rescue teams were also directly integrated into the organization of public safety response. Pertinent to this discussion, however, the advanced life support element of the Parisian EMS system, the Service d'Aide Médicale Urgente (SAMU) du Paris, maintained its own response alerting system and its own response assignment autonomy [12].

Given the police blockades and massive crowds, the protests posed significant challenges in terms of rescuing injured protesters and rescuers alike. Fortunately, the SAMU teams were clearly identified as being "neutral" medical personnel by the majority of demonstrators and they were even able to intervene more easily than the firefighters. Like the police, firefighters are paramilitary in nature and they report to the Ministry of the Interior versus the SAMU who branch under the auspices of the Ministry of Health.

Of note, during the demonstrations there was an appearance of improvised rescuers called "Street Medics." These unofficial volunteers appeared to accompany the extremist demonstrators but their skills and response equipment were not known or apparent. They had no direct coordination with SAMU medical rescue teams, but they did participate spontaneously in helping with the identification of first-aid needs and the extraction of the wounded in conjunction with the SAMU. This was an interesting and unplanned alliance that largely depended upon the interpersonal skills of the respective leadership involved.

Many injured protesters were treated onsite or they later presented spontaneously to the emergency department (ED) of any hospital near the demonstrations regardless of those facilities' capabilities. Consequently, inter-hospital transfers to appropriate specialty centers had to be organized subsequently to treat certain types of severe injuries, including ophthalmic, neurosurgical, or multiple trauma injuries. In contrast, members of the police forces who were wounded only received care from official rescue teams and they were transported directly to the designated appropriate facilities. Beyond exacerbating the day-to-day routine demand for ED services, the protests also disrupted and delayed responses to the everyday medical emergencies with the routing of ambulances being severely impaired causing delays in expeditious care for those being transported and overall compromising the immediate availability of ambulances [12].

Nonetheless, despite the massive scale of these gatherings and the extended number of protest months, there were no deaths of inner-city demonstrators. However, the blocking of road junctions in the medium-sized towns did lead to localized, intense violence. Several fatal accidents occurred when cars forced their way through blockades, killing (and extensively injuring) protesters.

In essence, these longstanding demonstrations of the yellow vests protestors constituted a *series* of mass gathering events that did require significant medical attention, but they also represented a particularly complex situation with unique challenges. These challenges arose from the difficulties in anticipating the evolving risks and threats and also from difficulties in coordinating the services across different chains of commands. It also emphasizes that violence can be perpetrated in what would otherwise have appeared, at first, to be peaceful rallies based on the historical experience. It also demonstrates that necessary police and security actions can obstruct adequate responses to the ill and injured and that hospitals and routine EMS responses can be impaired. Moreover, protesters were more confident with being rescued by medical personnel if they responded independently from the police. This is a difficult concern as traditional thinking would be to have EMS accompanied and protected by police or to use police and firefighters to help evacuate the sick and injured to a safer perimeter. Each situation therefore needs to be assessed according to such cultural, circumstantial and political factors.

Either way, it must be remembered that, even in political and terrorist circumstances, vulnerable populations can be involved and that they pose a higher risk of injury and medical complications. Therefore, special accommodations and associated planning need to be considered and implemented for these types of active attendees or uninvolved bystanders (see Chapter 18).

The January 6 US Capitol Riot in Washington, DC

Following the election of a new President of the United States in November 2020, many supporters of the out-going president, disappointed with the results, later held a rally involving many thousands of persons on January 6, 2021 in Washington, DC, the day on which the election results were to be certified. The rally was planned and permitted by officials and, as approved, was held at predesignated park area of the city. However, this political rally subsequently devolved into a violent clash when subgroups of attendees proceeded to march about a mile or more to the US Capitol (the main government building) where the US congress was known to be in session to certify the final election results [6].

In that respect, this incident had many similarities to the evolution of the Yellow Vests protests in France when imbedded extremist insurgents eventually controlled the narrative and created violence [5, 6]. The difference in the Washington, DC event was the rapid evolution of such violence over just a few hours' period. Whether it was a spontaneous mob-mentality attack on the Capitol building on the part of some, or, perhaps more likely, as a planned incident by some of the imbedded participating insurgent groups within the crowd, the national lawmaking government building was indeed violently attacked. At least 400 persons (and likely more) attacked the police who were protecting the building and the rioters subsequently entered the halls of the Capitol where more violence unraveled. Deaths occurred and many more injured, but, relevant to this discussion, access to medical care was delayed to some extent due to the unanticipated number of rioters and the unexpected degree of the violence. This created a very unsafe scenario for all public safety officials let alone the involved principals being guarded.

While the Parisian and Washington, DC examples were national, attention-garnering events, these types of scenarios stemming from civil unrest are not that uncommon particularly in the case of racial protests following highly publicized in-custody deaths or certain police-involved shootings. While such mass gatherings are comprised of extremely angry protestors, they are generally peaceful marches in the majority of cases. However, as previously described, these mass gatherings can devolve when a smaller contingent of opportunists might resort to looting, setting fires, or invoking violent assault. For both law enforcement and medical personnel, delineation of the perpetrators in these settings is not always easy. Regardless, for the medical care personnel, the task remains the same. In preparation, considerations for protection including body armor, helmets, and other precautions, need to be considered in some settings, even if the event is deemed a peaceful activity upfront. However, such considerations should also consider the experience of the French SAMU where being unassociated with the police was an apparent asset. The better alternative, as described later, may be to have specialized, trained tactical medics or physicians within the ranks of medical personnel, a concept that will be subsequently discussed in more detail.

While the previous two examples of civil unrest with mass gatherings infiltrated by extremists predominantly occurred in the capital cities of two nations, incidents of domestic civil unrest are also becoming more and more frequent in many other smaller communities. Unfortunately, even the most peaceful events can suddenly turn violent without warning, particularly when instigated by malicious organized groups or simply a "lone wolf" driving a vehicle into the crowd [4, 5]. As previously alluded, violence is more likely to occur when large segments of the crowd hold very strong differences in political or religious viewpoints.

One example was the "Unite the Right" rally in Charlottesville, a large city in the US state of Virginia on August 12, 2017 [4]. In this incident, hundreds of self-declared "nationalists" and their supporters gathered to rally and protest plans to remove a Confederate army statue. However, during the event, the "Unite the Right" protesters were then confronted by counter-protesters. The counter-protesters' attendance was indeed anticipated by authorities and concerns arose that clashes could be expected to break out. Exacerbating the tension, the "Unite the Right" rally was actually deemed to be unlawful, thus augmenting the anti-government sentiment. Authorities and medical personnel were thus prepared for such a confrontation.

Fortunately, upfront, the incident appeared to be relatively controlled despite the overt contentious behaviors. But, of note, as crowds were dispersing, a protester's vehicle purposely drove into a crowd of counter-protesters who had been marching through the downtown area and were now exiting. This attack resulted in a death and more than a dozen others being seriously injured. Complicating this event even further was that the State police later reported the crash of one of their helicopters monitoring the events, killing two troopers. Virginia's governor declared a state of emergency demonstrating that a small local civil unrest event can evolve into a major mass gathering event, result in significant numbers of deaths, and create a major state of crisis.

In this specific case, there was pre-event intelligence that some of the rally attendees had been known for creating violent skirmishes in other venues and that they were assembling in surrounding counties before heading to Charlottesville. In fact, the night before the rally, hundreds of these nationalists marched through the nearby University of Virginia grounds carrying burning torches likely to instill student fear or to promote a sense of defiance against the more liberal students' viewpoints. It was clear therefore that there was an intended confrontation and even an provocative enticement to engage. Accordingly, the coordination of such intelligence gathering was pivotal in terms of mass gathering medicine preparations.

In their developing a response plan, public safety planners anticipated the worst possible scenario. Their response considerations included the physical restrictions to the area of protest, whether they were involving mobile or stationary attendees. The goal was to secure evacuation routes, and to ensure rapid access/egress for transportation resources adjacent to the crowds but also keep them sequestered and protected. Redundant, secure, and clear communications became a vital asset between the event incident command (law enforcement) team, event medical staff, and local EMS, fire, and even the destination hospitals. Experience in Charlottesville and elsewhere has demonstrated that redundancy (back-up) in communication abilities is paramount as it is the single most common source of breakdown in event response. In this case, event security teams were also spread throughout the various pockets of crowds as a strategy to quickly mitigate individual eruptions of clashes.

In many respects, the plans were working well and violence contained. However, as previously described in the 2017 Manchester Arena bombing or the 2016 Dallas Police ambush, one must be continuously vigilant and assume that the potential for violence will still exist until the scene is completely cleared of all attendees. In the Charlottesville rally, the event was declared to be ended when the crowd was in the process of leaving, but not yet fully dispersed. In fact, with the event command being terminated, a unilateral decision was made to open some of the closed roads in order to facilitate more rapid exiting of the crowd. Unfortunately, that action then permitted the vehicle attack because the driver was then able to use one of the roads that was just opened to attack the crowd. Once again, this event became a clear reminder that "it's not over until it's over" in many of these situations of violence inflicted upon mass gatherings [1, 4, 7].

The Charlottesville incident also provided some positive medical care examples. With the early intel provided about the high-risk for violence, hospitals voluntarily discharged in-patients among those who could be. They expedited any admissions from the ED and also overstocked ED supplies. Nonemergent surgery cases were cancelled and staffing of nursing and security personnel was augmented. They added additional controls at all hospital access points and established a separate family waiting area. The EMS system even altered its usual transport patterns in a manner to safely send appropriate patients to alternative destinations to protect the trauma center's ability to absorb any injured patients coming from the event. At the same time, other area hospitals became part of the vital communication links and they were alerted to serve as back-up as needed. Coordination with the city's emergency operations center (EOC) was in place to facilitate in-the-moment rerouting of ambulance traffic to different hospital destinations should normal access routes be affected. In that respect, an EMS physician specialist was also made available to designate the most appropriate receiving hospitals as needed as well as to triage patients to appropriate medical care facilities not impacted by the event. This asset also had the added value of keeping EMS resources safe within their communities by not placing them in harm's way close to the event and recommending safe and appropriate transport elsewhere. Using this model during the Charlottesville "Unite the Right" rally, the majority of EMS patients in surrounding counties were successfully and safely protected from being transported into Charlottesville's zone of concern.

In fact, these strategies became very helpful. They kept local hospital resources open to receive patients from the rally once the truck-induced violence did erupt at the end of the rally. The near-empty trauma center ED and surgery suites were able to absorb the many major trauma patients almost simultaneously as they arrived. Due to the early intel regarding higher risk of confrontation, preemptive actions were taken which resulted in a smaller number of patients. Therefore, Charlottesville medical officials did not encounter the same immediate lack of resources experienced at first by Manchester three months earlier and Clark County two months later. Nonetheless, and most importantly, even though the event appeared to be over, planners and incident commanders need to be aware of such an unfortunate "finale" attack as that seen in Charlottesville, Dallas, and Manchester.

Risk Assessment of Civil Unrest and Terrorism

The relevance of the preceding examples is that all mass gathering events have risk but some have much higher risk than others. Prudent risk assessment is therefore one of the most important factors concerning a mass gathering. It makes it possible to prepare and dimension a response plan that has been adapted to fit the situation. Sparing resources for the surrounding community in terms of managing the day-to-day medical needs and budgetary prudence are both truly important, but a mass gathering plan must also avoid the underestimation of need. At the same time, there is a counter-position that planners should avoid accumulation of various unnecessary resources and equipment that would be costly and likely be ineffective in a mass gathering setting, and even provocative in certain situations. Therefore, the prior assessment of risks and the different scenarios that could lead to a possible violent event should be shared among all potential stakeholders with the omnipresent understanding that any event, even low risk scenarios, can always be a target for malfeasance.

In such planning, a variety of contexts may be considered:

- Any gathering of persons presents a potential risk for violence, particularly if it involves persons with deep-seated anger (justifiable or not), significant alcohol inebriation, extremist ideation, mob mentality, or any combination of these factors. Likely examples include protest demonstrations infiltrated by malevolent individuals, a political or trade union rally influenced by extremists or relatively spontaneous marches held in anger such as

racial or religious belief related fatal incidents. If the event is authorized by the police prospectively, this provides the benefit of some prior organization such as a more controlled designated and supervised route of protest and the organizers' abilities to optimize control over their own security services and staging.

A spontaneous manifestation of violence is more apt to occur whenever there is no identified organizer or entity responsible for guiding the process, though violence can still occur despite strong leaders [5, 6].

- However, even in the case of an authorized demonstration, as noted previously, the dispersal phase is the most sensitive. This phase is known to be associated with violent confrontation with protesters and the police, but it is also associated with opportunistic actions by perpetrators of mass attacks [1, 4, 6, 7]. Likewise, the eruption of provocateurs or uncontrolled elements who are not under the supervision of organizers can lead to unforeseen outbursts of violence. Positions of potential blind-sided attacks from various factions or high-positioned sniper elements also need to be considered [1–6].

- In contrast, most music concert performances or most sporting events with a cheerful, family-friendly audience are not usually predisposed to violence. However, it is also this type of gathering of "innocents" that is the preferred target for a terrorist attack. Within the current context of worldwide events, it can be considered that any large gathering of crowds, especially if widely advertised in the media, may be the target of a terrorist act. The terrorist attack is the most dangerous form of violence because it specifically relies on an aggressive strategy directed against the crowd. This strategy can be quite rudimentary, often called "low-cost terrorism." For example, an individual or pair of aggressors stabbing members of the public in a underground subway or perpetrating a random truck attack on a populated esplanade [9, 10]. More sophisticated scenarios are those using more complex strategies such as multiple, sequential coordinated explosions, and specifically those first aimed at the primary crowd site, but then targeting the evacuation routes provided for the crowd as surviving crowd members try to escape. It can also involve terrorist commandos using automatic firearms, or even targeted chemical attacks on those evacuating crowds. Terrorists may also block those exits, precipitating human stampedes that provoke crowd crushes and compressional asphyxia [13, 14]. As observed in the peaceful yellow vest protests or the January 6 US Capitol riot, the instigations of extremist provocateurs (e.g., "Black Bloc" or "Proud Boys") can also lead to outbursts of uncontrolled violence among those who would usually be law-abiding participants.

- This risk analysis is best carried out jointly by all the services likely to participate in the event or its direct supervision. If a severe risk is determined, preventive measures must be taken into account before the event and, if indicated, officials should consider postponement or canceling altogether. Global scoring risk tools have been developed for selected type of events (soccer matches, religious mass gathering) but none have been explicitly dedicated to civil unrest or terrorism and mass casualty [15]. However, risk tools can still be extrapolated from lessons learned, either directly or indirectly, from other mass casualty events such as stampedes and structural collapses [16].

Preparation and Planning Considerations

Planned Events and Coordination of All Services Involved

In large gatherings that may carry a degree of security risk, coordination between the different services involved in the organization, security, and rescue is important at all stages: preparation, in-progress, and feedback phases [17]. To better prepare for violence from civil unrest, protests and terrorism, all the various services mobilized during a mass gathering event (e.g., police, fire services, EMS, venue staff, fire marshals, government agencies) should have their own standard operating procedures for disasters and mass casualty incidents. In that respect, it is important to construct an effective choreography of these various entities. At the same time, contingencies for instant adaptability are also required to provide a more coordinated response to a rapidly evolving dangerous situation. These contingencies need to be anticipated and applied to both organized public events as well as any unauthorized, unplanned or unexpected demonstration or terrorist attacks. This coordination also needs to involve some delineation of what would be the organizer's responsibility and what would be the public authorities' responsibility.

In France, for example, these concerns are often addressed and specified at a national level. If the public attendance includes more than 50,000 persons, it is the state authorities (the "Prefect") who will take the overall lead and incident command and they will validate the proper organization of the preparations, and execute all other actions and logistics for ensuring the security and maintenance of public order. During such large gatherings, a common command post bringing together representatives from each of the various agencies and services is set up at the site, usually in a high level setting to provide an overview and better coordinate, in real time, event management. This includes the management of medical emergencies. Most other nations, including the United Kingdom, Australia, the US, and Germany have similar organizational models or even statutes covering very high-risk events such as Olympics, World Cups, and political conventions (see Chapter 14). In this common type of construct, all police, rescue, and emergency care teams, in and around the perimeter, communicate with (and report to) the site command post. Communications also include direct links to the broader communities' central headquarters and dispatchers so that the command post leaders can directly call upon outside reinforcements if needed and also trigger specific plans to respond to a terrorist attack. Most often, the services/agencies involved and/or the private companies that organize these events are accustomed to working together and usually carryout joint exercises well ahead of time, even for a singular event, or they will do so on a routine basis for recurring events such as weekly professional football or basketball games. This familiarity between the organizers and the public authorities make it more feasible to manage any evolution of the situation in real time and to immediately adapt with necessary measures in the event of natural disaster (e.g., earthquake, lightning), fire, explosion, weapon attack, structural collapse or any other potential mass casualty or mass evacuation incident.

In recent years, many governments provide resources such as bomb sniffing canines or personnel or check the site for radiation with the imminent threats of so-called "dirty bombs," let alone a suitcase nuclear device such as those portrayed in some popular action movies. One important consideration is that the command post itself could become a direct target of terrorists or simply become collateral damage from primary attack. Therefore, redundancy in communications and off-site back-up incident command centers (and staff) need to be planned as well. Accordingly, the same redundancy/back-up concerns and plans will apply to the medical assets for similar reasons. In addition, many terrorists are known to detonate that "come hither" bomb to bring in medical, fire, and law enforcement responders who later become victims themselves when a secondary larger bomb detonation or an automated weapon or chemical attack is launched [2].

Beyond terrorist threats, violence can erupt in sport stadiums such as that observed during professional football (soccer) matches [15]. After the phenomenon of hooliganism emerged, football stadiums in Europe, for example, have now organized strategies to protect matches and the public from such violent persons. In addition to preventive measures (e.g., filtering access, reinforced security checks) and the presence of numerous spotters and stewards, a specific coordinated command post for detecting such incidents is usually established within the stadium in which all services (including medical and security representatives) monitor the public visually (binoculars) or with closed circuit video systems. The goal is to detect early violent behavior, movements, and reactions of the crowd during the match that would trigger an early public safety response and perhaps begin to stage medical responders into a nearby position. This same video surveillance is also very useful in terms of rapidly identifying time-dependent medical emergencies such as a cardiac arrest or severe injury (e.g., fall from a higher level of the stadium or evolving crowd crush). In essence, the medical response system should be integrated into such a surveillance program.

Unauthorized Demonstration or Terrorist Attacks

In the event of unauthorized sudden formation of a protest demonstration or unpredicted terrorist threat or attack, the close coordination of police, EMS, and third party medical support is even more mandatory. As indicated in the stadium model, an incident command post (CP) is established and

representatives of the rescue teams (EMS, police, and fire) are imbedded. Outside such fixed venues, the CP could be the local police headquarters or emergency management operations center (EOC). The CP staff should be in constant contact with all the responding teams on-site. The CP also receives and assimilates the information transmitted by intelligence services, social networks and surveillance video cameras. When available, a mobile command post (specialized truck, van, or bus) dedicated to the incident commander may also be useful for on-site coordination, though potentially a target as well.

Incorporated Tactical Medical Response

During any demonstration or terrorist attack the first mission of the police is to maintain public order and contain perpetrators. To prevent more injuries, medical care transiently becomes a secondary concern, but hopefully becomes a closely aligned priority as soon as possible. Depending on local experience, firefighter rescue teams and/or EMS medical teams may be integrated into the police response either as tactical response teams (TRTs) or as trained operators imbedded directly into special weapons and tactics (SWAT) teams [18, 19]. Lead medical responders may also retain their autonomy in a well-positioned (but safe) standby locations awaiting directives to move in. Regardless, local coordination of the different services is a critical issue since the environment can remain unsecured and the situation continually evolving, especially during the early intervention of law enforcement or rescue forces. In many cases, the perpetrators may not be found for lengthy periods of time, thus compounding the safety concerns for would-be rescuers standing-by before moving in to treat patients. Accordingly, and depending on the scenario, preparations should also include consideration for the potential need for medical responders being protected from chemical attack, tear gas use, "Molotov cocktail," radiation threats, or any other hazardous material.

In the context of a terrorist attack, many countries first employ special police or military units such as SWAT teams to intervene on scene [18]. As mentioned, SWAT or designated counter-terrorist units may often have integrated physicians (Figure 20.1) or specially trained SWAT medics who are imbedded into their teams. These specialized responders can

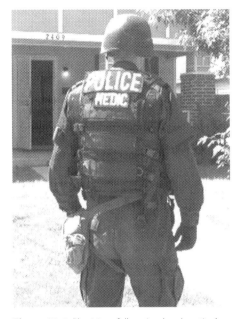

Figure 20.1 Physicians fully trained and routinely responding as a part of counter-terrorism and counter-riot police teams such as special weapons and tactics (SWAT) units can provide demonstrated life-saving functions at violence-ridden incidents such as terrorist attacks [19]

perform tactical medicine duties in which they apply military techniques and combat casualty care within a civilian environment [18, 19]. The primary mission of a tactical medicine specialist is to provide life-saving care under fire for members of the counter-terrorist unit or the victims of the attack. They can also carry out an initial triage of victims. As actual members of the SWAT team, they often carry firearms and they are garbed in tactical protective gear. They are trained in police procedures and they are able to defend themselves and their patients accordingly. They may often be sworn officers or carry the assigned status of deputy police officers, but most are invariably cross-trained as police officers and have emergency response vehicles, carrying SWAT team equipment and they are routinely deployed with the team which makes them more effective in a major event. These medical operators also help to optimize relations between the other emergency services and the police.

In several European countries, some US jurisdictions, Canada, Australia, and elsewhere, it is possible to deploy these specialized medical teams quite rapidly to the site of the violence, including physicians with prehospital and tactical experience. As a general notion, there are well-accepted arguments for not equipping most other EMS team members with bulletproof vests, helmets, or shields if they have not received tactical medicine training. Wearing and carrying such protective items can even be dangerous if it creates a false sense of security for the novice responder in terms of exposing themselves to the risk or even become perceived as "police" targets themselves by the perpetrators. However, doctors and medics who are trained and who are routinely imbedded with SWAT teams can provide invaluable life-saving actions in the so-called hot zones, but they also can provide some other services as well [19]. For example, once the scene is secured, these field-worthy physicians can become part of a strategy that can potentially facilitate triage and immediate life-saving specialized care if needed. The plan can also later include possible on-site treatment of those relatively stable persons whose in-hospital care can be transiently deferred when there is an very large number of casualties and many persons with severe injuries. Transportation to hospitals can also be medically regulated in a manner to address victims' specific needs allowing optimal triage to available and appropriate hospital facilities and not just those nearest to the scene or major to trauma centers when not truly indicated [20].

If an advanced ("far-forward") medical post can be feasibly established, damage control rescue procedures including control of hemorrhage (tourniquets, compressive bandage) can be performed on-site prior to transport if not performed immediately on-scene [21–23]. Mechanisms are now in play to deliver whole blood to such scenes using air medical or ground units and delivery by drones [12-23]. While it is much more preferable to use a load and go system for the most ill or injured, that strategy is still very dependent on the possibility of immediate access of and egress of ambulances and other transport-capable vehicles. As shown in the Clark County sniper incident, the chaos led to displacement of persons by private vehicles, police, and rideshare (Uber/Lyft) drivers [3, 24]. Take-home lessons were that all persons providing public transportation such as these rideshare drivers and police should all learn bleeding control practices such as use of tourniquets, let alone the public at large starting with adolescent school children [24].

At the onset of a terrorist attack or civil disobedience threat, the priority is to neutralize the aggressors, thus security forces (SWAT, military) are in the "leading" position. Once security is restored, the rescue, care, and evacuation of victims should become the leading priority and the other services are "contributing" to that reprioritized medical mission. While these concepts seem intuitive, it is the prospective, preplanned coordination that makes mitigation of these scenarios effective. The organization of large-scale exercises involving all relevant services playing out several complex scenarios is a worthwhile task. Those exercises can include table-top exercises that present multiple scenarios that involve different agencies (or services) each taking a turn as the lead agency for a given issue needing to be addressed. This is not only a good practice to play out several scenarios, but it can also help to educate each of the participants stemming from different disciplines to understand each other's respective critical roles, capabilities and concerns. It also gives opportunity to debate or understand unclear issues and contingencies long before the event. Most importantly, it allows the various on-site leaders to get to know each other ahead of time. This familiarity consistently strengthens team coordination and it creates a new level of trust and understanding that will become invaluable while responding to a real event.

The so-called "load-out" equipment for most responding medical rescue teams should not differ fundamentally from that of usual interventions. Such portable equipment is often placed in a well-balanced backpack with easy-to-access compartments to quickly manage casualties outside of the ambulance. However, in the case of terrorist attacks, it may be critical to have additional supplies for on-site teams that would allow them to rapidly implement hemostasis on many persons (e.g., tourniquets, compression bandages) and to do so on-site as needed. These additional hemostatic devices can be kept in supplemental storage slots on each response vehicle and/or brought to the scene en masse by nearby specialized vehicles stationed at multiple sites throughout the jurisdiction and always ready to respond immediately.

Beyond hemostatic devices, one piece of equipment that should be considered for carrying to the scene in additional batches are finger pulse oximeters which can provide important early and on-going information in far-forward or crowded conditions while patients are being evacuated from the scene (e.g., saturation, heart rate and regularity/pulse rise characteristics). These simple devices can be applied

rapidly and reused for the next round of evacuations. Most tactical responders or medical persons servicing mass gatherings will routinely carry several of these very useful tools.

Perimeters of Care and Evacuation

Defining the perimeter of care and evacuation circuits according to the specific risks is one of the basic principles of mass gathering medicine. In most mass gathering settings, the management of victims with traumatic emergencies has been well-described [16]. However, the intent here is to focus on the management of mass casualties caused by civilian unrest or terrorist attack. To prepare, plan and deploy an effective medical response, several factors must be analyzed.

Knowledge of the site and its preparation: If the care of victims takes place in a known site for a planned event, collecting points for casualties, places to provide emergency care, evacuation routes, and positioning of rescue teams dedicated to these missions are anticipated and planned with redundancies and back-up sites. Conversely, the incident may be an event with either a sudden focused gathering or a migrating demonstration with subsequent violence erupting at some point within the crowd. Therefore, anticipated treatment sites and evacuation routes become much more difficult to establish let alone maintain. Also, the plan may be adapted in real time accordingly to the evolving situation. Instant exchange of information provided by the on-site teams to dispatchers (on back-up radio or phone channels) or to the rapidly established (fixed or mobile) CP and incident commanders are paramount tasks though these communications are often difficult or compromised in the din of the crowd or apparatus noise. Texting tools can be very useful in these situations and video cameras observing strategic areas can also be helpful for the CP or incident commander. If the perpetrators have sequestered themselves in a building or some other known structure, site maps and floor plans may become invaluable and available electronically through fire marshals, the EOC, public works, or other agencies' information systems.

Site Security Constructs: In the context of outright terrorism or active shooter events, responding rescue teams may inadvertently enter into a dangerous area and become victims. Moreover, attacking rescuers is usually a part of terrorist strategy. In general, the majority of EMS teams today are not as well prepared for providing interventions in actively dangerous environments as they should be. In that respect, staging of EMS crews in a safer zone is typically established early on and the timing of eventual EMS access to the scene is controlled by the onsite tactical teams. In France, for example, a national doctrine has been adopted for defining the timing and locations (zones) for interventions in the event of a terrorist attack or a major unsecured threat [25]. Similar constructs have been applied elsewhere such as the National Association of EMS Physicians (NAEMSP) textbook of clinical practice and systems oversight [26]. The "red zone" is the unsecured scene where hunt and seek actions are being conducted or frank, active fighting is transpiring (Figure 20.2). Only trained and authorized law enforcement agencies enter this zone. They can include a medical first-responder team component as previously described who could be trained police officers, tactical medics, or even tactical physicians imbedded as part of the team and specifically trained in tactical, armed and protected medicine actions and response (Figure 20.1) [19]. Nonetheless, even these special operators with medical roles are usually just focused on simple rescue actions for injured police officers (e.g., tourniquets, airway, chest seal). They then can also identify the most severely injured (and yet still potentially salvageable) victims to allow their rapid extraction using

protected tactical team members. Though not a uniformly accepted strategy nor feasible in some scenarios, the basic strategy is to rapidly move such priority patients from the red zone site to a buffer zone called the orange zone – if not directly to transport vehicles in a relatively protected area. Classic rescue and care systems could be deployed to the immediate periphery of that orange zone into the so-called "green zone," which is deemed to be secured and protected (Figure 20.2). In this safer zone, teams can either rapidly transport the victims and/or set up an advanced medical post to provide immediately needed care and better organize the flow of transportation to the most optimal hospitals [2, 26, 27].

This three-zone organization sounds both logical and feasible, but, in real incidents, it is a theoretical construct and somewhat arbitrary in nature. When violence is unexpected, rescue teams may suddenly find themselves in the red zone under fire or exposed to chemicals or radiation. In this case, they should be instructed to leave the affected area as quickly as possible or find a refuge to protect themselves from the shooting, the chemicals or other threats and then communicate their position. This refuge will usually become a protected area and made a priority by the security forces and can evolve into a "sanctuary" to gather nearby victims. As soon as possible, a protected evacuation corridor will be opened to bring the rescue

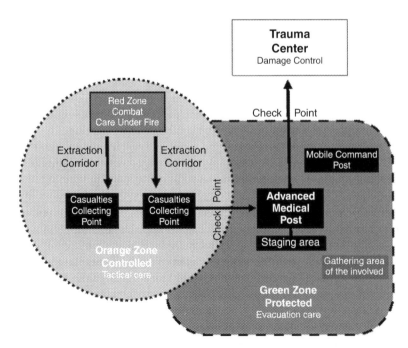

Figure 20.2 In a model of active shooters, perimeters of security are marked by an active under-fire Red Zone, an Orange (buffer) zone for extrication and casualty collection which extends to a Green Zones where patients can be triaged and transported as indicated or even treated on-site in advanced medical outposts

team and victims back to the evolving orange and green zones. This tactic requires control of communications, established procedures and training.

During the multisite 2015 attacks in Paris, for example, the zoning tactic was implemented along with establishment of an advanced medical post both at the Stade de France bombing site and at the Bataclan nightclub shootings. However, it was not feasible to do so for the migrating shooting incidents that moved along the 11th district café terraces. The terrorist use of a mobile commando operation with active shooters only allowed for the organization of protected casualties collecting points. Again, prospective planning, drills, communications, and coordination with police agencies is critical.

Evacuations

Control of evacuation routes and protection of transport to the hospital is a critical and often complex component of civil unrest and tactical medical responses. Panicked fleeing crowds can make it very difficult to access victims and this crowd scenario can considerably slow down evacuation of patients to a trauma center delaying definitive care. During a terrorist attack, ambulances evacuating victims can also become an easy target for assailants and even be hijacked for escape, further malfeasance, or even to seek entry into a hospital. It should be noted that standard ambulances do not provide sufficient protection against assault rifles or long guns and the oxygen tanks carried add an additional risk of fire and explosion. Most importantly, whether inbound or egressing, transport vehicles must not cross the lines of fire or cross the path of the aggressors. On-scene rescuers need to communicate that concern and routing for inbound units as well as those exiting. Uncontrolled and improvised transports (private vehicles, taxis, police) of the casualties to the nearest hospitals is also a risk. Certain health care facilities may not be adapted for major trauma management and, even if they are, they can be easily overwhelmed by mass casualties such as that seen in the Manchester arena and Route 91 Harvest festival tragedies [3, 7].

In the event of a planned gathering, the preparation of the event must include redundant and controlled evacuation routes and back-up routes in case primary routes are obstructed or destroyed. Therefore, the plan must provide for their securing those routes with barriers, checkpoints, control of

crossroads, and enough police to facilitate these purposes. Also, when safety within or around the site is compromised, the evacuations themselves must be protected. Starting from the advanced medical post or evacuation staging areas, ambulances need to be guarded and may need to be grouped in a convoy and escorted by police vehicles. In heavy fire conditions, SWAT tank-like armored vehicles (e.g., Bearcat^{TM}) might serve a purpose in effecting a desperate special evacuation from Red Zones.

Sequestered Evacuations

While safe and efficient traditional individual evacuations of patients to hospitals are one task for medical personnel and security teams to plan, one other consideration is the sequestering of the healthy or lesser injured mass gatherers to a controlled site. For forensic, public health, or other special circumstances, organizers may want to plan and facilitate movement of apparently uninjured attendees to another safe, secured site that is nearby and capable of holding large crowds, especially if perpetrators are not yet apprehended. This could also be appropriate if there is a serious concern for a bomb threat, exposure to something toxic such as a chemical or radiation substance thus prompting the need for further screening and security checks as indicated. In other situations this may apply to rallies or demonstrations and weather becomes an issue.

Communication Tools

Most of the previous discussions have repeatedly highlighted the pivotal component of communications. All responding departments, agencies, and services should have two-way encrypted portable radios, but most often the networks and portable stations of each service are different and they do not communicate well with one another. A common channel also invites overwhelming walk-over chatter and inability to communicate an emergency rapidly when other services are talking. Moreover, they may not be well-heard or transmitted in the din of the event and particularly with loud weapons and vehicle noise [2]. The local command post must be in contact with all stakeholders and responders and pass the necessary information on to all services. The posts must also be able to either send discrete messages or, on some occasions, trigger a general alert. The use of mobile ("cell") phones is not recommended in principle but, in practice, they may still be useful, especially for texting purposes. In the event of terrorist attacks, commercial Wi-Fi and mobile telephone networks may be shut off for security reasons such as the neutralization of the remote triggering of an improvised explosion device (IED). Messaging and groups of social networks (such as WhatsApp) or similar applications can serve as potential alternatives because they are known to most persons and are very easy to use. Variations of these networks, reserved for professionals and operating in specially secured modes, are being placed into practice.

In terms of messaging, one significant concern still remains, namely the messaging coming from within a hostage situation such as the protracted Bataclan or Pulse (Orlando) nightclub incidents or some other hostage crisis. One must be aware that the information being sent from victims' phones may actually be sent by the perpetrators using victims phones with misleading information or the messages may be sent from another site by terrorists to mislead responders and their decision-making.

Hospital Actions

Predesignated receiving hospitals should be able to cope with a mass casualty event, deploy a generic disaster plan and prepare for and establish a secondary triage area at that facility when overwhelmed. This type of organization has been described previously [28, 29]. As most civil unrest and terrorist attacks are unanticipated on a day-to-day basis, the following points should be considered:

- Receiving hospitals must be informed in advance of a violent manifestation or of the possibility of violence occurring and the risk analysis shared.
- Hospitals must continually check that their internal disaster plan is operational including redundant and secured access entrances to the ED, additional parking areas for emergency vehicles and the possibility for a protected additional triage zone at the entrance to the emergency department; this may also involve the need for chemical and radiological decontamination rinses.
- Obviously, back-up plans for mobilizing additional personnel and additional sites of care beyond the ED and operating theaters. Such plans must be tested routinely in unexpected disaster drills.

- Parking and staging of media with both external and internal site (e.g., auditorium) consideration and/or potential use of a pooled photographer [2].
- Prioritizing rapid notification of a violent event to hospitals can save precious time to establish preparations prior to arrival of the first victims, even if none or few eventually arrive.
- The ED team may also be the first to alert other agencies and in-hospital services if there is a spontaneous arrival of victims which may be the first sign of the crisis.
- Direct phone or electronic contact with EMS or police headquarters and dispatchers should be routine on a day-to-day basis and dedicated redundant applications can improve the alert.
- Hospitals may also need to upgrade specific skills as part of their preparations. For example, during the yellow vest demonstrations in Paris, it was necessary to provide additional ophthalmologic, burn, and facial trauma care to manage injuries caused by nonlethal weapons used by the police forces [11].
- Traceability of victims is a very important point as is the confidentiality of their medical chart because this type of event will probably give rise to an investigation and has legal implications
- Areas for identification and reunification with family members.
- The safety of the ED itself should not be underestimated. Screening of victims at the hospital entrance, whether EMS transported or not, should be part of the plan with purposeful exclusion of escorts and definitive separation of victims and potential aggressors [30].

Aggravation and Escalation of Violence

The sudden occurrence during a mass gathering of a violent act can be the prelude to a much more serious crisis. Indeed, a terrorist attack in a stadium can be the first act of a multisite attack as was the case in Paris. Likewise, a violent confrontation between protesters and police can escalate into a citywide riot.

- Reinforcements of medical responders at regional levels must be considered for a mutual aid response. Concentration of all principal forces at the first site of violence can deprive other potential sites from timely response of rescue teams [3].

- In the event of a terrorist attack risk of escalation is particularly high. As soon as the first attack occurs, all public safety services, including EMS, should be informed and prepare for a large-scale multisite attack; this pre-emptive strategy reduces the risk of a second attack such as secondary or time-bomb at the initial scene; secondly, the reinforcements can be rebalanced according to the needs of each site and this better ensures rapid response to the usual vital emergencies beyond and despite the crisis.

- In anticipation of overwhelming numbers of calls made to the public safety answering points (just for information), alternative triage and call handling plan plans should be considered and planned well ahead of time [31].

- For hospitals, anticipation of escalating violence is also part of the response plan. It is prudent not to completely saturate nearby hospitals and, instead, to use more distant hospitals for more stable victims to maintain possibilities for emergency treatment in the event of a second wave of injuries. This strategy was used successfully during the terrorist attacks in Paris [2, 8, 9]. Again, hospitals themselves can also be targeted by the terrorist attack and preemptive precautions must be implemented.

Coordination and All-Services Debriefing

All implemented measures and interventions linked to unauthorized or violent demonstrations will become the subject of a systematic debriefing carried out jointly by all the services with the purpose of analyzing the coordination and the lessons learned to better prepare for further incidents. The medical component is often a critical focus in such debriefings and after-action reports. Participation is an elemental aspect of mass gathering medicine practice.

Ethical, Political, and Social Considerations

Ethical Considerations

Ethical considerations are especially important within the context of a terrorist attack and multiple victims in a mass gathering. Would a terrorist be given priority for care and transport when there are many innocent victims or even injured emergency personnel waiting to be treated or transported [32]?

A conventional ethical viewpoint requires that medical care and transport priorities should always be based solely on strict medical parameters alone. However, in reality, on-site, social, and personal pressures would favor the prioritization of innocent victims and the rescuers. Rescue teams can even be challenged on-scene by bystanders and those accompanying the victims. Confusing matters further, during a terrorist attack, the precise and rapid distinction between a victim and a seriously injured terrorist can also be uncertain. In some cases, the victims may also be known to rescue team members.

In that respect, ethical training for rescue teams, both medical and security, including specialized doctors intervening in the field, is a necessary function.

The ethical standard of care should stand as long as caring for a terrorist or attacker does not impose an additional risk for EMS teams. Injured suicide bombers may detonate themselves upon contact with rescue teams or while medic personnel are rescuing an injured aggressor while under fire.

Whatever the circumstances, the medical management of a terrorist or an aggressor must still meet criteria of humanity and medical priority. Terrorists may be transported to a different facility than that accommodating the victims as along as it affords the same quality of care and constant police surveillance/oversight. Beyond ethical considerations, salvaging terrorists may also lead to important intelligence that will convict others perpetrating the event and prevent subsequent attacks. Also, it can be argued that saving the life of a kamikaze perpetrator contradicts the objectives and philosophies of terrorists. It preserves the proof that the rescue system could not be disabled by the attack and that rescuers continue to maintain impenetrable moral standards.

Other Political and Social Considerations

In the context of a political or social demonstration, it is possible that the emergency personnel may have sympathy (or antipathy) with the demonstrators. It is the responsibility of EMS managers to remind the team members to maintain professional neutrality, both in terms of attitude, actions, and verbal statements, particularly in a world filled with mobile phone videos, body cams, and media coverage. Moreover, the proximity and importance of coordinating close relations between EMS teams and police could cause protesters to doubt the neutrality of EMS and raise doubts about the quality and confidentiality of care that may be rendered. This could lead to uncontrolled evacuations of injured protestors, delay their care, and cause an unforeseen surge of patients into hospitals nearby or even those distant from the site. It can also lead to the emergence of unofficial volunteer rescue workers intervening among the demonstrators and sharing their motivation, but not necessarily having optimal competencies or experience with medical care in a tactical environment.

There are other sociological challenges turned medical challenges that could face the medical responders including what the protesters are wearing or carrying. These could include sharp objects, or signs that injure eyes or cause lacerations to other protesters or could even hurt the rescuer. Sometimes protesters can even carry hidden weapons or use pepper spray. Therefore, the rescuer must be prepared for self-treatment, "buddy-care" for fellow rescuers, and care of protestors and police alike. In recent years, protesters have been found to create new challenges for rescuers such as the use of superglue to stick their hands to surfaces ranging from doorways and coffeehouse countertops to live lanes on motorways and gallery oil paintings [33, 34]. Be it for climate change, animal abuse, or anti-oil protests, these pose new challenges for rescuers, particularly when immobilized protesters need to suddenly use toilets but are unable to use their hands to do so [33, 34].

The bottom line is that medical requests in mass gatherings can pose new challenges that can also conflict with sociological issues. The same ethical considerations should apply.

Psychological and Mental Well-Being

In closing, it must kept in mind that healthcare workers staffing a mass gathering event may not be familiar with or be routinely exposed to violence or even massive trauma, let alone multiple tragic casualties. As frequently mentioned in this chapter, being involved medically in violent rallies or terrorist incidents can lead to serious threats to one's mental well-being in both the short- and long-term [1]. Therefore, appropriate long-term monitoring and care of those participating on-site should become part of the planning and standard procedures for these types of mass gathering incidents [1].

Moreover, it should made clear that feelings of fear, anger, guilt, self-doubt, and second-guessing are "normal" human feelings in such tragedies. Accordingly, it should be articulated that that those emotions should be expected and that there are multiple mechanisms to deal with them [35]. In the meantime, heat-of-the-moment criticisms of others can be inappropriate and, in turn, those received from others should be taken in context for the moment. Immediate blaming of others and feelings of letting others down should be tempered and understood as typical reactions. Appropriate counseling services should be provided and constructed ahead of time with a series of options [35].

References

1. Pepe P. E., Metzger J. C. It Ain't Over Till It's Over: The Unfortunate Evolving Experience with Active Shooters. *Journal of Emergency Medical Services* 2018;**43**:43–48 (special supplement on 2017 *Lessons Learned*).

2. Pepe P. E., Anderson E. Multiple Casualty Incident Plans: Ten Golden Rules for Prehospital Management. *Dallas Medical Journal.* 2001;462–468.

3. Lombardo J., et al. Las Vegas Metropolitan Police Department report of the October 1 (2017) Mass Casualty Shooting event number 171001–3519. Aug 2, 2018. pp 1–187. www.reviewjournal.com/crime/homicides/read-the-final-report-from-las-vegas-police-on-the-oct-1-shooting/. Accessed September 21, 2023.

4. Heaphy T. J., Garney T. T., Dine K. C., et al. Final Report: Independent Review of the 2017 Protest Events in Charlottesville, Virginia. *Hunton and Williams, LLP* report: pp 1–207.

5. Lichfield J. How the Black Bloc seized French streets. *The Post.* December 16, 2020 https://unherd.com/2020/12/how-the-black-blocs-seized-french-streets/. Accessed September 21, 2023.

6. US Department of Justice. One year since the January 6 attack on the Capitol. Publication of the United States Attorney's Office. December 30, 2021. www.justice.gov/usao-dc/one-year-jan-6-attack-capitol. Accessed September 21, 2023.

7. Craigie R. J., Farrelly P. J., Santos R., Smith S. R., Pollard J. S., Jones D. J. Manchester Arena Bombing: Lessons Learnt from a Mass Casualty Incident. *BMJ Military Health.* 2020;**166**(2):72–75. doi: 10.1136/jramc-2018-000930.

8. Hirsch M., Carli P., Nizard R., et al. The Medical Response to Multisite Terrorist Attacks in Paris. *Lancet.* 2015;**386**(10012):2535–2538. doi: 10.1016/S0140-6736(15)01063-6.

9. Carli P., Pons F., Levraut J., et al. The French Emergency Medical Services After the Paris and Nice Terrorist Attacks: What Have We Learnt? *Lancet.* 2017;**16**:390(10113):2735–2738. doi: 10.1016/S0140-6736(17)31590-8.

10. 2016 Berlin truck attack: https://en.wikipedia.org/wiki/2016_Berlin_truck_attack. Accessed September 21, 2023.

11. Thakar H. J., Pepe P. E., Rohrich R. J. The Role of the Plastic Surgeon in Disaster Relief. *Plastic and Reconstructive Surgery.* 2009;**124**:975–981.

12. *Mouvement des gilets jaunes:* Yellow vests protests. https://en.wikipedia.org/wiki/Yellow_vests_protests. Accessed September 21, 2023.

13. de Almeida M. M., von Schreeb J. Human Stampedes: An Updated Review of Current Literature. *Prehospital and Disaster Medicine.* 2019 ;**34**(1):82–88. doi: 10.1017/S1049023X18001073.

14. Duan J., Zhai W., Cheng C. Crowd Detection in Mass Gatherings Based on Social Media Data: A Case Study of the 2014 Shanghai New Year's Eve Stampede. *International Journal of Environmental Research and Public Health.* 2020;**17**(22):8640. doi: 10.3390/ijerph17228640.

15. Khan A. A., Sabbagh A. Y., Ranse J., Molloy M. S., Ciottone G. R. Mass Gathering Medicine in Soccer Leagues: A Review and Creation of the SALEM Tool. *International Journal of Environmental Research and Public Health.* 2021;**18**(19):9973. doi: 10.3390/ijerph18199973.

16. Memish Z. A., Steffen R., White P., et al. Mass Gatherings Medicine: Public Health Issues Arising from Mass Gathering Religious and Sporting Events. *Lancet.* 2019;**393**(10185):2073–2084. doi: 10.1016/S0140-6736(19)30501-X.

17. Koski A., Kouvonen A., Sumanen H. Preparedness for Mass Gatherings: Factors to Consider According to the Rescue Authorities. *International Journal of Environmental Research and Public Health.* 2020;**17**(4):1361. doi: 10.3390/ijerph17041361.

18. Service médical du RAID (Recherche, Assistance, Intervention, Dissuasion) Feedback on terrorist attacks on November 13, 2015. Bataclan's Terrorist Attack Management by the Tactical Medical Support of the French Police. *Annales Françaises de Médecine d'Urgence.* 2016;**6**:3–8. doi :10.1007/s13341-015-0601-4.

19. Metzger J. C., Eastman A. L., Benitez F. L., Pepe P. E. The Life-Saving Potential of Specialized On-Scene Medical Support for Urban Tactical Operations. *Prehospital and Emergency Care.* 2009;**13**(4):528–531. doi: 10.1080/10903120903144940.

20. Carli P., Nahon M., Télion C. Attentats avec sites multiples – la stratégie du "camembert à Paris." *Journal Européen des Urgences et de Réanimation.* 2016;**28**:109–111. English abstract: https://doi.org/10.1016/j.jeurea.2016.05.007.

21. Tourtier J. P., Palmier B., Tazarourte K., et al. The Concept of Damage Control: Extending the Paradigm in the Prehospital Setting. Annales Françaises d'Anesthésie et de Réanimation. 2013;**32**(7–8):520–526. doi: 10.1016/j.annfar.2013.07.012.

22. Pepe P. E., Jui J., Roach J. P., Holcomb J. B. Non-Mechanical Hemostasis in Trauma Care. Part I: Evolving Prehospital Practices and the Role of TXA. *EMS World.* 2020;**49**:15–17.

23. Pepe P. E., Roach J. P., Winckler C. J. State of the Art Review: Prehospital Resuscitation with Low Titer O+ Whole Blood by Civilian EMS Teams – Rationale and Evolving Strategies for Use. In: *2020 Annual Update in Intensive Care and Emergency Medicine.* Vincent J. L. (ed.) Springer International Publishing: Berlin; 2020; pp. 366–376.

24. US Department of Health and Human Services (DHHS), Assistant Secretary for Preparedness and Response (ASPR) Technical Resources, Assistance Center, and Information Exchange (TRACIE). Mass casualty trauma triage: paradigms and pitfalls. July 2019 ; pp. 1–59. https://files.asprtracie.hhs.gov/documents/aspr-tracie-mass-casualty-triage-final-508.pdf. Accessed September 21, 2023.

25. Plan NOVI. https://fr.wikipedia.org/wiki/Plan_Novi. Accessed September 21, 2023.

26. Tan D. K., Siegler J. E. Tactical Emergency Medical Support. In: *Emergency Medical Services: Clinical Practice and Systems Oversight.* Cone D. C., Brice J. H., Delbridge R. T. (eds.). *National Association of EMS Physicians,* Wiley On-line Library, August 18, 2021; Chapter 107. doi: 10.1002/9781119756279.ch107

27. Baker D. J., Telion C., Carli P. Multiple Casualty Incidents: The Prehospital Role of the Anesthesiologist in Europe. *Anesthesiology Clinics.* 2007 ;**25**(1):179–188. doi: 10.1016/j.atc.2006.11.006.

28. Melmer P., Carlin M., Castater C. A., et al. Mass Casualty Shootings and Emergency Preparedness: A Multidisciplinary Approach for an Unpredictable Event. *Journal of Multidisciplinary Health.* 2019;**12**:1013–1021. doi: 10.2147/JMDH.S219021.

29. VandenBerg S. L., Davidson S. B. Preparation for Mass Casualty Incidents. *Critical Care Nursing Clinics of North America.* 2015;**27**(2):157–166. doi: 10.1016/j.cnc.2015.02.008.

30. De Cauwer H., Somville F., Sabbe M., Mortelmans L. J. Hospitals: Soft Target for Terrorism? *Prehospital and*

Disaster Medicine. 2017;**32**(1):94–100. doi: 10.1017/S1049023X16001217.

31. Marrazzo F., Spina S., Pepe P. E., et al. Rapid Reorganization of the Milan Metropolitan Public Safety Answering Point Operations During the Initial Phase of the COVID-19 Outbreak in Italy. *JACEP.* 2020;**1**:1–10. doi: 10.1002/emp2.12245.

32. Gold A., Strous R. D. Second Thoughts About Who Is First: The Medical Triage of Violent Perpetrators and Their Victims. *Journal of Medical Ethics.* 2017;**43**(5):293–300. doi: 10.1136/medethics-2016-103496.

33. Porterfield C. Activists Glue Themselves to a Van Gogh Painting in Climate Change Protests. *Forbes.* June **30**, 2022. www.forbes.com/sites/carlieporterfield/2022/06/30/activists-glue-themselves-to-a-van-gogh-painting-in-climate-change-protest/?sh=5a5251d76c88. Accessed September 21, 2023.

34. National Policing Improvement Agency (NPIA). Dealing with the removal of protestors. FASLANE 365 (produced in Consultation with the Ministry of Defence Police Divisional Support Group of Scotland), 2007: pp. 1–77.

35. Maloney L. M., Hoffman J., Pepe P. E., et al. Minding the Mind in EMS. *EMS World.* Part I. 2020;**49**:38–40; Part II: 2021;50:36–41; Part III: 2021;50:42–46.

Impact of Weather and Climate Change on Mass Gathering Events

John W. Martel and J. Matthew Sholl

Introduction

Meteorological phenomena play a notable role in the rate of patient presentation and types of medical complaints at mass gathering events (MGE) [1]. Multiple weather and climatological events can complicate MGE. Common pathologies include heat- and cold-related injuries, although less common but severe weather events such as lightning and storms can significantly impact these gatherings as well [2]. A variety of environmental considerations that impact mass gathering medicine have been extensively discussed in the literature and should be considered by MGE planners and Medical Directors. These include ambient temperature and humidity, indoor versus outdoor settings, and event geography [3]. It was more recently suggested that these attributes fall under a specific MGE environmental domain that incorporates features such as event geography and weather [4]. Weather has been collectively reported to be the most commonly measured variable in mass gathering research, and includes such elements as temperature, heat index, relative humidity, Wet-Bulb Globe Temperature (WBGT) (which is a composite index of overall heat stress exerted by direct sunlight including ambient temperature, humidity, wind speed, sun angle, and cloud cover), air quality, precipitation, as well as geographical attributes such as altitude, outdoor venue status, and local water availability [1].

While conventional MGE associated with cultural and recreational events may be impacted by meteorological and geographic considerations, there are also some MGE, as well as mass human migration and displacement, that occur specifically due to discrete severe weather disaster events, including hurricanes, tornadoes, flooding, and drought. Even planned annual cultural events like the Hajj in Saudi Arabia regularly pose several medical care challenges due to extremes in temperature, extensive sun exposure, low water availability, and infectious disease risk [5]. In addition to the

anticipated impacts of exposure to weather extremes and discrete severe weather events, the alarming rate of warming associated with global climate change presents an even more daunting challenge to mass gathering medicine. Human activity has been implicated in an estimated 1 degree Celsius increase in average global temperature since the onset of the industrial revolution by 2017, with a continued 0.2 degree Celsius increase per decade at the current rate [6]. Although there is concern for an increase in a variety of severe weather events, including drought, torrential rainfall, and more intense storm patterns, a common hallmark of these events includes humankind's increasing exposure to heat. It has been reported that heat waves across the globe have not only increased in frequency, duration, and cumulative temperature since the mid-twentieth century, but also adversely affect regions already experiencing a disproportionate impact of climate change [7–9]. These changes have already exerted a significant effect on human health, as demonstrated by recent estimations that climate change may be responsible for nearly 40 percent of heat-related deaths worldwide since 1999 [10]. In addition, sunny, high humidity environments may experience elevated WBGT that render evaporative cooling ineffective due to moisture-saturation of surrounding air to a degree that some subtropical regions are now near the limit of human survivability, especially where WBGT > 35 degrees Celsius [11].

Temperature Extremes and Related Illness

Epidemiology of Heat-Related Injury

Heat-related injuries and dehydration are particularly common reasons that patients seek medical care at MGE [2, 12]. While other weather-related events, such as cold or lightning, may also play a role in MGE, heat-related illnesses are the most common weather-related events impacting MGE and therefore should be a particular area of focus in planning and preparation for event organizers. It has been demonstrated that temperatures above 27 degrees Celsius increased patient presentation rate at an MGE; even a single degree increase from 20 degree to 21 degree Celsius led to a more than 10 percent increase in the number of patients requiring medical attention in large group settings [12]. The interface of ambient temperature and humidity is thought to be particularly important, as the number of patients presenting for medical care at another MGE increased by three per 10,000 patrons for every 10 degree Celsius increase in Heat Index [13]. The National Weather Service defines Heat Index as an "apparent temperature" measurement that reflects how hot a location feels when the Relative Humidity (RH) is factored into the actual air temperature [14]. Heat Waves are defined as periods of abnormally high temperatures accompanied by unusually high humidity that last for two or more days [15]. Independent of MGE, heat and heat related illnesses have a tremendous impact on human health. In the US alone there were over 700 heat-related deaths on average per year between 2004–18 [16]. Moreover, another study conducted over a similar timespan reported more than five million annual deaths globally due to extreme heat [17]. Heat burden is determined by location and geography as well as other features. For instance, radiant heat transferred by human-made structures such as pavement and buildings may occur within an Urban Heat Island (UHI) that renders urban areas up to 3.9 degrees Celsius warmer than adjacent rural areas during the daytime and up to 2.8 degrees Celsius warmer at night [18].

Pathophysiology and Treatment of Major Heat Injuries

The International Classification of Disease (ICD) published by the World Health Organization (WHO) details a number of heat-related disorders that are applicable to MGE medicine [19]. *Heat Cramps* generally occur following physical exertion and range in presentation from mild muscle fasciculations to severe muscle cramping. They are associated with perspiration-induced hyponatremia in the setting of heavy perspiration, inadequate hydration or

hydration with free water that does not contain electrolytes, and suboptimal environmental acclimatization in high heat/humidity environments [20, 21]. The painful involuntary muscle spasms have been attributed to hyperchloremic hyponatremia and symptoms improve following rehydration with salt-containing fluids but may worsen with free water intake [22]. Depending on clinical stability, patients experiencing heat cramps at MGE may be effectively managed with common electrolyte-containing sports drink products or isotonic intravenous fluids (IV) in more severe cases. In contrast, Heat Tetany may manifest as a combination of carpopedal spasm, extremity and circumoral paresthesias, and tetany immediately following brief but intense periods of heat stress. It is generally less painful in large muscle groups than heat cramps, and symptoms are thought to be associated with hyperventilation and resulting respiratory alkalosis. Care is supportive, and focused on patient cooling and respiratory rate slowing.

Extremity swelling and skin rash are common patient complaints in hot environments. Heat Edema is a transient swelling of the distal upper and lower extremities following heat exposure that is thought to be due to increased aldosterone secretion in the setting of dehydration that leads to excess water retention as a function of sodium conservation [23]. Symptoms usually resolve within a few days of onset as a result of environmental acclimatization. Compression stockings and extremity elevation are potential supportive measures. Diuretics are not indicated in this context. Heat Rash, known colloquially as prickly heat, occurs with obstruction of sweat ducts that results in inflammation, maculopapular rash, pruritus, vesicles, and localized swelling particularly in locations covered by tight clothing. Wearing loose clothing in high heat/humidity environments is an excellent preventative measure. Pruritus associated with vesicles is treated with antihistamine medications, and if there is evidence of superinfection and cellulitic change, antibiotic coverage for *Staphylococcus aureus* is important.

More severe heat-related illness may manifest as pre-syncope or syncope, escalating to the more classic and concerning heat exhaustion or heat stroke syndromes. Heat Syncope is thought to result from perspiration-induced dehydration that results in peripheral vasodilation and reduced venous return. It must be distinguished from cardiovascular, neurological, or metabolic causes by history. Treatment is similar to prior heat-related disease entities, and is centered around electrolyte-containing oral rehydration and cooling. Heat Exhaustion is generally thought of as a precursor of Heat Stroke, with a suite of additional symptoms beyond those of heat syncope. Headache, tachycardia, nausea, vomiting, dizziness, and malaise may be accompanied by hyperthermia (core temp 38.3–40°C). Treatment is largely supportive, with focus on rehydration with oral or IV fluids, active cooling measures, observation with serial vital sign measurements, and heat avoidance. Patients with refractory symptoms, vital sign abnormalities, or other clinical concerns require hospital transport for further evaluation.

Heat Stroke is a life-threatening syndrome clinically delineated from heat exhaustion by the presence of encephalopathy and is associated with core body temperatures above 40 degrees Celsius. This extreme hyperthermia results from a physiological failure to dissipate heat due to multiple factors including a cascade of cellular and systemic responses, thermoregulatory dysfunction, an acute-phase response, and a heat shock protein response [24]. The constellation of pathophysiologic responses results in the clinical manifestation of central nervous system (CNS) dysfunction and multisystem organ failure (MSOF) [25, 26]. Heat stroke has been further divided into *classic* and *exertional* subtypes.

Classic Heat stroke is considered to be passive, occurring in the context of exposure to extreme heat that is not adequately counterbalanced by physiological heat dissipation mechanisms. It disproportionately impacts elderly, young children, and chronically ill patients, and has been responsible for high mortality during several urban heatwaves in the United States; in July 1995 alone, there were 739 deaths in Chicago attributed to a five-day heat wave [27]. Heat waves are the single most deadly type of extreme weather event [28] and may lead to disproportionately high mortality among the elderly [29]. Rising average temperatures across the globe, increased heat wave incidence, and rapid urbanization that facilitates urban heat island development [30] all lead to the potential for increased incidence of heat related emergencies among vulnerable populations.

Exertional Heat Stroke is caused by episodic activity occurring within environments with high ambient temperatures. Onset of symptoms may occur in as little as sixty minutes depending on the nature of patient exertion and environmental conditions [31]. Although commonly associated with sports-related activities, exertional heat stroke may be encountered during other types of MGE. A variety of MGE factors such as dancing at festivals as well as alcohol and recreational stimulant drug use (e.g., methamphetamine, cocaine) increase the risk of morbidity and mortality associated with exertional heat stroke [32]. In severe cases, a hyperthermia-related inflammatory cascade may occur similar to that seen with systemic inflammatory response syndrome (SIRS) and lead to rapid clinical deterioration, disseminated intravascular coagulation (DIC), MSOF, and death [26, 33].

Independent of the causal factors in the MGE environment, care of heat stroke is focused on rapid cooling with a goal of decreasing core body temperature (CBT) to less than 39 degrees Celsius. Rapid cooling in exertional heat stroke generally relies on ice water immersion and is optimally initiated prior to EMS transport. It is considered the gold standard for rapid lowering of CBT in heat stroke as compared with other methods [34, 35]. Specifically, it has been shown to more effectively lower CBT in hyperthermic patients, is safe and effective in older patients, and should take priority, even over hospital transport, when operationally feasible [36, 37]. There are a variety of adjunct therapies that may be options when logistical challenges preclude access to cold water immersion. These include passive cooling, cool IV administration, topical measures (e.g., ice packs), and use of fans or water misting [38]. However, when risk for heat illness exists, event planners should attempt to include strategies for cold water immersion, rather than less rapid or effective methods of cooling. While patients suffering classic heat stroke will all require hospital transport, event planners may be more selective in transport decisions regarding exertional heatstroke. Transport decision should include features including, but not limited to, response to on scene treatment, persistence of symptoms, underlying past medical history, and potential for alternate diagnosis.

Prevention of Heat Related Injuries During Mass Gathering Events

Event organizers and MGE medical planners should consider strategies for prevention of heat related illness any time there is credible risk. There are numerous individual risk factors that may lead to decreased

Table 21.1 Features leading to increased risk of heat illness

Diminished cardiovascular reserve	Poor levels of cardiopulmonary fitness
Extremes of ages	Dehydration
Increased body mass index	Tight or poorly ventilated clothing
Poor heat acclimatization	Hypohidrosis
Excessive skin scars	Physical exertion
Use of medications that either increase heat production or compromise function of thermoregulatory centers, including:	
Alcohol	Calcium channel blockers
Alpha-adrenergics	Cocaine
Amphetamines	Diuretics
Anticholinergics	Laxatives
Antihistamines	Neuroleptics
Antipsychotics	Phenothiazines
Benzodiazepines	Thyroid agonists
Beta-blockers	Tricyclic antidepressants

heat dissipation, increased heat production, or maladaptation to heat stress. These highly individual features may be difficult for event planners to predetermine, while other risk factors, such as age, may be more easily discoverable. Events focused on elderly or other populations with decreased cardiovascular reserve should pay particular attention to preventive strategies for heat-related illnesses. A list of features leading to increased risk of heat illness can be found in Table 21.1.

Predictive Modeling

A variety of predictive tools exist to aid with identification of event-specific conditions that may lead to increased medical utilization rate (defined by patient presentation to on-scene medical resources or patient transport to hospitals) and are designed to help estimate risk associated with an MGE [2, 4, 39–41]. Most of the weather-related focus of these resources emphasize heat and heat-related factors, rather than other environmental conditions such as cold or lighting. In addition, these predictive models include heat-related features with other, nonenvironmental factors. For example, one such tool includes crowd size, crowd age, crowd intention, and presence of alcohol as elements of a combined patient risk assessment [41]. In review of multiple predictive tools, humidity, temperature, and heat index all appear to be the most reliable factors impacting patient presentation and hospital transfer rates [39]. While the accuracy of these models is uncertain and may lead to over or under estimation of patient impact [39], common features in many of the available predictive models that may lead to increased heat impact include:

(1) Ambient temperatures greater than 26.6 degrees Celsius [42]
(2) Heat Index greater than 32.2 degrees Celsius [41]
(3) WBGT (greater than 30°C for limitation of intense activity in acclimated, fit, healthy participants vs greater than 32.2°C for cessation of all activities) [43]

Multiple predictive tools exist for a variety of different contexts, including sporting events, concerts, and fairs. When applying any of the available predictive tools, using a context-specific predictive tool is advised and may lead to increased accuracy in predictive modeling. Even when applying context-specific predictive tools, event planners and medical directors should understand that no such tool has yet to demonstrate excellent accuracy and more research is necessary to develop externally validated predictive models [39]. There are online resources for predictive calculation of heat index using the NOAA Heat Index Calculator [44].

In addition to predictive modeling, event historical data may also be a useful resource for estimation of medical impact of an event. When available, this information may be more accurate than currently available predictive models and therefore should be incorporated into event planning [45].

Preventive Measures

Heat injury prevention relies on a sophisticated understanding of the current environmental conditions, familiarity with future weather conditions/weather forecasting, development of an on-site response and mitigation plan, and extensive knowledge of both the proximity and resource capacity of local healthcare facilities. In addition, experience suggests that active preventive measures may decrease the number of heat related injuries. Installation of cool water showers and ample access to cold water sources is postulated to have decreased numbers of heat related injuries in pilgrims during the Hajj [40]. Ease of access to other, similar resources, such as misting tents, cooling stations, or shaded areas may have similar effects.

In some cases, a venue site may be located remotely with complex transport to the most proximate health care facility. For instance, the annual Burning Man Festival site is located in the remote Black Rock Desert 120 miles from the nearest medical facility in Reno, NV, and may require complex transfer decisions based on availability of transport assets. Effective preparation essentially entails consideration of such factors through the construction of what tactical medical teams commonly term a Medical Threat Assessment (MTA) [46]. Constructing a similar document is a central component of pre-event planning and consists of several sections, including identification of routine threats, environmental concerns, EMS staging/transport, medical training and equipment, and familiarity with healthcare facility resources. Given that information can be disseminated both widely and rapidly via a variety of social media and broadcast platforms, clear messaging regarding anticipated weather-related issues and clothing/hygiene recommendations will help reinforce participant personal event preparation as well.

With regard to event planning and threshold for event postponement, it has been suggested that the risk of health injury was lowest for WBGT <27.8 degrees Celsius and increased between 27.8 and 30.0 degrees Celsius [47]. Some authors suggest that standardized WBGT cut offs may not account for regional variations in individual acclimatization that occurs with repeated exposures to heat. Instead of a single cut off, these authors suggest that the location of the event must be considered and implement a modification of threshold WBGT's based on the event location [43]. Occupational Safety and Health Administration (OSHA) offers an online text platform WBGT calculator [48] to assist in determining the WBGT. In addition, the University of North Carolina-Chapel Hill has constructed an online graphic WBGT tool that provides morning and afternoon estimates on a daily basis specifically for locations in the humid US southeastern region [49].

Ideally, extended events would not occur in open sunlight during hazardous WBGT conditions and would ensure plenty of shaded space and other preventive measures are available. Several options exist to help ameliorate WBGT where applicable. One such strategy is to consider starting athletic events (e.g., marathons, sports matches) earlier in the morning in order to finish prior to the onset of the warmest period of the day. Another is to hold more extended events (e.g., concerts) after dark when ambient temperatures are cooler. An additional option is to schedule events during cooler seasons as in the case of the FIFA World Cup Qatar 2022, which was moved to November–December 2022 rather than the typical June–July event timing,

Highly reflective, human-made surfaces are considered to be one of the most important determinants of heat island magnitude [50]. It has been reported that increasing reflectivity in urban environments, such as painting surfaces white, can reduce urban air temperatures by 1–3.5 degrees Celsius.[51] Although there is no specific MGE data available, the use of reflective surfaces may be effective in diminishing heat sinks and a key operational consideration for construction of MGE sites and medical facilities in warm environments.

Epidemiology of Cold-Related Injury

In comparison, cold-related injuries have historically exerted less strain on MGE medical resources [3, 52, 53]. However, of particular concern is cold or even cool weather in combination with wet conditions, and the influence of wind chill. Cold injury is not limited to environmental extremes and may occur even in warmer ambient temperatures. Another common mechanism for developing accidental cold injury is when individuals are wearing wet clothing, experience excessive perspiration, or are participating in water-based activities [54–56]. There are four main mechanisms of heat loss: (1) conduction (the direct transfer of heat from warmer to cooler objects); (2) convection (the transfer of heat to or from a gas or liquid that is in motion); (3) radiation (the transfer of heat in the form of electromagnetic energy); and (4) evaporation (the loss of heat by vaporizing liquids) [57]. Individuals may lose heat via conduction simply by sitting or lying on cold ground for extended periods in ambient temperatures less than 20 degrees Celsius by means of radiation if not wearing proper protective clothing, through evaporation when wearing wet clothing and/or undergoing physical exertion, and via convection if conditions are windy. Wind Chill is a term used to describe the relative colder conditions that individuals experience when wind blows on exposed skin to accelerate heat loss at a given temperature [58]. For an ambient temperature of 0 degrees Celsius with wind speed 15mph, the calculated wind chill is –6 degrees Celsius [59]. In addition, larger scale cold weather-related severe weather events such as snow and ice storms may lead to hazardous conditions, motor vehicle accidents, structural collapse, a potential for high patient numbers, and difficult conditions for providing care.

Pathophysiology and Treatment of Major Cold Injuries

Hypothermia (a systemic cold injury) occurs when CBT falls below 35 degrees Celsius and may be associated with focal cold injuries of varying severity ranging from minor cold injuries (such as chilblains) to major cold injuries (such as frostbite). An important consideration for MGE medical response is that populations accustomed to warmer temperatures may be less prepared than those living in colder climates [60]. This is an important consideration for events occurring in colder regions as well as transiently cold locations such as desert or humid temperate environments. Event planners and medical directors should not underestimate the potential for cold related injuries, even during warmer conditions. Prolonged exposure to wet conditions, even when temperatures are mild, may lead to significant numbers of cold injuries [56].

In mild hypothermia (core body temperature [CBT] 32–35°C) physiological compensatory mechanisms remain intact and work to counter heat loss. Hallmarks of the response include sympathetic discharge with associated increased O2 consumption, tachycardia, peripheral vasoconstriction, and vigorous shivering response. Moderate hypothermia (CBT 28–32°C) often presents with confusion, dysarthria, decreased fine motor skills, and ataxia as well as a reduced shivering response. In contrast, patients with severe hypothermia (CBT< 28°C) exhibit no shivering response, dramatic decrease in cognitive and neurological functioning, and increased hemodynamic instability (bradycardia, hypotension). Accurate measurement of core temperature may not be available or even feasible during a response to a mass casualty incident. Event medical responders should therefore be familiar with the clinical characteristics of each level of hypothermia [57].

Once identified, the key to treatment of hypothermia is prevention of further heat loss, rewarming, and, especially in moderate or severe cases, hospital transfer. Protection from further heat loss and passive rewarming are generally sufficient in mild cases with an intact shivering response, and consists of protection from cold, wet environments, removing wet clothing, providing vapor barriers and insulation as well as moving toward a warm environment, when available. Active external rewarming may be added, even in mild cases, to augment the shivering response. Shivering response augmentation has the advantage of increasing patient comfort and decreasing energy utilization. In the absence of a shivering response, active external rewarming measures are necessary, and in the MGE environment may consist of devices such as warm water bottles, blankets, and large heating pads (electric or chemical). It has been suggested that external heating sources should range 49–45 degrees Celsius in order to maintain efficacy while avoiding skin burns [61]. When external heat sources are used, they should be applied to the axilla, chest, and back (in that order) which are areas of highest conductive heat transfer [57]. Where resources permit, a combination of warm, humidified supplemental oxygen (up to 42°C) and IV (up to 40°C) may supplement the above techniques of rewarming and decrease heat loss association with respiration [62]. This should not be the primary means of rewarming however, as heat exchange through the respiratory system is not effective as a solitary rewarming method [57]. Warm showers or baths should be avoided as these both can increase peripheral blood flow, potentially leading to hypotension and cardiovascular collapse. In addition, small heat packs (such as those used for hand and feet warming) should not be used as a primary means of rewarming moderate to severe hypothermic patients. These devices do not offer sufficient systemic heat to appreciably rewarm the core and may cause local thermal burns as temperatures of these devices may exceed the above recommendations for maximum temperatures [57]. However, these devices may still have a role in MGE planning and preparation as they can help prevent localized cold injuries to the extremities and enhance patient comfort.

Patients with evidence of severe hypothermia should be handled gently as CBT in this case lowers the threshold for ventricular tachydysrhythmias. Should severe hypothermia be encountered and complicated by cardiac arrest, standard resuscitative measures such as CPR and airway management should proceed in the same manner as for non-hypothermic patients. Initial attempts at defibrillation should proceed as normal. If unsuccessful, subsequent attempts at defibrillation should be paused until the patient's CBT reaches 30 degrees Celsius. In addition, there is limited evidence on the effects of medications during hypothermic cardiac arrest and most experts recommend that vasopressor medications in particular be held until the patient's CBT reaches 30 degrees Celsius [57].

Extremity injuries are also common complications of cold exposure. Less severe manifestations include trench foot, chilblains, frostnip, cold urticaria. Trench foot is a soft tissue injury that occurs due to prolonged exposure to wet conditions above the freezing point. Feet appear pale with associated skin breakdown, and the condition is generally painless. Treatment is generally supportive and includes providing dry socks and footwear as well as rewarming where appropriate [63, 64]. Chilblains, Cold Urticaria, and Frostnip are nonfreezing superficial cutaneous injuries. Each is characterized by early paresthesias and numbness. Chilblains are erythematous lesions that form due to prolonged vasoconstriction in the setting of cold exposure, cold urticaria stem from a hypersensitivity reaction over exposed skin, and frostnip is considered a reversible frostbite precursor. In each case symptoms are self-limited, and treatment is focused on rewarming and supportive care [65, 66].

In contrast, Frostbite is a freezing injury characterized by formation of ice crystals that may lead to cell lysis and microvascular occlusion [66]. The degree of reversibility and ultimate severity depends on multiple factors including ambient temperature, duration of freeze injury, and exposure to freeze-thaw cycling [54]. Commonly affected areas include digits, distal upper and lower extremities, nose, ears, and face. Frostbite is commonly classified in four "degrees" based on acute findings as well as advanced imaging after rewarming. First degree frostbite presents with numbness and erythema. Patients will demonstrate white or yellow firm and slightly raised plaques in the area of injury and may have minor associated edema. Second degree frostbite presents with superficial blisters containing a clear or milky fluid surrounded by erythema and edema. Third degree frostbite presents with hemorrhagic blisters signifying deeper tissue damage. Finally, fourth degree frostbite presents with necrosis signifying injury that extends through the demis and involves subcutaneous tissues. As the above classification scheme requires rewarming and advanced imaging, some authors have proposed a simpler, two-tiered classification scheme for use in acute phases of care. Superficial injuries are inclusive of the acute findings noted in first- and second-degree frostbite, including pallor, waxy, firm skin as well as edema, erythema, and clear blisters. These injuries are suggestive that the patient will experience no to minimal tissue loss. Deep injuries include the acute findings noted in third- and fourth-degree frostbite, including hemorrhagic blisters and early necrosis. These findings suggest more extensive injury and are more likely to be associated with tissue loss [67]. Initial treatment for all types is similar and consists of active rewarming via warm water bath (37–39°C) or warm compresses in areas that may be more difficult to immerse. In the event that freeze-thaw cycle is a concern, it is recommended that the impacted areas remain frozen [67]. All cases should be placed in clean, dry dressings, and transferred to a local hospital for further evaluation. Although more severe cases may ultimately require surgical debridement after ultimate demarcation, early intervention is generally not indicated until the extent of irreversible damage is known [65].

If risk of severe cold injury exists, event planners and EMS System leaders should consider transport to facilities with advanced diagnostics and therapies, for example, thrombolytics in the case of frostbite or sophisticated rewarming capabilities in the case of severe hypothermia.

Prevention of Cold-Related Injuries During Mass Gathering Events

Predictive Modeling

As with heat-related injuries, a variety of tools exist to aid with prediction of environmental conditions. Specifically, there is an online resource for predictive calculation of wind chill calculator [68]. Fewer predictive models exist to help estimate risk of cold-related MGE injuries and less evidence exists regarding cut off temperatures at which event plans should be altered. The state of Minnesota's "Special Event and Mass Gathering Medical Care Plan" uses temperatures of 4.4 degrees Celsius and −17.7 degrees Celsius (inclusive of wind chill and the availability of onsite sheltering) as elements of a risk calculator along with additional event characteristics including peak attendance, ethanol consumption, crowd age, crowd intent, and transport time to hospitals. In this reference, intermediate risk is assigned to temperatures –17.7 degrees Celsius to 4.4 degrees Celsius and severe risk is assigned to temperatures less than 17.7 degrees Celsius [69]. With fewer available predictive models available to determine risk for cold-related injuries, event planners and medical directors should consider available historical experience to assist with planning and preparation.

Preventive Measures

As with planning and preparing for heat related injuries, understanding of the current environmental conditions, familiarity with future conditions through weather forecasting resources, development of an on-site response, and mitigation plans are key. While less evidence exists for the preventive possibilities of warming tents, sheltering, insulative layers, warm beverages, adequate nutrition resources, and other measures, focused empiricism would suggest these measures should hold some potential for averting cold injuries. The availability of such measures should be widely publicized during the event. Social messaging should focus on ensuring adequate insulative layers, removal of wet clothing and replacement with dry clothing, minimizing physical contact with cold ground (either sitting or laying down) for extended periods without adequate without insulation (clothing, blankets), minimizing skin exposure to the cold, donning dry, wind-resistant clothing, and staying out of the direct wind as much as possible.

Other Meteorological Phenomena That Adversely Impact MGE

Epidemiology of Lightning-Related Injuries

In addition to temperature, wind, and heavy precipitation, lightning strikes are one particular vulnerability posed by warm season outdoor MGE. Lightning flash and subsequent cloud-to-ground strikes can be difficult to predict and may lead to considerable morbidity and mortality ranging from cardiac arrest to secondary injury as a function of difficult evacuation conditions and stampede. It has been suggested that lightning occurs up to 100 times per second worldwide, and that more than 2,000 thunderstorms are active at any given moment across the globe [70]. A recent study suggested that cloud-to-ground lightning strikes might increase by as much as 12 percent per degree of warming (Celsius). Increasing average annual temperatures have led to a 50 percent increase in lightning strikes over the twenty-first century within the continental US alone [71]. Accelerated increase in ambient temperature and humidity anticipated with climate change are expected to power the moisture, instability, and uplift that drive thunderstorm formation.

A lightning strike can carry a voltage exceeding 10 million volts with up to 110 amperes of current, be as hot as 30,000 Kelvin, and may be either positively or negatively charged, thereby leading to risk both direct and alternating current injuries [72]. Fortunately, strikes involving direct contact with an object struck by lightning are the least common. Instead, most victims contact lightning via *splash* emitted laterally after an adjacent object is struck or from *ground current* that contacts an individual after traveling from the point of a ground strike. More than one individual may be impacted by a single strike [73]. Victims have up to a 30 percent mortality rate compared with other electrical injuries and it has been reported that up to three quarters may have chronic sequelae associated with the injury [74]. Many lightning injuries occur in rural, remote, and outdoor settings [75]. Victims are primarily males and approximately 30 percent of strikes are fatal [76]. Lightning injuries are the second most common weather-related cause of mortality, and deaths commonly occur as a result of current-induced dysrhythmia and diaphragmatic tetany leading to respiratory arrest.

Pathophysiology and Treatment of Lightning-Related Injuries

A wide variety of injuries are observed as a result of lightning strikes. Although severe burns are uncommon due presumably to the short duration of current exposure [77], there have been reports of full thickness burns at entry and exit points, although deep tissue necrosis rarely occurs [76]. However, given that skin tends to conduct electrical current to deeper tissues, the relatively small, well-demarcated burns at entry or exit points cannot be reliably used to estimate total body surface area (TBSA) affected [78]. Fern-like burn patterns (Lichtenberg Figures) and linear burns are common patterns. Most such burns are superficial and readily heal. Routine burn care is appropriate, including removal of burned and smoldering clothing to prevent further injury.

Other injuries that occur following current exposure include ocular cataract formation, rhabdomyolysis, renal failure, compartment syndrome [79] and transient paralysis and paresthesias referred to as *keuranoparalysis* that mimic traumatic spinal injury [75]. In addition, barotrauma secondary to blast wave exposure can result in ocular injuries, tympanic membrane rupture and deafness, solid organ injury [74, 77] as well as a variety of blunt trauma injuries due to falls or after contact with debris.

Most concerning is the disproportionate adverse impact that lightning strike has on myocardial tissue, including dysthymias, myocardial infarction and stunning, ventricular failure, cardiogenic shock, and cardiac arrest that require emergent management and Advanced Cardiac Life Support interventions. Lightning strike is essentially a massive direct current discharge capable of instantaneously depolarizing the entire myocardium and inciting a catecholamine surge [91]. This can result in life-threatening asystole due to myocardial depolarization, ventricular fibrillation (VF), and ventricular tachycardia (VT), in addition to the more common and transient occurrence of sinus tachycardia and atrial fibrillation.

Unlike standard triage, which minimizes care of cardiac arrest patients during mass casualty events, patients suffering cardiac arrest as a consequence of lightning injuries should have resuscitative resources directed toward their care. This concept is commonly known as Reverse Triage. It is recommended in the mass casualty response to cardiac arrest related to lightning strike as return of circulation commonly precedes the resolution of respiratory arrest related to direct CNS injury or diaphragmatic tetany. While evidence for the benefit of this practice is limited, available case reports and experience suggests that patients supported during the period between ROSC and resolution of respiratory arrest may survive if resuscitative measures are provided [81].

Preventive Measures to Avoid Lightning-Related Injuries During MGE

While there is evidence that lightning strike fatalities have decreased over the last thirty years due to a wide variety of protective protocols [82] and improved weather forecasting, there will always exist a degree of measured risk of lightning injuries in the outdoor MGE environment.

The 30–30 Rule for Lightning Safety at Outdoor Events is one tool that may be utilized to mitigate this threat [83]. Using this model, if there is a lightning to thunder "flash-to-bang count" under thirty seconds indicating the presence of lightning within ten kilometers, all activity should cease, and the crowd should be moved to designated shelter space. When available, participants should seek shelter in the largest available enclosed building away from doors and windows. No structure provides complete protection from lightning strikes, however the interior of large buildings are safest [81]. If not available, participants should seek shelter inside metal or hard topped vehicles with windows and doors closed. If neither option exist, participants should seek shelter in structures with hard roofing. Tents, tarps, or similar structures do not provide protection from lightning strikes [81]. In addition, open structures, such as overpasses, may protect against rain, but will not protect against lightning side splash or ground current and therefore should be discouraged as shelter options [81]. Some authors suggest that sheltering in structures such as deep caves may diminish but not eliminate risk of lightning strike [84]. Risk of lightning ground current may be exacerbated if the floor of the cave is saturated with water [85]. Long tunnels share similar characteristics as deep caves. Both structures should not be considered primary shelter options, as neither offer complete protection from lightning injury. When choosing shelter locations, event planners and medical directors should consider the potential size of the party requiring shelter and implement strategies to identify and access participants in case of medical emergency while the group remains sheltered. Larger group sizes, rapidity of evacuation, and limited sheltering resources all raise the potential for injuries during transit to shelters. Such injuries may be mitigated by ensuring shelter sizes that are able to accommodate the maximum size of anticipated participants as well as early and clear messaging once sheltering is deemed necessary.

In addition, there is a recommended thirty-minute pause prior to resumption of the event. These events remain difficult to predict and rapidly respond to given that the average lead time for a supercell thunderstorm, capable of producing tornado conditions, is approximately eleven minutes. For this reason, extra caution must be exercised in geographical areas with high heat islands and unstable weather patterns. It is crucial that event organizers and medical planners maintain situational awareness regarding risk of lightning strike. Once risk escalates, widespread messaging via diverse platforms (including social media) should occur directing attendees to seek shelter in predesignated sites, avoid sheltering under trees, and to refrain from using mobile phones and earbuds (intracranial injury risk) or carrying metallic objects (e.g., jewelry, keys) [82].

Beyond Conventional MGEs: Climate Crisis, Conflict, and Migration

While much of the discussion above has been geared toward planning for MGE and anticipating associated weather challenges, the progressive warming of Earth has also forced a revisioning of what defines mass gathering and requires evolution of the response to such events. Climate change is a well-documented complex agent of political instability and conflict [86]. The term global warming was introduced in 1975, and attributed pronounced environmental temperature increases to rising atmospheric carbon dioxide levels [87]. The terminology has since transitioned to climate change, and it is considered to be a driving force of resource competition, human conflict, and migration. A combination of climate change and biodiversity loss have been predicted to expose much of the world's population to increasing food insecurity, water scarcity, weather extremes, conflict, degrading environmental quality, and emerging or reemerging infectious diseases [88]. In 2010, it was reported that climate change would represent one of the most serious issues with respect to expansion of pathogens into new geographic regions [89]. The year 2020 was tied for the hottest year on record, and during this year alone, six Atlantic storms exceeded rapid intensification thresholds as a result of warming temperatures, leading to both more storm-related damage as well as leaving less time for populous areas to prepare or evacuate. In Central America, increasing storm intensity, drought, and environmental degradation have exacerbated political instability and increased the likelihood of large-scale human migration [90].

Climate change, exceeded only by infectious disease, is considered to be one of the two highest impact threats the world is facing over the next ten years [91]. Climate change places additional strains on already marginalized communities. Social supports and resources, including medical resources, may be scarce

at baseline and MGEs have the potential to disproportionately impact these communities further. Despite significant gains made in decreasing both extreme poverty and global hunger since the 1990s, food insecurity has risen dramatically in recent years in concert with climate change and conflict [92]. The majority of the world's population that experiences food insecurity resides in Low- and Middle-Income Countries (LMIC) disproportionately impacted by fragility and conflict, climate change, and economic crisis [93].

These issues are considered major forces driving migration in Latin America, Sub-Saharan Africa, and Southeast Asia, and may generate up to 143 million additional "climate migrants" by 2050 [94]. In 2017 alone, there was an estimated 86.5 million forcibly displaced persons worldwide, with approximately one third uprooted by sudden, severe weather events while the remainder considered a function of humanitarian crises often linked with slower onset events such as desertification, rising sea levels, shifting precipitation patterns and environmental pollution that combine to diminish biodiversity [95]. A looming global food crisis, vast economic and health disparities, political conflict, increasing weather-related disasters, and resulting large-scale human migration may place historic demands upon the resources of neighboring countries, regions that exist along mass migration routes such as Central America and Mexico, and High Income Countries (HIC) such as the United States and European Union [96]. The very definition of what comprises a MGE may change with time via the formation of large, slow-moving transnational gatherings that may travel together for weeks, months, or years before settling en masse near international borders for more extended periods of time. It will be important for nations that exist both along mass migration routes as well as those that serve as final destinations to have the ability to effectively respond to sudden large gatherings requiring shelter, food, hydration, and medical care resources for thousands of people at a time with short notice. For instance, in late 2021 up to 14,000 immigrants rapidly gathered to shelter under an international bridge in Del Rio, TX (population 35,000); the size and rate of formation for this gathering posed an unprecedented stress on the local resources available for humanitarian response as well as an associated sanitation crisis [97]. Without adequate planning and logistical support, the rapid evolution of large gatherings has the potential to disastrously outstrip local resources.

Summary

A variety of important environmental considerations impact the safe execution of mass gathering events that hinge upon both comprehensive planning and effective medical response. While it is impossible to eliminate all potential health threats associated with MGE that occur in a dynamic meteorological environment, it is possible to mitigate risk considerably by using a combination of event specific predictive tools and, when available, historic experience. In addition, the conventional concept of MGE as primarily cultural or recreational in nature is increasingly being questioned as climate change has rendered some areas of Earth nearly uninhabitable, spurred an increased degree of global resource inequity, and driven conflict that has led to the most widespread and sustained pattern of migration in human history. This challenges long held ideas of what constitutes MGE, and will require a forward-thinking, proactive approach to address an increasing number of human aggregations that present significant challenges for provision of care in the context of increasingly intense weather events.

References

1. Hutton A., Ranse J., Gray K. L., Turris S. A., Lund A., Munn M. B. Environmental Influences on Patient Presentations: Considerations for Research and Evaluation at Mass-Gathering Events. *Prehospital and Disaster Medicine.* 2019;**34**(5):552–556. doi: 10.1017/ S1049023X19004813.

2. Soomaroo L., Murray V. Weather and Environmental Hazards at Mass Gatherings. *PLoS Curr.* 2012;**4**: e4fca9ee30afc4. doi: 10.1371/4fca9ee30afc4.

3. Milsten A. M., Maguire B. J., Bissell R. A., Seaman K. Mass-Gathering Medical Care: A Review of the Literature. *Prehospital and Disaster Medicine.* 2002;**17**(3):151–162. doi: 10.1017/s1049023x00000388.

4. Arbon P. The Development of Conceptual Models for Mass-Gathering Health. *Prehospital and Disaster Medicine.* 2004;**19**(3):208–212. doi: 10.1017/ s1049023x00001795.

5. Aitsi-Selmi A., Murray V., Heymann D., McCloskey B., Azhar E. I., Petersen E., et al. Reducing Risks to Health and Wellbeing at Mass Gatherings: The Role of the Sendai Framework for Disaster Risk Reduction. *International Journal of Infectious Diseases.* 2016;**47**:101–104. doi: 10.1016/j. ijid.2016.04.006.

6. Intergovernmental Panel on Climate Change. Special Report on Global Warming of 1.5°C. www.ipcc.ch/ sr15/chapter/chapter-1/. 2018. Accessed July 1, 2021.

7. Kjellstrom, T. Impact of Climate Conditions on Occupational Health and Related Economic Losses: A New Feature of Global and Urban Health in the Context of Climate Change. *Asia Pacific Journal of Public Health.* 2016;**28**:28S–37S. doi: 10.1016/ j.ijid.2016.04.00610.1177/1010539514568711.

8. King A. D., Harrington J. The Inequality of Climate Change from 1.5 °C to 2 °C of Global Warming. *Geophysical Research Letters.* 2018;**45**:5030–5033. doi: 10.1029/2018GL078430.

9. Perkins-Kirkpatrick S. E., Lewis S. C. Increasing Trends in Regional Heatwaves. *Nature Communications.* 2020;**11**:3357. doi: 10.1038/s41467-020-16970-7.

10. Vicedo-Cabrera A. M., Scovronick N., Sera F., et al. The Burden of Heat-Related Mortality Attributable to Recent Human-Induced Climate Change. *Nature Climate Change.* 2021;**11**:492–500. doi: 10.1038/ s41558-021-01058-x.

11. Dangerous humid heat extremes occurring decades before expected. NOAA Research News May 8, 2020. https://research.noaa.gov/article/ArtMID/587/ArticleID/ 2621/Dangerous-humid-heat-extremes-occurring-dec ades-before-expected. Accessed July 1, 2021.

12. Kman N. E., Russell G. B., Bozeman W. P., et al. Derivation of a Formula to Predict Patient Volume Based on Temperature at College Football Games. *Prehospital and Emergency Care.* 2007;**11**(4):453–457. doi: 10.1080/00207450701537043.

13. Perron A. D., Brady W. J., Custalow C. B., Johnson D. M. Association of Heat Index and Patient Volume at a Mass Gathering Event. *Prehospital and Emergency Care.* 2005;**9**(1):49–52. doi: 10.1080/ 10903120590891976.

14. National Weather Service. "Heat Index Chart." www .weather.gov/safety/heat-index. Accessed December 5, 2021.

15. National Weather Service Glossary. "Heat Wave." https://forecast.weather.gov/glossary.php?letter=h. Accessed December 8, 2021.

16. Vaidyanathan A., Malilay J., Schramm P., Saha S. Heat-Related Deaths: United States, 2004–2018. *Morbidity and Mortality Weekly Report.* 2020;**69**(24):729–734. doi: 10.15585/mmwr.mm6924a1.

17. Zhao Q., Guo Y., Ye T., Gasparrini A., Tong S., Overcenco A., et al. Global, Regional, and National Burden of Mortality Associated with Non-Optimal Ambient Temperatures from 2000 to 2019: A Three-Stage Modelling Study. *Lancet Planet Health.* 2021;**5**(7):e415–25. doi: 10.1016/S2542-5196(21) 00081-4.

18. United States Environmental Protection Agency. Heat island effect. 2021. www.epa.gov/heatislands. Accessed August 15, 2021.

19. World Health Organization. International statistical classification of diseases and related health problems (ICD). 2021. www.who.int/standards/classifications/classification-of-diseases. Accessed 5 August, 2021.

20. Bergeron M. F. Exertional Heat Cramps: Recovery and Return to Play. *Journal of Sport Rehabilitation.* 2007;**16**(3):190–196. doi: 10.1123/jsr.16.3.190.

21. Schwellnus M. P., Drew N., Collins M. Muscle Cramping in Athletes: Risk Factors, Clinical Assessment, and Management. *Clinical Journal of Sports Medicine.* 2008;**27**(1):183–194. doi: 10.1016/j.csm.2007.09.006.

22. Lau W. Y., Kato H., Nosaka K. Effect of Oral Rehydration Solution versus Spring Water Intake During Exercise in the Heat on Muscle Cramp Susceptibility of Young Men. *Journal of the International Society of Sports Nutrition.* 2021;**18**(1). doi: 10.1186/s12970-021-00414-8.

23. Montain S. J., Laird J. E., Latzka W. A., Sawka M. N. Aldosterone and Vasopressin Responses in the Heat: Hydration Level and Exercise Intensity Effects. *Medicine and Science in Sports and Exercise.* 1997;**29**(5):661–668. doi: 10.1097/00005768-199705000-00012.

24. Lipman G. S., Eifling K. P., Ellis M. A., Flavio G. G., Otten E. M., Grissom C. K. Wilderness Medical Society Practice Guidelines for the Prevention and Treatment of Heat Related Illness: 2014 Update. *Wilderness and Environmental Medicine.* 2014;**25**: S55–65. doi: 10.1016/j.wem.2014.07.017.

25. Leon L. R., Bouchama A. Heat Stroke. Compr Physiol 2015;**5**:611–647. doi: 10.1002/cphy.c140017.

26. Epstein Y., Yanovich R. Heatstroke. *N Engl J Med.* 2019;**380**(25):2449–2459. doi: 10.1056/NEJMra1810762.

27. Whitman S., Good G., Donoghue E. R., Benbow N., Shou W., Mou S. Mortality in Chicago Attributed to the July 1995 Heat Wave. *Am J Public Health.* 1997;**87**(9):1515–1518. doi: 10.2105/ajph.87.9.1515.

28. Office of Climate, Water, and Weather Services. Weather fatalities 2018. National Weather Service. www.nws.noaa.gov/om/hazstats.shtml; 2019. Accessed August 15, 2021.

29. Yang J., Zhou M., Ren Z., Mengmeng L., Boguang W., De Li L., et al. Projecting Heat-Related Excess Mortality Under Climate Change Scenarios in China. *Nat Commun* 2021;**12**:1039. doi: 10.1038/s41467-021-21305-1.

30. Kravchenko J., Abernethy A. P., Fawzy M., Lyerly H. K. Minimization of Heatwave Morbidity and Mortality. *Am J Prev Med.* 2013;**44**:274–282. doi: 10.1016/j.amepre.2012.11.015.

31. Hosokawa Y., Adams W. M., Belval L. N., et al. Exertional Heat Illness Incidence and On-Site Medical Team Preparedness in Warm Weather. *Int J Biometeorol.* 2018;**62**: 1147–1153. doi: 10.1007/s00484-018-1517-3.

32. Nadesan K., Kumari C., Afiq M. Dancing to Death: A Case of Heat Stroke. *J Forensic Leg Med.* 2017;**50**:1–5. doi: 10.1016/j.jflm.2017.05.008.

33. Huisse M. G., Pease S., Hurtado-Nedelec M., Arnaud B., Malaquin C., Wolff M., et al. Leukocyte Activation: The Link Between Inflammation and Coagulation During Heatstroke – A Study of Patients During the 2003 Heat Wave in Paris. *Crit Care Med.* 2008;**36**:2288–2295. doi: 10.1097/CCM.0b013e318180dd43.

34. Proulx C. I., Ducharme M. B., Kenny G. P. Effect of Water Temperature on Cooling Efficiency During Hyperthermia in Humans. *J App Physiol.* 2003;**94**:1317–1323. doi: 10.1152/japplphysiol.00541.2002.

35. Casa D. J., McDermott B. P., Lee E. C., Yeargin S. W., Armstrong L. E., Maresh C. M. Cold Water Immersion: The Gold Standard for Exertional Heatstroke Treatment. *Exerc Sport Sci Rev.* 2007;**35**:141–149. doi.org: 10.1097/jes.0b013e3180a02bec.

36. Douma M. J., Aves T., Allan K. S., Bendall J. C., Berry D. C., Chang W. T., et al. First Aid Cooling Techniques for Heat Stroke and Exertional Hyperthermia: A Systematic Review and Meta-Analysis. *Resuscitation.* 2020;**148**:173–190. doi: 10.1016/j.resuscitation.2020.01.007.

37. Ito C., Takahashi I., Kasuya M., Oe K., Uchino M., Nosaka H., et al. Safety and Efficacy of Cold-Water Immersion in the Treatment of Older Patients with Heat Stroke: A Case Series. *Acute Med Surg.* 2021;**8**(1):e635. doi: 10.1002/ams2.635.

38. Bouchama A., Dehbi M., Chaves-Carballo E. Cooling and Hemodynamic Management in Heatstroke: Practical Recommendations. *Crit Care.* 2007;**11**(3): R54. doi: 10.1186/cc5910.

39. Van Remoortel H., Scheers H., De Buck E., Haenen W., Vandekerckhove P. Prediction Modelling Studies for Medical Usage Rates in Mass Gatherings: A Systematic Review. *PLoS ONE.* 2020;**15**(6): e0234977. doi: 10.1371/journal.pone.0234977.

40. Alkassas W., Rajab A. M., Alrashood S. T., Khan M. A., Dibas M., Zaman M. Heat-Related Illness in a Gathering Event and the Necessity for New Diagnostic Criteria: A Field Study. *Environ Sci Pollut Res.* 2021;**28**:16682–16689. doi: 10.1007/s11356-020-12154-4.

41. Hartman N., Williamson A., Sojka B., et al. Predicting Resource Use at Mass Gatherings Using a Simplified

Stratification Scoring Model. *Am J Emerg Med.* 2009;**27**:337–343. doi: 10.1016/j.ajem.2008.03.042.

42. Milsten A. M., Seaman K. G., Liu P., Bissel R. A., Maguire B. J. Variables Influencing Medical Usage Rates, Injury Patterns, and Levels of Care for Mass Gatherings. *Prehosp Disaster Med.* 2003;**18**(4):334–346. doi: 10.1017/S1049023X00001291.

43. Grundstein A., Williams C., Phan M., Cooper E. Regional Heat Safety Thresholds for Athletics in the Contiguous United States. *Appl Geogr.* 2015;**56**:55–60. doi: 10.1016/j.apgeog.2014.10.014.

44. National Weather Service Weather Prediction Center, Heat Index Calculator. 2020. www.wpc.ncep.noaa.gov/html/heatindex.shtml. Accessed 28 August, 2021.

45. Schwartz B., Nafzinger A., Milsten A., Luk J., Yancey A. Mass Gathering Medical Care: Resource Document for the National Association of EMS Physicians Position Statement. *Prehosp Emerg Care.* 2015;**19**(4):559–568. doi: 10.3109/10903127.2015.1051680.

46. Toffoli C. A. Optimizing Mission-Specific Medical Threat Readiness and Preventive Medicine for Service Members. US Army Med Dep J 2018; Jan-Jun (1-18):49-54.

47. Cooper E. R., Ferrara M. S., Casa D. J., et al. Exertional Heat Illness in American Football Players: When Is the Risk Greatest? *J Athl Train.* 2016;**51**(8):593–600. doi: 10.4085/1062-6050-51.8.08.

48. Occupational Health and Safety Administration. OSHA Outdoor WBGT Calculator. 2008. www.osha.gov/heat-exposure/wbgt-calculator. Accessed August 28, 2021.

49. Convergence of Climate-Health-Vulnerabilities. Wet Bulb Global Temperature (WBGT) Tool. University of North Carolina. 2021. https://convergence.unc.edu/tools/wbgt/. Accessed August 28, 2021.

50. Tong S., Prior J., McGregor G., Shi X., Kinney P. Urban Heat: An Increasing Threat to Global Health. *BMJ.* 2021;**375**:n2467. doi: 10.1136/bmj.n2467.

51. Memon R. A., Leung D. Y., Chunho L. A Review on the Generation, Determination and Mitigation of Urban Heat Island. *J Environ Sci (China).* 2008;**20**(1):120–128. doi: 10.1016/s1001-0742(08)60019-4.

52. Thompson J. M., Savoia G., Powell G., Challis E. B., Law P. Level of Medical Care Required for Mass Gatherings: The XV Winter Olympic Games in Calgary, Canada. *Ann Emerg Med.* 1991;**20**:385–390. doi: 10.1016/s0196-0644(05)81660-9.

53. Grissom C. K., Finoff J. T., Murdock D. C., Culberson J. Nordic Venue Medical Services During the 2002 Winter Olympics. *J Emerg Med.*

2005;**30**:203–210. doi: 10.1016/j.jemermed.2005.08.005.

54. Petrone P., Asensio J. A., Marini C. P. In Brief: Hypothermia. *Curr Probl Surg.* 2014;**51**(10):414–415. doi: 10.1067/j.cpsurg.2014.07.005.

55. Zafren K. Out-of-Hospital Evaluation and Treatment of Accidental Hypothermia. *Emerg Med Clin North Am.* 2017;**35**(2):261–279. doi: 10.1016/j.emc.2017.01.003.

56. Gocotano A. E., Dico F. D., Calungsod N. R., Hall J. L., Counahan M. L. Exposure to Cold Weather During a Mass Gathering in the Philippines. *Bull World Health Organ.* 2015;**93**(11):810–814. doi: 10.2471/BLT.15.158089.

57. Dow J., Giesbrecht G. G., Danzl D. F., Brugger H., Sagalyn E. B., Walpoth B., et al. Wilderness Medical Society Clinical Practice Guidelines for the Out-of-Hospital Evaluation and Treatment of Accidental Hypothermia: 2019 Update. *Wilderness Environ Med.* 2019;**30**(45):S47–S69. doi: 10.1016/j.wem.2019.10.002.

58. National Weather Service Glossary, "Wind Chill." 2009. https://forecast.weather.gov/glossary.php?letter=w. Accessed December 8, 2021.

59. National Weather Service, "Wind Chill Chart." www.weather.gov/safety/cold-wind-chill-chart. Accessed December 8, 2021.

60. Healy J. D. Excess Winter Mortality in Europe: A Cross Country Analysis Identifying Key Risk Factors. *J Epidemiol Community Health.* 2003;**57**(10):784–789. doi: 10.1136/jech.57.10.784.

61. Vanggaard L., Eyolfson D., Xu X., Weseen G., Giesbrecht G. G. Immersion of Distal Arms and Legs in Warm Water (AVA Rewarming) Effectively Rewarms Mildly Hypothermic Humans. *Aviat Space Environ Med.* 1999;**70**(11):1081–1088.

62. Danzl D. F., Pozos R. S. Accidental Hypothermia. *N Engl J Med.* 1994;**331**(26):1756–1760. doi: 10.1056/NEJM199412293312607.

63. Olson Z., Kman N. Immersion Foot: A Case Report. *J Emerg Med.* 2015;**49**(2):45–48. doi: 10.1016/j.jemermed.2015.02.040.

64. Michael T. P. Chapter 208: Cold Injuries. In: Tintinalli's Emergency Medicine: a Comprehensive Study Guide, 8th Edition. Tintinalli J. E., Stapczynski J. S., Ma O., Yealy D. M., Meckler G. D., Cline D. M. (eds.). New York: McGraw-Hill Education; 2016. https://accessemergencymedicine.mhmedical.com/Content.aspx?bookid=1658§ionid=109385692. Accessed December 10, 2021.

65. Jurkovich G. J. Environmental Cold-Induced Injury. *Surg Clin North Am.* 2007;**87**(1):247–267. doi: 10.1016/j.suc.2006.10.003.

66. Imray C., Handford C., Thomas O., Castellani J. Nonfreezing Cold-Induced Injuries. In: *Auerbach's Wilderness Medicine*, 7th Edition. Auerbach P. S., Cusing T. A., Harris S. (eds.), New York: Elsevier; 2016. pp. 222–234.

67. McIntosh S. E., Hamonko M., Freer L., Grissom C. K., Auerbach P. S., Rodway G. W., et al. Wilderness Medical Society Practice Guidelines for the Prevention and Treatment of Frostbite. *Wilderness Environ Med.* 2011;**22**(2):156–166. doi: 10.1016/j.wem.2011.03.003.

68. National Weather Service Weather Prediction Center, Wind Chill Calculator. 2020. www.wpc.ncep.noaa.gov/html/windchill.shtml. Accessed August 28, 2021.

69. State of Minnesota Special Event and Mass Gathering Medical Care Plan. 2015. https://mn.gov/boards/assets/Special%20Events%20and%20Mass%20Gathering%20Matrix%20-%202015_tcm21-28041.pdf. Accessed on 8 December, 2021.

70. National Oceanic and Atmospheric Administration. Science on a Sphere. Lightning Flash Rate. https://sos.noaa.gov/catalog/datasets/lightning-flash-rate/. Accessed December 10, 2021.

71. Romps D. M., Seeley J. T., Vollaro D., Molinari J. Projected Increase in Lightning Strikes in the United States due to Global Warming. *Science.* 2014;**346**(6211):851–854. doi: 10.1126/science.

72. Jensen J. D., Thurman J., Vincent A. L. *Lightning Injuries.* Treasure Island (FL): StatPearls Publishing; 2021. www.ncbi.nlm.nih.gov/books/NBK441920/. Accessed September 22, 2023.

73. Kubilius D., Rimdeika R. Simultaneous Lightning Injury in a Group of People: Case Report. *Burns.* 2012;**38**(3):e9–12. doi: 10.1016/j.burns.2012.01.011.

74. Ritenour A. E., Morton M., McManus J. G., Barillo D. J., Cancio L. C. Lightning Injury: A Review. *Burns.* 2008;**34**(5):585–594. doi: 10.1016/j.burns.2007.11.006.

75. Cherington M., Yarnell P. R., London S. F. Neurologic Complications of Lightning Injuries. *West J Med.* 1995;**162**(5):413–417.

76. Zafren K., Durrer B., Herry J. P., Brugger H., ICAR and UIAA MEDCOM. Lightning Injuries: Prevention and On-Site Treatment in Mountains and Remote Areas. Official Guidelines of the International Commission for Mountain Emergency Medicine and the Medical Commission of the International Mountaineering and Climbing Federation (ICAR and UIAA MEDCOM). *Resuscitation.* 2005;**65**(3):369–372.

77. Lederer W., Kroesen G. Emergency Treatment of Injuries Following Lightning and Electrical Accidents. *Anaesthesist.* 2005;**54**(11):1120–1129. doi: 10.1007/s00101-005-0910-6.

78. Moore K. Hot Topics: Electrical Injuries in the Emergency Department. J Emerg Nurs. 2015;**41**(5):455–456. doi: 10.1016/j.jen.2015.06.006.

79. Watanabe N., Inaoka T., Shuke N., Takahashi K., Aburano T., Chisato N., et al. Acute Rhabdomyolysis of the Soleus Muscle Induced by a Lightning Strike: Magnetic Resonance and Scintigraphic Findings. *Skeletal Radiol.* 2007;**36**(7):671–675. doi: 10.1007/s00256-006-0247-5.

80. Jost W. H., Schönrock L. M., Cherington M. Autonomic Nervous System Dysfunction in Lightning and Electrical Injuries. *NeuroRehabilitation.* 2005;**20**:19–23.

81. Davis C., Engeln A., Johnson E., et al. Wilderness Medical Society Practice Guidelines for the Prevention and Treatment of Lightning Injuries: 2014 Update. *Wilderness Environ Med.* 2014;**25**(4 Suppl): S86–95. doi: 10.1016/j.wem.2014.08.011.

82. Elsom D. M., Webb D. C. J. Deaths and Injuries from Lightning in the UK, 1988–2012. *Weather.* 2014;**69**:22–26. doi: 10.1002/wea.2254.

83. Zimmermann C., Cooper M. A., Holle R. L. Lightning Safety Guidelines. *Ann Emerg Med.* 2002;**39**(6):660–664. doi: 10.1067/mem.2002.124439.

84. Gookin J. Backcountry lightning risk management. 21st Annual Lightning Detection Conference. April 19–20, 2010, Orlando, Florida.

85. O'Keefe Gatewood M., Zane R. D. Lightning Injuries. *Emerg Med Clin North Am.* 2004;**22**(2):369–403. doi: 10.1016/j.emc.2004.02.002.

86. Mach K. J., Kraan C. M., Adger W. N., Buhaug H., Burke M., Fearon J. D., et al. Climate as a Risk Factor for Armed Conflict. *Nature.* 2019;**571**(7764):193–197. doi: 10.1038/s41586-019-1300-6.

87. Broeker W. Climate Change: Are We on the Brink of a Pronounced Global Warming? *Science.* 1975;**189**(4201):460–463. 189;4201:460–463. doi: 10.1126/science.189.4201.460.

88. Watts N., Amann M., Arnell N., Ayeb-Karlsson S., Belesova K., Boykoff M., et al. The 2019 Report of the Lancet Countdown on Health and Climate Change: Ensuring That the Health of a Child Born Today Is Not Defined by a Changing Climate. *Lancet.* 2019;**394**(10211):1836–1878. doi: 10.1016/S0140-6736(19)32596-6.

89. Cutler S. J., Fooks A. R., van der Poel W. H. Public Health Threat of New, Reemerging, and Neglected Zoonoses in the Industrialized World. *Emerg Infect Dis.* 2010;**16**(1):1–7. doi: 10.3201/eid1601.081467.

90. Office of the Director of National Intelligence. Annual Threat Assessment of the Intelligence Community. April 9, 2021. www.dni.gov/files/ODNI/documents/

assessments/ATA-2021-Unclassified-Report.pdf. Accessed April 12, 2021.

91. World Economic Forum. The Global Risks Report 2021 16th edition, Insight Report. 2021. www.weforum.org/reports/the-global-risks-report-2021. Accessed January 24, 2021.

92. Food and Agriculture Organization of the United Nations. The State of Food Insecurity in the World. 2015. www.fao.org/3/a-i4646e.pdf. Accessed January 24, 2021.

93. Food and Agriculture Organization of the United Nations. The State of Food Insecurity and Nutrition in the World. 2019. www.fao.org/3/ca5162en/ca5162en.pdf. Accessed January 24, 2021.

94. Rigaud K. K., de Sherbinin A., Jones B., et al. *Groundswell: Preparing for Internal Climate Migration.* World Bank: Washington, DC; 2018. h

ttps://openknowledge.worldbank.org/handle/10986/29461. Accessed January 24, 2021.

95. Podesta J. The Climate Crisis, Migration, and Refugees. July 25, 2019. The Brookings Institution. Washington, DC. www.brookings.edu/wp-content/uploads/2019/07/Brookings_Blum_2019_climate.pdf. Accessed January 24, 2021.

96. United Nations Development Programme. Human Development Report 2020, The Next Frontier: Human Development and the Anthropocene, December 15, 2020. http://hdr.undp.org/sites/default/files/hdr2020.pdf. Accessed January 24, 2021.

97. Flores R., Sanchez R. Thousands of Migrants Held in Squalor Under Texas Bridge. 2021. www.cnn.com/2021/09/17/us/texas-del-rio-migrants-bridge/index.html. Accessed January 24, 2022.

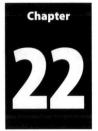

Occurrence of the Mass Casualty Incident at a Mass Gathering Event

Gregory A. Peters and Eric Goralnick

Introduction

The mass casualty incident (MCI) has been defined as "an event that overwhelms the local healthcare system, where the number of casualties vastly exceeds the local resources and capabilities in a short period of time" [1]. Mass gathering events (MGE) are particularly vulnerable to MCIs, given that mass gathering events include large numbers of potential patients in a setting that is typically marked by limited resources, barriers to accessing resources, or otherwise relatively decreased efficiency of services within an unusual setting. Therefore, the prospect of the MCI is a key consideration for any mass gathering event. The purpose of this chapter is to outline the foundational principles related to managing the occurrence of the MCI at a mass gathering event. In this chapter, we will address the following goals: (1) summarize the special challenges presented by the MCI in the setting of a mass gathering; (2) review the guiding principles for preventing and reducing risk of the MCI at a mass gathering; (3) review the proper framework for optimizing MCI readiness at a mass gathering; (4) describe the key principles related to MCI response at a mass gathering; and (5) outline the recovery process following the MCI at a mass gathering.

Special Challenges Associated with the MCI Scenario at Mass Gathering Events

The MCI marks the ultimate challenge for emergency medical services (EMS) at a mass gathering event. The MCI is defined by an acute mismatch between the supply of EMS and the demand for those services, and MGE tend to present a scene in which this balance is inherently strained by incidents that might otherwise be relatively minor in the context of routine EMS.

The number of patients involved in an MCI marks the most obvious way to measure the degree of challenge presented to emergency services and local agencies, but "MCI Multipliers" can also increase the degree of challenge for responders. "MCI multipliers" (Table 22.1) can multiply the magnitude of an MCI beyond its size (i.e., number of patients) and are often inherently associated with the MGE setting [2].

MGE tend to limit options for access and egress for emergency services personnel. First, MGE are often marked by local traffic that will delay both response time and transport time before and after the one-scene patient encounter, respectively. Second, MGE are often located in places with limited highway access points, particularly in the case of large temporary venues, which can further delay the delivery of definitive care. After contending with these factors to gain access to the venue (e.g., arriving at the entrance to an outdoor stadium hosting a concert), additional on-scene factors may prolong scene time. The need to maintain security can delay patient contact at multiple points prior to initiating the patient encounter. Efficient transport is typically limited at MGE (particularly in the absence of dedicated transport-capable units on standby assignment), such that emergency vehicles are unable to establish direct access to patients, requiring emergency responders to walk or use other slower alternative modes of transportation to complete travel to a scene (e.g., carts, bicycles, scooters), which also typically limits access to equipment and materials (which must be carried or transported via modes of transportation with less carrying capacity). Similarly, patient extrication can be complicated by crowding or an unusual setting (e.g., the extrication of a sick or injured passenger via the narrow aisle on an airplane that cannot accommodate typical EMS stretchers). In the case of structural compromise (e.g., stage collapse

Table 22.1 Mass casualty incident (MCI) multipliers typically associated with the mass gathering setting

1. Limitations to access/egress, with respect to direct patient contact and the greater scene
2. Other simultaneous incidents that drain available resources
3. Unfamiliarity with the scene, local facilities, or MCI practices among responders
4. Unfamiliarity with the scene, local facilities, or MCI practices among patients/bystanders
5. Self-deployment of bystanders as responders
6. Complications related to crowd management
7. Limited hospital resources or other strains on local receiving facilities
8. Limited emergency services resources or other strains on local agencies
9. Impediments to communication and need for communication between multiple agencies
10. Complicated assessment of scene safety for responders

at a concert), a deliberate insult (e.g., terrorist bombing), or a disaster within an enclosed setting (e.g., fire in a theater), mass gathering events are likely to include a greater number of patients, which complicates search and rescue efforts and translates to delayed extrication. Moreover, the "scene size-up" and safety assessment practices that mark a critical aspect of any emergency response tend to be extremely dynamic and complex at MGE, which can require the recruitment of additional emergency services personnel to secure the scene, necessitate frequent ongoing reassessments of a dynamic and poorly secured scene, present increased risk to responders, and introduce further delays to extrication and patient care. These causes of prolonged prehospital time can lead to increased severity of illness or injury, increased number of patients associated with an ongoing insult, and worse patient outcomes [3].

One key principle of MGE is to provide appropriate care to patients while protectively stewarding the resources of local emergency services agencies and receiving facilities. MGE often draw volumes of people from outside the local area, which can in some cases multiply the local population manifold times its number of permanent residents. For example, the population of Mecca in 2010 was roughly 1.5 million [4], but the Saudi Arabian government estimated more than 3.1 million attendants at the 2012 Hajj pilgrimage (the majority of whom traveled from outside the country) [5]; as another example, State College, Pennsylvania has only 42,000 permanent residents according to the 2010 US Census [6], but its Beaver Stadium alone has held as many as 110,000 spectators for Pennsylvania State University football games [7]. In cases of MGE such as these, if local resources such as hospital capacity and emergency services staffing are determined only by typical population statistics, even routine medical needs alone for

such volumes of visitors would easily overwhelm local resources. Unintended consequences of redistribution of EMS may also negatively impact routine care [8]. For example, an analysis of Medicare beneficiaries who were admitted to marathon-affected hospitals (eleven different city marathons) with acute myocardial infarction or cardiac arrest on marathon dates had longer ambulance transport times before noon (4.4 minutes longer) and higher thirty-day mortality than beneficiaries who were hospitalized on non-marathon dates.

The occurrence of the MCI in an ordinary setting tends to call for the mobilization of resources and activation of plans to rapidly increase hospital capacity and emergency response staffing (e.g., surge plans). However, the planning of a mass gathering within a region might already call for a surge in staffing at receiving facilities and the consumption of hospital capacity to accommodate the increase in routine patient volume, which can directly challenge a system's MCI management by depleting the local reserves upon which surge plans are predicated. Similarly, mass gatherings can threaten the exhaustion of local human resources in the out-of-hospital sector. For example, large numbers of local police might be deployed to routine mass gathering event-related duties such as securing the perimeter of an event and managing local traffic, and the introduction of an MCI in the absence of extensive mutual aid or other contingency planning can produce the dilemma to choose between the maintenance of these routine crowd management operations at a time when crowd management is especially critical, versus the reassignment of these personnel to securing a safe scene to facilitate direct response to the MCI itself. These common features of MGE can easily exacerbate the mismatch between supply and demand for resources and rapidly increase the magnitude of an MCI.

MGE tend to present an unfamiliar setting to patients, bystanders, and responders. Such events often draw attendants from outside the region, as well as outside personnel (e.g., EMS, law enforcement, and fire services from an outside service area) to assist in event-related operations. There are multiple challenges to MCI management that are introduced by the unfamiliar setting of a MGE. First, the MCI tends to present an unfamiliar situation to participants in the mass gathering, which can stimulate confusion, fear, and panic. These factors can create an unpredictable and unsafe scene, which can cause delays, additional casualties, and increased need for additional security and other emergency personnel. Moreover, patients in an unfamiliar setting and situation might underestimate or overestimate the need for attention to their injury or illness due to anxiety or concerns regarding the scene or receiving facility. For example, a patient with chest pain and significant risk factors might try to avoid a crowded and potentially dangerous emergency department (ED) during response to a mass shooting, whereas an otherwise young and healthy patient with minor injuries might seek ED transport from the scene of a multiple-vehicle collision because others are doing the same. Second, a scene that is unfamiliar to EMS can present additional complications. In these situations, familiarity with available supplies and equipment in the field is key, as well as familiarity with the communication system and incident command system (ICS). These situations can lead to suboptimal prehospital care (e.g., delays in patient contact, unsafe extrication due to inability to find appropriate equipment), as well as suboptimal assignment of receiving facilities (e.g., unfamiliarity with local hospital capabilities, such as burn, trauma, or pediatric centers). Preparation for these common issues can drastically improve MCI management at the mass gathering event.

The crowd itself at the MGE presents additional complications for MCI management that include safety risks for responders, the self-deployment of bystanders as responders, and the potential of a human stampede. Crowd management, also discussed in a separate chapter, will be covered but a few challenges warrant highlighting as it relates to MCI. The unfamiliar situation of the MCI coupled with a MGE, can lead to confusion, fear, and panic among the crowd, which can create a volatile and unsafe scene. Human stampedes lie at the most

extreme end of this spectrum and have massive potential to multiply the severity of any MCI. In addition, the self-deployment of bystanders as responders can present additional challenges if such bystanders are insufficiently trained for the incident at hand, poorly equipped, emotionally, or cognitively compromised (e.g., distracted, intoxicated, attending to a loved one), or nonadherent to proper scene-safety practices. These factors can interfere with patient care and jeopardize the safety of emergency services personnel.

Finally, MGE tend to introduce complications that impede communication during the response to an MCI. Temporary venues can have limited signage and poor infrastructure for mass communication with the crowd (e.g., lack of intercom systems) that can be critical for directing the crowd and maintaining order. High levels of noise can be associated with the crowd, or the MCI type itself (e.g., fire, weather, explosives), leading to impaired verbal communication. The MCI itself can lead to technical barriers (e.g., power outage), or the communication system can be strained by increased use (e.g., overwhelmed radio frequencies). Similarly, the typical use of online medical direction can be strained by rapid surges in demand from EMS in the field. MCI events often require efficient communication between multiple agencies in the field (e.g., fire, police, EMS), as well as communication between those agencies and local receiving facilities (e.g., updates regarding hospital capacity and capabilities), and the mass gathering setting can introduce personnel unfamiliar with proper practices (including how to communicate across the different communication systems used by these entities) in the absence of adequate preparation. A framework for approaching the various MCI multipliers associated with mass gathering events will be described later in this chapter.

Epidemiology and Classification

Discussion of the occurrence of the MCI at mass gathering events tends to call to mind recent famous incidents of this sort: notable examples include the 2015 Garissa University College Attack in Kenya, the November 2015 Paris Attacks, the 2004 República Cromañón Nightclub Fire in Argentina, the 2015 Mina Stampede during the Hajj at Mecca, the 2017 Las Vegas Shooting in the US, and the 2013 Boston Marathon Bombing in the US. In addition to such large-scale tragedies that generate international headlines, smaller MCIs frequently occur at MGE and require the swift execution of emergency response efforts that are often multidisciplinary and complex.

The most comprehensive report in the literature to describe the epidemiology of the MCI at mass gathering events was published by Turris, Lund, and Bowles in 2014 [9]. Turris et al. performed an extensive literature review spanning 1982–2012 that captured 290 mass gathering events at which ten or greater casualties associated with a single incident were reported in the literature. In decreasing order of prevalence, these MCI occurrences at mass gatherings were attributed to the following mechanisms: crowd management and control incidents (e.g., stampedes, riots; 162 of 290, 56 percent), fires and electrical injuries (15 percent), structural collapses (13 percent), deliberate insults (e.g., projectiles and explosives; 9 percent), motorized vehicle crashes (5 percent), and toxic exposures (2 percent). The authors also acknowledged extreme weather conditions as another common cause of the MCI at mass gatherings, but all such examples happened to be excluded from the study, primarily due to the relatively high minimum casualty criterion. These findings indicate the diverse nature of MCI occurrences at mass gathering events, and the preponderance of crowd-related incidents – which were most common at sporting events and religious gatherings in particular – highlights the potential for the MCI to multiply rapidly in severity and scale in the setting of a densely crowded and often unfamiliar setting. Therefore, mass gatherings will typically require preparation for a wide variety of possible incidents, and particular attention must be invested in effective crowd control practices.

Importantly, there is wide variation in the number of casualties used to operationally define the MCI for research, with many studies suggesting that as few as three patients associated with a single incident can be sufficient to overwhelm routine emergency response practices (particularly in the context of an intentional insult such as an active shooter incident). It is also helpful to recall that the special challenges associated with mass gathering events inherently add strain to emergency response efforts. Therefore, it would be reasonable to use a lower minimum threshold to define the MCI at MGE, which would of course yield a much greater incidence that would more accurately reflect the commonplace nature of relatively smaller MCIs that nevertheless present a difficult test for EMS at MGE and for local agencies (and likely result in

a different distribution of MCI mechanisms). Further study of this topic is needed, and researchers are currently working to establish integrated international databases to facilitate the study of MCI occurrences, including those at mass gathering events.

Finally, which patterns of illness and injury are associated with the MCI mechanisms that most commonly occur at mass gathering events? In the acute phase, trauma tends to account for the vast majority of patient needs [10]. These needs range from sprains and abrasions to hemorrhage, severe burns, crush injuries, and fractures that can be associated with altered mental status, airway compromise, respiratory distress, or hemodynamic instability. Polytrauma can rapidly consume human and other resources, both at the scene and at receiving facilities, especially in the context of the MCI. Despite limited research focused on the injury and illness patterns associated with the heterogeneous category of the MCI at mass gatherings, evidence in the literature suggests that the fairly vast majority of patients associated with MCI occurrences of this sort are traumatic in nature [10]. The MCI at a mass gathering is often marked by a minority of critically injured polytrauma patients, along with a majority of patients with minor injuries associated with falls, such as ankle sprains, abrasions, and other musculoskeletal or cutaneous injuries, but these patterns vary widely by specific MCI mechanism. Common injury patterns should be factored into planning as it applies to choose of equipment and materials (e.g., vehicles, extrication equipment, medical supplies), education and preparation of offline medical direction (e.g., medical training, protocols), and identification of appropriate receiving facility options (e.g., trauma centers, burn centers).

Although trauma accounts for the majority of the literature associated with the MCI at mass gatherings, acute illness must also be considered. MCI occurrences associated with infectious outbreaks – such as a cluster of fifty Legionnaire's disease cases associated with a single cruise ship – and widespread foodborne illness – such as nearly 300 hospital presentations for severe gastrointestinal symptoms associated with a single lunch at a local religious event – have been reported, particularly at prolonged events such as religious gatherings or cruises [11, 12]. Mass environmental exposures have been reported, such as at Woodstock 1994 when a precipitous drop in temperature of 30 degrees Fahrenheit occurred while heavy rain and hail poured over a crowd of 350,000 ill-prepared concert attendants and led to mass exposure to wet and cold conditions (and reports of emergency services personnel trudging through mud up to their knees), with EMS treating and transporting an estimated 150 patients per hour from the concert [13, 14]. Bioterrorism events and unintentional mass-poisonings, such as the Tokyo subway sarin attack in 1995, are less common but can carry grave consequences and present novel challenges [15]. Of course, psychological repercussions of the MCI can be experienced by patients, bystanders, on-scene responders, hospital providers, and even the public exposed through media, such as in the case of the Boston Marathon bombing in 2013 [16]. Finally, in the longer-term phase of MCI management, chronic conditions – such as diabetes mellitus and reactive airway disease – among a potentially larger than normal census of patients can consume local resources and should be factored into hospital planning as well.

A Framework for Approaching the MCI at a Mass Gathering Event

In 2002, New Zealand passed the Civil Defense Emergency Management (CDEM) Act to mitigate the nation's risk related to public hazards of all types by improving infrastructure for emergency services and planning for disaster management [17]. The 2002 CDEM Act introduced the "Four Rs" approach to CDEM – also known as the emergency management cycle – that has been adopted across the globe as a framework for approaching the MCI [18]. The emergency management cycle includes reduction (i.e., prevention, mitigation), readiness (i.e., preparedness), response, and recovery, as summarized in Figure 22.1.

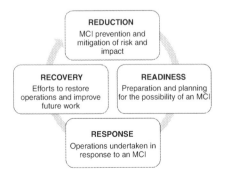

Figure 22.1. The emergency management cycle

This organizational framework will lend itself to the structure of this chapter, mapping onto the pre-, intra-, and post-MCI phases of management with explicit consideration of the special mass gathering context.

Reduction

In the four Rs paradigm, reduction refers to the process by which sources of risk are identified and analyzed in order to inform the prevention or mitigation of risk associated with particular hazards. Applied to the mass gathering context, the reduction phase of the emergency management cycle is an ongoing process that conceptually underlies the readiness phase, in which careful analysis of risks associated with the venue, the surrounding geography and environmental factors, the purpose and audience associated with the event, the sociopolitical context of the event, and the timing of the event (e.g., time of day, season, recent events) can inform the steps that must be taken to promote readiness and mitigate risk. The majority of hazard analysis and risk assessment should occur prior to initiation of the MGE, but should also continue throughout the event and be informed by post-event review practices, particularly for recurring events.

Environmental and Geographical Factors: In MGM, place and time for the event are often chosen by other parties, at best with input from experts in mass gathering medicine and public safety. In any case, any setting comes with sources of risk that should be identified and mitigated beforehand. Risk of environmental exposure is largely determined by choice of place and time but can be mitigated in some cases. For example, a report on 2011 Burning Man, an annual several-day music festival in the summer at Black Rock Desert in Nevada, described the anticipation of significant risk of heat and sun exposure, but only found eleven cases of hyperthermia among more than 50,000 attendants in part due to successful mitigation of environmental risk through preventative measures such as availability of potable water and ample access to protective shelter [19]. If a weather-related emergency is forecasted, such as a hurricane or extreme blizzard, reduction considerations must include not only the increased risk of MCI, but also the increased challenges for EMS that would respond. Unfortunately, alterations to the venue that would mitigate risk might be limited, but postponement can be considered in serious cases. For example, severe blizzards led to the postponement of multiple events during the 1984 Olympic Winter Games after discussion between event leadership and consultants in the domain of public safety and MGM [20].

Local geography must be considered as well. Complicated access or egress related to the MCI scene or greater venue can increase the magnitude of an MCI by delaying both patient contact and delivery of definitive care. The number and location of highway exits must be considered, and strategic deployment of traffic control can reduce the impact of an MCI. Similarly, access and egress within the venue directly factors into the impact of an MCI, and associated risk can be mitigated by clear signage and intelligent positioning of on-site medical facilities and casualty collection points. Finally, analysis of the surrounding geography, including available resources and impediments to accessing them, must be conducted and can further inform proper readiness. For example, the 2010 MV Mavi Marmara attack took place aboard a crowded Comoros-based ship nearly 200 miles off-shore, and diligent planning that accounted for the risk of such an incident – including plans for the dispatch of medically trained responders from nearby vessels – successfully reduced the impact of this MCI [21].

The 2010 Love Parade disaster in Duisburg, Germany demonstrates the powerful role that geographical and engineering considerations – particularly entrance and exit points – can play in the reduction of MCI risk [22, 23]. Event security corralled a tremendous crowd in Duisburg into one designated area leading to a large tunnel to enter the event, at which point they announced that no additional people could be admitted to the free-access music festival. This announcement induced extreme crowding from people who pushed into the area from outside in order to gain admission, which led to a panicked and turbulent rush toward the only available exit staircase in this area. Twenty-one crowd members were crushed to death and an additional more than 500 were injured, and critical analysis of this MCI has suggested that a larger staging area with adequate egress points might have prevented this disaster [23]. Crowd disasters are a critical problem in mass gathering medicine that will be discussed at length in the following pages, and planning related to the layout of an event can play an important role in reducing risk of such an MCI.

Crowd Management and Security: Crowd management represents a tremendous source of risk associated with any mass gathering event that must be addressed in the reduction phase of MCI management. Concerns related to crowd management include structural integrity of the venue, plans regarding capacity and seating, event security, traffic control, the purpose and audience associated with the event, and safety policies associated with the event. Public safety consultants should be involved in event planning as it relates to proper matching of the venue and seating plans with the nature of the event and expected attendants. Of course, a careful assessment of the proper maximum capacity of a venue and its structural integrity must be undertaken by experts. Reassurance against structural collapse is a prerequisite for planned events, in addition to forethought regarding the prospect of mass evacuation (i.e., does the venue lend itself to swift evacuation of all attendants?) or search and rescue operations. For example, emergency response to the 1990 Happy Land Social Club fire in the Bronx, NY in which eighty-seven people died was severely complicated by fire and building code violations that left the venue highly vulnerable to the disastrous impact of an act of arson [24]. Adherence to building and fire codes might have both reduced the risk of rapid structural compromise and facilitated safe evacuation of attendants, presenting a clear lesson to ensure that public safety guidelines are reviewed and followed.

Beyond the proper determination of maximum capacity for a mass gathering event, seating plans are also important. In general, evidence suggests that assigned seating events are safer than general admission events, particularly where the crowd is mobile [10, 25]. Assigned seating events have been associated with lower patient volume primarily driven by lower incidence of falls and minor injuries [25], and general admission events have been associated with greater rates of MCI, primarily driven by human stampedes [9]. Given the outstanding potential for a crowd-related MCI (e.g., human stampede) to grow exponentially in magnitude, implementing assigned seating might be one of the most important measures one can take to mitigate MCI risk at a mass gathering. In the words of Paul Wertheimer, a crowd control expert with more than four decades experience: "Standing room environments – often called festival seating – are the most dangerous and deadly crowd configuration at live entertainment events. It forces people in a crowd to compete against each other for the best location or best area to be. And in crowd safety, that's the last thing you want to occur" [26]. It is also important to note that the level of emotional activation among the crowd at religious and sporting events marks a key factor driving the high incidence of MCI associated with human stampedes, and that lack of assigned seating and other basic crowd control practices at religious events significantly increase risk. For example, a recent stampede at a religious gathering at Israel's Mount Meron in 2021 led to at least forty-five deaths, further underscoring the need for crowd management at such events [27]. Similarly, the Hajj in Saudi Arabia has been extensively analyzed as an extreme case study in crowd management due to its extreme size and its high incidence of human stampedes over the years, and evidence suggests that recent concerted efforts to implement effective crowd management interventions has saved lives, including measures such as the maximization of entrances and exits, controlled entry points with staggered admission, and establishment of unidirectional crowd flow to avoid dangerous crowding [28]. Therefore, assigned seating policies can mitigate both the risk of MCI occurrence and reduce strain caused by simultaneous drains on resources (i.e., routine patient volume). In either case, ticketed events in which capacity can be more accurately measured and managed lend themselves to more accurate risk and needs assessments, which promotes improved readiness. Plans for a mass gathering event must include an estimate of attendance, as well as the anticipated needs associated with it (e.g., differences in needs associated with a concert marked by crowd intoxication and mosh pits compared to a law school graduation event of the same size).

Event security lies at the foundation of MCI reduction for virtually all mass gathering events. An event with a secure perimeter and controlled entrances provides the best defense against overcrowding and violation of maximum capacity, entrance of disorderly attendants (e.g., significant intoxication or agitation), introduction of hazards (e.g., weapons, vehicles), and other unexpected changes that can impair MCI readiness. Security within the venue can further mitigate MCI risk by monitoring the crowd, establishing boundaries (e.g., separating courtside spectators from players at a basketball game), providing swift response to incidents (e.g., early interventions for altercations), securing the scene in the event of an MCI, facilitating orderly evacuation in the event of a disaster, deterring deliberate insults, and communicating directly with the crowd (e.g., providing instructions). These operations critically reduce risk and impact of the MCI at a mass gathering event. For example, analysis of the 2011 Vancouver Stanley Cup riot at a gathering of roughly 100,000 outdoor viewers for the Canucks' loss to the Boston Bruins suggested that insufficient "presence and visibility" of police due to significant under-deployment played a major role in the development of a chaotic MCI associated with dozens injured, dozens of arrests, and extensive property damage [29]. Moreover, evidence suggests that human stampedes present the deadliest threat at the undifferentiated mass gathering, and proper security presence appears to provide the best defense against the development and growth of the MCI associated with stampedes by maintaining an orderly crowd [9]. Therefore, ensuring sufficient numbers and preparation of public safety personnel marks a primary responsibility when planning any mass gathering event. Moreover, public safety personnel often contribute to traffic control, which can facilitate movement of emergency responders (e.g., designated emergency vehicle lanes) and reduce risk of motor vehicle collisions (a common type of MCI at MGE) [9].

The reduction phase of MCI management requires consideration of the purpose and audience associated with the mass gathering event. The purpose of the event can guide speculation regarding the nature of the audience and can also provide important data to guide planning independent of the crowd. For example, a protest or political rally would require a very different MCI readiness profile than a vacation cruise ship of the same size. Similarly, evidence suggests that different types of events are associated with different degrees and types of MCI risk. For example, religious and sporting events were associated with higher risk of deadly stampedes, whereas political and religious events were more strongly associated with deliberate attacks [9]. Of course, there is significant variation in needs even within these categories. For example, research has found that patient volume varies drastically within the heterogeneous category of mass gatherings for sporting events, including a greater than 200-fold increase in patient presentation incidence at recreational bike rides compared to rugby games [30]. Mass gathering planning therefore requires research specifically tailored to the characteristics of the event in question at a level more granular than the overarching category of event (e.g., the New York City Marathon versus a high school basketball game versus the tennis championship at Wimbledon). Moreover, events marked by hazardous performances, such as firework displays or air shows, require specific planning as it applies to standby assignments for emergency services agencies, equipment and supply inventories, and coordination with nearby hospitals (e.g., trauma centers, burn centers). These characteristics related to event purpose carry important implications for MCI reduction and readiness.

The nature of the audience at a mass gathering event presents additional factors that must be considered. For example, an event that anticipates a young crowd, such as a temporary amusement park at a town fair or traveling carnival, should prompt identification of local pediatric receiving facilities and coordination with them, as well as consideration of dedicated training for some emergency services personnel [31, 32]. Other relevant crowd characteristics include the degree to which the crowd is associated together and the degree to which it is prepared for an MCI. For example, a report from a roof collapse at a Norwegian military command center in 2000 demonstrated the immense degree to which self-rescue and rescue by fellow victims was critical to successful MCI management among a cohesive, highly trained, physically fit population of victims [33, 34]. Similarly, the MCI at a workplace or school populated by sober people acquainted with one another and their surroundings, and potentially also subject to regular safety drills, would likely be more amenable to MCI management than the crowd at a music festival. Proper risk assessment also requires knowledge of the policies associated with the event that affect the state of the crowd, such as whether the event is ticketed and whether the audience is mobile, as well as whether alcohol will be available at the venue. In particular, the literature highlights general admission rock concerts as a notable source of small MCI occurrences associated with crowd management issues attributed to "the likelihood of injury to the mobile and intoxicated spectator" [10]. A study that sampled blood alcohol content among random attendants at Major League Baseball games found that more than half of spectators in the twenty–to thirty-five-year-old age range were positive for alcohol and more than ten percent were intoxicated beyond the legal limit, with the majority reporting intent to drive a vehicle from the game [35]. Of course, rates of intoxication vary widely between events and can include the sale of alcohol

within the venue or intoxication from illegal substances. Research suggests that mass toxicologic exposures, such as a dangerous batch of an illegal substance distributed among a crowd, were most commonly associated with concerts [10]. Moreover, research suggests that events associated with particular subcultures marked by drug use, such as widespread use of 3,4-methylenedioxymethamphetamine (MDMA) at electronic dance music festivals in the 2010s, can significantly benefit from deliberate reduction strategies (e.g., extensive access to potable water and medical areas prepared to administer supportive therapy for MDMA use including intravenous hydration and antiemetics), thereby decreasing rates of hospital transport [36]. These matters critically factor into proper needs and risk assessments as it relates to event security, as well as availability of other emergency services agencies and resources.

Stewardship of Resources and Surge Planning: The MCI is defined by an acute mismatch between supply and demand for resources associated with an incident. The majority of reduction efforts apply to mitigating the likelihood or magnitude of demand associated with an incident (i.e., preventing the MCI or reducing its impact), but reduction efforts can also be directed at the supply end of the equation. In particular, analysis of the plan for a mass gathering and its contextual factors marks a critical step in MCI reduction to inform proper readiness practices, including the intelligent stewardship of resources and the design of surge plans. Appropriate management of resources both in the field and at hospitals will be discussed in depth later in this chapter.

Readiness

MCI readiness refers to the preparatory phase for the possibility of the MCI, which includes the development of operational systems, contingency plans, and educational programs that enable the public, emergency services, local hospitals, and other agencies to respond more effectively to the occurrence of an MCI. Whereas reduction efforts tend to focus on risk assessment and mitigating demand for resources, readiness efforts tend to be directed at the compilation and organization of resources in order to optimize preparedness to meet the challenges of MCI management once it arises at the mass gathering event. Proper readiness practices include effective reduction strategies coupled with the identification of stakeholders;

the development of MCI response strategies and explicit plans; and ongoing efforts to promote, enforce, and update these efforts.

Identification of Stakeholders: The first step in MCI readiness is to determine who needs to be involved in preparation. Stakeholders associated with the MCI at a mass gathering will vary widely based on the nature and context of the event as well as the MCI risk assessment profile associated with it, but some basic principles can provide a guiding framework for this phase of MCI preparedness. Key typical stakeholders include EMS; fire departments; police departments and public safety agencies (e.g., security companies); hazardous materials teams (HAZMAT); municipal, state, and federal officials (e.g., city council members, city mayor) and emergency management agencies (e.g., the city health department, the Federal Emergency Management Agency); transportation agencies; venue facilities and engineering services; communications, public relations, and media services; local hospitals (e.g., administrators, clinicians, pharmacists); and the subset of the public most likely to be affected by the MCI, including the crowd, special participants (e.g., representatives of a performing musician or sports team), and local civilians in the nearby area [37]. In an ideal scenario, all of these entities are connected with each other and integrated into greater emergency response networks (including national response assets for large-scale disaster management) that can enable rapid scalability of MCI management efforts as needed. Each of these domains represent a critical component of MCI preparedness efforts for mass gatherings that require active engagement, but several warrant particular attentions and will be discussed here.

In mass gathering medicine, engagement with local EMS, fire services, and HAZMAT teams should be routine and are critical to MCI readiness. EMS agencies are often directly associated with fire and HAZMAT services, but not always – EMS systems vary widely and can be a fire-based department, a police-based department, an independent municipal entity (i.e., "third service"), a hospital-based service, a volunteer service, or a private company under contract with a municipality or venue [38]. MCI preparedness requires the involvement of experts with intimate understanding of these local systems. Similarly, an understanding of the breakdown of various levels of training among EMS and fire personnel, including basic life support and advanced life support prehospital

providers, will be required to develop appropriate MCI readiness plans. EMS agencies must be prepared to provide on-scene medical treatment and transportation to definitive care in the event of both routine medical needs and occurrence of the MCI. Fire and HAZMAT services should also be involved to provide support to EMS as needed and be prepared to carry out scene safety, search, rescue, and other operations within their local scope of practice. Primary agencies might also need to communicate with secondary agencies and review mutual aid agreements to ensure that MCI response plans would not leave the surrounding public vulnerable to disruptions in routine service. Ultimately, fire department officials are often effective liaisons between these entities due to their close collaboration in routine service within most regions.

Police, venue security, and public safety officials represent another vital component of MCI readiness that has the power to both prevent MCI occurrence and play a central role in MCI response. These services must be engaged early in mass gathering planning to ensure that local regulations are met including those regarding building codes and maximum occupancy policies (often managed by fire department officials as well), and to establish plans for crowd and traffic management. The critical importance of crowd management – including both perimeter security (e.g., monitoring of capacity, screening for banned items, deterrence) and maintenance of an orderly crowd (e.g., surveillance, deterrence, early intervention for crowd incidents) – has already been reviewed in this chapter to demonstrate the need for extensive preparation on this front with the involvement of these agencies in concert with expert leaders. It is also important to note that police services vary widely in their training, particularly as it applies to emergency medical management. Therefore, it is important to understand the medical training associated with the police and public safety personnel deployed to the event, given that overestimation of their preparedness to render first aid or basic life support can complicate MCI management. Moreover, all emergency responders (as well as the crowd in ideal conditions) should know exactly how to express concerns and report emergencies to venue security and local police authorities, in order to maximize event security and ensure the establishment of scene safety in the event of an MCI.

MGM requires coordination with the local hospitals that will serve as receiving facilities for patients and potentially provide staffing, materials, guidance, and other forms of assistance that require advance planning. The Joint Commission requires that hospitals develop an explicit MCI plan to include strategies and ongoing training for management of both internal and external disaster scenarios, but additional planning is needed in the event of a mass gathering [39, 40]. For example, hospitals located near a football stadium with capacity for tens of thousands of spectators must be aware of scheduled mass gathering events and should incorporate such events into their MCI plans, which should in turn be integrated into the plans of related agencies (e.g., EMS). Key aspects of hospital MCI preparedness include plans for the assessment of hospital capacity, creation of surge capacity, mobilization and deployment of additional staffing and materials, communication within the hospital and with outside agencies, and establishment of modified triage practices among other operations [37]. Venue and event leadership will often partner with hospital systems to promote such planning and often arrange contracts that provide staffing and materials, including the assignment of emergency physicians to provide care and serve an on-site leadership role in medical operations [19, 41]. Depending upon the nature of the event and the associated risk assessment profile, the recruitment of additional physicians from other specialties might be helpful (e.g., orthopedic surgeons for a sporting event). Physicians who plan to serve at a mass gathering event should clarify whether their employer or another entity will offer arrangements regarding their liability associated with prehospital care provided at the event. Medical directors for mass gatherings should also consider the capabilities of nearby hospitals and consider networking with additional institutions to ensure that needs identified during the mass gathering risk assessment phase will be met by receiving facilities. For example, the literature has been clear that trauma centers [42] and pediatric centers [32] play a key role in MCI management when mass gatherings are likely to require such services. Moreover, coordination between EMS and local hospitals, especially in urban environments, can be key to ensure intelligent distribution of patients. This sort of preparation was cited as a critical driver of the success associated with management of the 2013 Boston Marathon bombing [43–45]. For these reasons and others, hospital-based stakeholders related to mass gathering events should be involved early in MCI readiness efforts.

Other important stakeholders include venue-based personnel and affected segments of the public. In addition to venue security that are included under the umbrella of public safety officials, MCI preparedness requires engagement with venue facilities and engineering services to ensure that the venue is set up in ways that optimize security and safety. The use of clear signage to indicate the location of entry and exit points, emergency supplies, emergency communication and information centers, and hazards has been shown to promote safety [46], and the intentional implementation of rules and policies to direct crowd flow into and within the venue has been reported as an effective measure to reduce risk of human stampede [28]. Moreover, venue and event management should consult with public safety personnel to understand the implications of their plans for MCI preparedness, including the use of assigned seating policies as a way to reduce risk and promote order [9, 25, 26]. Venue engineering personnel should also be recruited to design communication infrastructure that can support the needs of emergency responders and enable direct communication with the crowd when necessary. In addition to on-site interaction with the crowd through standing signage and live communication, the crowd's preparedness to respond to an MCI must also be considered. As previously discussed, the preparedness of a crowd to participate in MCI management must be considered (e.g., the swift response to the roof collapse at a Norwegian military command center in 2000) [34], and various interventions have been studied to try to promote public preparedness, such as MCI drills at large workplace settings, advisory messages at the beginning of events, and the promotion of educational programs for the local public. Ultimately, venue and event management will often make many decisions before involving experts in disaster preparedness and mass gathering medicine, but it is important to ensure that they understand the public safety implications of these decisions and to engage them early to ensure that event planning optimizes MCI preparedness to the furthest possible extent.

Finally, MCI preparedness always requires effective communication between all these stakeholders. Without the establishment of working infrastructure and orderly communication practices, most MCI preparedness efforts will be quickly undermined and overwhelmed. Planning before a one-time event and ongoing meetings between recurring events (e.g., the eighty-one home games at a stadium during a Major League Baseball regular season) that include key stakeholders are necessary to optimize MCI preparedness, as well as an effective strategy for interagency communication during the event with clear designation of roles and responsibilities. This consideration introduces the need for familiarity with the Incident Command System (ICS).

Incident Command System: A clear system for how the many components of MCI management come together in the event of an MCI marks one of the most important aspects of MCI preparedness. In the 1970s, California faced a series of devastating wildfires that prompted the Firefighting Resources of Southern California Organized for Potential Emergencies task force to create ICS after failure analysis indicated that poor responses were more attributable to insufficient organization and coordination rather than insufficient resources [47]. In other words, ICS is a resource management system used to integrate multiple entities under one chain of command and coordinate a complex set of operations in the event of an MCI, which arose from the realization that even an overabundance of supplies and personnel cannot be substituted for organized use of resources. Therefore, event leadership should be intimately familiar with ICS, and all emergency responders should have at least a basic understanding of ICS and their place within it as part of their preparation for their role.

First, every event should designate one incident commander (IC) to oversee general MCI management operations, typically a high-ranked official from the fire department with experience in using ICS. The IC will typically appoint a public information officer, a liaison officer, and a safety officer, who each belong to the command staff and directly assist the IC in their specific roles. Four additional functional divisions are formed as needed based on the scenario, each with a chief that reports directly to the incident commander: operations, planning, logistics, and administrative (financial). ICS provides an established but flexible framework to facilitate organized communication, multifactorial decision-making, and the formation of rank between various agencies in the event of an MCI. Major ICS role designations should be assigned in the readiness phase of MCI management, and clear plans should be in place to guide the activation of ICS. A generic ICS diagram is presented in Figure 22.2.

Triage Algorithms, Casualty Collection Points, and Venue Facilities: Mass gathering medicine planning should account for the need to triage patients in the face of both surges in routine volume and the occurrence of an MCI. In the setting of an MCI, triage might take place at three distinct points: initially at the scene, secondarily at a casualty collection point (CCP), and finally at the receiving ED. A CCP, or field treatment site, is a secure designated area stocked with medical supplies and staffed by medical providers near the MCI scene where patients can be organized and receive treatment, typically while awaiting transport for definitive care. The CCP serves as an intermediate link between the scene (which typically has limited resources and is often less secure) and the receiving facility (which typically requires transport via a motorized vehicle such as an ambulance). Initial on-scene triage will typically be performed by first responders who might have limited medical training, such as firefighters with an emergency medical responder (certified first responder) level of training, ideally at least under the supervision of an emergency physician or EMS provider. This process will often utilize a rapid and simple triage system, such as the aptly named simple triage and rapid treatment (START) triage system, to determine the priority of each patient for transfer to a CCP for further management, ideally by a higher level of medical care and with greater capabilities [48, 49]. START includes four categories of acuity.

- Expectant: Patients with injuries or in a condition deemed incompatible with life, for whom resuscitation will not be attempted. These patients are left at the scene until all other patients are addressed.

- Immediate: Patients in life-threatening condition but who have the potential to survive. These patients are typically taken to the CCP immediately or potentially have resuscitation initiated at the scene if it is safe to do so.

- Delayed: Patients in serious condition without any immediate life-threat. Yellow patients will be brought to safety and then taken to the CCP after the Red patients.

- Minor: Patients in stable condition who typically are mobile with a Glasgow Coma Score (GCS) of 15. Green patients can often be instructed to participate in their own care, including to bring themselves to a higher level of care.

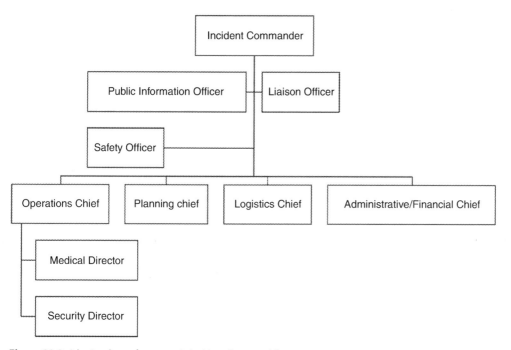

Figure 22.2 A basic schema for a generic Incident Command System

START assessment is typically based on a very rapid patient assessment that includes initial impression (e.g., injury burden), coupled with assessment of mental status (i.e., alert–verbal–painful–unresponsive or AVPU assessment), respiratory rate, and pulse rate. Importantly, JumpSTART was developed as an adjustment to START primarily to account for the handling of pediatric patients in the MCI setting, which can also be used in the initial on-scene phase of MCI management [50].

Next, triage will often be repeated at the CCP depending upon the magnitude of the MCI and other factors such as scene safety and availability of resources for treatment and transport at the scene. CCP triage will often use a slightly more thorough system, such as the sort–assess–lifesaving interventions–treat/transport (SALT) system [49, 51]. SALT uses the same color-priority classification system as START, but adds additional steps to standardize treatment (primarily management of threats to airway–breathing–circulation) and transport under the algorithm. Ultimately, treatment is provided to the fullest extent possible until transport can be arranged in order of medical priority. Importantly, any of these triage systems can be used at the initial scene as well, and even again at the ED, particularly if the ED is strained

by the MCI to the extent that it must abandon a more resource-expensive routine system, such as the emergency severity index (ESI) [52]. In the case of a particularly austere environment, the Secondary Assessment of Victim Endpoint (SAVE) algorithm can be used at CCPs as a simple system to guide the stewardship of limited transport capabilities [53]. The START then SAVE approach ultimately sorts patients into three categories based on expected mortality: those who will not survive regardless of transport, those who will survive regardless of transport, and those who will likely die without transport but will likely survive with the administration of definitive care at a hospital. MCI readiness must include decisions regarding the triage algorithms that will be used ahead of time, as well as a system to determine when retriage of patients might be appropriate.

At a permanent venue such as a stadium, CCPs are typically positioned at designated field treatment sites that are included in standing venue facilities, regularly stocked with medical materials, and staffed by medical providers for routine needs at the mass gathering. CCPs should have the capability to provide security from the MCI mechanism. MCI readiness might require contingency planning for additional or alternative CCPs. CCP preparation at these sites should account for the possibility of the MCI when assigning staffing and determining resource allotment. At a temporary venue such as a concert in a park or at a political rally, CCPs should be established by emergency responders in advance or as early as possible to avoid confusion at the scene and delays in treatment and transport. The CCP is particularly important in austere settings in which response times are expected to be delayed or in settings at which transport via standby units will not be readily available.

Preparation and Scalability of Resources: Alongside preparedness to orchestrate a coordinated response across multiple entities (i.e., ICS), the availability and scalability of resources in the event of an MCI at a mass gathering lie at the foundation of MCI readiness. Key resources can be categorized into human (i.e., staffing) and nonhuman (e.g., equipment, supplies) resources. Akin to the MCI surge plans in place at hospitals [40], mass gatherings should be associated with a plan for the swift enactment of a surge plan that can efficiently increase the scale of available resources, typically through coordination with partnering entities that include EMS, fire, police, local hospitals, and national emergency response assets (as well as other stakeholders previously mentioned). At the MCI scene, emergency responders should be sufficiently prepared to establish safe treatment areas (i.e., CCPs) and provide stabilizing interventions while arranging transport for definitive care. Medical and public safety officials at the mass gathering should be equipped with sufficient personnel to secure a scene and CCPs and provide life-saving interventions while awaiting further support and should have explicit plans for obtaining those additional human resources. Temporary partnerships associated with the mass gathering (e.g., agreements with local fire and EMS agencies), coupled with integration into larger networks (e.g., familiarity with state and federal agencies), will often be necessary to prepare for an MCI. CCPs should have standing inventories of critical supplies, and there should be a plan for material replenishment that includes dedicated personnel responsible for repleting and increasing stocks of supplies at CCPs from a central inventory or from external sources (e.g., incoming from outside agencies or facilities). In some cases, the source of supplies will provide inventory management personnel to facilitate the organization and distribution of supplies, referred to as a vendor-managed inventory [54]. National emergency response assets often use this model,

such as the Strategic National Stockpile initiative managed by the Centers for Disease Control and Prevention, through which critical supplies are delivered to a disaster along with inventory management personnel [55]. Event leadership must be familiar with such options in order to develop effective plans for the rapid compilation of needed supplies and the integration of those supplies into existing inventories in an organized fashion. Hospitals will of course also need surge plans to support the scene as needed and provide definitive care to transported patients, but these plans lie outside the scope of this chapter. Mismanagement of supply inventories marks a classic pitfall in MCI management that can be mitigated through the establishment of effective information systems (e.g., organized stock rooms with dedicated inventory management or digital inventories) and preformed plans for the integration of new materials into these systems.

Training and Regular Review: The maintenance of MCI readiness through regular training and review marks a critically important ongoing process that factors into the success of any MCI response. MCI readiness maintenance can be sorted into two categories: practices associated with a recurring mass gathering event (e.g., a season of sporting events, an annual marathon or music festival), or practices associated with a cohort of disaster responders who might be activated for a one-time event (e.g., EMS agency, fire or police department, hospital). In the first case, MCI readiness is associated with a specific mass gathering event, including its stakeholders and its setting, which is associated with the major benefit of specific preparation that can be informed and refined by ongoing risk analysis and operations reviews. In the second case, preparation is limited to generic MCI readiness, but is still critically important to ensure that responders understand their role and position within ICS as well as how to adapt communication and resource management in the event of an MCI. MCI readiness training among emergency services and hospitals can promote positive team dynamics within entities and help an MCI occurrence feel less unfamiliar to responders. Moreover, interprofessional simulation training can improve communication in the event of an MCI and promote collaboration between professions (e.g., physicians and nurses) and agencies (e.g., hospitals and EMS).

Maintenance of MCI readiness can be broken into two interacting phases: review and training. The review process refers to regular meetings by mass gathering stakeholders (e.g., EMS agency or ED administrators) at which risks are assessed, prior mass gatherings or MCI occurrences are reviewed, external evidence is presented and discussed, and plans are critically appraised and updated. For example, stakeholders associated with the season of a National Football League team's venue will send expert representatives to regular meetings at which data from prior games and seasons are reviewed, changes at the venue or in the greater surrounding context (e.g., new state EMS protocols or changes in local hospital capabilities) are discussed, new ideas from the literature or other football stadiums are presented, and plans for MCI response and training are carefully reviewed and edited as needed. Even outside the context of a specific mass gathering event, interdisciplinary meetings between MCI stakeholders (e.g., EMS agencies, local police and fire, hospital administrators, and governmental agency officials) provide key opportunities to ensure that leaders are updated with respect to partnering entities and to ensure that MCI plans are properly integrated into one another across domains of emergency services.

MCI training should be an ongoing process that is informed by review procedures and can also provide useful feedback that can be subject to review. MCI drills can identify critical weaknesses and gaps in MCI readiness in a low-stakes environment that can stimulate quality improvement efforts. The review process should yield a risk assessment that identifies likely hazards associated with a mass gathering or MCI response entity, which can lend itself to the intelligent curation of MCI readiness curricula and selection of drill scenarios. Training can come in various forms, from tabletop exercises to full-scale interdisciplinary simulations. These maintenance practices should cover key aspects of MCI response, for example including communication tests, cardiopulmonary resuscitation practical training, and didactic coverage of ICS. Mass gathering medicine leaders should utilize both types of training (i.e., standing MCI training associated with entities and dedicated MCI training associated with a particular mass gathering) and be sure to coordinate review efforts with all stakeholders.

Response

Response to the MCI is defined as the actions taken within the immediate time frame of an MCI, particularly in response to the primary insult and ongoing developments that arise during MCI management. Proper MCI response is predicated upon sufficient readiness but also requires additional competence and coordination to execute plans. MCI response is driven by careful evaluation of the MCI both initially and on an ongoing basis, swift mobilization of resources at the scene and receiving facilities, effective communication between stakeholders, orderly operations at the scene, and establishment of information systems to facilitate efficient response and recovery.

MCI Assessment: In the same way that initial assessment and frequent reassessment of a trauma patient using the ABC paradigm is critical to Advanced Trauma Life Support, one must use a systematic approach to evaluate the magnitude of an MCI at a mass gathering. The METHANE system for MCI reporting can be used as a brief, easily recalled method for MCI assessment [56, 57]:

M: Major incident recognition and declaration, including communication with key stakeholders.
E: Exact location of incident identified and reported.
T: Type of incident classified (e.g., multiple vehicle collision versus chemical exposure).
H: Hazards identified, including those currently present and those with potential to arise.
A: Access points, egress points, CCPs, and rendezvous points selected.
N: Number and nature of casualties estimated and described.
E: Emergency services currently present and those to be requested (e.g., two current fire alarms with request for one additional alarm, request for HAZMAT service).

These characteristics of an MCI should be assessed, frequently reassessed, and reported to key stakeholders. MCI assessment should initially focus primarily on those factors that inform scene safety and proper formation of organized command, then transition to assessment of the type and magnitude of disaster to identify and anticipate needed services and supplies, then move on to evaluating basic quality measures to ensure that appropriate progress is being made (e.g., rate of EMS transports, estimated number of victims to be rescued). Frequent reassessments are key to MCI response to ensure that proper adjustments are being made to maximize safety and efficiently manage limited resources. Regular discussions coordinated by the IC among leadership (i.e., ICS division chiefs and representatives of key agencies) at the MCI command center provide the advantage of a multifactorial MCI assessment that is less likely to miss key issues and more likely to promote a cohesive, holistic response.

Communication: Clear and organized communication practices lie at the cornerstone of successful MCI response. Upon the occurrence of an MCI at a mass gathering, the MCI must be declared to all stakeholders. The METHANE paradigm provides a useful mnemonic to organize the basic assessment of an MCI for an initial report [56, 57]. Declaration of the MCI should include communication with EMS, fire, police and public safety officers (e.g., venue security), receiving hospitals, greater disaster response assets (e.g., state or federal agencies), and any other stakeholders currently involved or requested to meet the demands of the MCI. Similarly, these stakeholders should have organized channels through which they can feed back information to the MCI command division. For example, local receiving facilities should provide regular status updates to the scene command division that can facilitate the intelligent distribution of patients to acute care facilities, including their estimated capacity to accept patients and any current or anticipated limitations.

In addition to communication among leadership to facilitate large-scale coordination of operations, direct communication on a smaller scale is also important. Transporting EMS units should continue to communicate with a centralized dispatch and continue to provide notifications to receiving facilities. Emergency services should have direct lines of communication with public safety officers to facilitate efficient movement of patients and resources in a safe manner and to enable the reporting of new hazards that might develop at the scene. Under ICS, the command division will often include the designation of a liaison officer and a public information officer. The liaison officer should utilize a systematic approach to measure the effectiveness of communication between entities and have contingency plans to overcome communication barriers or otherwise improve communication as needed. Moreover, the liaison officer should organize rendezvous points or interagency conversations to ensure that communication is optimized and that operations are properly integrated. The public information officer will oversee the dissemination of updates to the public and work with public safety officials to ensure that the crowd at the mass gathering is properly informed and instructed to maximize safety and facilitate recovery practices that will follow.

Prehospital Operations: Prehospital operations include all activities that occur outside the hospital setting, including all operations that take place at the mass gathering and transportation between the MCI scene and receiving facilities. Mass gathering events are a time limited phenomenon – in contrast to hospitals that have standing capabilities and routine operations – that require extensive planning in order to establish readiness for an effective prehospital response to an MCI. Therefore, most of the prehospital MCI response was covered under the Readiness section of this chapter, but a few points regarding MCI response warrant special attention. The Major Incident Medical Management and Support system and the Joint Emergency Services Intra-operability Programme have recommended the CSCATTT mnemonic to guide the approach to prehospital MCI response [57]:

C: Command

S: Safety

C: Communications

A: Assessment of the scene

T: Triage

T: Treatment

T: Transport

Establishment of ICS is a critical first step to MCI response that must be preemptively facilitated through readiness procedures (e.g., specific planning, training), such that chain of command and integration of operations across agencies should occur rapidly and seamlessly upon declaration of the MCI. As in all prehospital operations, the safety of patients, bystanders at the mass gathering, and responders must remain the primary priority. Under ideal conditions, a rapid scene assessment and establishment of a secure scene will have already been undertaken by first responders while the MCI is declared, and ICS is formed. The establishment of a safe scene, secure CCPs, and clear routes between key points (e.g., the scene, patient transport sites), all require a proper scene assessment, effective communication, and a properly integrated chain of command. It is also helpful to note that these practices must be established early but also constantly maintained and frequently reassessed. Following the execution of these first four steps, triage, treatment, and transport can take place. Triage was covered in the Readiness section of this chapter because EMS should always have a plan for MCI triage prior to the occurrence of the MCI. Treatment and transport rely on effective triage, communication, and information systems. Information systems should be developed to accomplish multiple key objectives, including prehospital inventory management, patient registration and documentation, and hospital capacity monitoring. These information systems can be as simple as a board with hand-written tallies or as sophisticated as an electronic system that is integrated between agencies and hospitals. Mass gathering leadership should ensure that readiness procedures account for all aspects of the CSCATTT paradigm, and in the event of an MCI should ensure that all activities under CSCATTT are properly managed and integrated.

Transportation of Patients to Acute Care Facilities: Effective transportation of patients to acute care facilities for definitive care marks the final critical step in prehospital MCI response from the perspective of a given patient. Mass gathering events, especially those of a large size, will often arrange to have one or more standby units assigned to the event with transport capabilities. However, an MCI scenario will typically exhaust the reserve of standby transporting units, even for the most prepared events. Proper planning will include a surge plan for transporting units, such that additional transport-capable units are designated for reassignment to the mass gathering without significant disruption in routine service to the surrounding area, particularly in the case of an MCI. If an MCI is marked by particularly high acuity, such as in the case of a mass shooting, nonmedical transport might be utilized. The literature suggests that a "scoop and run" approach to gunshot victims by nonmedical police units, particularly in urban environments associated with short transport times, can provide a timely and effective option at the scene of an MCI [58, 59]. For example, Philadelphia instituted formal protocols for the use of nonmedical police transport of violently injured patients in the late 1990s in the face of rising firearm injuries and intense strain on the supply of available EMS units [59, 60]. An MCI at a mass gathering can consider the use of such practices, particularly in the case of critically injured patients that outnumber available transporting EMS units in a setting marked by short transport times. Civilian transport of such patients has also been reported but are less likely in the mass gathering setting and should not be incorporated into plans. EMS can also consider transporting multiple patients per trip, particularly in the case of those who require definitive care but are not in critical condition. For example, at 1994 Woodstock, the decision was made to reassign mass gathering medical personnel to transporting units (i.e., a third provider was assigned to each ambulance) and transport as many as five patients per trip [14]. Close communication between EMS and MCI command should be in place to guide such decisions, including the request for additional EMS units, the use of nonmedical transport, or the adaptation of EMS transport operations.

The selection of receiving facilities can be critically important to MCI response, particularly in a setting associated with multiple local options. Trauma is by far the most common cause of the MCI at a mass gathering [9], so local trauma centers should be notified when an MCI is declared as they will likely receive most MCI patients in a common scenario. It is often helpful for MCI command to actively request initial estimates and regular updates from receiving facilities regarding their capacity to accept additional MCI patients, in order to properly inform centralized EMS dispatch operations that will direct transporting units in a coordinated fashion. For example, the 2013 Boston Marathon bombing has been subject to study as a successful case of MCI management, with much of its success attributed to the fact that the attack occurred at a central location in Boston among the city's six adult or pediatric trauma centers and a total of ten teaching hospitals at roughly similar distances, managed via intelligent distribution of patients across them [43]. In particular, a designated officer with expertise in prehospital systems worked with a physician to optimize the coordinated dispatch of transporting EMS units to various EDs, which enabled the transport of 30 patients initially triaged as red (i.e., patients in life-threatening condition who receive the highest priority for transport) within eighteen minutes after the explosions while minimizing strain at each receiving trauma center [43–45]. Applying this lesson, MCI response should include a centralized dispatch unit that can coordinate the intelligent transport of patients to receiving EDs, particularly in the case of a mass gathering held in an urban setting associated with multiple local hospitals. In more austere settings, greater time might need to be invested in prehospital treatment on-scene to optimize patients for longer transport times, likely to a smaller number of receiving facilities.

Hospital Operations: From the single patient perspective, delivery of definitive care at the hospital after successful prehospital management marks the final step in MCI response. Given that most MCIs are marked by trauma, trauma centers will likely receive most patients associated with a common MCI, particularly those who are most critically injured. Fortunately, most trauma centers should be fairly well-resourced at the time of MCI and will be required to have MCI plans in place per the Joint Commission [39, 40]. However, MCI response relies upon prompt notification of potential receiving hospitals and swift activation of MCI plans. Hospital-based response to an MCI typically includes operations geared toward the creation of increased capacity (i.e., beds), reallocation of resources (e.g., postponement of elective surgeries to increase operating room availability), establishment of increased security (especially in the case of an MCI associated with a deliberate attack), institution of surge staffing, and the mobilization of supplies (e.g., blood products). The hospital-based response marks a critical component of MCI management that is very complex and subject to significant variation across contexts and therefore lies beyond the scope of this chapter.

Preparation for Recovery: The final stages of MCI response led to the final phase of the emergency management cycle: recovery. Recovery will be covered in the following section of this chapter, but in general is predicated upon information related to MCI response. The recovery phase of MCI management relies upon the documentation and record keeping practices undertaken during MCI response in order to inform future analysis and research, as well as the identification of affected individuals and agencies in order to provide important services and support. The maintenance of information systems and documentation are sometimes neglected when MCI responders are overwhelmed but should always be prioritized to avoid problems that are likely to unfold later in their absence.

Recovery

In the aftermath of the MCI, the recovery phase begins. MCI recovery includes activities that take place immediately following the MCI at the scene, in the medium term at the scene and affected hospitals, and in the long term potentially throughout the entire community. An MCI can exert a major effect on local services, local resources, and community psychological well-being. Moreover, patients affected by an MCI are associated with ongoing needs that can continue to strain hospitals and local systems. Mass gathering leadership should be prepared not only for response to the MCI, but for the recovery phase that will follow it.

Community Support: The occurrence of an MCI can affect entire communities, from the families of victims to an entire nation. In order to meet the needs of communities affected by an MCI, particularly in the acute phase, the primary type of support comes in the form of information. For this reason, effective information systems are critical parts of readiness and response activities that facilitate MCI recovery. Mass gathering leadership should have a system in place to register and track patients, particularly those who are transported to hospitals. Smaller events, such as one-time outdoor concerts, might rely on EMS agencies for this information, whereas a football stadium that hosts a National Football League season might use its own venue-based information system to log routine patient care associated with events and can use this system for the occurrence of an MCI. These electronic medical record systems can facilitate the flow of information between patients and hospitals, especially in the case of patients who cannot communicate on their own behalf. This includes family reunification, as well as the collection of collateral and background information associated with patients to facilitate hospital care (e.g., medication lists). Family reunification can also apply to bystanders evacuated from a mass gathering, especially children, the elderly, or others who might have barriers to reaching their families. These family reunification efforts are predicated upon a well-planned and organized operation that lends itself to the identification and location of patients.

In the case of a particularly high-impact MCI, such as one associated with prolonged rescue and recovery operations or an act of terrorism, the affected community can be quite large and even span an entire nation. The media, from local to global markets, might report on the MCI and can be directed to a public information officer or other personnel with experience in media relations. In general, it is best to streamline these interactions such that information from the MCI flows to the media through one individual or committee, rather than in a disorganized bottom-up fashion that can lead to conflicting reports and misinformation. Such cases can stimulate a swell of volunteerism, for which it can be helpful to establish a task force for the coordination of volunteer efforts. Disorganized engagement of volunteers can compromise safety and disrupt ICS. In the absence of resources to dedicate to these endeavors, coordination with experienced leaders from partnering agencies, such as from local hospitals, police departments, and fire departments can assist in these large-scale interactions with the affected community.

Demobilization and Responder Debriefing: Return to normal operations within the prehospital sector can be a complex process with significant variation in duration. MCI scenes can be marked by ongoing rescue and recovery operations or the attraction of community members that require prolonged responses by police, fire, and other agencies. Even in cases associated with excellent preparedness, an MCI can disrupt routine EMS, hospital, and other operations in the surrounding community. Hospitals that take on increased capacity to respond to an MCI can face strains on staffing and critical shortages of supplies, such as medications for chronic conditions. For these reasons, demobilization after an MCI can require as much coordination and planning as mobilization. It is often helpful to reach out to federal agencies (such as the Federal Emergency Management Agency) during the recovery phase of MCI management to benefit from the expertise of experience officials and to rely on federal resources and sophisticated networks to replenish resources, receive additional personnel, and coordinate the offloading of strain on overwhelmed entities.

Responder debriefing marks a particularly important aspect of demobilization. Responder debriefing includes intellectual analysis of the MCI toward quality improvement, as well as psychological debriefing to help affected parties manage stress and psychological trauma associated with the MCI.

Critical Review and Analysis: Tying into reduction and readiness activities, critical analysis of an MCI marks a critical aspect of MCI management. All parties involved in an MCI should be involved in review activities on some level in order to learn powerful firsthand lessons and benefit from the experience they had in engaging with the MCI, even if it is limited to a debriefing session or statement led by their respective entity leaders. These operations are particularly important for recurrent mass gathering stakeholders, such as those associated with an annual marathon or lengthy sporting event season, given that they are most likely to be called upon to respond to an

MCI in the same setting if one occurs. Critical review procedures benefit significantly from accurate and reliable record keeping and organized data management during MCI response, which can inform lessons and guide research and quality improvement efforts. The lessons and findings associated with this work should be disseminated to all affected entities and potentially reported in the literature for peer review and broader dissemination.

Psychological First Aid and Critical Incident Stress Management: An MCI can cause stress and psychological trauma among all stakeholders involved, including prehospital responders, hospital workers, victims, families, bystanders, and the greater community. Psychological first aid is a concept that has been introduced into the disaster literature to describe "a systematic set of helping actions aimed at reducing initial post-trauma distress and supporting short- and long-term adaptive functioning" [61]. Professionals with training and experience in the provision of psychological first aid can be assigned to attend or cover call for a mass gathering in preparation for an MCI, or be recruited after the fact to assist in immediate MCI recovery. All the aforementioned stakeholders associated with an MCI can benefit from psychological first aid, from the IC to mass gathering attendants without medical needs.

MCI responders – both prehospital and hospital-based – are usually the most organized sector of stakeholders in that they have standing channels of communication within their agencies that can be used for debriefing. Critical incident stress debriefing or critical incident stress management (CISM), which refers to a broader set of related concepts, refers to a short-term psychological intervention used for secondary victims of an incident (e.g., the firefighters who respond to a derailed train, rather than injured passengers) to minimize the negative psychological impact of a specific crisis [62, 63]. CISM activities are often conducted among small homogenous cohorts of responders associated with a critical incident, such as among a single firehouse following a lethal fire. Key objectives associated with CISM include the minimization of disruption to the personal lives and professional function of responders (i.e., rapid and sustainable return to service), the reduction of likelihood to develop post-traumatic stress disorder or other long-term consequences among responders, and the restoration of a functional unit (e.g., a firehouse) and maintenance of group cohesion and performance. Potential responders to MCIs, such as prehospital workers and ED providers, should be made aware of the benefits associated with CISM and potentially harmful effects of unaddressed incident-related psychological trauma beforehand, such as during initial training (e.g., including within an emergency medical technician curriculum). CISM can also include further opportunities to engage within an MCI responder community or to continue serving those affected by an MCI, which can promote coping with incident-related trauma via sublimation. Coping strategies can vary widely between people and agency leaders should prioritize the establishment of open and accessible channels through which responders can express concerns and request psychological assistance.

Civilian stakeholders associated with an MCI include patients, family members, bystanders, and the greater community. Hospitals typically serve at the frontlines in the recovery process for patients and their loved ones, and they can easily find their routine staffing for psychological and social services overwhelmed by the increased demand associated with the MCI. Greater agencies and networks can be contacted to assist with these needs, such as FEMA. Additional support for patients and families can come from external sources (e.g., new fundraisers and groups founded to assist victims of an MCI), which typically collaborate with hospitals to connect with clients. Bystanders present at the mass gathering who directly witness the MCI and other MCI survivors who do not require hospital admission can have significant needs for psychological assistance but might be more difficult to engage. Events that require attendant registration might facilitate the identification of such individuals. In cases associated with a sufficiently secured scene or an organized mass evacuation from the venue, work can be done in the immediate recovery phase while such individuals are still located in one place to integrate them into a communication network or provide instructions to engage in future communications after the fact (e.g., announcement of a website or social media page to access updates or report concerns). In the absence of such options, bystanders are shifted into the general community, who might also be affected by the MCI, including though media coverage of the incident [16, 64]. Local advertisements and networking through local communities (e.g., schools, churches) might be used to reach such individuals, otherwise they

will be left to seek assistance through routine channels in the healthcare system. Proper interventions early in the MCI recovery phase can serve to decrease strain on mental health resources later and potentially mitigate longer-term psychological repercussions, including increased incidence of post-traumatic stress disorder and complicated grief reactions [64, 65].

Conclusions

MCI management in the context of a MGE requires cooperation and coordination among a diverse array of stakeholder entities across the span of the emergency management cycle. In the introduction of this chapter, the epidemiology of the MCI at mass gathering events was reviewed and the special challenges associated with such incidents – including key MCI multipliers – were discussed. The emergency management cycle, which provides the conceptual framework for the four Rs paradigm, was described and used to provide the format for this chapter. Key considerations related to the prevention of MCIs and reduction of their risk and impact were presented, with particular attention dedicated to MCI risk assessment and a recommended set of effective measures that can be used to promote crowd management within the mass gathering setting. MCI readiness lies at the core of MCI management. MCI readiness relies upon the critical initial step to identify and engage all stakeholders associated with the mass gathering event and the particular MCI scenarios associated with the event's risk assessment profile. Proper MCI readiness also requires specific plans for the establishment of command (i.e., ICS), effective channels for communication, regular drills and other training operations, and the compilation and organization of needed staffing and supplies. MCI response, predicated upon effective readiness procedures, was reviewed including frameworks to guide the assessment and reporting of an MCI and the organization of operations across the various sectors in which MCI response must occur. Finally, the MCI recovery process was described and recommendations for the provision of effective community support and psychological first aid were provided. These phases of the emergency management cycle tend to rely upon each other and should all be considered by leaders associated with any MGE.

References

1. DeNolf R. L., Kahwaji C. I. *EMS Mass Casualty Management*. Treasure Island, FL: StatPearls Publishing; 2022. www.ncbi.nlm.nih.gov/books/NBK482373/. Accessed February 21, 2022.

2. Heightman A. J. Many Factors Contribute to the Successful Management of a Mass Casualty Incident. *JEMS: EMS, Emergency Medical Services – Training, Paramedic, EMT News*. 2012. www.jems.com/operations/many-factors-contribute-successful-manag/. Accessed February 21, 2022.

3. Newgard C. D., Schmicker R. H., Hedges J. R., Trickett J. P., Davis D. P., Bulger E. M., et al. Emergency Medical Services Intervals and Survival in Trauma: Assessment of the "Golden Hour" in a North American Prospective Cohort. Annals of Emergency Medicine. 2010;**55**(3):235–246.e4.

4. Brittanica. Mecca | Definition, History, Pilgrimage, Population, Kaaba, City, & Facts | Britannica. 2022. www.britannica.com/place/Mecca. Accessed February 21, 2022.

5. Almukhtar S. To Get All the World's Muslims to Hajj, It Would Take at Least 581 Years. *The New York Times*. 2018. www.nytimes.com/interactive/2018/08/23/world/middleeast/hajj-attendance-expansion.html. Accessed February 21, 2022.

6. Census Bureau. U.S. Census Bureau QuickFacts: State College Borough, Pennsylvania. 2020. www.census.gov/quickfacts/statecollegeboroughpennsylvania. Accessed February 21, 2022.

7. Snyder S. Beaver Stadium. Penn State. 2016. https://sites.psu.edu/slspassion/2016/04/15/beaver-stadium/. Accessed February 21, 2022.

8. Jena A. B., Mann N. C., Wedlund L. N., Olenski A. Delays in Emergency Care and Mortality During Major U.S. Marathons. N Engl J Med. 2017 Apr 13;376(15):1441-1450 www.nejm.org/doi/10.1056/NEJMsa1614073. Accessed October 4, 2019.

9. Turris S. A., Lund A., Bowles R. R. An Analysis of Mass Casualty Incidents in the Setting of Mass Gatherings and Special Events. *Disaster Medicine and Public Health Preparedness*. 2014;**8**(2):1–7.

10. Milsten A. M., Maguire B. J., Bissell R. A., Seaman K. G. Mass-Gathering Medical Care: A Review of the Literature. *Prehospital and Disaster Medicine*. 2002;**17**(3):151–162.

11. Bajaj S., Dudeja P. Food Poisoning Outbreak in a Religious Mass Gathering. *Medical Journal Armed Forces India*. 2019;**75**(3):339–343.

12. Kak V. Infections on Cruise Ships. *Microbiology Spectrum*. 2015;**3**(4).

13. Florida R., Goldfarb Z. Woodstock '94. Peace, Music and EMS. *JEMS*. 1994;**19**(12):45–48.

14. Dress J. M., Horton E. H., Florida R. Music, Mud & Medicine. Woodstock '94: A Maniacal, Musical Mass-Casualty Incident. *Emergency Medical Services*. 1995;**24**(1):21, 30–2.

15. Riedel S. Biological Warfare and Bioterrorism: A Historical Review. *Proceedings (Baylor University Medical Center)*. 2004;**17**(4):400–406.

16. Keudell A. von, Koh K. A., Shah S. B., Harris M. B., Smith M., Rodriguez E. K., et al. Mental Health After the Boston Marathon Bombing. *The Lancet Psychiatry*. 2016;**3**(9):802–804.

17. CDEM. Civil Defence Emergency Management Act 2002 No 33 (as at 01 June 2018), Public Act 3 Purpose – New Zealand Legislation. 2002. www.legislation.govt.nz/act/public/2002/0033/51.0/DLM149795.html. Accessed January 27, 2022.

18. CDEM. National Civil Defence Emergency Management Strategy. 2008. www.civildefence.govt.nz/cdem-sector/plans-and-strategies/national-civil-defence-emergency-management-strategy/. Accessed February 21, 2022.

19. Bledsoe B., Songer P., Buchanan K., Westin J., Hodnick R., Gorosh L. Burning Man 2011: Mass Gathering Medical Care in an Austere Environment. *Prehospital and Emergency Care*. 2012;**16**(4):469–476.

20. Rutty M., Scott D., Steiger R., Johnson P. Weather Risk Management at the Olympic Winter Games. *Current Issues in Tourism*. 2015;**18**(10):931–946.

21. Glassberg E., Lipsky A. M., Abramovich A., Sergeev I., Hochman O., Ash N. A Dynamic Mass Casualty Incident at Sea: Lessons Learned from the Mavi Marmara. *Journal of Trauma and Acute Care Surgery*. 2013;**75**(2):292–297.

22. Dörries B. Violent Allegations Against the Organizers of the Love Parade. Süddeutsche.de. 2010. www.sueddeutsche.de/politik/loveparade-rainer-schaller-heftige-vorwuerfe-gegen-veranstalter-der-loveparade-1.980628. Accessed February 21, 2022.

23. Helbing D., Mukerji P. Crowd Disasters as Systemic Failures: Analysis of the Love Parade Disaster. *EPJ Data Science*. 2012;**1**(1):7.

24. Bird J. Fire in the Bronx: Austerity, Quality of Life, and Nightlife Regulation in New York City Post-1975. *Journal of Urban History*. 2020;**46**(4):836–853.

25. Baker W. M., Simone B. M., Niemann J. T., Daly A. Special Event Medical Care: The 1984 Los Angeles Summer Olympics Experience. *Annals of Emergency Medicine*. 1986;**15**(2):185–190.

26. Sanchez R. "Beyond Your Control." The Recipe for a Deadly Crowd Crush. CNN2021. www.cnn.com/2021/11/06/us/what-is-a-crowd-surge/index.html. Accessed February 21, 2022.

27. Kershner I., Nagourney E., Ives M. Stampede at Israel Religious Celebration Kills at Least 45. *The New York Times.* 2021. www.nytimes.com/2021/04/29/world/middleeast/israel-mount-meron-stampede.html. Accessed February 5, 2022.

28. Ganguly S., Friedman M. Mass Gathering Medicine: Lessons from the Hajj. *Emergency Physicians Monthly.* 2015. https://epmonthly.com/article/mass-gathering-medicine-lessons-from-the-hajj/. Accessed February 5, 2022.

29. Davies G., Dawson S. E. The 2011 Stanley Cup Riot: Police Perspectives and Lessons Learned. *Policing: International Journal of Police Strategy and Management.* 2015;**38**(1):132–152.

30. Delany C., Crilly J., Ranse J. Drug and Alcohol Related Patient Presentations to Emergency Departments During Sporting Mass-Gathering Events: An Integrative Review. *Prehospital and Disaster Medicine.* 2020;**35**(3):298–304.

31. Thierbach A. R., Wolcke B. B., Piepho T., Maybauer M., Huth R. Medical Support for Children's Mass Gatherings. *Prehospital and Disaster Medicine.* 2003;**18**(1):14–19.

32. Bernardo L. M., Veenema T. G. Pediatric Emergency Preparedness for Mass Gatherings and Special Events. *Disaster Management & Response.* 2004;**2**(4):118–122.

33. Rostrup M., Gilbert M., Stalsberg H. A Snow Avalanche in Vassdalen. *Tidsskrift for den Norske Laegeforening.* 1989;**109**(7–8):807–813.

34. Romundstad L., Sundnes K. O., Pillgram-Larsen J., Røste G. K., Gilbert M. Challenges of Major Incident Management When Excess Resources Are Allocated: Experiences from a Mass Casualty Incident After Roof Collapse of a Military Command Center. *Prehospital and Disaster Medicine.* 2004;**19**(2):179–184.

35. Wolfe J., Martinez R., Scott W. A. Baseball and Beer: An Analysis of Alcohol Consumption Patterns Among Male Spectators at Major-League Sporting Events. *Annals of Emergency Medicine.* 1998;**31**(5):629–632.

36. Friedman M. S., Plocki A., Likourezos A., et al. A Prospective Analysis of Patients Presenting for Medical Attention at a Large Electronic Dance Music Festival. *Prehospital and Disaster Medicine.* 2017;**32**(1):78–82.

37. Hendrickson R. G., Horowitz B. Z. Disaster Preparedness. In: *Tintinalli's Emergency Medicine: A Comprehensive Study Guide.* Tintinalli J. E., Ma O. J., Yealy D. M., et al. (eds.). New York: McGraw-Hill Education; 2020. accessmedicine.mhmedical.com/content.aspx?aid=1166526002. Accessed February 21, 2022.

38. Pozner C. N., Zane R., Nelson S. J., Levine M. International EMS Systems: The United States: Past, Present, and Future. *Resuscitation.* 2004;**60**(3):239–244.

39. Persoff J., Ornoff D., Little C. The Role of Hospital Medicine in Emergency Preparedness: A Framework for Hospitalist Leadership in Disaster Preparedness, Response, and Recovery. *Journal of Hospital Medicine.* 2018;**13**(10):713–718.

40. The Joint Commission. Emergency Management. 2022. www.jointcommission.org/resources/patient-safety-topics/emergency-management/. Accessed February 5, 2022.

41. Boyle M. F., Lorenzo R. A. D., Garrison R. Physician Integration into Mass Gathering Medical Care: The United States Air Show. *Prehospital and Disaster Medicine.* 1993;**8**(2):165–168.

42. Cryer H. G., Hiatt J. R. Trauma System: The Backbone of Disaster Preparedness. *Journal of Trauma and Acute Care Surgery.* 2009;**67**(2):S111.

43. Biddinger P. D., Baggish A., Harrington L., d'Hemecourt P., Hooley J., Jones J., et al. Be Prepared: The Boston Marathon and Mass-Casualty Events. *New England Journal of Medicine.* 2013;**368**(21):1958–1960.

44. Gates J. D, Arabian S., Biddinger P., Blansfield J., Burke P., Chung S., et al. The Initial Response to the Boston Marathon Bombing. *Annals of Surgery.* 2014;**260**(6):960–966.

45. Leonard H., Cole C., Howitt A., Heymann P. Why Was Boston Strong? Lessons from the Boston Marathon Bombing. Ash Center Policy Briefs Series, Harvard University. 2014. https://dash.harvard.edu/handle/1/42372460. Accessed February 5, 2022.

46. Rahmat N., Jusoff K., Ngali N., et al. Crowd Management Strategies and Safety Performance among Sports Tourism Event Venue Organizers in Kuala Lumpur and Selangor. *World Applied Sciences Journal.* 2011;**12**:47–52.

47. Williams J., Freeman C. L., Goldstein S. *EMS Incident Command System.* StatPearls Publishing; 2021. www.ncbi.nlm.nih.gov/books/NBK441863/. Accessed February 5, 2022.

48. Kahn C. A., Schultz C. H., Miller K. T., Anderson C. L. Does START Triage Work? An Outcomes Assessment After a Disaster. *Annals of Emergency Medicine.* 2009;**54**(3):424–430.e1.

49. Clarkson L., Williams M. *EMS Mass Casualty Triage.* StatPearls Publishing; 2021. www.ncbi.nlm.nih.gov/books/NBK459369/. Accessed February 5, 2022.

50. Romig L. E. Pediatric Triage: A System to JumpSTART Your Triage of Young Patients at MCIs. *JEMS.* 2002;**27**(7):52–8, 60–3.

51. Cone D. C., Serra J., Burns K., MacMillan D. S., Kurland L., Van Gelder C. Pilot Test of the SALT Mass Casualty Triage System. *Prehospital and Emergency Care*. 2009;**13**(4):536–540.

52. Wuerz R. Emergency Severity Index Triage Category Is Associated with Six-Month Survival. *Academic Emergency Medicine*. 2001;**8**(1):61–64.

53. Benson M., Koenig K. L., Schultz C. H. Disaster Triage: START, then SAVE – A New Method of Dynamic Triage for Victims of a Catastrophic Earthquake. *Prehospital and Disaster Medicine*. 1996;**11**(2):117–124.

54. Coleman C., Hrdina C., Casagrande R., Cliffer K., Mansoura M., Nystrom S., et al. User-Managed Inventory: An Approach to Forward-Deployment of Urgently Needed Medical Countermeasures for Mass-Casualty and Terrorism Incidents. *Disaster Medicine and Public Health Preparedness*. 2012;**6**:408–414.

55. CDC. Strategic National Stockpile. Public Health Emergency. 2021. www.phe.gov/about/sns/Pages/default.aspx. Accessed February 6, 2022.

56. Gamberini L., Imbriaco G., Ingrassia P. L., et al. Logistic Red Flags in Mass-Casualty Incidents and Disasters: A Problem-Based Approach. *Prehospital and Disaster Medicine*. 2022;**37**(2):1–8.

57. Lowes A., Cosgrove J. Prehospital Organization and Management of a Mass Casualty Incident. *BJA Education*. 2016;**16**(10):323–328. https://doi.org/10.1093/bjaed/mkw005

58. Van Brocklin E. "Scoop and Run" Can Save Lives. Why Don't More Police Departments Try It? *The Trace*. 2018. www.thetrace.org/2018/11/scoop-and-run-gunshot-victim-police-transport/. Accessed February 11, 2022.

59. Jacoby S. F., Reeping P. M., Branas C. C. Police-to-Hospital Transport for Violently Injured Individuals: A Way to Save Lives? *The ANNALS of the American Academy of Political and Social Science*. 2020;**687**(1):186–201.

60. Van Brocklin E. Where Cop Cars Double as Ambulances. *The Trace*. 2018. www.thetrace.org/2018/11/philadelphia-police-scoop-and-run-shooting-victims/. Accessed February 11, 2022.

61. Ruzek J., Brymer M., Jacobs A., Layne C., Vernberg E., Watson P. Psychological First Aid. *Journal of Mental Health Counseling*. 2007;**29**:17–49.

62. Mitchell J. T. Critical Incident Stress Debriefing (CISD). www.info-trauma.org 1995;10.

63. Everly G. S., Flannery R. B., Mitchell J. T. Critical Incident Stress Management (CISM): A Review of the Literature. *Aggression and Violent Behavior*. 2000;**5**(1):23–40.

64. Pfefferbaum B., Newman E., Nelson S. D., Nitiéma P., Pfefferbaum R. L., Rahman A. Disaster Media Coverage and Psychological Outcomes: Descriptive Findings in the Extant Research. *Current Psychiatry Reports*. 2014;**16**(9):464.

65. Heir T., Hussain A., Weisæth L. Managing the After-Effects of Disaster Trauma: The Essentials of Early Intervention. *European Psychiatric Review*. 2008;**1**:66–69.

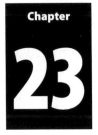

Chapter 23

Touring Medicine

Paul E. Pepe, Gerald W. (Jerry) Meltzer II, L. Scott Nichols, Stephen E. (Jake) Berry, and Peter H. Hackett[*]

Introduction

> True Riches Cannot Be Bought.
> One Cannot Buy the Friendship of
> a Companion
> to Whom One is Bound Forever By Ordeals
> Suffered in Common
> > *Excerpt from Antoine de St. Exupery's*
> > Wind, Sand and Stars *(1939)*

Consider the hypothetical situation that you are going on a long-awaited holiday trip or even a "dream vacation." Perhaps it is a honeymoon or twenty-fifth anniversary getaway. Maybe you're planning an adventurous overseas trip with college or work companions. Regardless of your age group, socioeconomic status, or destination, you have budgeted and already spent, relatively speaking, quite a bit of money. You also have already committed a significant amount of time planning each detail for a busy itinerary including flights or trains between different destination cities or countries. You think that you have identified the "perfect" places to stay and even have a well-conceived plan of action for many attractive tourist activities, sightseeing side-trips, and even some special local events while traveling through those destinations.

After a very long, somewhat exhausting flight and getting through immigration and customs, you've arrived at your lovelier than expected accommodation, take a short nap, and then set out on "day one" of your very special adventures. You even took advantage of an intriguing restaurant recommendation in your favorite search engine and it turned out to be such a great first evening. These were auspicious beginnings on the first stop of your journey.

On the third morning of what is already an unparalleled memorable trip, you rapidly develop the worst abdominal pain of your life. Trying to wait it out in your hotel room, you cancel the afternoon trip that you had planned, while your spouse, partner, or companions go ahead. The problem is, the pain becomes even worse over the next three hours. You suddenly have a chill and rapidly develop a fever as well as a terrible headache, muscle aches, terrible nausea, and possibly a blotchy rash. So should you call for an ambulance? How do you find one? Where will they transport you? Is there an emergency department (ED) or any hospital that will know how to handle this? Will they have computerized tomography (CT) scanners or magnetic resonance imagery? Will they have the right antibiotics or surgeons if needed? Will they practice the same kind of medicine that you would have had in hospitals using best practices in your home setting? Will they speak English (or your native language) well enough? The tourist book did not cover those questions and the embassy is in another city and the number is difficult to find. It's also the weekend. So now what? Also, what is the 911 or 999 equivalent number in this country?

While set up as a hypothetical, similar types of events do happen to many travelers. They are not that uncommon during important business or personal travel regardless of age, gender, home country, or occupation. It could be a mishap with a motorbike you rented that collides with the distracted truck driver who did not see the stop sign in Kuta (Bali), Quezon City (Philippines), or the road to Kamari beach in

[*] *The authors express their deepest gratitude to Doctors Aileen M. Marty and Michael T. Osterholm for their special support of mass gathering medicine and touring staff members, including most of the authors, over the past two decades. They also extend their gratitude to Sequel Tour Solutions for their unparalleled vision, leadership, inspiration and guidance in the support and development of touring medicine.*

Santorini (Greece). It could be a bicycle bump and flip in Mumbai (India), Amsterdam (Netherlands), or an intersection on the northside of Chicago (United States), or a gout attack in Dublin (Ireland) or Orlando (United States), or a very painful need for a root canal on a Sunday morning in Tokyo (Japan) or Seattle (United States). It could even be a crushing chest pain that feels like a vice tightening while in Santa Clara (United States) or Bergen (Norway). It could also be an abrupt loss of movement on the left side of your body in Auckland (New Zealand) or Sao Paolo (Brazil) or a sharp, unrelenting pain inside your cheek in Singapore or a pus-forming and extremely painful nailbed infection in Brisbane (Australia). How about an unrelenting, terrible cough in Seoul (Korea) or Glasgow (Scotland)? It may also be a sudden onset of a fast erratic heartbeat in the Peloponnese (Greece) or Madison Square Garden in New York City (United States). Where do you go? Who can you really trust, especially when your life may be at risk?

At the same time, and more commonly, the traveler will experience a newly acquired medical condition which is not as threatening at first glance because of mild symptomatology. However, that international (or even domestic) visitor may still need important medical information for reassurance or contingencies. Perhaps you are visiting London and you get sniffles and a mild sore throat. The COVID antigen test that you brought with you turns positive. Where would you go if you got worse, or you would simply like an anti-viral prescribed right way, and especially when 999 (UK Ambulance Service) would not seem to be an appropriate choice? Also, the closest medical facility recommended by the hotel on a google search does not sound like the best choice. Likewise, what if you are on a day trip sixty kilometers northeast of Marrakesh (Morocco) and your companion develops a very purulent eye infection or you are in Cape Town (South Africa) and have sudden lower back pain and some loss of feeling on one side of your right leg?

Beyond such unanticipated events, what if another tourist tells you that there was a rumor on social media about a new outbreak of dengue fever when you are visiting Mumbai (India)? What if there is a news media report in Sydney (Australia) that the air quality is going to be terrible that day due to nearby wildfires? It even smells smoky when you first walk out of the hotel. Should you stay inside the hotel or try to venture out? Likewise, wherever you are, is the water safe to drink or the ice cubes okay to use, especially in the hotel (or elsewhere)?

How would the altitude in Aspen (United States) or Mexico City (Mexico) manifest itself among different people and what should you do to prevent or mitigate the sickness? What if the next country in your itinerary across South America has an endemic yellow fever outbreak and the country to be visited next will not let you enter if you have been to that endemic region and you have no proof of inoculation? In fact, where would you procure that scarce vaccine? [1, 2]

****

The authors pose this somewhat excessive list of questions and conditions because they represent just a biopsy of the actual medical challenges, or very similar challenges, that they have *routinely* experienced while in those cited cities during tours with major entertainment artists or related travel. Moreover, most of these medical challenges were observed within the immediate past few years. The scenarios presented in the opening paragraphs were quite real for several of the typical core members of a touring team, often numbering about 150–200 persons (or more) for the tours with which the authors have been respectively involved for many years. Just having that number of travelers within such a major touring group obviously increases the odds of these various occurrences. Also, the length of the tours, several months at a time, increases that risk much further, not to mention the number of many ongoing tours conducted over a decade's time for a given artist. However, as described in great detail in this discussion, the nature of the travel, the work schedule, the proximity of tour personnel – and many other pertinent factors – will further accelerate the risks. These health and safety concerns even include dedicated tour members' hesitancy to abandon their posts to seek help for conditions that could later deteriorate and rapidly worsen. While the reticence to leave and receive medical care might be due to a very understandable loyalty to their duties, it is always frustrating to know that earlier intervention might have mitigated the problem.

Accordingly, having an expert, veteran touring medical specialist embedded into the touring team – and one who understands such nuances and how to manage them – has been found to be invaluable. Not only is such a specialist able to recognize and address such concerns, but the experienced and well-connected touring physician specialist will have prospective medical contingency plans for each city and for each venue (Figure 23.1). Such plans, usually established weeks or even months in advance, itemize

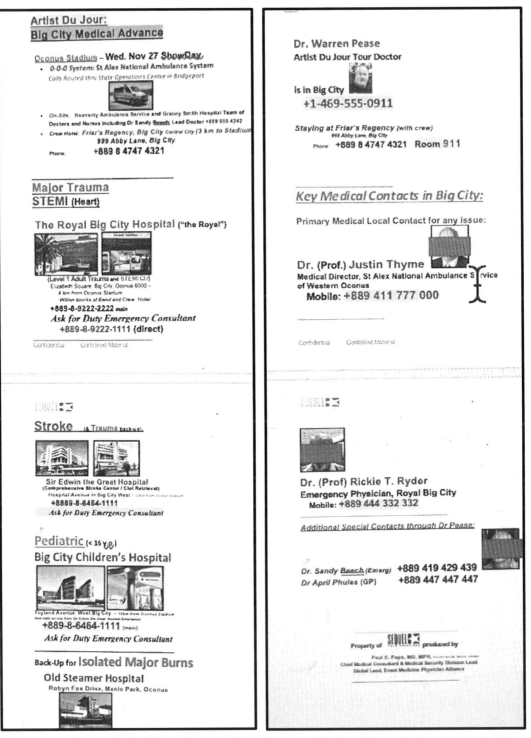

Figure 23.1 Mock-up of a Medical Advance Plan set up for scrolling on mobile phone (but combined here in two columns) – note: faces of actual contacts are covered purposely here, but is usually shown on this plan for rapid recognition on-site. There is also color-coding of the various conditions (stroke, brown; trauma/burns, red; pediatrics, orange; STEMI, green) for rapid reference.

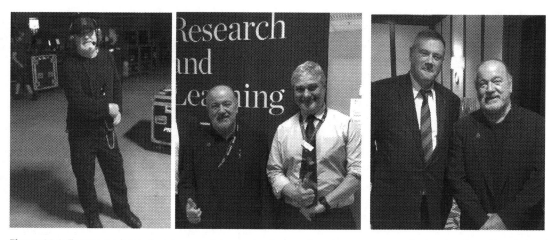

Figure 23.2 Touring medicine physicians usually have extensive experience in emergency medical services (out-of-hospital medical care), emergency medicine, and providing medical care in austere environments as well as experience in critical care medicine, travel medicine, epidemiology, protective medicine, and tactical medical response. They also develop close contacts and networks with similar specialists in major cities across the globe (pictured here are Dr. Paul Pepe, backstage in "all blacks" outfit in St Louis and later with counterparts in Melbourne, Australia, and Paris, France, Drs. Peter Morley and Pierre Carli, respectively).

the best local physicians in a given specialty who will be available to manage the respective medical care needs as well as several "point-person" expert physicians to contact when a relatively urgent condition arises, or even a critical life-threatening emergency arises. For many tour physicians, this point of contact has been the local emergency medical services (EMS) medical director(s) or the lead doctor(s) at the proximal trauma center and/or critical care center, especially if that contact (or a trusted surrogate) is to be working at the event (Figures 23.1 and 23.2). Refer to Table 23.1 for a list of suggested duties and responsibilities for touring physicians.

In proactive consultation with those local medical leaders, the medical advance work will include a plan for designating which hospitals would be the best facilities for each type of emergency threat as well as backup plans as indicated. The touring medical specialist also understands and anticipates potential threats such as local air quality concerns, endemic diseases and toxic drugs currently being peddled as well as emerging public health threats and contingencies for multiple casualty incidents (MCIs). Also, prior to travel, the crews are advised of appropriate vaccination requirements for the cities where performances will occur and also the preferred prophylaxis (if any) for potential threats. Beyond providing day-to-day minor care services, the on-site touring medical specialist will be capable of managing the first phases of life-threatening emergencies and

also provide any related communications with receiving doctors and staff, the family, and the tour directors as well as ensuring follow-up and providing continuity of care as indicated from one site to another or even arranging local follow-up for the patients when they return "back home." In essence, the touring doctor can be a major risk manager and a major risk reducer.

Regardless of the types of touring entities that engender mass gathering events, similar medical challenges may arise, be it for professional rugby or football teams traveling across Australasia or between Europe and South-Central America. The same is true for international tours for motorsports or tennis stars, and even heads of state and popes. Although there is, of course, the markedly increased risk for sports medicine related issues in athletic events, the entertainment tours are being singled out here because they bring along a flurry of additional challenges and circumstances that markedly increase the risk for a wide scope of illness and injury, either at each individual event site, or also as the tour moves from one city to another or, more often, one country to another.

Inherent Primary Medical Risk Factors in Touring Medicine

On a recent tour jointly served by several of the authors, the show crews found themselves in six different countries, many thousands of miles apart, over a fifteen-day period. Beyond different languages, cultures, politics, and religions in each of those countries, there were also extremes in climate where on one day the event was being held in bitter cold wintry weather and then, the next day, the crew arrives in a tropical nation with temperatures exceeding 86–88 degrees Fahrenheit (30–31°C) and oppressive dew-points (>65–70°F).

This example of every third- or fourth-day country-to-country schedule provides an initial basic level of insight into what differentiates tour medicine from most other mass gathering medicine "practices." The nomadic challenges of frequently moving from one time zone, climate and culture to another are compounded by an intensive work schedule, a lengthy travel day and the attendant compromise to the numerous crew members' sleep time and exercise time (if any) [3–21].

The need to travel together in very close proximity also creates attendant risks such as fully occupied, relatively long daily shuttle bus rides (e.g., hotel to the venue and back), commercial air travel on packed airline flights every few days and then working together in what are often cramped makeshift workspaces at the venue or stage areas [22].

For some, their rigorous schedule is also the ultimate challenge that they confront health-wise. For most crew members, the work can generate an internal sense of pride aided and abetted by the deep-rooted notion that they are part of a remarkable mission generated and stewarded by a multifaceted team comprised of the most talented professionals in each of their respective realms of duty and expertise. The extraordinary work ethic and loyalty to the mission is palpable. After spending the evening of the performance conscientiously accomplishing their various duties, tasks and chores for the show, the majority of the production team pitches in and begins to pack up and "load out" the entire stage, equipment, lighting towers, monitors and innumerable other components. Each of these pieces are tirelessly and repeatedly rolled out in relatively heavy freight cases, as rapidly but as safely as possible. The sooner the job is done, the sooner the team can get out and get some sleep (Figure 23.3). Physically, the load-out involves demanding labor and some risks. Various mishaps can and do happen. The process for most major tours typically starts just before midnight (i.e., within minutes of the performance ending and audiences still departing). While each of the crew members already have had fourteen to fifteen hours on the job that day, for many of them, their duties then progress well into the early morning hours. After those additional post-show hours, they may then travel back to the hotel for a possible pre-dawn "nap" before they usually need to embark on a very long travel day. That travel day, in a sense, launches the next work cycle. Accordingly, the touring physician witnesses and observes a very special culture and a unique team with a strong intrinsic work ethic, perceptible fortitude, and also a strong unspoken sense of pride and loyalty to completing a "best in show" mission. Even after the actual performance has ended, one still witnesses a highly choreographed and very interactive group of professionals efficiently de-constructing the stage, packing up and moving out and loading the various bins of cargo rapidly into transporting trucks. That post-show event makes this touring culture very special, but also very challenging health-wise on many levels [3–22]. Ironically, the imbedded tour physician, as a fellow nomad, not only faces many of the same risks and conditions, but also the additional risks of being on-call round-the-clock for one or two hundred souls who, regardless of time zone, typically can get sick or call for help in the wee hours of the morning or first thing before breakfast, right at dinner time or suddenly on an airplane. For the touring doctor, it can mean several months of "tour dyssomnia" for want of a better description.

In the following discussion, and to create context regarding a touring physician's role and practice, the authors will first provide a tedious detailing of a typical touring crew's workweek cycle while describing the span of the team members' variable ages and backgrounds. The discussion will include their relative risks, typical maladies (mostly described in the Introduction), and what preventive measures should be taken prior to touring (e.g., vaccinations, medical examinations, medications, and prescriptions). It then will discuss the impact of the various climates, environments, endemic diseases, and public health threats that the crew and band may encounter as well as the nuances of providing care to these intrepid crew members devoted to the mission. It will also address the unique issues of dealing with artists or management teams as well as navigating some unusual medical requests while in a country where the tour practitioner is not licensed to practice medicine and often faces logistic restrictions for optimal evaluation of a patient.

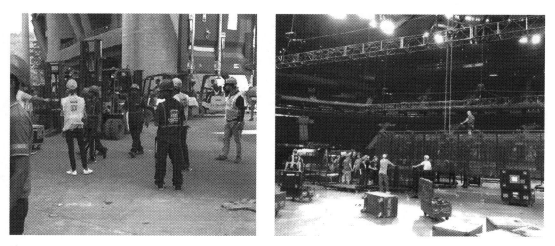

Figure 23.3 One of the major tasks of well-versed, high performance production crews is to choreographically move heavy equipment, in and out of stadiums and arenas every few days over several months, especially during late night hours after the show. These pieces include stage ("steel") skeletons, towers, large screens, lighting towers, massive speakers, barricades, monitors, video cameras and dozens of other apparatus and cargo. Although injuries are always a potential concern, the rigorous late night work hours after a long day of work can contribute to limited sleep and exercise time, thus predisposing to additional health risks that are compounded by an aggressive travel schedule from one city (or country) to another

As a central theme of the discussion, the authors will also review how the tour physician can better address the solutions to the questions posed at the beginning of this chapter, especially in terms of highly coordinated medical advance work. It will also discuss the role of the tour physician in collaborating with venue medical staff regarding care of the audience and venue staff, especially on show days (Figure 23.4). This interaction can often include preparations for MCIs, terrorist assaults, and unanticipated public health threats. It also involves medical support on-site when the tour physician is not licensed in the state, province or country of the tour performance.

The discussion will also begin to address how the tour physician can help the tour by serving as the infectious disease prevention professional, air quality specialist, and first-aid training instructor for the entire crew in an effort to ensure widespread basic cardiopulmonary resuscitation (CPR), automated external defibrillation (AED), choking, and bleeding control skills. It also includes being a medical equipment compliance watchdog ensuring the well-known and highly visible presence (and maintenance) of AEDs, tourniquets, pulse oximeters, and various other tools and interventions that pivotal team members will use. In the end, a "straw man" working job description will be offered as well as a strong

recommendation that we begin to train and mentor future event medicine (EVM) specialists [23]. That training and accompanying apprenticeship will hopefully help to facilitate how those protégés will know how to fit into this unique "loading dock lifestyle" and learn to humbly standby and serve each and every team member whenever needed.

Among the multitude of talented and world-renowned touring crew professionals doing their respective jobs in producing the tours, the tour physician is just one more adept technician who ensures that the show that "must go on, and will indeed go on. In that respect, the prospective medical practitioner learns to becomes one of many dozens of highly skilled and respected specialists, each providing their respective talents, be it in rigging, video, engineering, monitoring, lighting, audio, creative imaging, and many other tasks including those who are performing the entertainment for mass gathering audiences. In that respect, the touring production crew, band and managers comprise a family of sorts. Similar to a cohesive special operations military unit or a well-drilled disaster deployment team, they possess a mutual respect, esprit de corps, and history together. Regardless of their status in other settings, those new to that inner circle must earn that same degree of mutual respect and trust over time.

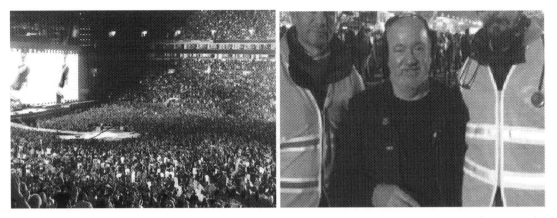

Figure 23.4 Many major tours will routinely encounter 75,000 to 100,000 audience members as well thousands of stadium workers, vendors, and many other support staff, all adding to an increased likelihood of medical events occurring during a given show. There is also an elevated risk for multiple casualty incidents (MCIs) from various precipitating events. In conjunction with tour security teams, tour physicians have a role in coordinating MCI planning and triage efforts with local emergency medical services, police and other public safety teams

The Work Cycle and Work Duties as Key Factors in Touring Medicine: Day One

Conceptually, like any other business traveler, the fresh work cycle begins with the travel day. A seasoned business traveler might simply envision that the trip begins with taxi or rideshare travel to the airport. After several minutes of going through priority security checkpoints and a brief wait until boarding the aircraft, there may be a three- to four-hour commercial flight to some domestic destination and a subsequent taxi/rideshare or bus/underground to an accommodation or meeting site. In contrast, for many logistical reasons, that scenario is much more protracted in the touring world.

For the touring crew, the flight is usually set for later in the afternoon on the day following the lengthy show day schedule and attendant overnight load-out process. However, when considering the large-scale migration of a typical major tour's crew size moving in unison, the schedule dynamic has to be adjusted and lengthened. This dynamic includes a very early arrival at the airport becoming a requirement in order to check in as many as 100 to 150 persons and their obligatory load of checked baggage as well as the time required to get this large contingent through security checkpoints in ample time, especially with unpredictable passenger traffic. At times, if all goes well, downtime at the airport can be lengthy. For reasons stated, that is an expected part of the job, but a longer travel day also can create an welcome opportunity for more relaxed networking, socializing, shopping, or browsing.

Nonetheless, even before that earlier timing for check-in, there is often lengthy travel to the airport in many large cities, often amplified by road traffic conditions. Bus rides to the airport can take over an hour or more in some venues. However, even before that transiting could take place, the combined luggage for those 100+ team members had to be steadily loaded ahead of time into one of several buses. Again, for such a large contingent, it adds in more time and early loading is encouraged. Fortunately, similar to post-show load-out, that process typically occurs with a collaborative good citizenship mindset to help ensure the team's timely departure from the hotel.

So, despite the overnight production load-out, the return to the hotel with perhaps only a little time to briefly nap, one must allot time for wake-up, clean-up, dressing and finishing one's packing before hopefully partaking in a departing breakfast and lining up for the hotel checkout before loading the luggage. Therefore, the travel day actually has a very early start despite the length of the previous (show) day and incumbent overnight post-show labors. This day often begins six to eight hours prior to a 2pm or 3pm flight departure for the next city or country.

Then, of course, upon arrival at that next destination, many hours later, there are the typical (long) lines at passport control, followed by the collective wait for everyone's checked luggage to be delivered and retrieved at the baggage claim area. After a rolling-luggage walk to the bus, often in a parking area at some distance away from the terminal, there is resumption of the loading baggage campaign, followed by another hour-long trip to the hotel during rush hour followed by the mass check-in process for over a hundred persons. After a brief visit to one's room, there may be subsequent lobby rendezvous meetings to explore dining in the new destination city or, in some cases, travel to the performance venue (stadium or arena) to begin their roles in the assembly and construction of various aspects of production. This activity sometimes occurs to ensure the timely build-up of "steel" (stage backbone) elements or lighting and audio consoles or it may be conducted to ensure that critical freight and equipment essentials have arrived as well as confirming that power, security, proper access, and other key elements of production are falling into place. Therefore, the travel days are (relatively) long for some and much longer for others.

Regardless of role, the schedule for most of the touring team would be considered quite imposing and rigorous for the average person, no matter their age, depth of calluses, or underlying physical condition. For these exceptionally talented and mission-oriented folks, however, it is simply what is expected. In that respect, they would likely find this tedious discourse on travel days a little perplexing and unclear as to its purpose. However, for the prospective touring physician, this perspective is essential to understanding these prospective patients. It helps to emphasize the exceptional time commitment that the touring job entails on a "light day." It is also written to enlighten readers and prospective tour doctors in terms of what they may expect to observe and participate in on such lengthy workdays beyond the medical care duties.

The "on-the-road again" setting is nothing like anyone's typical personal experience unless they had served in some analogous role such as volunteer team physician accompanying a high school rowing team traveling *en masse* to a national regatta in another state or country or if the practitioner had experience playing or working with a college football team, accompanied by coaches, cheerleaders and band members, to a distant opponent's stadium.

Day Two in the Typical Work Cycle: Main Load-In Day

By the next day (the formal "load-in" day), most of the entire crew is well in motion, from physical labor tasks to highly technical tasks. Hopefully after a good breakfast at the hotel, the work day often starts with a staggered schedule of shuttles taking subdivision members (e.g., lighting crew members, videographers,

"backline" technicians) to the venue. Depending on the locale and the venue, the ride from the hotel to the venue can often be less than a half-hour in Rome, walkable in New York, or greater than an hour in Luzon (Philippines). Once at the venue, there is a lot of movement, activity and moving parts, cables, fences, and likely very hot outdoor conditions depending on the site as many tours take place in the summer and an open stadium evening show.

By midday, the site is buzzing with high-visibility (high-viz) vests and hardhats (Figure 23.3). There is a well-practiced and long-established orchestration of the production team. Such teams are the best-in-the-business riggers and carpenters, stage managers, audio techs and lighting teams, videographers and monitor engineers, as well as an effective, hard-working catering group and information technology (IT) specialists. Around the venue, there are top-notch steel crews, power crews, climbing crews, barricade crews, merchandisers, stage and dressing room wranglers, and a cadre of experts in the assembly and function of various high-technology jumbo screens and their eventual operation during the show. Working "down under" (below the stage) are the most respected and skilled backline technicians, great musicians themselves, unloading an array of guitars, drums and keyboards, fine-tuning them – and staging a cadre of backup instruments for each song. Not to be outdone, there are very talented creative teams and animators, best-in-the-industry security teams and a hard-working cadre of production office specialists and usually a globally known production director. At every step, there are eagle-eyed on-site tour directors conducting a myriad of business-related and administrative tasks along with their veteran tour promotion team members. The list can go on. For the purposes of this discussion, however, the roster can also include the "Tour Medical Consultant" (or whatever title is assigned). As subsequently described in more detail, that physician is responsible for arranging, advising, facilitating, and optimizing the various aspects of health security and expert medical care for these many industrious souls hailing from various home bases around the globe.

The detailed list of crew members being described here is also a purposeful device to begin to indicate (for prospective tour medicine practitioners) the potential breadth of activities and personnel for whom they will be expected to attend and advise as well as to begin to allude to their various risks. On the larger, veteran circuits, the age of these various crew members can be quite variable, ranging from young adult men and women in their twenties to the bulk of the crew who usually are experienced veterans in their thirties, forties, and fifties as well as several "senior" team members in key leadership and oversight roles. As expected, many older members will be taking various medications and dealing with some typical middle-aged diseases, but, like any other collection of personages, even the younger cadre may have some underlying chronic or congenital conditions. They also can be young and quite healthy and yet incur and experience all of the conditions described in the opening paragraphs – among many other illnesses and injuries seen around the globe.

Nonetheless, what can make this pool of potential patients a little more complex may be their national origins, backgrounds and home bases. These A-list touring specialists can be quite diverse, hailing from multiple nations. Sometimes historical information can be lost-in-translation due to language or cultural differences, though these challenges are usually minor. However, the types of medications, remedies, or reported underlying conditions may fall outside of the practitioner's usual lexicon and experience [24]. Some persons may be using special prescriptions or they have preferably chosen to receive treatment suggestions from alternative sources or friends that may be in contrast to accepted practice. Overall though, it also creates a learning environment for the medical practitioners even if it does not change their own practice preferences or advice to others.

In addition to the on-site crew stemming from the tour, there are also local venue security and management teams and a long list of other building caretakers, contractors, cleaners, and maintenance crews for that venue.

By nightfall on day two, the team is usually still on-site working to make sure that everything is ready for the upcoming day, simply known as "show day." At this point, with a few key exceptions, such as the on-site tour promoters, tour director and related teams, the majority of the band's main entourage will usually not have arrived on-site at the venue. On other occasions, they may perform an evening sound-check on this preshow day and thus most of the crew members will remain on-board into the evening. For the on-site production team, however, most will eventually get that night off and hopefully catch up on sleep although, quite often, this preshow evening is a cherished time to relax, imbibe, socialize, and network with their companions-in-arms and others. Again, depending on the artist, the tour size and the particular tour culture, all of these scheduling practices may change, unpredictably.

Show Day

On day three, "show day" in this sample schedule scenario, the various crew members will once again be shuttled back to the venue. Depending on the priority, they may be shuttled to the venue in a staggered fashion to finalize tasks during the morning hours and into the afternoon. Accordingly, the tour physician's schedule may depend on the timing and location of the situation or logistics with respect to local support such as local doctors willing to come in and see patients at the venue. The touring clinician may encounter medical requests at the hotel or even escort crew members to a clinic or receiving facility for the purposes of conducting an excision of an infected cyst or facilitating MRI imaging on a knee. In other situations, they may be called to venue early on to attend to someone needing more urgent attention or to a band member's suite.

Sometime in the mid-afternoon or later, and depending on the artist, the band members and their entourage will likely beginning to arrive. The preshow warm-up rehearsals and sound checks will typically take place in the later afternoon. Then, as last-minute preparations are underway, most of the tour components will hopefully get a chance to secure a preshow meal at catering before show time.

In large A-list tours, there may be fifty or more personnel in the entourage who often travel separately from the production crew. This usually includes an assigned security member for each of the band members or, minimally, for some of the primary talent. It will also entail other personal and family security team members, wardrobe specialists and grooming assistants. It also includes the tour manager and assistants, the artists' management team, the band members themselves and accompanying family members, chaplains, personal trainers, physiotherapists, road manager, photographers, videographers, travel assistants, publicists, accountants, artist relations director(s), ticketing liaisons, creative directors, choreographers, business managers, and so on. Back-up singers and dancers may or may not travel separately. Opening act bands will typically travel separately, but most of these components will all arrive on show day adding to the growing mix of potential patients not to mention the army of various staff, ushers, venue security teams, vendors, merchandisers, ticket managers, runners (shuttle drivers), parking lot managers, local police, fire, and EMS.

Simply put, there are even more potential patients arriving on (or sometimes before) show day. Like the other production team members, these additional tour members may need advice or have a relatively minor medical issue such as onset of lower back pain, a zoster outbreak, a paronychia, a chalazion, a new bump felt on their skin, an unexplained rash, sialolithiasis, a likely fixed drug eruption from recently ingested ibuprofen, or just a classic sore throat with white patches. Particularly for those constantly wearing fitted earpieces, cerumen impact can be very common and a chronic cough can become a frequent occurrence in this close-knit, well-congregated group where adenoviruses love to spread as they often do in other recently gathered populations [25, 26]. Though less often a problem, there could be accompanying children or grandchildren who may have some chronic issue such as being a known diabetic who may require some assessment and reassurances for the parents. Adding to the mix, visiting VIPs, elected officials, movie stars, and personal friends of the artists will also be in attendance, sometimes joining into the entertainment and sometimes attending the show as special guests. While the need for medical attention for VIPs is relatively infrequent, interactions can be more complex (see Chapter 14 and subsequent comments in this chapter).

Oftentimes, because the crew had been so busy over the prior days with their various time-dependent tasks and also because the entourage may not have been on-site or even in the city of the performance for three days, a common time for requests for medical counsel and advice can be in the late afternoon hours just before showtime. Complicating this time frame is the very tight window of opportunity available for the respective tour members requesting help. Triage of priority patients involves juggling logistics. At times, finding those persons who are asking for help by text or through supervisors can be challenging. Accordingly, this preshow period could be an optimal time for having other trusted local doctors on-site to help expedite the process and more efficiently attend to all those requests under the concurrent time pressures. Also, in touring medicine situations, the medical actions may require

someone with medical licensure in that jurisdiction. Strategies for recruiting those trusted local associates are detailed later in this discussion.

Quite often, it is not the patients themselves but their supervisors or personal assistants that alert the tour doctor to attend to an ill or injured tour member. As discussed in greater detail in Chapters 4 and 14 and subsequent discussion here, team members themselves can be reticent or even become outright stoic about taking time out for medical attention. Concerned about not performing or completing their assigned tasks, these professionals often put their sense of mission over their personal needs. Therefore, sensitivity to that mindset must be anticipated and balanced patiently with good medical practices. Also, while the touring practitioner may set up a "clinic site" at the venue for seeing patients and ensuring privacy, very often, one may need to go to the band member or a family member in their secured dressing room areas, or more frequently, to see a sound engineer, personal assistant or backline technician at their respective posts. In contrast to standard medical practice today where patients usually travel to see the doctor, in this setting, house calls, or more appropriately, "back of house" calls are the norm.

The show itself is obviously intensive, hard work for the entire crew and their individual assignments as well as the security team, especially the security liaisons interacting with venue personnel, arranging motorcade ingress and egress and organizing last minute contingencies. The tour leaders and the tour staff members who are handling VIPs, special audience members and the media are in full swing. Managing last minute requests from the band are always front and center. On the medically related front, security teams have a very high-level focus on safely admitting the audience who may attempt to rush in to gain optimal positions in an open, first-come, first-choice general audience setting. Similarly, managing the packed-in crowds in front of the stage continues to be an issue throughout the performance. Also, many of the audience members may have been waiting, sometimes for days, outside of the stadium in heat, in cold, in rain, or even snow at times, to gain their cherished positions near the stage. That exposure to the elements and lack of sleep may not only affect their medical vulnerability, stability and resilience entering the venues, but also throughout the performance. As it is now show day, the venue medical personnel will largely manage these in-house circumstances, but the touring physician, as an extension of the tour brand and mission to support the fans, may often look in on these super fans awaiting entry to assess their well-being and ensure local medical teams are aware of their status.

Meanwhile, as the evening approaches, backstage activities are in full force from wardrobe and videographers to lighting/audio personnel and the litany of engineers and technicians, let alone the band, their managers and stage crews. As there was meticulous attention to detail in assembling the production on everyone's part, there is a similar perfectionist-driven mentality that guides each professional in terms of their part in the flawless execution of the performance. At the same time, despite this obvious intensity and accompanying pressures, flawless performance to exceed the fans' expectations is still the reason for the mission. It is a joy for each of the tour members to consider themselves a pivotal cog in the entertainers' artistry. Beyond the joy of the music itself, a successful performance is a brief but priceless reward for the entire crew, entourage and management. As one production crew member's embossed tee shirt might proudly read, "No Pressure, No Diamonds."

Then again, at the end of the show, in typical team-oriented mindset, the strenuous tear-down and load-out process begins once again, rolling into the wee hours of the night. Then the next multiday cycle dawns all over again.

Although the mentioned three-day turnaround may be common, some of the various city or country stopovers may also allow for an extra day or two for some well-deserved downtime. This mini-break can allow for special sightseeing and becoming the tourists themselves, sometimes by boat, often by foot, by bike, or just by the poolside. Nevertheless, the risks originally described for any tourist in the opening lines of this chapter still exist and the term "accidental tourist" can take on new meaning for the day-off adventurers. Also, once they are back on the job, the schedule and the consequential effects on human physiology still remain challenging. Also, there are other health risks in the world of touring beyond the work cycle.

Health Challenges Beyond the Work Cycle for Music-Industry Nomads

Given the obvious physiological stressors of the work cycle that can compromise sleep, exercise, and eating habits for many, it is logical that there is an ensuing compromise to immune systems [5–21]. This risk is further exacerbated by the close quarters in which these many dozens of persons may travel together on shuttle buses or airport coaches [22, 25]. Likewise, they may work in close proximity to each other within small indoor temporary office spaces, locker room areas, trailers, or even shared overnight sleeping coaches. Beyond the touring lifestyle, one problem that still continues throughout the world today is an individual who is coughing frequently in the presence of others and often without an attempt to suppress its expulsion. While less of issue than it was before COVID-19, one can still find unsuppressed coughers in many public places, work environments, airline flights, and municipal transportation today who, in fact, do infect others. Even without a frequent cough, persons talking freely (and very often in high volumes in a noisy bar or during a crowded bus ride) may expire more infection-laden breaths that can spread to others, especially sitting closely together during a poorly ventilated half-hour shuttle ride to the venue or on the return trip [22, 27].

One might better appreciate today the need for such team members to travel separately and to wear protective type (N95, KN-95) masks, especially if coughing, either on that bus or in any other close quarters indoors. However, even in the general population, and particularly in eating establishments or cafeterias, compliance with (appropriate) mask-wearing can be resisted, politically, sociologically and philosophically. Thus, health security risks can be further elevated in these circumstances.

In fact, as it is in many other work environments, and well before COVID-19, it has been common to watch a respiratory-pharyngeal type of infection spread rapidly across an entire cadre of production team members or band members. Today, there is more sensitivity to this concern and associated good practices, but good hygiene habits can always be improved. This concern constitutes another important oversight role for the touring physician including recommendations for infection control policies, monitoring compliance and appropriate circumstances for isolation. Also, to protect the mission, an important role can be to recommend vaccinations as indicated going well beyond the usual COVID and influenza guidelines.

Catering areas also create potential sources of cross-contamination with mutually handled cafeteria-line ladles, serving spoons, food covering lids, and shared table space. For some tours, there may have been shared space for dining with local working crews, guests and others. As a result, there could be well over 200–300 guests passing through a typical catering set-up, further adding to the risk. While better controlled today, there are also the usual potential risks encountered in these settings promulgated by servers using less than optimal hygienic practices or by food-borne illnesses related to contaminated food being transported in to the caterers in some locales or climates. Just one bad batch of a single food item (e.g., the chicken dish or the side salad dish) can conceivably cause a mini-MCI.

Prior to the COVID-19 pandemic, the use of hand sanitizers was negligible and, despite knowledge about infectious agents such as noroviruses wreaking havoc on cruise ships [22], it was never emphasized enough in terms of how important it was to use hand sanitizers before handling the ladles, serving spoons and food coverings. Presanitizing or wearing disposable gloves was never emphasized (i.e., to avoid passing pathogens onto to others). Similarly, an under-utilized practice is sanitizing hands after going through the buffet line to better protect that individual from any contamination that did occur from others less compliant with gloving or sanitizing. Noncompliance with these procedures can be especially threatening if there was sneezing/ coughing into the food area, even by mildly ill persons while in line. While procedures have now improved, there is still a large degree of laxity and this becomes an additional risk to other crew members. Losing pivotal staff or a band member to illness creates subsequent compromise to the delivery of key functions and the mission altogether. It also can create additional work for others picking up the slack. Again, this public health challenge can constitute another health security task for the touring medicine physician serving as the de facto public health officer.

External Factors and Preemptive Medical Considerations

Beyond some of the more team-related (internal) factors of work schedule, venue factors, job duties, travel, proximity, food-related issues, and even illness or injury while on a day off, there are also external factors that may need to be considered, particularly for an entertainment tour working mostly in outdoor venues. More specifically, these include air quality and climate-related working conditions, altitude, civil unrest, and endemic diseases or exposures to insect or animal-related threats including snakes, ticks, and mosquitoes. The list could go on.

Air Quality Is Not a Simple Air Quality Index Reading

Air quality is a perennial threat in some nations or regions and it may even preempt a decision to travel to such destinations. However, air quality issues (or civil unrest or new epidemics) may arise unexpectedly just prior to a tour that may have been planned years in advance. These threats are obviously a major concern with much at stake ranging from tour revenues and local economies to avoiding profound disappointments to tens of thousands of fans, many of whom will have traveled some distance to attend a long-awaited performance by their favorite artist, or even to attend several performances at a multishow / multiday destination. When attendees are outside in a stadium and being exposed to heavily polluted air or if there has been heavy wildfire smoke permeating the local atmosphere, often laden with very fine particulates, there is risk to the audience as well as the touring crew [28]. The audience is typically ventilating more frequently and more deeply than usual with enthusiastic singing, shouting, cheering, and also because of the adrenaline-stoked excitement that can prompt deeper and more frequent breaths. More importantly, the entertainers, and particularly the lead singers, will be aggressively running about large stadium stages, breathing more deeply and frequently due to the exercise-driven physiological demand [29]. Simply put, the active loud singing will pull in larger amounts of polluted air. Anyone with reactive airway disease or other risks can certainly be affected both on-stage or in following days [29]. Again, the same applies to the audience and also the crews who may have been working hard all day in that environment and during peak ozone periods in some environments. Knowing the air quality index (AQI) is one thing, but the type of pollution (forest fire, industry pollution, particulate matter size) can carry specific risks and ascertaining knowledge of any increased emergency department visits or calls to local pulmonary physicians or local health ministries may provide additional caution – or reassurances – depending on the findings [29–31].

Paul E. Pepe, Gerald W. (Jerry) Meltzer II, L. Scott Nichols, Stephen E. (Jake) Berry, and Peter H. Hackett

Elevation

Altitude illness can be either quite apparent or quite subtle depending upon the individual and often depending on the elevation [32, 33]. One can expect a myriad of manifestations across a variety of persons. Previous studies have even associated the increased risk of early symptomatology among the younger populations, but they can also recover and acclimatize faster. The usual signs and symptoms like bronchorrhea, trouble sleeping, and generalized malaise and headache can potentially augment the usual risks for the workforce and their job performance. Fortunately, the general audiences and local crews assisting the tour are less likely to have issues unless they are visitors from sea levels or from any significantly lower altitudes.

Popular high-risk venues for tours are Mexico City (7,349 feet above sea level), Bogota (8,661 ft), Johannesburg (5,751 ft), and Denver (5,279 ft), but, occasionally, there are visits to special sites or festivals (Aspen, USA, 7,908 ft or Telluride 8,750 ft) which can be even more challenging for the unacclimatized. As expected, finger pulse oximeter saturations will be lower with higher elevations, this includes in-flight experiences where cabin pressures are usually pressurized to the equivalent of 5,500 to 6,500 feet and sometimes at higher elevation equivalents. At significant altitudes or flying above 30,000 feet, low readings like 93 percent or 94 percent might be expected. Therefore, a lowish pulse oximeter reading is not necessarily reflecting a disease process. At the same time, it also does not rule out illness. Clinical assessment and experienced acumen remain the most important allies and another rationale for having knowledgeable tour doctors in the ensemble.

One high altitude issue is dehydration. The longer the flight, the longer the exposure and risk. Commercial flight cabins are not only pressurized to a (relatively) high altitude, but the air is quite dry. Similar to higher elevations, it can predispose to more insensible human volume losses, especially with the diuresis from concomitant ethanol intake by the air traveler or visitor to high altitudes. Subsequent evolving dehydration without frequent water intake will likely incur and exacerbate issues. Those insensible losses will be augmented in singing performers and others engaged in excess exercise and ventilatory demand [33]. Such politely stated admonitions about pre- and inflight alcohol intake, dehydration, and sometimes nebulous altitude symptoms should be emphasized to the crew members, performers, and all of their guests and family members.

Endemic Diseases and Emerging Threats

The tour doctor may be called into the tour administration to assess the need for disease prophylaxis at an upcoming destination [34]. It may also involve a request to directly find and obtain that proposed protective measure for the entire crew. Typically, someone in a risk management role may have seen some social media message reporting something like a malaria epidemic at the next stop on the tour. For this very circumstance, tour physicians develop a travel medicine acumen and are quite facile at ascertaining the actual risks. This capability can involve doing homework ahead of the tour and establishing local connections prospectively regarding any need for mass prophylaxis such as yellow fever inoculation or, in the case of malaria, with substances such as Malarone^{TM}, both adult and pediatric tablets (atovaquone and proguanil) [34]. In most cases, such prophylaxis is not without risk (or expense) and, depending on the specific time and place, the relative risk of not providing prophylaxis may be low, especially with shorter stays in the larger cities where the risk for the malaria or yellow fever may be lower.

Nonetheless, instead of simply dismissing the need for action altogether, the tour physician could suggest alternative strategies in such cases. For example, though not yet entirely proven to date, one could still recommend the vigilant use of something like N,N-diethyl-meta-toluamide (DEET) while working outside in the areas of concern. Beyond providing a pragmatic action plan. this approach may carry a greater benefit as malaria and mosquitoes are not the only concern. Depending on the venue, mosquitoes may carry dengue fever viruses, West Nile, zika, yellow fever, and many other pathogens and there are other threats, including tick-borne illness, for which DEET could be helpful.

At the same time, having an open mind is important. Thorough investigation *through numerous credible sources* (such as the same conscientious approach recommended for air quality) should be conducted. This would involve consulting with other travel medicine experts, infectious disease specialists, health authorities and boots-on-the-ground emergency department leaders. Therefore, having prospective contacts is important in pretour resource-gathering. *Shoreland Travax*^TM (authors have no conflicts of interest) is one additional resource traditionally used by VIPs and even public officials for ascertaining such information. Embassies can also provide some insights but with less reliability in terms of rapid access to information in an emergency.

Beyond mosquito and tick-borne concerns, various tropical parasites are common in some venues and water quality can be a universal problem as well as ventilation systems with outbreaks of Legionella and fungus-related disease being reported in more and more places, especially for certain susceptible persons [35]. Both globally and in one's own country, having a better working knowledge of toxicological, environmental and public health threats can put these uncommon threats on the radar screen for consideration and faster mitigation.

Preemptive Interventions and Pretour Advisories and Preparations

Also, developing a working knowledge of endemic and evolving epidemics in communities to be visited is an important preemptive task to accomplish long before the tour to ensure they have appropriate vaccinations prior to the tour for high-risk threats such as recent diphtheria-pertussis-tetanus, influenza, COVID-19, or the virus du jour. Tetanus is a common disease in some countries and the risk for lacerations and burns can be high in some aspects of the tour tasks. For some venues, vaccinations against hepatitis are strongly recommended, particularly hepatitis A and B as well as ensuring completion of many childhood vaccinations. Polio outbreaks were beginning to arise in 2019 (e.g., Philippines) and, since then, it has begun to arrive in other countries including nations on the other side of the globe such as the United States (U.S.) and United Kingdom [36–37]. Pretour advisories can also include recommendations for the tour members to see their personal healthcare providers before beginning the tour to better ensure that they will have precise copies of prescribed medicines (for countries with strict regulations regarding prescriptions) as well as an adequate supply of those medications which might not be available elsewhere. Knowledge of the medications that are considered illegal in certain countries is critical such as the case of medical marijuana-related compounds in the Russian Federation resulting in criminal charges, conviction, and lengthy incarceration.

In addition, having awareness of any local civil unrest or even political antipathy for the tour itself should always be an underlying concern prompting need to establish an MCI plan with local public safety agencies and particularly EMS. Not only would a clinician want to facilitate appropriate evacuations, but also ensure adequate supplies of hemostatic devices (tourniquets and pressure dressings) and also relevant training for key members of the crew, if not all crew members [39].

To summarize many of the preceding sections, there are many health risks that can predispose the nomads of touring to injury, diminished resilience, and even situational compromise to immune systems. These risks not only emanate from the rigorous work schedules, travel-related factors, and typical communal dining factors associated with entertainment tours, but also environmental and public health threats as well as tendencies for these professionals to stoically work through their own personal issues for the benefit of the mission.

Better Defining the Role of the Touring Physician and Regulatory Concerns

Obviously, maintaining confidential records of significant interventions or medical advice rendered is a priority, whether they were provided to staff, celebrities, or audiences. Beyond the usual documentation of medical care/advice rendered, this confidential documentation also helps to validate the extremely busy role of the physician working in the world of touring medicine. Keeping logs of the cases will readily demonstrate the breadth and volume of need. Until seeing the volume and depth of need, many tour promoters had not yet appreciated the clear need for the touring medical professional nor, more importantly, the differences in outcomes for those becoming ill or injured. Even when not directly providing care to the patients because of licensure and regulatory issues in some states, provinces or nations, the referral and the consultation provided should be documented, as well as the de facto co-involvement in decision-making that optimized the outcomes.

One issue about practicing medicine in the touring setting is as basic as whether or not the physician has a medical licensure to practice medicine in the jurisdiction of the venue. For example, a US physician is unlikely to be licensed to practice medicine in Singapore or Rome. Therefore, the role of the touring physicians may be more of a screening and consulting process in which they coordinate and enlist a known and trusted licensed physician in the respective country, state, or province, whether a known colleague or another trusted leader in the community.

Often a reliable contact is the jurisdictional EMS medical director for the city or region covering the event or one near the event. The metropolitan EMS medical directors (aka, medical "Eagles") global alliance is a very influential collaborative group of leading emergency physicians who, collectively, are responsible for the EMS protocols for the 911 system responses to over 110 million Americans and tens of millions of citizens in many others nations [40–42]. Each member of this cohesive team assesses and determines the best hospital destinations for various types of emergency patients within their respective jurisdictions and they also perform related follow-up quality assurance However, they also share and exchange, on a weekly basis, the most progressive best practices and novel experiences and insights. Accordingly, they have now been used routinely in recent years by all of the authors. This collaboration facilitates several goals. First, the jurisdictional EMS medical director is usually highly experienced with both in-hospital and out-of-hospital care. They are also generally the local experts and decision-makers in terms of setting destination policies for patients calling the public safety answering point (PSAP) for ambulance response (e.g., 911, 999, 112, 000, or 111). They would likely have the best working knowledge of where to take a severe stroke patient or a ST-elevation myocardial infarction (STEMI) patient or where to go for major adult trauma, an orthopedic injury or any pediatric emergency, dental emergency, or serious burns. The secondary gain is establishing mutual familiarity with any predetermined plan for mutually agreed hospital designations as previously noted. This working alliance also is exceptionally important in the event of an ensuing MCI to better ensure that the response is coordinated. It also allows for better follow-up, particularly if it involves artists or tour members. In addition, even if the local medical protocols used by contracted medical providers hired by the venue may have called for transport to the nearest facility, that jurisdictional EMS medical director can, for appropriate reasons, override that policy in advance (or in real-time) for indicated appropriate reasons, even if it was his or her own protocol. Most importantly, that physician and his or her team are typically highly respected emergency physicians or they would not be in that position. Most of them work in, or have worked in level I trauma center equivalents and/or tertiary care centers for the region. Accordingly, they can provide the best on-site medical care and on behalf of the touring medicine practitioner who, in turn, can still advise and assist that local medical leader as permitted. Most of the time, the touring physician is the one who is likely to assess and determine the care that the patient likely needs to receive, but then will refer the case to the local specialists for their "second (validating) opinion" and any intervention as indicated. This is analogous to a knowledgeable cardiologist determining a patient's likely need for a cardiothoracic surgeon's intervention (e.g., bypass surgery) and calling one in for their additional opinion and surgical care. Or, more simply, it is analogous to an internist diagnosing a likely appendicitis and referring the patient care over to the abdominal surgeon. As a result, the title of "tour medical consultant" works well for this paradigm. It also works quite well for most tours based in the United Kingdom, certain Commonwealth countries, and Ireland where the term, consultant, is usually defined as a respected senior physician or surgeon in the National Health Service (NHS), somewhat akin to a "Professor" moniker elsewhere.

Naturally, if a true critical emergency arises such as the need to perform CPR, use an AED, provide choking assistance, or stop overt bleeding, those interventions should be performed as needed and some basic interventions and prescriptions can be rendered if provided within the practitioner's home country, even if the tour is not located in his or her home state or province. Two of the authors who, over the years, respectively have served as the touring physicians for two of the largest-attended entertainment tours worldwide, are both licensed in multiple states and most national pharmacies will accept their prescriptions in any state as they have national practitioner numbers and US Drug Enforcement Agency (DEA) certifications. That same advantage may not apply for other countries, however. One resolution is to have a carry-along bag with a supply of commonly used medications and specialized tools (including an ear canal fiber-optic and simple suture kits), keeping in mind the drug policies of the countries to be visited. Clearly, having the local physician point person(s) involved and credentialed as local staff is optimal, particularly within the more rigid regulatory jurisdictions.

One consideration for transporting medical equipment and supplies could be to place them in a rolling cargo cabinet that could be transported with all other tour equipment. This also allows for additional equipment that would be transported in personal luggage. For example, while best suited for sports-related mass gatherings, one suggested assessment tool could be a portable point-of-care ultrasound (POCUS) machine. POCUS can serve dozens of on-site purposes ranging from facilitation of peripheral venous catheterization to detecting a pneumothorax, retinal detachment fracture, or gallstone. The cabinet can also hold a supply of many additional tourniquets or bags of fluids for intravenous infusions or portable electrocardiographic devices. Also, as there is likely room available in the cargo carriers, the tour could bring along neuroprotective CPR equipment (active compression-decompression device, impedance threshold device and an automated head elevation device) as part of the set-up [43,44].

Strategies to Enlist Additional Trusted Physicians on Show Day

In terms of routine contingencies such as a possible large volume of medical requests late on show day or a sudden crowd emergency, explosion, or other need for additional on-site medical support, there are multiple strategies including having many supplemental medical staff on-site.

Many venues provide their in-house medical support for the audience at large using the local EMS paramedics from the governmental entity that usually makes 911-type responses on a day-to-day basis for that community. However, some venues may enlist other services such as a hospital or private ambulance services that may or may not staff an EMS-oriented medical director or EMS fellow. The venue may hire a private ambulance service or create a hybrid of public and private services. Others contract or receive donated services from a local hospital with doctors, nurses and medics staffing several first aid rooms. Oftentimes, those entities will enlist multiple doctors. Therefore, the on-site support could come from these physicians already at the venue. The touring staff needing medical care could be referred to their stations, but, in reality, the logistics and difficulties in tour members leaving their posts have already been discussed. Also, the

venue doctors may not be able to assist on days other than show days or they may be too busy at their own posts to assist.

Using the strategy referenced previously, the on-site support doctors might preferably be the trusted local EMS or ED leaders who, at the recommendation of the tour physician, are prospectively recruited, vetted and credentialed by the tour security team and would remain on-site before and during the event. These doctors would be permitted to attend and enjoy the main entertainment itself but still are considered to be "on-call" and recognized as working staff prepared to respond as needed. In other words, they would not be drinking alcohol and they would be constantly monitoring their texts or other alerting systems amidst the noise of the event. These medical personnel can be remunerated for their stand-by time or, more often, these invaluable clinicians can be allowed to enjoy the music festivities at no cost as a guest of the production including the privilege of bringing a companion guest.

Plan B would be to have numerous other qualified medical persons stand by on a similar "on-call" mode, but outside the site. The problem with that approach is the potential for limited access if a violent situation has occurred and the venue is in lockdown. Other hurdles could be overcoming peri-event traffic or lack of the specialized credentials needed to get into the venue. There could be a combination of plan A and B, but having additional high-level medical staff credentialed and on-site, ready to go to work is much more optimal. This approach is not only much preferred by many tour physicians, but, again, it is even better if the on-site physician(s) could include the local jurisdictional medical authorities (physician medical directors) for the responding EMS ambulance system (i.e., 999, 911, 112, 000, 111, etc.) who can help to oversee ambulance routings, on-site MCI management or help organizers with specialized information about best destinations/options for their artists, crews and others who may need some type of specialized care (e.g., dentist) or prescriptions.

It should also be noted that some countries technically do not permit the provision of medical care outside of a medical facility, such as Japan, and so it can be somewhat difficult to have proper care provided on-site. That particular nuance becomes another issue to navigate particularly in terms of artists or dedicated

Paul E. Pepe, Gerald W. (Jerry) Meltzer II, L. Scott Nichols, Stephen E. (Jake) Berry, and Peter H. Hackett

crew members unwilling to leave their posts. Therefore, the concept of having a knowledgeable "navigator" at the venue has, at the very least, improved the situation given these circumstances.

In addition to having the local surrogate (the talented local physicians) present at the venue, it is also wise to develop a team approach for the tour physicians by having multiple touring specialists imbedded on the tour. Even if strapped with the same regulatory restrictions, the additional doctors can provide some downtime for the principal tour physician. This approach has worked quite well for one of the larger tours and it allows each of the doctors, from time to time, a break to return to their primary practices or it allows them to become more efficient, get more sleep and take turns being on-call and working around the clock as is often the case on large tours. As exhausting as the job can be for the crew, it can be even more challenging for the conscientious tour doctor. One recent methodology for accomplishing the touring doctor team has been the apprenticeship model in which a highly qualified emergency doctor becomes an event medicine physician in-training who is guided and mentored by a veteran touring doctor [23]. This creates efficiencies, redundancy in case of illness or indisposition (e.g., death in the family), and camaraderie in co-investigating and diagnosing a medical illness together which actually helps the patients with amplified medical consultation.

With some entertainment tours, these imbedded physicians may be housed with the band and entourage and even travel in conjunction with the band similar to the White House physicians for the US President. However, due to the size and higher volume needs of the production crews, other tour physicians tend to stay with the crews and arrive into the destination cities alongside them. With the concept of the apprenticeship and multiple doctors, those duties could be split, thus helping to cover both aspects of the tour even more effectively.

Of note, medical liability insurance is available for EMS physicians practicing in the US that covers them for EMS duties including this specialized type of practice. Also of note, it is understood that specialists in EMS practice are rarely (if ever) sued for malpractice and the insurance premium costs are very reasonable and even better if the group approach is used.

Medical Advance Work

The Optimal Receiving Facilities for Various Conditions

As previously alluded, a pivotal role of the touring medicine specialist is to identify the most trusted and knowledgeable physician resources in the tour's various destinations and then conjointly identify the optimal places for treating the various members for whom the touring specialist is responsible. This plan would be a working strategy for the entire tour personnel ranging from the lead singer, audio engineer, and tour accountant to the tour director, creative animator, and laundry handler. While some special adaptations might be arranged for the celebrities' privacy, security and related logistics, the basic care plan would apply to everyone for whom the tour practitioner is responsible (Figures 23.1 and 23.5).

As mentioned, the medical advance plan would be akin to that used by the US White House Medical Unit team members who, in conjunction with the US Secret Service, identify a designated hospital to be used in a given city where the US President is to be visiting. For various security reasons, usually one designated facility is chosen, usually a major trauma center. In touring medicine, the hospital designation may be a more comprehensive and tailored plan in terms of better fitting the designated destination to the underlying emergency (Figure 23.1).

As indicated in the previous discussion, the identified hospital destinations could involve designated trauma, burn, STEMI, cardiac resuscitation, stroke, and pediatric care centers. All of these centers may be different facilities or the same. The working medical advance plan document would not only include the main designated trauma center, but it would also include a notation of backup facilities in case of an MCI or a sudden emergency at that planned receiving facility. It would also include a separate burn center destination if different than the trauma center and/or pediatric trauma center.

Despite the medical condition-alignments and backup planning for receiving facilities, keeping last minute decision-making as simple as possible is a paramount goal. If there is a reasonably equal choice between two trauma centers equidistant from the venue, the logical choice would be the one that is also closest to the artists' or crew's hotel or the one that also has the burn center or the one that is also capable of handling the STEMI and stroke cases. In general, decision-making for destinations may also be divided or separately designated according to the location(s) of the overnight accommodations for the band members, entourage and main production crew (which can be quite different and far apart from each other, let alone the venue).

In one city, all cases of trauma, stroke, STEMI, burns, and even children may go to one location close to the venue, whereas additional facilities would be added into the plan if appropriate hospital destinations are much closer to the overnight accommodations. If the artists and entourage members are staying at a significant distance from the venue, a backup plan may need to be created for them including where to go along the route of travel. For example, if the venue for a Manila show is the Philippine Arena and the artists, entourage or crew are staying in the city center some 40 kilometers away (with some of the world's most challenging traffic), then alternative destinations in the city center would be optimal for such time-dependent emergencies. Similarly, if the show is being performed in Tampa, but some of the tour members are staying closer to Orlando, an alternative trauma center in Orlando might be the best choice for that group during the time that they are in that vicinity. In addition, the plan should also consider major trauma destinations along the ground travel route to and from the venue as needed. Furthermore, one would also want to designate closer optimal receiving facilities for nontraumatic emergencies such as STEMI and stroke, closer to this alternate accommodation site.

In rare instances, the patient, be they band or crew members, may have critical medical records for an underlying condition at certain hospital making that facility the most optimal destination depending on the circumstance. Having that contingency addressed ahead of time with the local EMS authorities would be encouraged, especially if local protocols would call for the nearest appropriate facility.

Atypical Medical Conditions and Contingencies

In addition to these choices for time-dependent life-saving emergencies, an optimal medical advance plan would also include knowledge of access to special categories of specialists for other types of medical problems. This type of issue might include how to urgently and discretely identify an endodontist on a Sunday morning in Tokyo or finding a top-notch otorhinolaryngologist late in the evening in Boston, or a pulmonary fibrosis specialist in Sao Paolo on Friday at 5pm Brazilian time. Some crew members or entourage members may have very specialized chronic conditions that may flare during the tour. While ensuring that all information is kept extremely confidential, prior knowledge of such conditions for all of the tour members would be very useful to the tour physician.

Therefore, ascertaining this information can become part of the duties of the touring medical specialist. However, as later discussed, many individuals are less apt to disclose their conditions for various understandable reasons. However, not having that knowledge may confound appropriate treatment. For example, before administering a drug like Paxlovid[TM] (nirmatrelvir tablets; ritonavir tablets) to a patient testing positive for COVID-19, the clinician would have needed to know about underlying conditions or other medications that might interact with the treatment. As in the case of US President Joseph Biden in July 2022, the attending physician put a brief hold on President Biden taking his usual anticoagulant and statin medications while also suggesting safer interim alternatives for the five-day treatment such as aspirin and perhaps dietary considerations. As another example, it would be helpful in both medical and logistical decision-making to know that the fifty-four-year-old man being evaluated for a near-syncopal episode after quickly standing up in a very hot environment is taking a beta-blocker, especially when the heart rate was found to be relatively normal. Among a myriad of other circumstances, early knowledge of prior experiences with underlying eosinophilic esophagitis (EoE) or sarcoidosis would be important. Collation of such conditions could be part of a separate "off-the-record" (very confidential) plan that the clinician could share with the patient and/or, in an emergency situation, a close confidante already familiar with the underlying condition(s). However, these personal conditions would not be disclosed a priori in terms of the formal medical advance plans being discussed here which are typically circulated in electronic document form to the designated inner circle of security and management personnel who are responsible for the escort and transportation of tour personnel including band members.

Paul E. Pepe, Gerald W. (Jerry) Meltzer II, L. Scott Nichols, Stephen E. (Jake) Berry, and Peter H. Hackett

The Strategic Medical Advance Plan Document

To optimize the rapid action and transport according to the medical advance plan, the working documents should be easy to read and easy to rapidly scan through on a smart mobile phone (Figure 23.1). Accordingly, this e-document can include color-coded designations for trauma (e.g., red), stroke (e.g., brown), STEMI (e.g., green) and major burn (also red) and pediatrics (e.g., orange). By knowing the color code, one can rapidly scroll down to the color for the condition (Figure 23.1). The information for each designated facility would include the phone numbers to the ED and, if applicable, the charge nurse number or consultant on duty number as well as security numbers and even a directions link and possibly photograph links. While it would be preferable to have immediate access and accompaniment of the touring medicine specialist or associate(s), those doctors may be in a situation where communications are poor or they could be working at another location at some distance from the individual who needs an immediate evaluation. The e-document therefore provides a surrogate directive for where the patient should be taken, even if it involves an ambulance service.

If judged safe to do so, it may also be faster to directly transport the patient to the designated facility if only just a few minutes away rather than await an unpredictable time-frame or distant ambulance response. Accordingly, in some plans, to expedite privacy and access, the accompanying clinician, tour associate or security team member may be instructed to bypass the main ED entrance and go to an alternative entrance. Having photographic images of that alternate entrance can assist in that process for those special purposes (Figure 23.5). This system has been used most often when the touring physician is busy at the venue managing crew issues and the patient is still at the hotel or somewhere in transit at some distance away.

Another contingency to consider in terms of great distances and traffic is the availability of air medical rescue when the venue is at distance such as that engendering an hour or more of travel time. Again, landing zones at the receiving facility may need to be established and cleared as indicated and the crew configurations vetted and discussed in terms of persons who would accompany the patient.

The Local Medical Point Person

Beyond the hospital or medical facility designations, the medical advance document should also include the designated point person (e.g., the local lead physician) and additional backup point persons. In most cases, these would be the very persons who helped the tour physician to design the destination selections and who are empowered to override current ambulance destination policies as needed. As stated before, in most situations, these points of contact are preferably the local EMS system medical directors responsible for medical oversight of the PSAP (e.g., 911, 999) and public ambulance services. In other cases, it may be other trusted local contacts of the tour physician or direct communications with ED medical directors or chief medical officers. Whomever becomes the responsible point person(s), their names, mobile telephone, photo headshot, and emergency contact numbers should be included in the medical advance plan. Multiple contacts should be established to create redundancy and failsafe planning.

The photograph would preferably be a current headshot that shows a close resemblance to how the local doctor will appear and present themselves on-site to the tour security team. It may also be used by the credentialing team if they need it to add a photograph into the security credential. This photograph request would apply to all physicians brought in to support the tour at the venue or asked to attend certain individuals off-site if possible. Having this contact is critical in case of the tour physician's inaccessibility or when the care is being delegated to the local physician(s).

In several recent scenarios, when the tour physician was out of communication on a later arriving flight or positioned with the band, the plan was easily followed by security and production teams. In each case, the local physician contact and hospital transport were rapidly enacted. This created a seamless and extremely effective expedited care of the patient. A sample plan, with such planned destinations and contacts, is attached (Figure 23.1).

Hospital Site Visits

Whether in Auckland, Minneapolis, Omaha, or Dublin, hospital site visits can be a critical aspect of the tour physician's activities (Figure 23.5). Not only does this gain familiarity with the facility set-up, the best place to discretely enter the hospital, and the

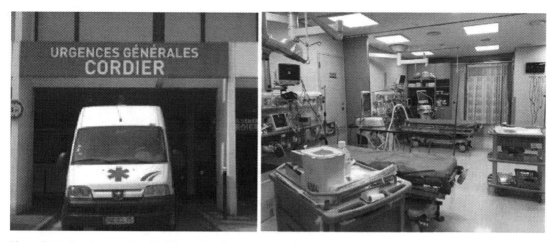

Figure 23.5 Site visits to regional facilities and local emergency medical services teams designated by the medical advance plan can be invaluable, particularly in terms of establishing direct communications to receiving hospital medical staff and security teams as well familiarity with the fastest and most private access to the planned bed sites and surgical and catheterization suites as indicated

location of resuscitation rooms, imaging areas, and surgery suites, but, importantly, it also creates relationships and acquaintances with the staff and how their system works. Oftentimes, the tour physician may ascertain (or even personally know) the ED physicians working on-shift, particularly on the night of the show. This also helps with a contingency for the principals or accompanying celebrities who want to visit the patient (e.g., the artist or their special guests). The tour doctor can help to plan the likely ED room where the patient can be securely placed with privacy ensured along with additional space for others accompanying the VIP such as security, publicists, personal assistants, and family.

Oftentimes, the hospital can provide contact information for patient advocates and direct "charge nurse" or emergency consultant's direct telephone lines or mobiles. In the case of the potential for a celebrity becoming the patient, prior contact with public information officers (PIOs), security chiefs, emergency department leadership and administrators on duty (AODs) can be quite useful, but it also can help to create an expedited evaluation and care for other key personnel needed back to be on-duty for the show without compromising any priority of care for the other patients from the general public also needing that facility.

This site visit activity is similar to the advance site visits conducted for heads of state to ensure that the facility's cited clinical resources are in place and to meet the key personnel and analyze security requirements. One might question if that is also a necessary function for an entertainment tour. For one thing, there have been occasions when the tour was told that specific equipment or interventions would be available at a given hospital, but the site visit revealed that a key intervention (e.g., embolectomy for stroke) is only available at certain times or on certain days. Likewise, one might find outdated diagnostic tools or long-expired medications or even inoperative equipment. At other times, the touring practitioner may be the one observing and learning about advanced techniques and care strategies that can be taken home and even used to enhance care for the tour.

Perhaps more to the point, the execution of the plan is most important. Among several dozens of relevant anecdotes, the following example from a recent world tour of a major entertainment artist helps to demonstrate the spectrum of benefits. In this case, a key member of the production staff, in his sixties, was ready to board a shuttle bus with others at his hotel loading dock for transportation to the venue. However, he was having difficulties and did not look quite right to his colleagues. The tour physician, still in his hotel room, was instantly contacted by mobile. Arriving at the loading dock within just a couple of minutes, he quickly noticed a facial droop and other indications of a likely stroke. The doctor rapidly checked for pink mucous membranes within the lower eyelids while observing comfortable breathing and feeling a strong, regular pulse. He asked the patient to take a deep breath (which he did) and raise the other arm (done with ease). Then knowing that the designated comprehensive stroke center was actually within walking distance based on the tour doctor's earlier hospital site visit on the day of arrival, he asked the bus driver if he knew the place and how to get there quickly. With a positive response, others were ushered off the shuttle quickly with the exception of security team members. While enroute, a pharmacy-bought finger pulse oximeter placed prior to shuttle departure continued to indicate excellent peripheral oxygenation and a normal regular heart rate while the tour doctor called the direct line to the ED charge nurse. Based on the site visit and subsequent communications, the charge nurse immediately knew who was calling, received the relevant information and immediately acknowledged that she understood what the needs would be and that she would initiate the appropriate alerts. In this case, the tour physician had also made site visits to the local EMS teams several days before and had a good working knowledge of their excellent capabilities including the superb quality of their medical directors and their first-class protocols for stroke management. However, the medical advance planning predicted the more timely arrival on the ready-to-go shuttle. By the time the public PSAP could be called and EMS would have been able to respond and start their appropriate on-site care, the patient would already be at the anticipated ambulance destination. The tour physician's boots-on-the-ground experience with such cases (over several decades) provided a very sanguine and appropriate decision in this situation. Also, getting to the hospital more rapidly is one thing, but, more importantly, knowing where and how to call ahead of time (largely based on the routine site visit) was a key action and one that expedited the actual care.

More specifically, arriving some four minutes after departing the hotel loading dock, the patient was met at the ambulance bay with an ED team and stretcher. He was in the resuscitation room within another minute or two where the alerted neuro-interventionalists were standing by and expeditiously facilitated the evaluation, imaging, and subsequent interventions. Following the subsequent indicated management, the patient recovered quite well despite the original significant neurological insult.

Although it would be a major disappointment for everyone to have this beloved crew member withdrawn from the tour, it was still agreed by all that it would be best for him to return back home, some 8,400 miles away, once safe to do so. In the interim, per the patient's request, the tour doctor was asked to be the one to break the sensitive news to his wife back home and hopefully provide her with reassuring information despite the obvious seriousness of the situation. After speaking to the spouse, subsequent actions included establishing contact with the chair of neurology at the patient's hometown university medical center. This contact was made early on to ensure timely continuity of care and to facilitate early medical record transfer. Later, the tour doctor also coordinated a plan to have a well-known band member discretely escorted in to visit the patient using a private access point and secured elevator. There was also subsequent coordination of the visit between the patient, his doctor and the tour director who was responsible for financial obligations and arranging safe travel home. Follow-up visits were made to ensure progress, and further assure the patient (and his wife).

Again, this case represents one of many others with similar challenges and medical decision-making, but it also nicely illustrates the value of creating an advance plan, making the site visit, and knowing how the system works. It also illustrates one pivotal role of the veteran tour physician who has the clinical experience, command of the relevant variables and knowledge-based confidence to make rapid and rational risk-benefit decisions. The case also demonstrates the important function of helping to optimize the patient's continuity of care and sensitively informing (and knowledgeably reassuring) loved ones, friends and colleagues in accordance with the patient's wishes. Unlike the general tourist who wonders how and where they should go to deal with a sudden emergency in a foreign country thousands of miles from home, the medical advance plan and early site visit here not only addressed those issues well ahead of time, but it also significantly expedited the actual care and longterm outcome.

Just to place more perspective on the frequency of tour members' going to the hospital and the role of the tour physician's early site visits, the described stroke case was not the only visit to that particular hospital in that particular city. Just as the tour physician was arriving at the airport of that city, one person already on-site at the venue had to be taken to that same hospital (per the proscribed medical advance plan) and he was admitted and managed for an acute abdomen. Several days later, one of the crew members had their foot run over by a heavy cargo roller (about 2 am during the post-show load-out). The tour physician used the same approach as the stroke patient calling ahead to the charge nurse. Stewarding the evaluation as a known entity to the staff, that patient was admitted to the ED, attended, examined, x-rayed, and discharged within forty-five minutes of arrival, just in time to get back to the hotel and ready for departure to the airport and travel to the next country later that day. As in the case of the stroke patient, the tour physician also read the x-rays directly with the attending ED physician and obtained copies of the imaging. This helped to facilitate a continuity of care contingency in case of a worsening condition and especially in light of an indeterminate atypical finding on the x-ray. In other words, from arrival to departure, the local hospital and staff becomes an extension of the tour physician's duties. Also, because the tour clinician was able to reciprocate during the visit with formal lectures and/or impromptu discussion on research activities and best practices, everyone benefitted from the mutual respect and generosities. And that was just the first international city on the tour – visits further escalated as the tour progressed.

Continuity of Care Is Another Important Function

As illustrated in the stroke scenario, a key function of the touring practitioner is to monitor an evolving illness or to see if a treatment is working over the ensuing week as the tour moves from one city or country to another. For example, several days after returning to the tour following a short break home, a crew member noticed a painless, nonpruritic elevated area on his lower back when toweling after a shower. Upon examination, the tour doctor observed a nearly pathognomonic erythematous target lesion about six inches (fifteen centimeters) in diameter. The history reveals that the patient and his family do indeed reside in a wooded area known to have ticks. Considering the potential severity of a Lyme disease threat, follow-up of the empiric antibiotic treatment (with before and after photos) is exceptionally important while on the road with a paucity of available diagnostics. With the exception

perhaps of a local paramedic's twelve-lead electrocardiographic tracing and a thorough history, review of systems, and physical examination, follow-up is essential. If the lesion begins to heal quickly, over just a few days, it bodes well but worsening (or no improvement) would prompt taking the time to seek a more definitive diagnosis and management. Having someone to ensure that continuity of care during the tour is critical, not only to confirm or reformulate the original diagnosis, but also to avoid delays in subsequent definitive care as indicated. Similar concerns might exist for the classic erythematous and painful throat with white patches. Treated with a standard or alternative drug by the local doctors in one country, such a condition requires close monitoring and particularly if it does not resolve within several days. Also, for those with a chronic condition, it is important to have an experienced clinician who can monitor the waxing and waning of the condition and circumvent the telling and retelling of past medical history to strangers and thus better expedite and help determine the best care strategy at any given time. The embedded doctor also can obviate the need to go to a medical facility for someone presenting with something unusual but not life-threatening such as likely sialolithiasis. While it may be somewhat painful and disconcerting for that person, the largest concern for them often is that they just want to know what is happening to them and to get some reassurances. The touring doctor can provide those answers and reassurances as well as a working management plan. Also, having someone who can closely monitor the condition and its tolerance can help to determine if further intervention is warranted, especially for a team member who is otherwise reticent to go into a hospital or other medical facility largely because of job obligations.

Role with the Venue and General Public in Attendance

In general, the touring physician will defer management of the audience to the local medical teams typically staffing or contracting with the venue to provide medical care and also interact with the local ambulance services. However, as inferred previously, it would be of great benefit to coordinate plans with those on-site teams in conjunction with the local responding EMS in case of emergency and in case of the need to transport a tour member to the designated

Paul E. Pepe, Gerald W. (Jerry) Meltzer II, L. Scott Nichols, Stephen E. (Jake) Berry, and Peter H. Hackett

hospitals to avoid any last minute controversy or even confrontation about hospital destinations. It also better prepares everyone for potential MCIs and familiarity if a major emergency incident does occur, be it in the audience or in the back of house. One other reason for a close interface is to observe and appreciate the competency of the staff for quality assurance purposes on behalf of the tour. If there are significant weaknesses identified – and there have been from time to time – similar to concerns about a hospitals' shortcomings, the tour can make or recommend adjustments for future shows. Care of the audience is a priority for most artists and the knowledgeable tour physician can sensitively and discretely help to identify issues in a constructive manner akin to security teams identifying potential weaknesses to mitigate problems on future visits to that venue.

Accordingly, tour physicians should always do their best to attend the tour's security briefings which most often occur a day or two before the show. This participation is enacted to establish familiarity and coordination with the medical leadership at the venue. There are similar internal briefings to attend involving the EMS and venue medical staff working on show day. Attendance at those briefings helps to have all of the paramedics, nurses and doctors become acquainted with the tour doctor and mutually learn key aspects of the medical advance plans and the doctor's role. The tour doctor can also make offers to be available to assist in a difficult cases. Experience has shown that the tour doctor can be asked to do so quite frequently. These interactions not only assist patients, but also provide teachable moments, camaraderie and better working relationships for the future.

Training and Equipping the Tour Members with Basic First Aid Skills

Several of the authors have respectively set up mechanisms to train all tour members in high-performance basic CPR, use of automated external defibrillators (AEDs), and use and choking interventions as well as basic interventions to stop severe bleeding (e.g., direct pressure, tourniquets) and check oxygenation and glucose (Figure 23.6). Sometimes with the help of local training institutions with a dedicated teaching site, resources can be provided to help expedite the skills training for all of the tour personnel. Depending on the circumstances or available equipment, one strategy would be to stagger a group of sessions with

a dozen or so persons in each session. Each session realistically can take no more than a half hour to successfully provide well-retained information and muscle memory. In addition to the training, the best available AEDs can be identified, secured, or recommended through the touring physician and several should be acquired and placed in visible and easily accessible locations where everyone knows their whereabouts at all times such as a highly visible, "in your face," and readily accessed position on or under the stage or in a similar position in the dressing room areas after being brought in (and taken out again) by the team security members who also make the AEDs available at the hotel, the motorcade, and aircraft for the artists and entourage. Similar considerations are made for the crews with the security office team and/or production office holding additional AEDs. Other recommended rapid-availability of equipment includes finger pulse oximeters to distribute to numerous appropriate persons and particularly security staff and other designated rapid-responder personnel. This can also include several easy-to-carry tourniquets and glucometers. Beyond acquiring AEDs and the other equipment, the tour physician should also ensure that AED batteries and pads are not expired or about to expire and likely do so before the tour with the understanding that shipping certain types of batteries is not allowed across certain borders or by air freight.

In a recent tour, shortly after tour physicians were revisiting the latest AED and CPR update issues on a show day, one of the crew members experienced a sudden cardiac arrest after boarding an airport shuttle the next morning. However, the patient was rapidly saved by other crew members using basic CPR and an AED, including one involved in the update discussions the night before. The young crew member experiencing the cardiac arrest was a husband and father, who fully recovered thanks to the quick action of colleagues, immediate availability of AEDs, and medical quality assurance initiatives.

In addition to the usual "doctor's bag" equipment and medications, one can also consider providing items such as chewable aspirin, an epinephrine injector (e.g., "EpiPen"), albuterol, diphenhydramine and perhaps a wireless otoscope, blood pressure cuff, and other basic over-the-counter (OTC) medications such anti-inflammatories and acetaminophen to a select number of responsible tour members. Also, use of neuroprotective CPR equipment (as previously

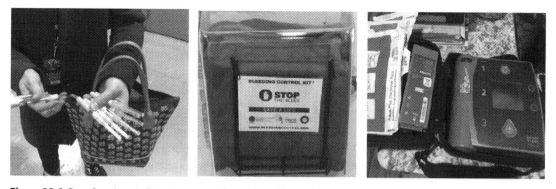

Figure 23.6 Part of touring medicine is to ensure the rapid availability of AEDs, resuscitative equipment and coordination with local medical teams regarding rapid availability of resuscitative and emergency medications. They also ensure the training of key staff (e.g., tour security teams), if not all tour members, in the latest methods for performing basic CPR, choking rescue, AED use, and hemorrhage control

described) is also a basic skill that can be performed by the average first responder [43,44].

Special Nuances of Dealing with the Talent, VIPs, and a Dedicated Crew

The touring physician may be called upon to respond to a medical need of the artists themselves or perhaps crew members right at the time of performance. This unique nuance of music-related mass gathering medicine is discussed in some detail in Chapter 14 discussing "VIPs," but some highlights are also worth reinforcing within the context of touring medicine duties.

If called upon to see the artist, family, or celebrity guest, one should sensitively assess the comfort level of the "VIP." Many artists are in good physical condition and typically well-maintained by physical therapists and trainers also imbedded in the tour. The need for evaluation by the tour physician may be frequent in some cases or rare in others. Creating trust can take some time and involve some intangible factors including personal rapport. Even if the responding clinician is a renowned and respected medical professional within the medical community at large, VIP encounters will often entail an entirely different realm of culture and expectations including the presence of other (nonmedical) persons being in attendance during any evaluation. Also, in early encounters, the VIP and confidantes may not be as willing to disclose underlying conditions to those not in the inner bubble. Managers, publicists, or family members may insert themselves into what typically would be a private assessment and mutual decision-making

visit in the outside world between a clinician and a patient. It is therefore incumbent upon the medical professional to have patience, sensitivity, and situational awareness during each encounter and to adjust his or her level of engagement based on the VIP's comfort level at the time as well as the acuity of the medical condition and the understanding that the clinician's index of suspicion for undisclosed conditions should remain high.

The tour physician should also be aware of a typical reticence to concede to a hospital transport or even recommendations to receive further evaluation at the time of the event. Beyond personal stoicism or wanting to avoid disruption of tight schedules, transport to a medical facility will be perceived as something that might engender embarrassing news stories and social media speculation in this era of mass communication, rumor-spreading, and optics. Therefore, the tour practitioner needs to first be patient, gain trust over the long run and not attempt to coerce the principal into accepting transport, but rather use a more patient demeanor of diplomacy and perhaps some reliance on others to help with informed decision-making and encouragement as indicated.

While the "optics" and privacy concerns for the principal involved can be significant, there are also similar issues for the accompanying entourage. Declining care or transport is also common among those serving the artists such as a longstanding touring crew member working for a popular entertainer and assigned to a pivotal task for the artists. As noted previously, unyielding loyalty to mission will often override or complicate what would otherwise be appropriate standards of care and medical decision-making.

Paul E. Pepe, Gerald W. (Jerry) Meltzer II, L. Scott Nichols, Stephen E. (Jake) Berry, and Peter H. Hackett

Discussions on how to manage such scenarios are outlined in some detail in Chapters 4 and 14. Nonetheless, to illustrate such a case here, during a live performance at a famous stadium being streamed out to hundreds of millions, a pivotal crew member took ill. He had been developing progressive dyspnea throughout the day and was found to have hypoxemia (SpO2 86–88%) and some (regular rate) tachycardia on finger pulse-oximeter readings. This was offset to a large extent with a nonbreather mask and oxygen supply (achieving 91–92 percent), but the situation remained quite concerning as it was ascertained that the person had a surgical abdominal procedure only a week earlier. Physical exam remained unremarkable except for possible "99" muffling at the right posterior base. He was afebrile and was alert and oriented and was performing his job superbly. Having the full capacity and absolute resolution to remain on duty, the tour doctor and local EMS captain stayed with the patient at his post with a cardiac monitor pads and leads attached and intravenous access placed along with nearby AED, and an ongoing oxygen supply for the next two hours. Despite the concerning differential diagnosis, he did remain stable throughout the performance and received CT-angiography of the chest within a half hour of the show ending. This action was again facilitated by the medical advance planning and accompaniment by the tour doctor. In the end, he was found to have fairly significant atelectasis that took a day or two to fully rerecruit, but his loyal dedication to the mission did require a creative and patient approach to manage the problem and keep the patient as safe as possible. Such "mission-first" situations are not infrequent, and they can be unsettling for a prudent medical professional. However, compassion, respect and appreciation for that dedication to the mission should still be admired within the context and strategies for managing the situation.

Medical Standards and Ethical Challenges

Some artists, staff, or family members may request to see a medical professional for atypical or social media-promulgated treatment such as certain vitamin or hormone injections or unusual intravenous infusions. The practitioner may be asked to provide or order some alternative therapy, pain medications, intimacy-related pharmaceuticals, or anxiety/depression medications. Such therapies may even

have been prescribed by other doctors or a primary care physician either in the country of the event or in their home nation. For years, many of these requests (and repeated requests) were reinforced through the acquiescence and "courtesies" rendered by the classic "rock doc" who, for the most part, was ready and willing to provide whatever was asked. However, for that very reason, they did develop an unfavorable reputation among the top-notch security and production contingents, largely based on their own sense of integrity and professionalism. With the advent of the trained and mentored event medicine (EVM) physician specialist, that unfortunate legacy may soon be in rear-view mirror [23].

One other issue is that the odd requests may often be filtered through surrogates (e.g., personal assistants), an awkward situation in which direct access to the requesting patient is not considered to be necessary. This, of course, disallows the standard professional communication and evaluation of medical need and necessity as one would usually expect in prudent day-to-day medical case management.

It is clear that most medical professionals wish to please every patient and none would want to disappoint any of them, let alone a famous person. Nonetheless, maintaining ethical standards and maintaining one's integrity in medical decision-making should always persevere and perhaps become an upfront understanding for all in terms of the tour physicians roles and responsibilities. Strategic and compassionate ways to communicate the reason for not granting the request can be found, especially when coupled with a sincere willingness to help in another way. Alternative solutions such as contacting the person's usual physician or referral to an appropriate local specialist at the current site or next city may also be suggested. In the end, one should consider the wise premise about whether or not they would administer the requested therapy to his or her own family members. Realistically, the practitioner should also consider if their medical licensure (and thus source of livelihood) could be in the balance.

While supplemental oxygen is requested frequently, it is unlikely to create any significant washout and oxygen toxicity for the very brief time that it is typically used backstage. So while some requests like this may seem questionable at the first, it should also be recognized that the entertainers using the oxygen will typically report that they felt better after the "therapy." So while they are likely enjoying a placebo effect largely due to their anaerobic activity going back into an aerobic state, the risk level is probably negligible and the close availability of supplemental oxygen may serve some other purpose, especially in the event of a true emergency. In essence, there can be tough calls at times. Some requests may be reasonable to fulfill, while others may not be so tolerable.

Regardless of these ethical and philosophical issues, extreme discretion and confidentiality need to be paramount. The touring medical professional must avoid any interaction with the media or anyone else, including colleagues if they are not directly involved in the case. If explicitly asked to make a public statement by the patient, their empowered family member or the patient-authorized representative, the media commentary should always be provided with the explicit approval of what could be revealed. Again, suggested tactics are provided in Chapter 14 and in other commentary [45].

Recap of the Potential Roles and Duties for the Touring Medicine Practitioner

As emphasized throughout this chapter, touring medicine is not an activity reserved for the show day and it is not targeted for the talent alone. The doctor should preferably be on-site during the tour setup and rehearsal period which can be as much as two weeks or more in advance of the first show and those duties should continue on until the last remaining tour members have departed. Many times, there even will

be follow-up at their home bases and often involving referral to medical teams at those home cities.

In terms of direct supervisor reporting lines, there are several existing models, the simplest of which is that the tour physician may be hired directly by the artist's manager. In this model (used by one of the authors), the physician primarily provides care for the artists, but will then also extend care to the management and production team as well. In another model (which has been used by the other authors), the tour physician is integrated into the tour as of part of the security team, serving as the division lead for health security. In this role, this tour physician, also a tactical responder and veteran of "protective medicine" service, can function in both medical and specialized health security roles previously described. This can include duties serving directly in stage-side assignments during performances and making choreographed appropriate movements with the artists. In this configuration, the practitioner can promptly assist in any medical crisis occurring on-stage or backstage.

Regardless of reporting mechanisms, event medicine overall is an evolving practice within the house of medicine and it has significant overlap with touring medicine [23]. However, touring medicine clearly has its unique aspects and nuances. Just as EMS was an offspring of the emergency medicine specialty and now a formal subspecialty unto its own, it did so by identifying its newly identified competencies. Many of the numerous special competencies, concerns and tasks for touring clinicians have been outlined in this discussion and they can be roughly itemized as suggested in Table 23.1.

Table 23.1 Suggested duties and responsibilities for touring physicians:

(1) **Serve as the embedded (on-site) medical / health security / risk reduction consultant for the A, B, C, and D components of the tour's overall enterprise** – where A = Administration/Management staff; B = Band (and entourage); C = Crew (majority of the production team) and D = domicile entities (local venue teams of ushers, security personnel, audience, and community at large). This can be accomplished largely through close communication and integration within the tour security lead and security team leaders for the A, B, and C components:

    (a) These duties include preparatory and operational tasks conducted **before, during, and after the tour.**

- When the tour physician is a known and trusted entity, one should confidentially ascertain, whenever feasible: the current health and potential medical needs of the team members within each of the A, B, C components; attempt to provide ongoing wellness checks and continuity of care; call-ahead preparations, medical appointments / evaluations in the next countries / cities / venues, as indicated.
- Provide follow-up care and assistance to the A, B, C team members who have become ill or injured, or for those who have departed or need to depart the tour for medical reasons.
- Provide pretour advisories regarding vaccination needs, anticipated prophylaxis and precautions for certain endemic and potential threats for A, B, C components.

Table 23.1 (cont.)

(b) Provide medical advance plan, local medical contacts, and ascertain potential health threats for the A, B, and C tour members.

(c) Work with local authorities to prepare coordination for multiple casualty incidents (MCIs) such as explosion, fire, stampede, terrorist attack, sudden weather assault with coverage for A, B, C components as well the D components.

(d) In essence, provide all-cause medical risk reduction to the business entity.

(2) Strategic Medical Advance Planning and Liaison to Local Medical Services

(a) Preplan and establish optimal medical advance plans for local medical care including optimal hospital destination contingencies – in terms of predesignating the highest quality and most appropriate medical facilities that are optimal for a heart attack, or a stroke, or severe trauma or childhood services, burns, orthopedic injuries, dental emergencies, and other urgencies. This should include site visits to those key facilities and local EMS crews once arriving in the destination city.

(b) Identify and Preplan Local Medical Point Persons – often the local emergency medical services (EMS) medical director or other community medical leader – these point persons would be preidentified reliable, trusted local medical contacts who can discretely facilitate and expedite the best available medical care in a trustworthy, caring manner either on-site or at the most appropriate medical care facilities. They would be able to help to formulate the medical advance plan and also help to identify, in real time, the best potential dispositions for health problems that arise and also to attend to tour staff at the venue or hotel as indicated (or assign a surrogate). They can also assist medical oversight on-site during load-in and show days as needed, and would particularly be of help for optimally managing potential multiple casualty incidents (MCIs) – and other critical events that may involve the EMS system.

(c) Serve as medical liaison for confidential medical communications and for facilitating continuity of care – being able to make early assessments and communicate those findings to the local medical care professionals who may be treating tour personnel while also protecting the privacy of those sick or injured tour personnel on-site or at medical facilities. This includes accompanying the very sick or injured to any indicated facility and helping them to navigate the local system and also help to facilitate/guide the most appropriate medical care decisions and dispositions given the need to be traveling to another destination (tour physician can bridge that continuity of care).

(d) Foster close working relations with local public safety and contingency disaster planning staff – meetings and briefings with local security and venue medical personnel, both at the show day team gatherings and in earlier venue security briefings as well as meetings with local public safety and hospital personnel during site visits, especially in terms of preparations for mass casualty events, unexpected catastrophes and complex terroristic threats/attacks, including applicable local hospital and EMS system site visits. Meetings with local tactical (Special Weapons and Tactics) teams and law enforcement is highly recommended if the tour physician has tactical / special operations skills.

(e) Assessment and Ongoing Monitoring of Endemic, Environmental and Other Threats to Health

- Garnering Medical Intel and Contingencies – for ongoing epidemics, endemic diseases, air quality, altitude, insect/animals threats, water quality, and also considerations for preventive care for crew protection before and during the tour. Also continue to assess and monitor for unanticipated public health threats or emerging infectious diseases (EIDs) to be encountered by the tour and also ensure the most up-to-date protective measures.

- Maintain, as best as possible, a working knowledge of the local environment including local toxicological, environmental, and biological threats at each venue and identify and secure contacts to experts in these threat arenas as indicated.

- Collaborate with health officials such as the Center for Infectious Disease Reporting and Policy (CIDRAP), BioWatch, the US Centers for Disease Control and Prevention (CDC) and the World Health Organization (WHO) to anticipate and/or manage EIDs or local endemic concerns and particularly to address any proactive (pretour or intra-tour) immunization or prophylaxis requirements or recommendations for the various international sites and potential individual needs.

(3) Recommend and Provide the Most Up-to-Date Advances in Medical Emergency Training and Useful Portable Medical Equipment for Touring Personnel including:

(a) the most up-to-date methods and training in CPR, choking reversal, AED use, Stop-the-Bleed techniques and use of important adjuncts such as pulse oximeters, tourniquets, glucometers, and methods to simplify/expedite related training.

(b) maintain and ensure up-to-date monitoring of devices such as automated defibrillators (AEDs) and any expiration dates on batteries and electrode pads as well as the same for emergency medications such as chewable aspirin, epinephrine injectors, albuterol inhalers, and other similar treatments.

(c) Consider take-along portable devices such as point of care ultrasound, neuroprotective CPR devices (43,44) and oxygen tanks and possibly whole blood.

Final Reflections on the Loading Dock Lifestyle

Touring medicine duties can be arduous. As previously detailed, the work and travel schedule in themselves would be extraordinarily demanding for the average person. Also, the pressure to perform each individual's task with perfection is clearly pervasive. Touring physicians not only share many of those same health risks, immune system challenges, exposures and drive to support the mission flawlessly, but their relative risks can also be amplified by many a sleepless night spent at the latest destination's tertiary care center.

The escorting, navigating, and stewarding of medical care and hospital management of multiple tour members, sometimes back to back during a given night, may only be an episodic event. However, when such random and suddenly occurring worknights do occur, they can become very stressful overnights, not only because of the work ethic and caring of a conscientious physician, but also because of the concerned worries that are experienced by any family member when their loved one has become significantly ill or injured. Indeed, the crew is *family* and a uniquely bonded one at that. Once accepted and trusted by this respected family of tour specialists, the tour physician becomes enmeshed in the camaraderie of their joint mission. Like foxhole companions of sorts, attachments become strong.

Regardless of one's competence and experience, the nuances of touring medicine are outside of most clinicians' comfort zone. Despite the usual professional stressors and omnipresent uncertainties in the realm of any medical diagnosis, challenges are amplified when attempting to deliver optimal health care in unfamiliar lands, cultures and environments. Also, many of the tasks are best fitted for general practitioners and not necessarily fitting the bailiwick of the typical core group of touring medicine doctors (appropriately) emanating from backgrounds in critical care, EMS, travel medicine, tactical medicine, and emergency medicine. So why do it? The quick answer: the artist, the touring professionals, and, above all, the audience.

Many of us grew up becoming cynical about how, in our society, some people such as movie stars, athletes, entertainers, and other celebrities have made so much money and yet often squander those resources while teachers, nurses, and paramedics, so important to us all, continue to be underpaid and underappreciated despite their critical roles.

However, when a touring physician has the privilege of serving a special talent whose philosophy and sincere love for their audiences are not only quite evident, but also quite inspiring, that medical professional has the true privilege of witnessing firsthand the impact their performances on the lives and happiness of their fans. Standing behind the barricade stage-right or walking along the fence line at the B-stage, one can clearly observe and experience the joyfulness and elation that the performer(s) bring to those fans. And those fans are not "fanatics," but rather everyday people whose lives have been made a little more fulfilled because of the music they love. Becoming just one small cog among a team of professionals who support the mission of those inspiring artists and whose mutual hope is to somehow achieve perfection in the art of bringing joy to others is exceptionally rewarding. For a health professional, saving lives is an essential duty, but improving the quality of life for others is paramount (46). To be part of a team that regularly achieves that goal, across the globe, has been a privilege and a treasured memory – very much worth the rigorous price of admission!

References

1. Lucey D. R., Donaldson H. Yellow Fever Vaccine Shortages in the United States and Abroad: A Critical Issue. *Annals of International Medicine.* 2017;**167**:664–665.

2. Gershman M. D., Angelo K. M., Ritchey J., et al. Addressing a Yellow Fever Vaccine Shortage. *Morbidity and Mortality Weekly Report.* 2017;**66**:457–459. www.cdc.gov/mmwr/volumes/66/wr/mm6617e2.htm. Last accessed September 21, 2023.

3. Janse van Rensburg D. C., Jansen van Rensburg A., Fowler P. M., et al. Managing Travel Fatigue and Jet Lag in Athletes: A Review and Consensus Statement. *Sports Medicine.* 2021;**51**:2029–2050.

4. Hebl J. T., Velasco J., McHill A. W. Work Around the Clock: How Work Hours Induce Social Jetlag and Sleep Deficiency. *Clinics in Chest Medicine.* 2022;**43**:249–259.

5. Roenneberg T., Foster R. G., Klerman E. B. The Circadian System, Sleep, and the Health/Disease Balance: A Conceptual Review. *Journal of Sleep Research.* 2022;**31**(4):e13621. doi: 10.1111/jsr.13621.

6. Rusu A., Ciobanu D., Vonica C. L., et al. Chronic Disruption of Circadian Rhythm with Mistimed Sleep and Appetite: An Exploratory Research. *Chronobiology International.* 2021;**38**:807–816.

7. Smithies T. D., Eastwood P. R., Walsh J., Murray K., Markwick W., Dunican I. C. Around the World in 16 Days: The Effect of Long-Distance Trans-Meridian Travel on the Sleep Habits and Behaviours of a Professional Super Rugby Team. *Journal of Sports Science.* 2021;**39**:2596–2602.

8. Charest J., Samuels C. H., Bastien C. H., Lawson D., Grandner M. A. Impacts of Travel Distance and Travel Direction on Back-to-Back Games in the National Basketball Association. *Journal of Clinical Sleep Medicine.* 2021;**17**:2269–2274.

9. Born J., Lange T., Hansen K., Mölle M., Fehm H. L. Effects of Sleep and Circadian Rhythm on Human Circulating Immune Cells. *The Journal of Immunology.* 1997;**158**:4454–4464.

10. Lange T., Dimitrov S., Born J. Effects of Sleep and Circadian Rhythm on the Human Immune System. *Annals of the New York Academy of Sciences.* 2010;**1193**:48–59.

11. Opp M. R., Krueger J. M. Sleep and Immunity: A Growing Field with Clinical Impact. *Brain, Behavior, and Immunity.* 2015;**47**:1–3.

12. Patel S. R., Malhotra A., Gao X., Hu F. B., Neuman M. I., Fawzi W. W. A Prospective Study of Sleep Duration and Pneumonia Risk in Women. *Sleep.* 2012;**35**:97–101.

13. Cable J., Schernhammer E., Hanlon J. C., et al. Sleep and Circadian Rhythms: Pillars of Health: A Keystone Symposia Report. *Annals of the New York Academy of Sciences.* 2021;**1506**:18–34.

14. Moldofsky H. Central Nervous System and Peripheral Immune Functions and the Sleep Wake System. *Journal of Psychiatry and NeuroScience.* 1994;**19**:368–374.

15. Karlsson B., Knutsson A., Lindahl B. Is There an Association Between Shift Work and Having a Metabolic Syndrome? Results from a Population Based Study of 27,485 People. *Occupational and Environmental Medicine.* 2001;**58**:747–752.

16. Dimitrov S., Lange T., Tieken S., Fehm H. L., Born J. Sleep Association Regulation of T Helper 1 / T Helper 2 Cytokine Balance in Humans. *Brain, Behavior, and Immunity.* 2004;**18**:341–348.

17. Besedovsky L., Lange T., Born J. Sleep and Immune Function. *Pflugers Archiv.* 2012;**463**:121–137.

18. Kolla B. P., Auger R. R. Jet Lag and Shift Work Sleep Disorders: How to Help Reset the Internal Clock. *Cleveland Clinic Journal of Medicine.* 2011;**78**:675–684.

19. Baker F. C., Driver H. S. Circadian Rhythms, Sleep, and the Menstrual Cycle. *Sleep Medicine.* 2007;**8**:613–622.

20. Almeida C. M., Malheiro A. Sleep, Immunity and Shift Workers: A Review. *Sleep Science.* 2016;**9**:164–168.

21. Segerstrom S. C., Miller G. E. Psychological Stress and the Human Immune System: A Meta-Analytic Study of 30 Years of Inquiry. *Psychology Bulletin.* 2004;**130**:601–630.

22. Kak V. Infections in Confined Spaces: Cruise Ships, Military Barracks, and College Dormitories. *Infectious Disease Clinics of North America.* 2007;**21**:773–784.

23. Pepe P. E. and Nichols L. S. Event Medicine: An Evolving Subspecialty of Emergency Medicine. In: *2013 Yearbook of Intensive Care and Emergency Medicine.* Vincent J. L. (ed.). Springer-Verlag: Berlin Heidelberg; 2013; pp. 37–47.

24. Persaud N., Jiang M., Shaikh R., et al. Comparison of Essential Medicines Lists in 137 Countries. *Bulletin of the World Health Organization.* 2019;**97**:394–404C. doi: 10.2471/BLT.18.222448.

25. Dela Cruz C. S., Pasnick S., Gross J. E., Keller J., Carlos W. G., Cao B., Jamil S. Adenovirus Infection and Outbreaks. *American Journal of Respiratory and Critical Care Medicine.* 2019:**199**:13–14.

26. Hoffman J. Adenovirus: Ocular Manifestations. *Community Eye Health.* 2020;**33**:73–75.

27. Fitzgerald N., Uny I., Brown A., et al. Managing COVID-19 Transmission Risks in Bars. *Journal of Studies on Alcohol and Drugs.* 2021;**82**:42–54.

28. Graham, A. M., Pringle, K. J., Pope R. J., et al. Impact of the 2019/2020 Australian Megafires on Air Quality and Health. *GeoHealth.* 2021;**5**:e2021GH000454. doi: 10.1029/2021GH000454

29. Kargarfard M., Poursafa P., Rezanejad S., Mousavinasab F. Effects of Exercise in Polluted Air on the Aerobic Power, Serum Lactate Level and Cell Blood Count of Active Individuals. *International Journal of Preventive Medicine.* 2011;**2**:145–150.

30. Thaller E. I., Petronell S. A., Hochman D., Howard S., Chhikara R. S., Brooks E. G. Moderate Increases in Ambient PM2.5 and Ozone Are Associated with Lung Function Decreases in Beach Lifeguards. *Journal of Occupational and Environmental Medicine.* 2008;**50**:202–211.

31. Pope C. A., et al. Particulate Air Pollution as a Predictor of Mortality in a Prospective Study of US Adults. *American Journal of Respiratory and Critical Care Medicine.* 1995;**151**:669–674.

32. Hackett P. H., Roach R. C. High-Altitude Illness. *New England Journal of Medicine.* 2001;**345**:107–114.

33. Billaut F., Aughey R. J. Update in the Understanding of Altitude-Induced Limitations to Performance in Team-Sport Athletes. *British Journal of Sports Medicine*. 2013;**47**:i22–i25.

34. US Centers for Disease Control and Prevention. Malaria information, by country. www.cdc.gov/malaria/travelers/country_table/i.html. Last accessed September 21, 2023.

35. Forster V. Legionnaires' Disease Outbreak in NYC Kills 1 Person and Sickens 19. www.forbes.com/sites/victoriaforster/2022/05/28/legionnaires-disease-outbreak-in-nyc-kills-1-person-and-sickens-19/?sh=363465f34edc. Last accessed September 21, 2023.

36. World Health Organization Western Pacific. Polio Outbreak in the Philippines. 2019. www.who.int/westernpacific/emergencies/polio-outbreak-in-the-philippines. Last accessed September 21, 2023.

37. Goodman B. New York Adult Diagnosed with Polio: First US Case in Nearly a Decade. www.cnn.com/2022/07/21/health/new-york-polio/index.html. Last accessed September 21, 2023.

38. Mandavilli A., Ward E. Britain Declares National Incident After Polio Virus. June 22, 2022. www.nytimes.com/2022/06/22/health/uk-polio-london-poliovirus.html. Last accessed September 21, 2023.

39. Scerbo M. H., Mumm J. P., Gates K., et al. Safety and Appropriateness of Tourniquets in 105 Civilians. *Prehospital and Emergency Care*. 2016;**20**:712–722.

40. www.UsEagles.org. Last accessed September 21, 2023.

41. Gates H. Gathering of Eagles – Part I: Better Ways to Handle Familiar Problems. *EMS World*. www.hmpgloballearningnetwork.com/site/emsworld/article/12333659/gathering-of-eagles-part-i-better-ways-to-handle-familiar-problems. Last accessed September 21, 2023.

42. McVaney K. E., Pepe P. E., Maloney L. M., et al. The Relationship of Large City Out-of-Hospital Cardiac Arrests and the Prevalence of COVID-19. *EClinicalMed (The Lancet open access publication)*. 2021;**34**:e100815.

43. Moore J. C., Pepe P. E., Scheppke K. A., et al. Head and Thorax Elevation During Cardiopulmonary Resuscitation Using Circulatory Adjuncts Is Associated with Improved Survival. *Resuscitation*. 2022;**179**:9–17.

44. Bachista K. M., Moore J. C., Labarère J., et al. Survival for Non-Shockable Cardiac Arrests Treated with Non-Invasive Circulatory Adjuncts and Head/Thorax Elevation. *Critical Care Medicine*. 2024;**52**:(in press).

45. Pepe P. E., Pepe L. B., Davis R. M., Mann P., Whitmeyer R. EMS Physicians as Public Spokespersons. In: *Emergency Medical Oversight: Clinical Practice and Systems Oversight*, 2nd Edition. Cone D. C., Brice J. H., Delbridge T. R., Myers J. B. (eds.). Hoboken, NJ: Wiley and Sons, Inc.; 2015; pp. 146–159. Companion Website: www.Wiley.com\go\Cone\NAEMSP

46. *American College of Emergency Physicians* Creative Careers: Exploring Unique Career Options for Emergency Physicians. *ACEP Now*. 2023;**42**:12.

Infectious Disease and Mass Gathering Medicine

Vivek Kak and Mehekmeet Bhatia

Introduction

Aristotle had said that "Man by nature is a social animal" and thus given to meet in herds to celebrate or travel. While other animals may travel in large herds like the wildebeest across the Serengeti or meet around watering holes, humans tend to gather in masses to celebrate events such as sporting feats and religious ceremonies. These mass gathering events involve multiple individuals gathering in a specific place over a period of time for various events including religious events, sporting events, or music festivals to name a few. These events involving multiple individuals with differing infectious risks meeting in proximity have been linked to a number of outbreaks of disease and even epidemics [1]. Often these infections can start as outbreaks when cases exceed an expected level in a given space at a specific time, however if these gatherings are huge there exists the potential of the outbreaks becoming epidemics when these cases expand to a much larger part of the population. A pandemic is said to have occurred when infections spread across multiple countries. When an infection establishes itself permanently within the population it becomes an endemic [1].

The development of an infection and its spread in the context of a mass gathering is related to the presence of individuals with differing immunity and different potential infections in proximity. The conditions that favor the acquisition of an infecting organism include the behavior of the host, the underlying environment, and the host immune status. While traditionally the focus often is on the host acquiring the infection, the environment where the infection is acquired is often the most important risk factor that leads to development of an infection [2]. An outbreak typically starts with an individual case with subsequent dissemination of the infection occurring based on risk factors including international travel, crowded living conditions, and host immunity. This chain of transmission involves an interaction between an infectious agent, susceptible host, reservoir, portal of entry, mode of transmission, and portal of exit, and in theory any of the six elements can be intervened on to break the chain [1]. Infections can however differ widely in their presentation, producing symptoms in some hosts and an asymptomatic carrier state in others [3]. Some carriers never experience symptoms, whereas others can transmit the infection before developing symptoms, termed as incubatory carriers. Convalescent carriers can transmit the infection after recovering from their illness, and chronic carriers continue to harbor the infection months or years after the initial illness. In any carrier state, the host is asymptomatic and therefore unaware of their potential to transmit the infection [3]. As such, they may not follow traditional precautionary measures, such as washing their hands, that a symptomatic host would, which results in a wider spread of infection, sometimes escalating to the point of an outbreak.

The development of a symptomatic infection within a host is contributed by both host and pathogen specific factors with host characteristics such as a weakened immune system, age, genetic factors, socioeconomic factors, and comorbidities which may increase host susceptibility. Concomitantly people living in marginalized communities and crowded living conditions have less access to hygienic conditions and preventive healthcare overall, making them more likely to be exposed to infectious pathogens. During mass gatherings, the population is composed of individuals with a wide spectrum of age, differing immune systems, and coming from various different communities, thus there is always the possibility of an individual patient (either a carrier or a symptomatic host) introducing an infectious agent into a mass gathering, leading to the development of infectious illnesses that may emerge as an outbreak and thus have the potential to develop into epidemics. An exception to this general rule is sporting events such as triathlons, mud-races where the contestants may be exposed to conditions which could already harbor infectious agents and thus have a point source of an outbreak.

The introduction of an infectious agent within a mass gathering can also be through a common source outbreak where each case is exposed to the same source, such as those associated with contaminated food sources. A propagated source outbreak refers to transmission from one person to another through a variety of vectors including, for instance, person-to-person contact (e.g., syphilis) or vector-borne (e.g., yellow fever outbreak through mosquitoes). In a mixed outbreak, transmission starts with a common source, which is then propagated secondarily by person-to-person contact, such as the introduction of typhoid within a gathering and then being propagated by patients and carriers. These outbreaks are propagated by common sources at various points in time, but involve sufficient contact between vectors and human hosts, as well as among human hosts, resulting in a wide net of infection. Thus, outbreaks affecting mass gatherings result from both common and propagated sources, making it challenging to identify the source given its dynamic nature.

In the current era of globalization, national borders are not a barrier to the spread of infections with infectious disease outbreaks easily able to transform into endemics given ease of migration and travel. Thus, various global religious and sports events such as the Hajj, Kumbh Mela, and the Olympics, can function as point sources of introduction and subsequent dissemination of infectious diseases including multidrug resistant bacterial infections [4].

We will briefly discuss the current literature about infectious diseases seen in the context of mass gatherings and discuss preventive measures that could minimize the impact of infections among mass gatherings.

Epidemiology

Respiratory Illnesses

The most common infectious outbreaks during mass gatherings are those involving the respiratory tract. There are multiple epidemiologic studies highlighting the incidence of respiratory infections occurring on outbreaks incurred during religious events including the Hajj, the Kumbh Mela, and sporting events.

The Hajj is an annual Islamic pilgrimage with at least two million pilgrims from around 185 countries and involves pilgrims retracing the footsteps of the Prophet Mohammed and undertaking the same rituals [5, 6]. The pilgrimage starts out in Mecca, Saudi Arabia, making stops in several cities in the vicinity, and finally ending at Mecca [6]. The presence of two million people gathering in closed spaces leads to the potential for multiple infectious agents having an opportunity for airborne agents to spread [5]. The warm and humid environment in addition to congested traffic adds to the risk of transmission [6]. The majority of infectious diseases occurring during the Hajj involve the respiratory tract. In a large retrospective analysis, the incidence and risk factors of pneumonia among hospitalized pilgrims in Medina, Saudi Arabia, from 2004 to 2014 was analyzed. In their study they found that the most common bacterial pathogens found among bacterial pneumonias, with *Staphylococcus aureus* being the most common pathogen detected (36.1 percent), followed by *Klebsiella pneumoniae* (29 percent), *Haemophilus influenzae* (24.3 percent), community acquired *Methicillin Resistant Staphylococcus Aureus* (6.5 percent), *Pseudomonas aeruginosa* (3.1 percent), and *Streptococcus pneumoniae* (1 percent) [7].

In terms of the viral pneumonias, Sheikh et al. (1998) showed that among all patients evaluated by complement fixing antibody for various viral pathogens in the 1991–92 season, Influenza A was the most common virus detected in both Hajj seasons (22 percent) followed by Adenovirus (37 percent). Influenza B and parainfluenza 1 were seen in 3.9 percent and 2.6 percent cases, respectively [8]. This data reinforces the importance of vaccination in preventing the acquisition and spread of influenza pneumonia, as well as maintaining basic hygienic practices such as washing hands and covering the face while sneezing or coughing.

In these studies, many patients with respiratory infections were over fifty years of age, with diabetes mellitus being the most common comorbidity (34.8 percent) followed by cardiovascular disease (23.3 percent), asthma (7.8 percent), and COPD (7.1 percent). The authors raised concern that special education regarding infectious disease awareness and prevention be provided to pilgrims above fifty years of age and those with comorbidities given the morbidity burden in these groups. These data have implications for public health and health care measures directed at preventing and better managing bacterial pneumonia in the Hajj pilgrims, especially as related to vaccinations [8].

The Kumbh Mela is another religious mass gathering event based in Hindu ritual held every four years in India over a period of few months which involves the spiritual cleaning of body and soul. The events and rituals are situated by the multiple large rivers including the Ganges in Haridwar, Godavari in Nasik, Kshipra in Ujjain, and Ganges in Prayagraj (Allahabad). Though routed in Hinduism, the event typically welcomes visitors from all religions including international travelers. The rituals involve both drinking from and bathing in the water that is frequently contaminated due to open defecation and lack of cleaning on a regular basis. As such, much of the infectious disease burden results from contaminated water. In addition to poor sanitation, the crowded conditions can and do lead to increased rates of respiratory infections during this event [9, 13, 14]. The Mela also attracts pilgrims from multiple differing socioeconomic statuses, with generally low vaccination rates and awareness of preventive practices. As such, droplet borne diseases including measles, chickenpox, pertussis, mumps, and influenza have been frequently reported at this event [9]. As part of a twenty-three-day observational study conducted by the Harvard School of Public Health during the 2013 Mela, there was an uptick in upper respiratory infections two days after the Mela had started. There is also a rising concern for the incidence of multidrug resistant tuberculosis in the setting of low vaccination rates and crowded living conditions, both of which are seen among the pilgrims at Kumbh Mela [9, 10].

More recently, the Kumbh Mela was termed as a "super spreader event" with a surge of COVID-19 cases in multiple cities in Northeastern India [11]. The Indian government postponed the 2021 event to April 2021 and reduced the duration of the event to 30 days instead of 100 days. Despite the decrease in duration of the event there was a large congregation of people from all across the country leading to an uptick in the number of COVID-19 cases during the event, first reaching 100,000 then escalating slowly to above 400,000 soon after the event ended [12]. There were multiple variants identified during this surge and this led to the surge of COVID-19 cases in India with Haridwar city, a center for the Kumbh, reporting an increase of 276 percent, from 37 to 144 cases per day. This surge was worsened by most attendees not performing mitigation efforts at the Kumbh Mela such as

hand hygiene, social distancing, and wearing masks and a lack of vaccination in the majority of Indian population.

Apart from the religious events, national and global events have also historically resulted in respiratory infection outbreaks. During the Eighth Micronesian Games that took place in 2013, six new cases of measles were reported prior to the opening games. There have also been reports of measles outbreaks during the XXI Olympic Winter Games in 2010 in Vancouver, Canada, and the Italian Super Cup in 2011 [15]. The majority of affected individuals had not been vaccinated reiterating the importance of vaccination in preventing vaccine preventable diseases. The incidence escalated to 251 up to three months after the games had ended. The Sochi 2014 Olympics reported respiratory and gastrointestinal infections affecting 58 percent of the athletes. Similarly, during the 2016 Olympics, the US athletes who had traveled to Rio de Janeiro, Brazil had tested positive for several tropical, mosquito borne infections including West Nile virus, Dengue fever, and Chikungunya [16].

Gastrointestinal Infection

There have been numerous outbreaks of gastrointestinal infections at mass gathering events. The presence of proximity of individuals, close living quarters, common food supplies all facilitate the spread of gastrointestinal infections at such events. Traditionally cholera was often a big concern at huge mass gathering events such as the Hajj as it led to significant morbidity and mortality and was of great public health concern in 1989 Hajj. However, with improvement in sanitation and better diagnosis and management the incidence of gastroenteritis has become less common at least in the last two decades.[17] The data from a tertiary care center in Makkah during the 2003 season showed 2.4 percent prevalence of gastrointestinal disease which included noninfectious illnesses such as chronic liver disease along with gastroenteritis. Data from the same healthcare center in 2005 showed a 11 percent prevalence of gastrointestinal disease in hospitalized pilgrims, and gastroenteritis being much less common. Data from the 2008 season was reviewed and included 4,136 pilgrims who presented to 13 different primary health care practices in Mina. The dataset was primarily outpatient and showed gastrointestinal disease in 13 percent of pilgrims, with 3.8 percent cases of gastroenteritis and 1.2 percent of diarrhea.

In terms of the etiology of diarrhea, a study suggested parasitic infection was diagnosed more commonly compared to viral and bacterial among patients who had gastrointestinal infections [17]. *E. histolytica* and *Giardia lamblia* were the most detected parasites, followed by *Cryptosporidium* spp and *Ascaris lumbricoides*. As for viral illnesses, data was obtained from pediatric patients between 2002 and 2003 at the main hospitals of Jeddah, Makkah, and Riyadh. Rotavirus was most detected (6 percent) followed by norovirus (3.5 percent), astrovirus (1.9 percent) and adenovirus (1.4 percent). In a more recent data set from 2013, astrovirus was commonly seen in 6.6 percent of cases. There is limited data on food borne infection during the Hajj. The data set from the 2012 Hajj season showed some evidence of *Tropheryma whipplei* in Hajj pilgrims. Among 129 rectal swabs obtained from French pilgrims all were negative before pilgrimage. Among nine pilgrims that underwent rectal swab testing two (20 percent) were positive for *Tropheryma whipplei*.17

Despite a lower prevalence of gastrointestinal infections during the Hajj, compared to respiratory infections, antibiotic resistant diarrhea is still a significant public health concern. Close to 50 percent of pilgrims from various nationalities have reported the use of antibiotics for diarrhea from 2012 to 2016. These include 45–48 percent of Indian pilgrims, 53 percent French pilgrims, 58 percent Iranian pilgrims, and 61 percent Malay pilgrims [5].

As part of a study on French pilgrims during the 2013 pilgrimage, there was a significant increase in *Escherichia coli* resistant to ceftriaxone being found in returning pilgrims with an increase from 10 percent to 32 percent before and after the Hajj [18]. Another analysis during the 2015 Hajj season including pilgrims from two hospitals in Makkah documented antimicrobial resistance toward beta lactams, the most common being amoxicillin-clavulanate especially in *Klebsiella pneumoniae*. The presence of quinolone resistance, especially toward ciprofloxacin, was found among multiple organisms especially among *Escherichia coli*, *Acinetobacter baumannii*, methicillin resistant *Staphylococcus aureus*, and *Klebsiella pneumoniae*. The presence of aminoglycoside resistance especially to tobramycin was also found only in *Escherichia coli*, *Acinetobacter baumannii*, and *Klebsiella pneumoniae* [19]. The emergence of multidrug resistant pathogens in the bowel in the setting of inappropriate antibiotic use calls for better prevention

and management of gastroenteritis as well as respiratory infections. This can be accomplished through limiting risk factors of drug resistance including misuse of antibiotics and limiting access to antibiotics without a prescription.[5]

The Kumbh Mela held periodically in India in the past was often associated with large outbreaks of gastrointestinal illnesses. The association of cholera with Kumbh was widely prevalent in the past dating all the way to the eighteenth century. The development of the 1867 cholera pandemic started from the Kumbh mainly due to the large crowds bathing multiple times in unsanitary water [20]. The disease outbreak exploded with cases increasing to thousands within a month, and then rapidly spreading across national borders to Afghanistan, Persia (Iran) in 1867 and 1868, Turkey and Kiev in 1869, and eventually to Russia and Europe resulting in over a million deaths. The last cholera outbreak in India was reported in 1906 that occurred despite diligent sanitary measures. It was felt that this was due to a hesitation in drinking chlorinated or treated water due to superstition, failure of affected patients to clean their soiled garments, drying up of rivers and drinking from polluted water beds [9].

With the development of modern sanitation procedures at sporting events the occurrence of gastrointestinal infections at sporting events have been less common. There have still been occurrences of viral gastroenteritis as evidenced by the norovirus outbreak at the 2018 Pyeongyang Winter Olympiad, though the event primarily affected security staff. Occasionally there have been reports of bacterial gastroenteritis outbreaks such as a *Salmonella* outbreak at an international youth ice hockey competition in Riga, Latvia in 2015 [4].

The prevention of these infections involves safe and clean disposal of sewage and prevention of sewage contamination of the water supply and controlling potential deficiencies in food and water handling as well ensuring that food handlers are not infected and ensuring vaccination especially against *Salmonella typhi* among participants among mass gatherings in areas where typhoid is endemic.

Meningococcal Disease

The development of meningococcal disease was often the most serious infection reported at mass gathering events especially the Hajj leading to the recommendation for meningococcal vaccination among Hajj pilgrims. Despite this recommendation, meningococcal disease is still prevalent among Hajj pilgrims, particularly disease caused by serogroups not covered by vaccination. A study of international pilgrims from 2014 showed a 3 percent carriage of *Neisseria meningitides* after the Hajj, most isolates being serogroup B which is not one of the isolates covered by the traditional recommended vaccination. Part of the issue is that many countries worldwide continue to use the polysaccharide vaccine which, unlike the recommended meningococcal vaccination, does not cover serogroups A, C, Y, and W-135. Therefore, common serogroups such as W-135 continue to be prevalent among Hajj pilgrims, as seen in 27 percent Turkish pilgrims from 2010 Hajj compared to 13 percent before the pilgrimage.

As part of a literature review of meningococcal disease at mass gatherings between 2002 and 2011, invasive meningococcal disease was found in sixteen Hajj pilgrims and one Umrah pilgrim [21]. There have been reports of development of invasive meningococcal disease at the 2015 World Scout Jamboree in Japan.

The key to prevention of meningococcal disease at mass gatherings includes ensuring vaccination against meningococcal disease using the current approved vaccines and minimizing crowding at events and ensuring proper infection prevention methods such as hand washing and covering coughs.

Sexually Transmitted Infections

The development of sexually transmitted infections (STIs) has been reported commonly during sports gatherings. This may be due to the nature of participants and spectators at these events being of a younger age compared to the participants at gatherings at pilgrimages. In the 2014 FIFA World cup in Brazil, 1586 travelers were seen at HIV reference centers and 28 were found to be HIV positive including 3 with acquired immunodeficiency syndrome (AIDS), while 9 individuals had acute symptomatic HIV infection suggesting acquisition at the sporting event. There have also been cases of Human Papilloma Virus (HPV) and human herpes virus (HHV-2) coinfections with HIV have also been reported at the event [22]. The number of cases of bacterial STIs at mass gathering is generally underreported though news reports at Rio Olympic games in 2016 showed a vast increase of commercial sex workers at the event with likely corresponding increase in number of STIs.

Prevention and Planning

The key to preventing epidemics at mass gathering events involves implementing a multimodal approach involving limiting the introduction of infectious agents into the gathering and then limiting the potential spread of any contagious diseases. An excellent example of this was implemented in February 2020 to limit the introduction of COVID-19 at the Kingdom of Saudi Arabia (KSA) where there was a temporarily suspension of the entry of pilgrims to the KSA for Umrah [23, 24]. In addition, the KSA also banned the entry of persons from countries affected by COVID-19. The Saudi government did resume the Umrah pilgrimage after three months though only select devotees were then allowed entry. The Saudi government only allowed entry of pilgrims aged twenty to sixty-five years who were relatively healthy, nonpregnant, and had negative results on the COVID-19 PCR screen. The pilgrims quarantined for two weeks prior as well as after the event. During the event, the pilgrims were assigned in small groups to safe hubs and were required to follow preventive practices including social distancing and masks, along with designated tracks. After the event, pilgrims underwent additional COVID-19 PCR screens prior to returning to their home countries. As a result of this plan there were no reported cases of COVID-19 during the Umrah pilgrimage. Though Umrah hosts a small number of participants compared to the Hajj, the attendees are of a similar demographic particularly those of older ages and several comorbidities. The KSA prevention plan is therefore much applicable to larger mass gatherings at least as related to prevention of COVID-19.

The Olympic games in Japan were also postponed to 2021 and a strict preventive plan was implemented for participants and spectators.[24] The participants were required to be screened twice within three days prior to their arrival in Japan, then rescreen upon arrival and were required to quarantine for three days upon arrival, and quarantine for fourteen days if they refused daily screening. The participants were screened after the Olympics and before leaving Japan. During the events there was an emphasis on strict preventive measures including hand hygiene, social distancing, and masks. The participants who tested positive during the games were isolated and kept away from the games during the infectious phase. All players were prohibited from using public transportation, and spectators were prohibited from watching games in-person to enforce strict social distancing measures [12].

Previously in 2004, a large outbreak of cholera was averted successfully during Kumbh Mela in India [25]. The presence of diarrhea cases was reported early through a telemedicine system implemented at the main hospital in Prayag City in Northern India. The system implemented daily reporting of hospitalized patients as well as outpatient cases of diarrhea. The information was relayed to the local reference laboratory, where the microbiology department analyzed stool samples and rectal swabs and found *Vibrio* in 22.6 percent (seven of thirty-one) of samples. The information was rapidly relayed to the main hospital in Prayag City, and the health department soon after implemented strict hygienic measures at the event. This was successfully followed by a swift decrease in the incidence of diarrhea cases in the Kumbh attendees [25].

Meticulous risk assessment and preventive planning was also demonstrated by the Serbian government during two large sporting events in 2009 [18]. During the twenty-fifth Universiade and the tenth EXIT festival the government had expected an uptick in influenza (H1N1) cases in the setting of international travel. The Serbian government had relayed to all traveling countries that they reconsider their travel plans if presenting with flu-like symptoms. Serbia had considered cancelling the event if 1 percent of the attendees were diagnosed with H1N1 influenza, one reported case of acute respiratory distress syndrome, or one death. National surveillance strategies were implemented such that daily reporting took place to identify the first cases of influenza. Early detection strategies included public education about the presentation of influenza, a 24/7 telephone line to report suspected cases, posters at the airport showing the presentation of influenza and help line contact numbers. The event sites were distributed with similar posters and helpline contact numbers. Mobile teams at the event site were established to identify any suspected cases and early cases were stratified into travel-related or domestic and any positive cases led to contact tracing to identify any potential spread of cases. All confirmed cases were isolated at designated sites at both events with patients not requiring hospitalization being self-isolated. All critically ill confirmed and suspected

cases were transferred to isolation facilities at a designated central hospital. This multimodal approach led to early detection of influenza cases, early and adequate treatment, and mitigated uncontrolled spread.

The role of vaccination in preventing disease at mass gathering events is underappreciated. All participants at mass gatherings should consider getting vaccinated against yellow fever if they are traveling to endemic areas such as Africa or Central and South America. In addition, we also recommend routine vaccination with inactivated influenza vaccine, pneumococcal vaccine, coronavirus vaccine and against varicella virus and MMR (measles, mumps, and rubella) in patients with no contraindications to live virus vaccinations. The participants should also consider vaccination against *Neisseria meningitidis* [22]. Despite the known data about use of vaccination in preventing invasive meningococcal disease vaccination rates among travelers have also been lagging for meningococcal disease [21]. It is much more beneficial to be vaccinated several days prior to the mass gathering event given a seven-to-ten-day lag in the development of protective antibodies. Vaccination against meningococcal disease is particularly recommended in travelers from endemic areas such as Africa and in adolescents. Given prior outbreaks of invasive meningococcal disease during the Hajj and Umrah, Saudi Arabia as of 2018 has mandated meningococcal vaccination in travelers. As of December 2018, all travelers to Saudi Arabia above two years of age who are Hajj or Umrah pilgrims, seasonal workers or anticipating contact with pilgrims must provide proof of polysaccharide or quadrivalent conjugate ACWY vaccine given within ten days to three years for polysaccharide vaccine, and within five years for conjugate vaccine [21].

There is also a need for real-time surveillance of infectious disease at mass gathering events, with data collection and analysis, advanced molecular genotyping, and phenotyping to identify genetic risk factors and establishing a global community to promote dialogue among various countries about infectious disease outbreaks [4].

The prevention of infectious diseases at these events thus involves a multipronged approach involving vaccination of attendees, screening of attendees for infectious agents with isolation, and isolation of infected individuals. The mass gathering organizers should ensure adequate adherence to infection prevention measures such as ensuring multiple hand washing stations, adequate sanitation and sewage facilities, and ensuring safe and clean food preparation. Once an infection is identified, the infection should be rapidly identified and patients appropriately isolated to prevent dissemination of the infection. This approach while not eliminating infections can prevent an outbreak developing into an epidemic.

Conclusion

Mass gatherings historically have resulted in infectious disease outbreaks with significant associated morbidity and mortality, the most recent one being the COVID-19 outbreak as part of the Kumbh Mela. Given the ease of travel locally and internationally, an outbreak at a mass gathering can lead to development of a pandemic. The development of meticulous preventive plans that include vaccinations well ahead of travel, basic hygienic practices, and easy access to health care should be pursued aggressively as part of mass gatherings. There should be communication among event planners and local health authorities to report emerging cases, isolate and treat the affected persons to limit transmissibility. The prevention of infectious diseases at mass gatherings involves adequate pre-event planning, ensuring a clean and hygienic event, and early diagnosis of infections at the event.

References

1. Krämer A., Akmatov M., Kretzschmar M. Principles of Infectious Disease Epidemiology. In: *Modern Infectious Disease Epidemiology*. New York: Springer; 2009; pp. 85–99.

2. Kak V. Infections in Confined Spaces: Cruise ships, Military Barracks and College Dormitories. *Infect Dis Clin N Am.* 2007;**21**:773–784.

3. Casadevall A., Pirofski L. A. Host-Pathogen Interactions: Redefining the Basic Concepts of Virulence and Pathogenicity. *Infection and Immunity.* 1999;**67**(8):3703–3713.

4. Memish Z. A., Steffen R., White P., Dar O., Azhar E. I., Sharma A., Zumla A. Mass Gatherings Medicine: Public Health Issues Arising from Mass Gathering Religious and Sporting Events. *Lancet.* 2019;**393**(10185): 2073–2084. doi:10.1016/S0140-6736(19)30501-X

5. Hoang V. T., Gautret P. Infectious Diseases and Mass Gatherings. *Current Infectious Disease Reports.* 2018;**20**(11):1–12.

6. Ahmed Q. A., Arabi Y. M., Memish Z. A. Health Risk at the Hajj. *The Lancet.* 2006;**367**(9515):1008–1015.

7. Shirah, B. H., Zafar, S. H., Alferaidi, O. A., Sabir, A. M. Mass Gathering Medicine (Hajj Pilgrimage in Saudi Arabia): The Clinical Pattern of Pneumonia Among Pilgrims During Hajj. *Journal of Infection and Public Health.* 2017;**10**(3);277–286.

8. El-Sheikh S. M., El-Assouli S. M., Mohammed K. A., Albar M. Bacteria and Viruses That Cause Respiratory Tract Infections During the Pilgrimage (Haj) Season in Makkah, Saudi Arabia. *Tropical Medicine and International Health.* 1998;**3**(3); 205–209.

9. Sridhar S., Gautret P., Brouqui, P. A Comprehensive Review of the Kumbh Mela: Identifying Risks for Spread of Infectious Diseases. *Clinical Microbiology and Infection: The Official Publication of the European Society of Clinical Microbiology and Infectious Diseases.* 2015;**21**(2):128–133. doi:10.1016/j.cmi.2014.11.021

10. Maurya A. K., Singh A. K., Kumar M., Umrao J., Kant S., Nag V. L., Kushwaha R. A., Dhole T. N. Changing Patterns and Trends of Multidrug-Resistant Tuberculosis at Referral Center in Northern India: A 4-Year Experience. *Indian Journal of Medical Microbiology.* 2013;**31**(1):40–46. doi:10.4103/0255-0857.o108720

11. Shukla S., Khanna R., Ahmed Y., Memish Z. A. (2021). Conducting Mass Gathering Events During the COVID-19 Pandemic: A Case Study of Kumbh Mela 2021 as a Potential "Super Spreader Event." *Journal of Travel Medicine.* 2021. taab160. Advance online publication. https://doi.org/10.1093/jtm/taab160

12. Rocha I. C. N., Pelayo M. G. A., Rackimuthu S. Kumbh Mela Religious Gathering as a Massive Superspreading Event: Potential Culprit for the Exponential Surge of COVID-19 Cases in India. *The American Journal of Tropical Medicine and Hygiene.* 2021

13. McConnell J., Memish Z. The Lancet Conference on Mass Gatherings Medicine. *Lancet Infectious Diseases.* 2010;**10**:818–819.

14. Memish Z. A., Stephens G., Al Rabeeah A. Mass Gatherings Health. *Lancet Infectious Diseases.* 2012;**12**:10.

15. Heywood A. E. Measles: A Re-Emerging Problem in Migrants and Travelers. *Journal of Travel Medicine.* 2018;**25**(1):10.1093/jtm/tay118. doi:10.1093/jtm/tay118

16. Memish Z. A., Steffen R., White P., Dar O., Azhar E. I., Sharma A., Zumla A. (2019). Mass Gatherings Medicine: Public Health Issues Arising

from Mass Gathering Religious and Sporting Events. *The Lancet.* 2019;393(10185):2073–2084.

17. Gautret P., Benkouiten S., Sridhar S., Al-Tawfiq J. A., Memish Z. A. (2015). Diarrhea at the Hajj and Umrah. *Travel Medicine and Infectious Disease.* 2015;13(2):159–166.

18. Loncarevic G., Payne L., Kon P., Petrovic V., Dimitrijevic D., Knezevic T., Coulombier D. Public Health Preparedness for Two Mass Gathering Events in the Context of Pandemic Influenza (H1N1) 2009-Serbia, July 2009. *Eurosurveillance.* 2009;14(31):19296.

19. Haseeb A., Faidah H., Baksh A. R. et al. Antimicrobial Resistance Among Pilgrims: A Retrospective Study from Two Hospitals Makkah Saudi Arabia. *International Journal of Infectious Diseases.* 2016;47 (C).

20. Bryceson A. D. (1977). Cholera, the Flickering Flame. *Proceedings of the Royal Society of Medicine.* 1977;70(5):363–365.

21. Muttalif A. R., Presa J. V., Haridy H., Gamil A., Serra L. C., Cané A. Incidence and Prevention of Invasive Meningococcal Disease in Global Mass Gathering Events. *Infectious Diseases and Therapy.* 2019;8(4):569–579.

22. Lima L. R. P., da Silva A. D. S., da Cruz Gameiro E. R., Fernandes J., Lanzarini N. M., de Oliveira R. C., Cunha, R. G. Sexually Transmitted Infections in Mass Gathering: Brief Review. *Virus Rev Res.* 2016;21.

23. Ebrahim S. H., Memish Z. A. Saudi Arabia's Drastic Measures to Curb the COVID-19 Outbreak: Temporary Suspension of the Umrah Pilgrimage. *Journal of Travel Medicine.* 2020;27(3).

24. Gautret P., Al-Tawfiq J. A. COVID 19: Will the 2020 Hajj Pilgrimage and Tokyo Olympic Games Be Cancelled?. *Travel Medicine and Infectious Disease.* 2020;34:101622.

25. Ayyagari A., Bhargava A., Agarwal R. et al. Use of Telemedicine in Evading Cholera Outbreak in Mahakumbh Mela, Prayag, UP, India: An Encouraging Experience. *Telemedicine Journal and E-Health.* 2003;9(1):89–94.

Chapter 25

Toxicology and Mass Gathering Medicine

Abigail Kerns, Brian Nao, and John C. Maino II

Introduction

Toxicology is the field of science which examines the effects of chemicals, substances, or situations on people, animals, and the environment. A mass gathering is any organized event with greater than 1,000 attendees. These events can be for any purpose, including daily commutes on public transportation. Mass gatherings are also often related to sporting, religious, or music events. Resources in these settings are often limited. There is a paucity of evidence and guidelines for care of intoxicated individuals in mass gatherings. Available literature is largely anecdotal and descriptive related to personal experiences and solutions to problems, as much of the available literature has been contributed by the experiences of emergency department providers who have responded to such events.

Mass gatherings may be subject to changing conditions and variables that can result in an increase in the number of intoxicated or sick individuals. Heat index and weather conditions should be considered. Planners should also consider the event location, and if conditions are sheltered or exposed. Events with a long duration may result in a greater number of patients requiring care. Certain mass gatherings may attract a specific age demographic that can influence care requirements [1]. The event type may play a role in what type of toxicological exposures occur. For example, ethanol and drug use are frequently associated with sporting and music events, while dance raves are associated with substances that aim to broaden perception, heighten energy or sexual function, or provide a novel experience [11]. Lastly, consideration should also be given to the distance of a mass gathering to a major health care receiving facility. Small emergency departments near the venue may be poorly equipped for a surge of sick patients.

Toxicologic exposures in the setting of mass gatherings can be either intentional or unintentional. Recreational substances including ethanol, marijuana, and other substances of abuse are frequently encountered in mass gatherings. Understanding basic principles of specific substances can aid in management. For the purposes of this chapter, we will categorize substances of abuse as stimulants/hallucinogens or central nervous system depressants.

Stimulants/Hallucinogens

Cocaine (Coke, Snow, Blow, Crack): Benzoylmethylecgonine is the chemical name for cocaine. Cocaine can be found in various forms. Cocaine base (*crack*) is a rock crystal that vaporizes when heated, allowing it to be inhaled. The salt form is a white powder than can be snorted or dissolved in water and injected. Onset of symptoms is rapid. If inhaled, users experience near-immediate effects lasting five to ten minutes. If snorted, onset of symptoms is slower, but effects may last fifteen to thirty minutes.

Immediate effects of cocaine use include euphoria, increased energy and alertness, and reduced need for sleep. Adverse effects can include paranoia, hallucinations, and agitation. Vital sign abnormalities include hypertension, tachycardia, and hyperthermia. The effects of hypertension and vasoconstriction increase risk of acute myocardial infarction, aortic dissection, and stroke. Cardiac dysrhythmias can occur. Cocaine use also increases risk of seizures. In the setting of inhalational use, risk of diffuse alveolar damage ("crack lung") has been reported.

3,4-methylenedioxymethamphetamine (MDMA, ecstasy, Molly):3,4-methylenedioxymethamphetamine (MDMA) is an amphetamine-like substance originally developed as an appetite suppressant in 1965. Currently, its main use is for recreational purposes. MDMA stimulates release and prevents reuptake of serotonin, dopamine, and noradrenalin. MDMA induces feelings of euphoria, empathy, and intimacy, along with heightened sense of awareness. Due to its amphetamine-like properties, individuals may be able to stay awake for long periods of time.

MDMA is typically found as small tablets that can be swallowed or crushed. It may also be found in capsule form, often known as "Molly." Less commonly, it is inserted rectally or smoked. It is often mixed with other drugs such as cocaine, benzodiazepines, caffeine, or lysergic acid diethylamide (LSD). If ingested, peak levels are reached within one hour and last three to six hours.

MDMA toxicity can mimic that of serotonin toxicity. Patients may appear agitated or delirious and can experience headache or palpitations. Intoxicated individuals can have hyperthermia with extreme thirst, which may increase intake of free water. MDMA also increases production of antidiuretic hormone (ADH). These effects can result in profound, life-threatening hyponatremia [18]. Physical exam findings may include tachycardia and hypertension, with mydriasis and flushed skin. Akathisia, hyperreflexia, and muscle rigidity can occur. Severe toxicity can result in rhabdomyolysis with renal and hepatic failure. Fatal arrhythmias have occurred in the setting of MDMA use.

MDMA has been featured in the media over recent years due to its use at electronic dance music festivals. The *Los Angeles Times* reported twenty-five drug-related deaths over a ten-year period associated with rave parties from three Los Angeles-based promoters. Most deaths were related to intoxication with MDMA in otherwise healthy individuals age fifteen to twenty-five years old [9].

Methamphetamines (Speed, Ice, Crank, Meth): Methamphetamine is a sympathomimetic amine that acts as an indirect neurotransmitter. It exerts its effects by promoting the release epinephrine, norepinephrine, dopamine, and serotonin in the brain. Methamphetamine can be ingested as a pill, snorted intranasally, or injected. Clinical effects can include paranoia, agitation, and psychosis. Other short-term effects can include increased wakefulness and physical activity. Intoxicated individuals may experience diaphoresis or palpitations. They may have hypertension, tachycardia, or dysrhythmias. Coma and death can occur in severe toxicity [14].

Prescription Stimulants (Adderall, Ritalin): These prescription medications are frequently used by college-aged students as study aids. Their stimulant effects increase abuse potential [14].

Lysergic acid diethylamide (LSD, acid) and natural hallucinogens: Lysergic acid diethylamide (LSD) is a synthetic hallucinogen synthetized in 1938. Naturally occurring hallucinogens include psilocybin and *N,N*-Dimethyltryptamine (DMT). Hallucinogens are used for their ability to distort reality and allow the user to feel more connected with music and other stimuli. Toxicity can result in severe agitation, particularly at high doses [21].

Ketamine (Special K, Vitamin K, Cat Valium): Ketamine is an anesthetic that derived from phencyclidine (PCP). Its dissociative effects and hallucinatory potential have increased its appeal as a party drug. It can be ingested or smoked in liquid or powder form. Onset of symptoms is rapid and typically lasts forty-five minutes. Users may have tachycardia or palpitations and hypertension. Respiratory depression can occur at high doses. Its dissociative effects and anterograde amnesia have resulted in its use with drug-facilitated sexual assault [14, 19].

Amyl Nitrites (Poppers): Amyl nitrites are inhalants used to enhance sexual pleasure. They are vasodilators that can result in profound hypotension and cardiovascular collapse at high doses. Severe toxicity can result in coronary ischemia or stroke with increased intracranial pressure. Management is typically supportive or related to secondary-organ ischemia [14, 24].

Methylenedioxypyrovalerone (Bath salts) and Mephedrone (Diablo, Meow Meow, Eric 3): Methyldioxypyrovalerone (MDPV) and mephedrone are synthetic cathinones, also known as "bath salts." Synthetic cathinones are stimulants and may be used to increase energy, sociability, or sex drive. Synthetic cathinones are manufactured in powder forms that can be ingested, snorted, smoked, or injected. Adverse reactions include panic attacks and paranoia with psychosis. Toxicity may increase risk of violent tendencies or trauma [25].

251-NBOMe (Legal LSD, N-Bomb): 251-NBOMe is a new psychoactive substance used for its psychedelic and hallucinatory effects. Users may seek to enhance the visual and auditory experience of concerts or other events. It is manufactured by clandestine labs in the form of blotter paper, powder, liquid, or tablet. It can be taken orally, sublingual or buccal, smoked, or snorted intranasally. Toxicity may present with agitation or seizures. Vital sign abnormalities may include hyperthermia, tachycardia, and hypertension. Mydriasis may be noted on physical examination. Severe toxicity can result in rhabdomyolysis, disseminated intravascular coagulation, and multiorgan failure [26].

Central Nervous System Depressants

Ethanol: Ethanol is one of the most frequently used substances at mass gatherings. It is classified as a central nervous system depressant, but may paradoxically decrease inhibition at relatively lower doses. Ethanol is responsible for a large number of visits to local emergency departments following mass gatherings [3]. Ability to bring one's own ethanol or purchase from a vendor may also contribute to the number of intoxicated individuals [5]. The effects of ethanol on an individual may vary by gender, weight, and amount of food recently consumed. Demographics of a specific mass gathering event may impact the effects of ethanol on surrounding health services.

Ethanol is typically ingested and is primarily absorbed by the duodenum, with a small amount of absorption occurring in the stomach. Following consumption, peak levels can be reached in thirty to ninety minutes on an empty stomach. Alcohol dehydrogenase rapidly metabolizes ethanol in the liver [4].

Symptoms are often dose-related, and individuals may have varying responses to the same dose. Common signs and symptoms of ethanol intoxication may include slurred speech, nystagmus, headaches, drowsiness, impaired judgment and memory, decreased coordination, and decreased perception. Nausea and vomiting may be present. Individuals may exhibit disinhibited behavior early in intoxication. At higher doses, individuals may become unconsciousness which can progress to coma [6]. Vital sign abnormalities may include tachycardia and hypotension secondary to peripheral vasodilation and volume loss [4].

Cannabis/cannabinoids: Marijuana is one of the most commonly used recreational substances and its recent legalization by some states is likely to result in increased use. The dried buds of the plant *Cannabis sativa* contain delta-9-tetrahydrocannabinol (THC), the chemical primarily responsible for the substance's psychoactive properties [7]. THC content varies widely between marijuana products. Structural analogs of THC have also been recently developed. These chemically synthesized products often have higher binding affinity for cannabinoid receptors and can

lead to a more severe intoxication and less predictable effects.

THC is often inhaled or ingested. Psychotropic effects occur within seconds to minutes of inhalation and last several hours. Ingestion results in a slower onset of symptoms, which can take thirty to ninety minutes [8]. Signs and symptoms are nonspecific and include both central nervous system (CNS) stimulation and depression. Individuals may experience euphoria or dysphoria. Common symptoms of CNS stimulation include anxiety, agitation, and paranoia, while psychosis/hallucinations and seizures are rarer. CNS effects can result in depressed consciousness, which can progress to coma. Other nonspecific symptoms can include slurred speech, impaired coordination, headache, nausea, and vomiting. Physical exam findings may include dry mouth or conjunctival injection, and while individuals may present with tachycardia and hypotension, bradycardia and orthostatic hypotension have been documented. While there is no direct association of acute coronary syndrome with cannabis, case reports have described cardiac events following use of cannabis [8]. Cannabis intoxication may be challenging to diagnose. If inhaled, cannabis odor on clothing may suggest exposure [8].

Gamma-hydroxybutyrate (GHB): Gamma-hydroxybutyrate was synthesized in the 1960s as an anesthetic. It was available in health stores as a reported athletic enhancer prior to being banned in 1990. Its medical use is not limited to the treatment of narcolepsy. Illicit GHB is made in clandestine labs and sold on the dark web. It is marketed as a club drug due to its euphoric effects that increase sociability and sexual feelings. At high doses, central nervous system and respiratory depression can occur. Individuals may be amnestic to events, which has resulted in its use in drug-facilitated sexual assault.

GHB is manufactured in powder form and is water-soluble. It has a slightly salty taste that can be masked with alcohol. Co-ingestion with ethanol increases risk of central nervous system and respiratory depression. Patients may have hypotension. Severe hypothermia can occur [19, 16, 17, 23].

Benzodiazepines, Rohypnol ("Roofies"): Benzodiazepines are sedative-hypnotic medications with many medical indications. Rohypnol (flunitrazepam) is a benzodiazepine that is not legal in the United States, but remains available in some countries in Europe and Latin America. Physical effects are similar to other benzodiazepines, but it is ten times more potent than diazepam. Onset of action varies by specific agent, but frequently effects are seen within fifteen to twenty minutes following ingestion and last several hours.

Common effects of sedative-hypnotics include anxiety reduction, relaxation, and sedation. Due to its strong potency and amnestic qualities, Rohypnol is used for drug-facilitated sexual assault. It comes in green oblong tablets that produce a blue color in drinks. Clandestine labs manufacture white pills that can be taken whole or crushed and snorted. These illicit pills may not result in color change if placed in drinks [17].

Opioids: While opioid abuse has reached epidemic proportions in recent years, its use is relatively uncommon at mass gatherings. The classic triad of opioid toxicity includes depressed mental status, decreased respiratory rate, and miotic pupils. Individuals with opioid toxicity may not present with all three findings, and use should be considered in any individual with depressed mental status. Miotic pupils are a classic finding, but often pupils will be normal depending on specific agent or other co-ingestions.

Nitrous Oxide (Whippets, Laughing gas): Nitrous oxide is a dissociative anesthetic gas also used in automotive and food industries. It is placed in an inhaled delivery system such as a balloon, gas cylinder, or whipping cream canister. Users experience euphoria. Discharge of the gas is endothermic and may result in frostbite of the oral or nasal cavity. Adverse reactions include psychosis, tachycardia, myocardial infarction, seizure, and stroke [27].

General Management Considerations

A generalized approach should be used to evaluate the intoxicated patient with concerns for instability [19]. Initial assessment should focus on assessment of airway, respiratory, and cardiovascular status. Cardiac monitoring and pulse-oximetry should be used. Vital signs and a rapid bedside glucose level should be performed. Treatment is mainly supportive with emphasis on cardiovascular and airway support. Priority should be placed on airway protection in sedated or obtunded patients. Patients may require intravenous fluid resuscitation. Patients with nausea or vomiting can be treated with antiemetics, such as ondansetron. Intravenous fluid hydration should be considered in the setting of volume depletion. If

patients do not respond to basic supportive measures, they will require transfer for definitive management. Transfer to higher level of care should be considered in patients with evidence of respiratory compromise, cardiovascular instability, severe hyperthermia, or mental status changes that fail to improve with basic measures [33].

Patients may present with agitation. If symptoms are mild, they may require a quiet, comfortable area until effects wear off. Some individuals require a quiet, protected shelter to rest and recover from the effects of substances [32]. Such "respite" centers can be easily staffed by nurses and security staff and provide a solution to the overburdening volume of patients in on-site care. If patients are severely agitated, benzo-diazepines or antipsychotics may be considered to facilitate care. Vital sign instability such as hypertension and tachycardia often improve with management of anxiety and agitation but can be managed with labetalol if severe. If cocaine toxicity is suspected, beta adrenergic receptor blocking medications should be avoided due to concern for unopposed alpha stimulation [19, 20]. Patients should be assessed for hyperthermia, which can be managed with external cooling, such as ice packs. Patients may be at risk for rhabdomyolysis, which can progress to disseminated intravascular coagulation and multiorgan failure in severe cases [26]. In patients presenting with depressed mental status, a trial of naloxone can be considered in suspect opioid toxicity. Small doses should be provided initially with increasing doses can be considered if there is lack of response [22].

Patients with mental status changes should be assessed for causes other than intoxication. Hypoxia, hypothermia, and hypoglycemia can present with mental status changes. Ethanol intoxication can mimic many other conditions and further workup for metabolic derangement, infection, or alternative etiologies should be considered in the appropriate clinical setting [4]. Patients should be broadly assessed for traumatic injuries, particularly in the setting of hallucinogen use.

Patients may present with complaints that may seem unrelated to drug intoxication. Cocaine is associated with vasoconstriction of blood vessels and can result in coronary ischemia or cerebrovascular accident. Individuals with severe headache or neurologic changes should be assessed for intracranial hemorrhage or ischemia [27]. Substances that are inhaled, such as marijuana or crack cocaine, may result in pulmonary injury. The presentation of sharp, pleuritic chest pain or subcutaneous emphysema should raise concern for pulmonary injury. If an individual inhales and coughs while attempting to hold their breath with marijuana use, pneumothorax or pneumomediastinum can occur [7]. Specific agents may also have side effects that should be assessed for. For example, discharge of nitrous oxide gas is an endothermic process that may result in frostbite of the oral or nasal cavity.

The ultimate goal of on-site care is to administer first aid and provide spectators with a positive experience while avoiding delays in transferring patients to outside facilities. Patient disposition will ultimately depend on clinical status. On-site care also provides stabilization and triage in the event of a mass casualty incident. If the volume of individuals requiring care surpasses the ability of on-site care centers, the sickest individuals should be transferred to the nearest emergency room. Event planners should anticipate toxicologic concerns prior to mass gatherings. For example, those planning music festivals should anticipate a preponderance of heavy alcohol use. Electronic music festivals have been associated with MDMA and other stimulants. Planners should also consider factors such as weather and temperature, event type, location, and duration. Crowd density, attendance numbers, and demographics should be considered when allocating resources [28, 29]. The number of individuals in attendance does not always correlate with medical requirements [30]. It is important to have resuscitation areas for the rare but potential life-threatening respiratory or cardiovascular events. For less severe injuries, first aid tents or booths can be placed in strategic locations. Transport for the immobilized patient should also be available to and from the venue [31, 29].

Special Considerations

Chemical Terrorism: Mass gathering events may be targets for chemical terrorism events [35]. The 1994 sarin gas attacks in Japan involved sarin solution heated to a gaseous state and blown by a fan. The attack resulted in 7 deaths and 660 injured victims. A second attack occurred in 1995 when vinyl bags with sarin were punctured with an umbrella tip allowing passive dispersal. This attack resulted in 13 deaths and 5,500 affected individuals. These attacks prompted Japan to employ countermeasure plans

[36]. Agents used in chemical terrorism may be easily accessible. Food and water supplies are a potential source [37]. Ricin is a chemical warfare agent that is easily extracted from the castor bean [38]. Industrial chemicals such as halogens, hydrogen sulfide, cyanide, and phosgene are also readily accessible [39].

Preparation for chemical warfare attacks involves consideration of accessibility to antidotes. For example, high potency fentanyl analogues were used in the Dubrovka Theater hostage crisis. Naloxone is an antidote that should be used in cases of suspected opioid toxicity. Cyanide is another potential chemical warfare agent. It is a gas that blocks cellular respiration, which results in depressed consciousness, hyperventilation, and nausea. Higher doses can result in cardiovascular collapse, respiratory failure, and death. If recognized promptly, hydroxocobalamin is an effective antidote. Nerve agents include organophosphates, such as sarin. These are cholinesterase inhibitors that lead to accumulation of acetylcholine at synapses. Symptoms are those of a cholinergic crisis and include miosis, hypersalivation, rhinorrhea, sweating, defecation, fasciculations, paralysis, seizures, bronchoconstriction, and bradycardia. The antidotes are atropine and pralidoxime.

Identifying a chemical terrorist attack involves recognizing an unexplained cluster of illnesses, atypical smells or smoke, and, in the case of explosions, casualties out of proportion to the trauma incident. A hot zone or exclusion area starts where dead bodies are first found. The decontamination area extends 100 meters indoors and 200 meters outdoors. A safe zone outside this area should be demarcated. Proper use of personal protective equipment is essential. Transport vehicles are to be designated as contaminated. Undressing and decontamination may be considered depending on the setting. Since most toxins result in respiratory compromise, airway and oxygen support should be available [40, 41, 42, 43].

Carbon Monoxide: Carbon monoxide (CO) exposure can occur related to automotive racing or congested campsites with generators placed too close to recreational vehicles or tents [44]. Headache, dizziness, nausea, weakness, and chest pain should prompt consideration of CO intoxication. A handheld pulse co-oximeter can be used. Prevention by education, along with surveillance of campsites for potential issues, can be valuable. Removal from the exposure site is first-line therapy. Exposed individuals should receive 100 percent oxygen until asymptomatic along with normalized CO levels. Anyone with significant levels, symptoms, pregnancy, or older age should be considered for transfer for further studies, oxygen, and monitoring [45].

Conclusion

Toxicology is the field of science that helps us understand the harmful effects that chemicals, substances, or situations can have on people, animals, and the environment. A mass gathering involves the congregation of a large group of people involving more than 1,000 people, often for the purposes of religious, political, sporting, or entertainment purposes. Ethanol and cannabis are the most commonly used substances at mass gatherings. Electronic dance music and rave parties are associated with drugs such as ecstasy, which are taken to heighten the experience. Toxicity from recreational substances can result in profound respiratory depression, cardiovascular collapse, and central nervous system depression. Co-ingestions and product contamination can result in unpredictable clinical presentations. Management should emphasize assessment of airway, breathing, and circulation, followed by supportive care. Measures such as antiemetics and fluid hydration can be administered. Many individuals will improve with conservative measures, but some may require transfer to a higher level of care. Individuals with mental status changes should be broadly assessed for vital sign abnormalities, hyperthermia or hypothermia, hypoglycemia, and trauma.

Mass gatherings may be the target of chemical terrorist attacks. The Japanese subway attacks are an example of the significant morbidity and mortality that can occur in such an event. Preplanning and risk assessment should take place in any setting that poses potential risk. In the event of an attack, pattern recognition and identifying potential toxic agents should occur without delay. Antidotes should be readily available and accessed. A hot zone can be demarcated as the margin of the deceased, followed by a decontamination zone, and finally the safe zone. Personal protective equipment should be provided for personnel that enter contaminated areas.

References

1. Milsten A. M., Maguire B. J., Bissell R. A., Seaman K. G. Mass-Gathering Medical Care: A Review of the Literature. *Prehospital and Disaster Medicine.* 2002;**17**(3):151–162. http://pdm.medicine.wisc.edu

2. American Addiction Centers Editorial Staff (February 9, 2022). Substance Use At Live Music Events. American Addiction Centers. drugabuse.com

3. Ruest S., Masiakos B., Camargo K. Substance Use Patterns and In-Hospital Care of Adolescents and Young Adults Attending Music Concerts. *Addiction Science and Clinical Practice.* 2018;**13**(1):1–9. doi:10.1186/s13722-017-0105-x

4. www.uptodate.com/contents/ethanol-intoxication-in-adults?search=acute%20alcohol%20intoxication&source=search_result&selectedTitle=1~150&usage_type=default&display_rank=1

5. Bullock M., Ranse J., Hutton A. Impact of Patients Presenting with Alcohol and/or Drug Intoxication on In-Event Health Care Services Literature Review. *Prehospital and Disaster Medicine.* 2018;**33**(5):539–542.

6. The Truth About Alcohol. Foundation for a Drug-Free World. 2015. www.drugfreeworld.org/course/lesson/the-truth-about-alcohol/what-is-alcohol.html. Accessed September 1, 2023.

7. Cannabis (marijuana): Acute intoxication. UpToDate. www.uptodate.com/contents/cannabis-marijuana-acute-intoxication?search=acute%20cannabis%20intoxication&source=search_result&selectedTitle=1~150&usage_type=default&display_rank=1. Updated May 22, 2023. Accessed September 1, 2023.

8. Takakuwa K. M., Schears R. M. The Emergency Department Care of Cannabis and Synthetic Cannabinoid Patient: A Narrative Review. *International Journal of Emergency Medicine.* 2021;**14**:10.

9. Romero D. EDM's "Summer of Death" Reporting Is More Than Just Tabloid Raving. Electronic Music. *The Guardian.* September 23, 2016. www.theguardian.com/music/2016/sep/23/edm-summer-of-death-los-angeles-tabloid-raving-:~:text=EDM%27s%20%27summer%20of%20death%27%20reporting%20is%20more%20than%20just%20tabloid%20raving,-There%20have%20been&text=In%202010%2C%20around%20the,American%20football%20games%20held%20there. Accessed September 21, 2023.

10. Ruest S. M., Stephan A. M., Masiakos P. T., Biddinger P. D., Camargo, C. A., Kharasch, S. Substance Use Patterns and In-Hospital Care of Adolescents and Young Adults Attending Music Concerts. *Addiction Science Clinical Practice.* 2018;**13**(1):1–9.

11. Fox J., Smith S., Yale A., Chow C., Alaswad E., Cushing T., Monte A. Drugs of Abuse and Novel Psychoactive Substances at Outdoor Music Festivals in Colorado. *Substance Use Misuse.* 2018;**53**(7):1203–1211.

12. Krul J., Sanou B., Swart E. L., Girbes A. R. Medical Care at Mass Gatherings: Emergency Medical Services at Large-Scale Rave Events. *Prehospital and Disaster Medicine.* 2012;**27**(1):71–74. doi:10.1017/S1049023X12000271.

13. Sanchez D. The Top Music Festivals In the World (Ranked by Amount of Drugs Used). *Digital Music News.* April 16, 2018. www.digitalmusicnews.com/2018/04/16/top-music-festivals-drugs/

14. Top 10 Most Dangerous Party Drugs. Northpoint Washington. www.northpointwashington.com/blog/top-10-dangerous-party-drugs/. Updated May 1, 2019. Accessed September 1, 2023.

15. Klega A. E., Keehbauch J. T. Stimulant and Designer Drug Use: Primary Care Management. *American Academy of Family Physicians*, copyright 2018. www.aafp.org/atp.

16. Krul J., Sanou B., Swart E. L., Girbes A. R. Medical Care at Mass Gatherings: Emergency Medical Services at Large-Scale Rave Events. *Prehospital and Disaster Medicine.* 2012;**27**(1):71–74. doi:10.1017/S1049023X12000271.

17. Thomas W. Rave Drugs and Club Drugs. *American Addiction Centers.* November 29, 2021.

18. Grange J. T., Corbett S. W., Downs D. M. The Games: What Can the Sports Medicine Community Learn from Raves? *Curr Sports Med Rep.* 2014;**13**(3):155–162. doi:10.1249/JSR.0000000000000060.

19. Klega A. E, Keehbauch J. T. Stimulant and Designer Drug Use: Primary Care Management. *American Academy of Family Physicians*, copyright 2018. www.aafp.org/atp

20. Nelson L. S., Odujebe O. Cocaine: Acute Intoxication. UpToDate. www.uptodate.com/contents/cocaine-acute-intoxication?search=acute%20cocaine%20intoxication&source=search_result&selectedTitle=1~150&usage_type=default&display_rank=1. Updated July 17, 2023. Accessed September 1, 2023.

21. Delgado J. UpToDate. Intoxication from LSD and other common hallucinations. www.uptodate.com/contents/intoxication-from-lsd-and-other-common-hallucinogens?search=lsd%20intoxication&source=search_result&selectedTitle=1~150&usage_type=default&display_rank=1. Updated May 23, 2022. Accessed July 2023.

22. Stolbach A., Hoffman R. S. UpToDate. www.uptodate.com/contents/acute-opioid-intoxication-in-adults?search=acute%20opioid%20intoxication%20in%20adults&source=search_result&selectedTitle=1~150&usage_type=default&display_rank=1. Updated August 17, 2023. Accessed September 1, 2023.

23. Krul J., Girbes A. R. J. Gamma-Hydroxybutyrate: Experience of Nine Years of GHB-Related Incidents During Rave Parties in the Netherlands. *Clinical Toxicology.* 2011;**49**(4): 311–315. doi:10.3109/15563650.2011.576253

24. Perry J. UpToDate. Inhalant misuse in children and adolescents. www.uptodate.com/contents/inhalant-abuse-in-children-and-adolescents?search=amyl%20nitrite&source=search_result&selectedTitle=1~18&usage_type=default&display_rank=1. Updated August 11, 2023. Accessed September 1, 2023.

25. Synthetic Cathinones ("Bath Salts") Drug Facts. *National Institute on Drug Abuse.* July 2020. https://nida.nih.gov/research-topics/commonly-used-drugs-charts - bath-salts.

26. Zawilska J. B., Kacela M., Adamowicz P. NBOMes-Highly Potent and Toxic Alternatives of LSD. *Frontiers in Neuroscience.* 2020;**14**:78. doi:10.3389/fnins.2020.00078

27. Kleinkopf, K. Nitrous Oxide: The Popular Drug at Music Festivals. Struggling with Addiction. November 29, 2021. https://strugglingwithaddiction.com/nitrous-oxide-the-popular-drug-at-music-festivals/

28. Chan C. H., Friedman M. S. Onsite Medical Care, Resuscitation Increasingly Important at Mass Gathering Events. *ACEP Now* (April 11, 2017) www.acepnow.com/article/onsite-medical-care-resuscitation-increasingly-important-mass-gathering-events/

29. Grange J. T., Corbett S. W., Downs D. M. The Games: What Can the Sports Medicine Community Learn from Raves? *Curr Sports Med Rep.* 2014;**13**(3):155–162.

30. McQueen C., Davies, C. Health Care in a Unique Setting: Applying Emergency Medicine at Music Festivals. In: *Open Access Emergency Medicine.* Yorkshire: Dove Medical Press; 2012; 69–73.

31. Hewitt S., Jarrett L., Winter B. Emergency Medicine at a Large Rock Festival. *Journal of Accidental and Emergency Medicine.* 1996;**13**:26–27.

32. Hunter C. L., Thundiyil J., Ladde J., et al. Emergency Care at a Music Festival: A First Person Report. *Emergency Medicine.* 2017;**49**(6):248–257.

33. Gahlinger P. M. Club Drugs: MDMA, Gamma-Hydroxybutyrate (GHB), Rohypnol, and Ketamine. *American Family Physician.* 2004;**69**(11):2619–2627.

34. Day N., Criss J., Griffiths B., Gujral S. K., John-Leader F., Johnston J., Pit S. Music Festival Attendees' Illicit Drug Use, Knowledge and Practices Regarding Drug Content and Purity; a Cross-Sectional Survey. *Harm Reduction Journal.* 2018;**15**(1):1–8.

35. Santos C., El Zahran T., Weiland J., Anwar M., Schier J. Characterizing Chemical Terrorism Incidents Collected by the Global Terrorism Database, 1970–2015. *Prehospital and Disaster Medicine.* 2019;**34**(4):385–392.

36. Okumura T., Seto Y., Fuse A. Countermeasures Against Chemical Terrorism in Japan. *Forensic Science International.* 2013;**227**:2–6.

37. Khan A. S., Swerdlow D. L., Juraner D. D. Precautions Against Biological and Chemical Terrorism Directed at Food and Water Supplies. *Public Health Reports.* 2001;**116**(1):3–14.

38. Gomes Raffagnato C., Abdalla de Oliveira Cardoso T., de Vasconcelos Fontes F., Montez Carpes M., Cynamon Cohen S., Americo Calcada L. Chemical Terrorism: Risk Modeling Proposal for Attacks Involving Ricin in Mass Gatherings in Brazil. *Saude Debate/Rio de Janeiro.* 2019;**43** (Especial 3):152–164.

39. Casillas R. R., Tewari-Singh, N., Gray J. P. Special Issue: Emerging Chemical Terrorism Threats. *Toxicology Mechanisms and Methods.* 2021;**31**(4);239–241.

40. Emmett S. R., Blain P. G. *Chemical Terrorism.* New York: Elsevier Ltd; 2019.

41. Ciottone G. R. Toxidrome Recognition in Chemical-Weapons Attacks. *The New England Journal of Medicine.* 2018;**378**(17):1611–1620.

42. Markel G., Krivoy A., Rotman E., Schein O., Shrot S. , Brosh-Nissimov T., Dushnitsky T., Eisenkraft A. Medical Management of Toxicological Mass Casualty Events. *IMAJ.* 2008;**10**(11):761–766.

43. Chapter 15 – Chemical, Biological and Radionuclear Risks to Public Health. *The WHO Manual for the Public Health Management of Chemical Incidents* (pp. 140–148). www.who.int/environmental_heal th_emergencies/publications/Manual_Chemical_Inc idents/en/

44. Bacon J. 4 Die at Faster Horses Festival in Michigan, Including 3 of Suspected Carbon Monoxide Poisoning. *USA Today*, July 18, 2021.

45. Pasquier M., Dami F., Carron P.-N., Yersin B., Rignel R., Hugli O. Mass Casualty Triage in the Case of Carbon Monoxide Poisoning: Lessons Learned. *Disaster Medicine and Public Health Preparedness.* 2017;**12**(3):373–378. doi:10.1017/dmp.2017.65

Chapter 26

Medicolegal Considerations in Mass Gathering Medicine

Bruce D. Gehle

Introduction

You are employed by a small emergency medicine group and are asked by your eight-year-old son's soccer league director if you will accompany the team to a tournament occurring the coming weekend and be available in case "anyone needs medical attention." You agree to go as a volunteer, or you agree to do it but only if there is a contractual arrangement with your emergency medicine group and you attend as an employee of your group. However, what if you cannot attend, because you have previously agreed to serve as a volunteer medical director for church event that weekend, or as an employed medical director overseeing medical direction services at a college football game that same weekend? Can you be sued if someone claims they received negligent medical care at any one of these events? What are your liability risks for direct care versus as a medical director? How does your volunteer or employment status impact your liability risk? What should you do to mitigate your liability risk and protect yourself? Are there any other medicolegal concerns other than medical malpractice?

The answers to all these questions are varied and complex–there is no "one size fits all." The answers are varied because medical negligence laws, both statutory and common law, are different to some degree in every state, even though the standard elements of a medical negligence claim are the same. The answers are complex, because even if everyone agrees on basic facts, the laws are not always clear, with room for interpretation case by case, and of course the purported "facts" themselves can leave room for interpretation.

In order to analyze the particular risks, first there must be an understanding of the essential elements of a liability claim, as well as of the nuances of Good Samaritan laws, medical directorship laws and agreements, as well as professional liability insurance. Most claims will be in either the category of negligence in providing direct medical care or for negligence in administrative actions and decision-making. Claims of negligence for providing direct medical care will be subject to a traditional medical malpractice/professional liability analysis, while claims of administrative negligence will undergo a more traditional negligence analysis with consideration of any statutory immunities or conditions. Liability insurance considerations are applicable to both types of claims, but an understanding of the specific coverage available in a particular policy is important for providers, because a policy may cover one type of claim but not another.

Can I Be Sued?

One of the most common preliminary questions clinicians ask when assessing risk is "can I be sued?" The often unhelpful but accurate answer to such a "can" question, which is always a question of possibility, is almost always going to be "yes." The legal threshold for filing a lawsuit (as opposed to the threshold for actually prevailing in a lawsuit) against another person for alleged negligence, whether ordinary negligence or medical malpractice, is very low. Essentially all a plaintiff needs to have is a "good faith" basis to file a suit – which essentially means an assertion of facts which, if accepted as true (which is the presumption a court would initially make), would meet the required elements for recovery in a lawsuit. The remedies for persons who feel they are "wrongfully sued" are limited and difficult to prove. If you believe you are the victim of a legally inappropriate lawsuit and choose to take the accuser to court for filing the lawsuit, you would need to prove that the accuser was liable for "malicious prosecution," that is to say, that there was no conceivable factual or circumstantial basis for the claim, *and* that it was filed with the intent to cause harm to the defendant. An additional practical problem for countersuing is that most plaintiffs do not have any assets to recover if you do win your suit. You would likely spend lot of money, and even if you won, you would simply just be out a lot of money; a quintessential pyrrhic victory. Some states have additional prerequisites for plaintiffs in medical malpractice cases, for example Virginia, which requires that a plaintiff obtain an opinion from a qualified expert that the defendant breached the standard of care resulting in harm to the plaintiff *prior to serving the lawsuit* on the defendant [1]. Even with that last caveat, very few barriers or deterrents (other than the requisite approximately $300 filing fee) exist to instituting civil litigation in the United States.

Given that it is very easy to file a suit, a more relevant question for clinicians is whether you can be *successfully* sued, that is to say, is the plaintiff likely to obtain a monetary settlement or win a judgment or verdict. Fortunately, although the threshold for filing a suit is quite low, the odds of a plaintiff obtaining a settlement are also low, and the available data supports that odds of a plaintiff obtaining an actual jury verdict or judgment are very low. Although not all liability concerns for mass-gathering medicine are medical malpractice related, that is most likely the area of primary liability concern for clinicians practicing in this realm. There is good data from closed claims databases about medical malpractice claims resolutions, which highlight the previous point. The Medical Professional Liability Association (MPLA) compiles closed claims data from participating members of its professional liability insurer trade organization. This information represents national data, and from 2016 to 2018, 64.7 percent of all closed claims against their insured health care providers were dropped, withdrawn, or dismissed, 24.2 percent were settled, and only 0.7 percent represented plaintiff's verdicts [2]. Unfortunately, there are no databases specifically consisting of claims related to mass-gathering events. These MPLA numbers show that all things being equal, fully two-thirds of all medical malpractice cases go nowhere, and the providers will not experience adverse consequences. Even in the event of a settlement or judgment, the provider's insurer pays the amount owing, and the only real adverse consequences for a provider are if National Practitioner Data Bank or Medical Board reporting is required.

The available MPLA data does specifically identify claims as those made against medical directors, director medical care providers, and/or volunteers, but in all likelihood the claims were for direct medical care, because they implicated the provider's malpractice insurance. As we will discuss below, malpractice claims (successful or otherwise) are much less likely to be brought against volunteer clinicians or against medical directors who are not providing direct patient care.

Medical Malpractice 101

Medical malpractice cases are state civil lawsuits and are governed by the jurisdiction and laws of the particular state in which they are filed. Many important laws peculiar to medical malpractice vary from state to state, for example, statutes of limitations, Good Samaritan laws, expert witness qualifications, damages caps, pre-suit certifications, and limitations on the collateral source rule. However, the four elements required to prove a claim for medical malpractice, which are derived from English common law, are the same in all fifty states: (1) duty, (2) breach of the duty, (3) causation, and (4) damages. The definition of each of these elements is governed by state law, and certain factual scenarios may result in different outcomes depending on the state in which the claim is brought.

In the vast majority of claims and states each of the four elements needs to be established by the plaintiff (i.e., the plaintiff has the "burden of proof") by what is called the "preponderance of the evidence." Preponderance of evidence generally is defined as "more likely than not," or, put another way, if one were to put all the evidence the plaintiff presented on one side of a scale, and the defendant's evidence on the other side, if the scale tipped ever so slightly (e.g., 51 percent) to the plaintiff's side, then the plaintiff would prevail. This burden being on the plaintiff is important, because in theory, a defendant would not have to put on any evidence at all and they would win the case. That said, "preponderance of the evidence" is a relatively low burden of proof when compared to the "beyond a reasonable doubt" required in criminal cases. The higher standard reflects the more severe consequences of a criminal trial (loss of individual liberty) versus a civil trial (loss of money).

Duty

The commonly accepted point at which a provider has a legal duty for which they can be held legally accountable is at the establishment of a doctor-patient relationship [3]. Typically this relationship is established when a patient agrees to be seen by the physician and the physician agrees to care for the patient and commences the encounter (e.g., by asking the patient for a history or beginning the examination). In some states a duty may be found even in the absence of a physician–patient relationship if an alleged injury was simply "foreseeable" [4]. Often times the answer is not clear cut, and a court may leave the question of a doctor–patient relationship up to a jury.

Although defining the commencement of a doctor–patient relationship can be hard depending upon the facts, it is helpful to at least define situations where such a relationship is clear and where it would not be clear. At a mass gathering event a doctor-patient relationship would be clear when the patient is brought to the provider for care and the provider begins to obtain a history either from the patient or the patient's accompanying friends or family if the patient is incapacitated or unable to communicate. However, if the provider at the event is never made aware of a particular patient or their plight, then the provider will not be held to have a duty. Importantly, simply because the provider is either an organizational volunteer or employed clinician for the purpose of being available for care at an event does not mean the provider automatically has an individual duty to everyone at the event. The duty for medical malpractice purposes is individual to the provider, and again, only commences when the provider undertakes care of a particular person.

For an example of commencement of legal duty, consider being an on-site employed health care provider (employed by a company who is contracting with the college) working at a local college's football game. You are in the medical tent and receive a call that someone has fallen and gotten "hurt" in one of the seating sections near to you, and you immediately leave to see the patient. Once you arrive, the patient is awake and not able to communicate clearly, and he appears intoxicated to you. A woman who says she is his girlfriend is also there, and she says he was drinking bourbon both prior to and during the game, and he fell and hit his head on the concrete trying to catch a commemorative t-shirt thrown into the crowd by the cheerleaders. You do a neuro check, which is normal, and you examine an apparent injury to the patient's head. There is a three- to four-inch scalp laceration that is bleeding, but it does not seem to be deep enough to require stitches. You clean out the wound and apply Steri-strips and a bandage. You give instructions to the girlfriend to take him home but to keep an eye on him, and if he starts to bleed more or exhibits seizures, repeated vomiting, convulsions, or is unable to be woken up, that she should call 911 immediately and get him to the hospital. When you get back to your medical tent, you document everything in a patient note.

In this example your legal duty the particular patient as a provider likely commenced at the time you arrived at the patient's side and begin taking a history. That was the moment you exhibited specific intention to care for the young man, and although he was noncommunicative, his consent to your care would likely be implied. Depending upon the specific facts and the jurisdiction should a suit be filed, an argument could be made that the relationship was established at the time you first took the call and took action to go see the injured person, so if you stopped along the way for a cup of coffee, you might be responsible for any harm caused by your delay in getting to the patient. The call-in shows intent to have the patient treated, and your actions evidence your intention to care for the patient, even though you have not yet seen him.

If the facts were slightly altered, such that you were only at the same football game as an attendee sitting next to the young man with the scalp laceration, you would have no legal duty to act in the vast majority of states. You would not have to do anything and would not be liable for any adverse consequences even if you could have done something. Notably, there are three states that do mandate a "duty to act" in such situations, but they are a distinct minority [5]. However, once you do decide to intervene and assist, then you will have assumed a legal duty as a "rescuer." Even though you would be a true volunteer in this instance, once you attempt to undertake to help in a given situation, then you are obligated to act reasonably. If you are a healthcare provider, "reasonably" would be defined as acting within the standard of care. As discussed below, the Good Samaritan statutes would make it less likely you would ultimately face any liability repercussions if a bad outcome occurred, but you would still have a duty to act within the standard of care. Without meeting the prerequisite of a legal duty, no liability claim will be successful against a health care provider for malpractice.

Breach

Once established, the "duty" is to act within the "standard of care." The standard of care in a particular instance can vary state by state (some states say standard of care is defined at the state or local level, others at the national level) as well as case by case. There is no legally accepted or required "standard of care" written in any textbook or journal, or expressed in any classroom or operating room which legally mandates a jury to agree with it. The standard of care in every case is what the jury determines it should be in that particular case based upon the evidence presented. In almost all instances an expert witness will be necessary to explain to the jury what the standard of care is, and there will be expert witnesses on both sides of the case. The jurors are charged with listening to the facts, listening to what the experts on each side say a "reasonable prudent practitioner in the same field of practice or specialty" [6] should have done, and then the jury decides who they want to believe. Experts can show the jury literature, videos, educational materials, and so on, but the jury is not required to adopt the opinions expressed in those materials, no matter how authoritative they may seem. If the jury finds that the standard of care was not followed, then that is a "breach" of the standard of care, which is the second prerequisite for a successful malpractice liability case.

Continuing with the example introduced in the previous "Duty" section, if the patient you saw at the game goes home, suffers a massive brain hemorrhage and dies, and then his family sues you, it is likely they will find an expert to argue that standard of care required that you sent their loved one immediately to a hospital for a head CT. The question would be what a reasonable prudent clinician with your training and experience should do under the same or similar circumstances. The plaintiff would not likely argue that you needed to *ensure* a CT at the event, but they would have an expert who would point to facts in support of the opinion the patient needed to go straight for a CT, for example, the distance the patient fell, the surface he hit, the size of the laceration, any other injuries, slurred speech, and so on. The defense would have

an expert likely counter those points by arguing that the patient did not lose consciousness, that the cut was not deep, and that you left him in the hands of sober friends who knew what to do and were capable of doing it. A jury would ultimately decide who to believe.

The argument over whether a breach occurred is a true battle of the experts, and with no mandated legal authorities, will be determined on a case by case basis, although it is important to remember that the plaintiff has the burden of proof.

Causation

Simply a breach of the standard of care is not relevant unless the plaintiff can also show that the specific breach actually "caused" some harm to the plaintiff. Causation is the third element required to prove a medical malpractice claim, and it is also a battleground for the experts, because of the specialized knowledge required to make a medical link between a breach of the standard of care and a particular health outcome. There is one area of exception and that is when causation is within the realm of understanding of a layperson, for example, "lack of consent" cases (where a physician is alleged to have completely failed to obtain any consent for medical care, as opposed to simply obtaining inadequate informed consent, which requires expert testimony to prove).

Again, the plaintiff will need to establish this causation element by the preponderance of the evidence in order to prevail, so in addition to relying upon their experience, and perhaps outside authorities such as journal articles or texts, the plaintiff's expert will need to cite to specific evidence in the record to support their position. In the continuing example of the person with the head injury at the football game, the plaintiff's expert(s) would need to show that if the patient had gotten to an emergency department promptly, that he would have undergone a CT scan, and that his death would have been prevented. The defense expert will try to rebut those arguments by claiming the "die was already cast" at the time of the fall, and even if the patient had a CT he would still very likely have died. The defense may also make additional arguments, such as the CT would have taken too long to get in order to make any difference. As with the standard of care question the jury will make the determination as to who is correct.

Damages

The final element required for a successful medical malpractice claim is actual damages or harm. The plaintiff must be able to prove that the breach of the standard of care caused a particular harm to the plaintiff. Even if the evidence is overwhelming that the standard of care was violated, but if for any reason harm was avoided, then the plaintiff cannot recover (e.g., a "near miss"). Plaintiffs who claim they are just suing over what "could have happened," will lose. Harm that is purely theoretical or speculative is not going to be recoverable.

In the ongoing example the death of the young man would be the obvious harm, but what does that mean medicolegally and how does the harm translate into money damages? There are usually two types of damages recoverable in a medical malpractice suit, economic and noneconomic. Economic damages are theoretically objectively determinable: past and future medical bills, past and future lost wages and any other items suggested in a life care plan, such as home modifications and special assistance. Noneconomic damages include "pain and suffering" and loss of consortium, which are not defined by any legal guardrail and are up to a jury to determine as it sees fit. In most states damages for wrongful death are limited than if you have to compensate an injured person for a lifetime of medical bills, lost wages and pain and suffering. In a wrongful death case the economic damages would include the medical bills prior to death and the expected wages he would have earned if he had lived (usually proven by experts and actuarial tables). Non-economic damages would depend greatly on the state's laws. In some states the only recovery for wrongful death is lost earnings or lost earning capacity [7], while in others the decedent's survivors are entitled to their loss of companionship [8]. One irony of malpractice cases is that if the patient had not died, but had lived and required significant medical care for the rest of his life, then he would likely be able to recover a higher award at trial due to the significant amount of economic damages he could claim even though death would seem to be the ultimate harm.

Good Samaritan Laws

What are commonly referred to as "Good Samaritan" laws may come into play for a clinician sued as a result of treatment rendered at a mass-gathering event if they provide treatment as (1) a volunteer in (2) an emergency situation. These laws are generally understood as providing immunity from suit to providers who treat an injured person out of the goodness of their hearts, and not due to any employment reason or expectation of compensation or reward. Good Samaritan laws are state-specific and are limited in their application and provide immunity from ordinary negligence or malpractice claims. Good Samaritan laws change liability risk significantly if the prerequisites for application of the law exist.

A recent decision from Virginia lays out the historical evolution of these Good Samaritan statutes and their interpretation: *Stoots* v. *Marion Life Saving Crew, Inc.* [9]. In *Stoots* the plaintiff sued a number of volunteer paramedics and the designated emergency response agency of their local county, MLSC. The Virginia state code (Va. Code Section 8.01–225) provides that anyone rendering emergency care "in good faith" and "without compensation" will be immune from civil suit. The court first noted that under the common law (law that developed by judges over centuries as opposed to statutory law which is developed by legislatures) that most state codes did not create any legal duty on a person to act to help or "rescue" in an emergency. If one did act in an emergency, they were required to act reasonably or with ordinary care. To encourage volunteer rescue efforts, a majority of states passed Good Samaritan statutes to remove fear of liability as a disincentive to render aid in an emergency.

Kentucky's Good Samaritan law lays out the standard requirements most states have for application of these protections.

Nonliability of Licensees and Certified Technicians for Emergency Care

(1) *No physician* licensed under Kentucky Revised Statutes (KRS) Chapter 311, registered or practical nurse licensed under KRS Chapter 314, person certified as an emergency medical technician by the Kentucky Cabinet for Health and Family Services, person certified by the American Heart Association or the American Red Cross to perform cardiopulmonary resuscitation, or employee of any board of education established pursuant to the provision of KRS 160.160, who has completed a course in first aid and who maintains current certification therein in accordance with the standards set forth by the

American Red Cross *shall be liable in civil damages for administering emergency care* or treatment at the scene of an emergency outside of a hospital, doctor's office, or other place having proper medical equipment excluding house calls, for acts performed at the scene of such emergency, *unless such acts constitute willful or wanton misconduct.*

(2) Nothing in this section applies to the administering of such care or treatment where the same is rendered for remuneration or with the expectation of remuneration. KRS 411.148. *(Emphasis added)*

Virginia's law couches the liability hurdle to be proving the defendant did not act in "good faith," which the courts have interpreted to mean "bad intent or dishonest motives," which is essentially the "willful and wanton conduct" seen in Kentucky's and other state statutes.

A. Any person who:

1. In *good faith*, renders emergency care or assistance, *without compensation*, to any ill or injured person (i) at the scene of an accident, fire, or any life-threatening emergency; (ii) at a location for screening or stabilization of an emergency medical condition arising from an accident, fire, or any life-threatening emergency; or (iii) en route to any hospital, medical clinic, or doctor's office, shall not be liable for any civil damages for acts or omissions resulting from the rendering of such care or assistance.

Va. Code Section 8.01–225(A)(1). (Emphasis added)

The first point to note about Good Samaritan laws is that they do not prevent a provider from being sued, rather they make it harder for a plaintiff to prevail in a claim for medical malpractice. In most states for a Good Samaritan law to apply the situation must be an "emergency," that is to say, the patient must be at risk of imminent harm or death. Also, the provider must be voluntarily providing their services for free, not as a result of employment or with expectation of compensation or a reward of any kind. Most importantly, the plaintiff will have to prove that the provider was not only negligent, but that the provider was "grossly negligent," or not acting in "good faith," or intentionally or recklessly (i.e., "willfully and wantonly") injured the plaintiff. The specific bar is set state by state and would be fleshed out in court decisions. This higher bar is a significant deterrent to bringing a claim against a Good Samaritan.

Whether an action or inaction is deemed "gross negligence" or "willful and wanton" will be a decision left up to the jury in a medical malpractice case. The guidance for what is ordinary negligence would be a "breach of the standard of care" by the health care provider. To be grossly negligent, there must not only be a breach of the standard of care, the plaintiff must also establish that the breach was so outside the bounds of reasonable care as to be considered reckless. Common examples of gross negligence include providing medical assistance while knowingly intoxicated or acting well beyond the scope of medical training and experience. As with ordinary negligence cases an injury must occur as a result of the alleged grossly negligent conduct for a suit to be successful.

It should also be noted that there are certain states which have what are referred to as "duty to act" laws, which require individuals (not just medically trained persons) to assist in an emergency or face a criminal penalty:

Duty to assist.
A person at the scene of an emergency who knows that another person is exposed to or has suffered grave physical harm shall, to the extent that the person can do so without danger or peril to self or others, give reasonable assistance to the exposed person.
MINN.STAT.ANN. 604A.01

These laws provide the same immunities from claims of general negligence, but again do not protect individuals or health care providers from findings of gross negligence or injury due to reckless action or inaction.

Some examples where Good Samaritan protections are likely to apply: You are a volunteer assistant coach on your daughter's field hockey team and one of the players suffers a laceration on her leg after a hard collision with another player. You go on the field to help to assess her laceration, which is bleeding badly, and you bandage her up. Later she develops a bad infection in her leg which results in reduced function and tissue loss. The appearance of her leg is permanently altered, and she is embarrassed about how she looks in addition to the loss of functionality. Absent evidence of gross negligence with your attention to her wound, you would be immune from suit under the Good Samaritan statute. A fact that might change the outcome would be if there had been visible dirt in the wound and you bandaged it up without attempting to clean it out, because this would demonstrate a knowing disregard of a danger to the patient, and could be interpreted as "reckless."

Another example would be if you are a physician attending a rock concert simply as a regular concert-goer and find yourself next to a person who appears to be choking and you can't get them up to do a Heimlich maneuver. They are on the ground and you determine that they need an emergency tracheostomy. You quickly pull out your pocket knife and perform the tracheostomy correctly, and the person survives but suffers permanent damage to their vocal cords. You are sued with the claim that a tracheostomy was unnecessary and that you should have put more effort in attempting a Heimlich maneuver, which they allege would have "more likely than not" eliminated the obstruction without any resultant harm. Although you may not have made the "best" decision and be possibly negligent, your decision was not entirely unreasonable, and so you likely would be protected from a negligence claims by the Good Samaritan statute. If instead you had chosen an obviously dirty knife, when with little effort you could have procured a clean one, or had spit on it to "clean" it prior to performing the tracheostomy and the patient developed a serious infection, then you might be considered grossly negligent or reckless, because you intentionally chose an unsafe option.

One final and practical deterrent to lawsuits against Good Samaritans is that the plaintiff is also asking the jury to essentially punish a health care provider who stepped in to help during an emergency. It is possible that jurors may perceive this as a "cheap shot" by the plaintiff to attempt to get money from someone who obviously had good intentions, and make it nearly impossible for the plaintiff to prevail. Also, jurors may put themselves in the shoes of the plaintiff and think that if they were ever in a similar predicament, they would hope someone would come help. Jurors might also be concerned that allowing a plaintiff to win a lawsuit against a volunteer would deter future volunteers and be unsafe for not only themselves, but society in general. There is no available data to support this theory, but it is a consideration a plaintiff's lawyer has to take into consideration when deciding whether even to take on a particular case against a Good Samaritan, and no doubt is a disincentive for them to do so.

In summary, Good Samaritan laws reduce the risk of liability in very limited circumstances thus making it safer for a provider to choose to volunteer and provide medical assistance in an emergency. The most significant change is in the degree of negligence or recklessness that the plaintiff has to prove in order to prevail. Although they do not alter the requirements of establishing duty/breach/causation/damages, or the "preponderance of the evidence" burden of proof, they typically require the plaintiff to establish that the provider was not only negligent, but "grossly" negligent or acted willfully (intentionally tried to harm the plaintiff) or wantonly (recklessly).

Health Care Decision-Making

The need to obtain consent from persons prior to treatment is not obviated by the fact that a clinician is a volunteer or a Good Samaritan, or because the patient is an attendee at a mass gathering. Care rendered without consent is considered a legal "battery" and can be the basis for a lawsuit against the individual care provider. Assuming the patient is capable of making health care decisions (e.g., is not a minor or incapacitated), they have a right to consent prior to any medical interventions upon their person.

There are two standards for obtaining informed consent in the United States depending upon the state in which the alleged negligence occurs. About half the states follow a "subjective" standard and the other half follow the "objective" standard. The "subjective" standard requires the health care provider to inform the patient of the risks, benefits, and alternatives to the medical intervention that a "reasonable person in the same or similar circumstances as the particular patient" would want to know. The "objective" standard requires the health care provider to inform the patient of the risks, benefits, and alternatives to the medical intervention that a "reasonable health care provider [physician/nurse]" would inform a patient under the same or similar circumstances. The subjective standard is patient-centric, requiring the fact finder to get into the head of the patient, whereas the objective standard is provider-centric and asks the fact finder to not just look at the particular patient or provider, but what a "reasonable" provider would do. As providers attending mass-gathering events it is not so important to know which standard the state you are in follows, because often the information will be the same, but do realize that you do need to obtain consent before undertaking any medical intervention, just as if the patient were in your office or at the hospital.

One important exception to the consent doctrine is known as the "emergency exception," which allows a provider some flexibility in the event the patient is not capable of consent, no surrogate is reasonably available, and immediate care or treatment is needed to prevent serious injury or death. Given that providers at mass-gathering events will often be managing emergency situations, this exception may come into play. Generally, it is advisable to try to get consent from a surrogate if readily available (e.g., spouse, or parent if the patient is a minor), but if any delay will cause harm to the patient this exception allows providers to act without delay. In order to protect themselves from potential litigation claiming lack of, or inadequate, informed consent, providers should be sure to document why an emergency existed and any other circumstances precluding them from obtaining patient or surrogate consent.

Bringing consent into our examples, the choking patient who needed the tracheostomy would presumably be unable to consent, and the provider could proceed under the emergency exception. The fact that harm to the patient was imminent without action would justify moving forward without consent. If, however, the patient was able to communicate, any medical intervention such as stitches, medications, or transportation to a medical facility would require patient consent. To protect yourself, you would want to document that the patient was advised of the risks, benefits, and alternatives of the proposed intervention and elected to proceed in order to protect yourself.

A final area of concern when it comes to consent issues is when a patient refuses the care you recommend. This is called an "informed refusal." If, for example, you were examining a patient at a football game who had recently taken a hard fall and hit his head, and you recommended that the patient be taken to the closest emergency department for evaluation, and the patient refused to go, then what should you do? You cannot force a patient to go in these circumstances, so if he has friends or family with him, you could talk to them to help you persuade the patient to go to the hospital. Sometimes, however, that may not work in which case you need to protect yourself, and the recommended practice Is to document that you advised the patient of his diagnoses and the risks, benefits, and alternatives of your recommendation, but that the patient specifically refused. You do not need to obtain a signature of the patient, but you do need to document the refusal in order to protect yourself.

Licensure

It can be surprising for physicians to learn that their state medical licenses only provide them with legal authority to practice medicine in that one state. Medical school curricula and training have been similar across the nation for decades now, but licensure is still governed state by state under the jurisdiction of state medical boards [10]. Each state also has a law requiring anyone who practices their particular health care profession in that state, be it medicine, nursing, and so on, to have a license issued by their state board [11]. Failure to comply with this requirement is a felony [12]. The key question then is whether what the health care professional is doing constitutes the "practice of medicine" within that particular state.

There is no federally applicable definition of the "practice of medicine" so each state has crafted its own definitions with general agreement on the base definition, but with predictable variability when it comes to the details. Some states do not require an out of state provider to be licensed if all they are doing is providing a consultation across state lines. Other states agree, but only if the consultations are infrequent. Some states allow limited licenses for telehealth encounters (a consequence of the COVID-19 pandemic), but also limit the care to telehealth services [13]. Federal law, the "Sports Medicine Licensure Clarity Act" [14] allows providers practicing within the scope of their specialty to travel and practice medicine in states where they are not licensed with college and professional sports teams. The same act also requires their malpractice insurance to cover them. There are no uniform exceptions to clinicians who travel for other large public events, for example, rock concerts or political rallies. In those instances providers will need to check with the state medical board for the states in which they can envision being asked to provide care in order to determine whether they need to be licensed.

How do Good Samaritan and licensure laws interact? If you happen to undertake a Good Samaritan activity in a state in which you are not licensed, you should not face any civil or administrative liability. Many state laws contain exceptions to their licensure laws for emergency care provided for free [15].

There are also insurance considerations for licensure. Most medical malpractice policies have an exclusion to their obligation for coverage if you were required to be licensed when performing clinical care but you are in fact unlicensed. This is further reason to sort out licensure requirements before you undertake clinical care at a mass-gathering event occurring outside the state of your licensure, so you are not in a position of facing a felony charge (which not only includes potential fines and jail time, but is expensive to defend and can impact your ability to stay licensed in other states) or being denied coverage for a malpractice case by your professional liability insurer.

Health Information Portability and Accountability Act

Although they are not medical malpractice cases, Health Information Portability and Accountability Act (HIPAA) violations can result in significant fines and sanctions for providers and their employers. State and federal (HIPAA) privacy laws apply to the relationships any health care provider has with someone they care for at any type of mass-gathering event, just as if they were treating the patient in their office or at the hospital. HIPAA sets the floor for what is protected personal health information (PHI), which can only be disclosed by a health care provider with the patient's authorization unless an exception applies [16]. States can make their own privacy laws stricter than HIPAA and if there is a conflict between the two, the more strict of the privacy laws will apply [17]. Violations of HIPAA result in fines and potential disciplinary actions [18]. HIPAA does not allow a private right of action for suit, but state privacy laws may. Regardless, you want to be sure you do not share PHI about a patient with a third party unless you are confident an exception applies.

The most common exception to the authorization requirement likely to be implicated when providing care at a mass gathering is for persons "involved" in the patient's care [19]. For example, if a young man comes to a medical services tent in the company of a friend, and he is intoxicated and has a facial laceration from a fall, you may talk to the friend about his condition unless he objects or gives you reason to believe he would object. You are entitled to rely upon your professional judgment in these instances. If, however, the young man shows up alone for treatment and then leaves, and a friend shows up later asking about him, you cannot disclose information without his authorization unless you have a reasonable basis to believe the friend is involved in his care. The same risk management strategy applies here as for the

situations described earlier: document your interaction and make a note as to why you felt it was appropriate to talk to the friend. Regardless, always remember that whether you are seeing the patient as a volunteer, as an employee of an organization, or even as the patient's personal physician, HIPAA will still apply.

Administrative Liability: Medical Director

The role of Operational Medical Directors (OMDs) for a mass gathering brings up unique liability concerns. First there is traditional medical malpractice liability as discussed above for instances where an OMD is directly involved in caring for a patient or perhaps is consulted by an EMS provider for treatment advice which is then relied upon to the patient's detriment. The additional area of liability concern for an OMD is for alleged negligence (or violations of law) in the OMD's administrative responsibilities. For example, a patient injury or number of patient injuries at a mass-gathering event could lead to claims against the OMD for poor or unsafe systems, or for poor hiring, credentialing, or supervising of the emergency services personnel. The analysis and risks of these claims are very different.

For direct claims of negligence the first question for an OMD is whether they are working as a paid employee or contractor, or they are working without compensation, that is, a volunteer, because the liability risks are different. For an employed or compensated OMD, their direct patient care liability would be analyzed as described above for a traditional medical malpractice claim. If, however, the OMD is uncompensated, then depending upon the state they are in, they may be immune from lawsuits or liability as long as they act in "good faith" and are not "grossly negligent" or engaging in "willful misconduct," as described in the following statutory example from Virginia:

> B. Any licensed physician serving without compensation as the operational medical director for an emergency medical services agency that holds a valid license as an emergency medical services agency issued by the Commissioner of Health shall not be liable for any civil damages for any act or omission resulting from the rendering of emergency medical services in good faith by the personnel of such licensed agency unless such act or omission was the result of such physician's gross negligence or willful misconduct.
>
> *Virginia Code Section 8.01–225(B).* [20]

The above statute clearly protects OMDs from traditional medical malpractice claims, and arguably would protect them from civil claims for administrative failings as well. However, if the OMD was fined or administratively sanctioned, this statute would not provide protection, because it only applies to "civil damages," which are money damages awarded in personal injury suits – not governmental fines or penalties.

Another area of concern for liability of OMDs is whether they can be held vicariously liable for the actions of the emergency services workers (EMTs) under their supervision. In other words, can the OMD be liable as if they were acting as the EMT and causing the alleged harm, simply due to the fact that the EMT works under the OMD? In most instances this is not likely to be the case, because the OMD him or herself does not actually employ the EMT. Under traditional vicarious liability analysis, it is the entity which employs an individual that can become vicariously liable for the individual's actions. So, while the company who pays the EMT could be sued and held vicariously liable, the OMD could not. Note that this is distinguishable from a claim of "supervisory negligence," where the allegations would be that it was the failure to supervise the EMT that caused the harm.

Due to the OMD's role in supervising EMTs there is liability risk of a claim for negligent supervision, that is, the OMD knew of deficiencies with the processes or with individual emergency care providers yet did nothing to address those deficiencies and someone or some group of persons were injured. Such claims are not cognizable in all jurisdictions in the United States, but in states allowing such claims, if there is a bad outcome as a result of EMT care, it is fair to assume a jury could find that the OMD with their superior knowledge, training, and responsibilities should have foreseen the potential harm and was in a position to do something about it. The plaintiff, however, will also have to establish a causal link between the OMD's alleged poor supervision and the specific harm suffered.

In addition to any common law duties with respect to any direct patient care provided by the OMD, the administrative legal obligations of OMDs are often formalized in state codes or regulation [21]. Generally, the obligations include: (1) establishing protocols, policies, and procedures; (2) verifying that the qualifications and credentials for EMS personnel meet state law requirements; (3) overseeing the performance of EMS personnel; (4) responsibility for a quality management program; and (5) interacting with governmental authorities and agencies to ensure protocols and policies are in line with state and local laws. OMDs could be sued for failure to adequately perform any of these obligations, but again, to succeed with such a claim for personal injury, a plaintiff would have to establish a causal link between the failure to comply with statutory obligations and the plaintiff's injuries, which would likely be very difficult to do.

The previous example of the young man with the choking incident at a football game is useful to identifying the liability risks of a nonvolunteer OMD. If the OMD is not the one directly providing care to the young man, but rather it is an EMT under the OMD's supervision, the OMD would not be directly liable to the young man, because the OMD does not have a physician–patient relationship with him and therefore no legal "duty" to the young man. If, however, the EMT had called the OMD for treatment advice, and the OMD had provided the advice, then the OMD would likely be held to have an "implied duty" to the patient and potential liability if the advice was relied upon to the alleged detriment of the patient. The OMD would also not be vicariously liable for the actions of the EMT if the EMT performed her duties, because the OMD does not personally employ the EMT (the company who does, however, would have vicarious liability). The OMD's responsibilities regarding credentialing and developing a plan for the event could theoretically be a source of liability, but a plaintiff would have to tie an alleged failure in that regard to an actual injury, and the state where the injury occurred would have to recognize "negligent credentialing" as a valid claim (many states do not recognize this cause of action) [22]. In other words, the plaintiff would have to establish that (1) the OMD should not have credentialed the particular EMT, and (2) that had that particular EMT not been present, the injury to the patient would not have occurred. If an OMD's event plan was alleged to be deficient, again, the plaintiff would have to prove that the alleged deficiencies caused the plaintiff's harm, which would be a high bar. Finally, in the event any type of negligence claim was made against an OMD for the personal injury, it would likely be made against the OMD in their capacity as an employee of whatever entity was responsible for the event, and the plaintiff would look to that organization, as opposed to the OMD independently, for recovery, because the organization is much more likely to have "deeper pockets," that is, greater insurance coverage and assets.

Insurance coverage for OMD's personal liability is not always clear, and OMDs should seek assurances of coverage prior to undertaking OMD responsibilities. Professional liability insurance policies that OMDs have for medical malpractice claims may only cover claims arising out of direct patient care, whereas liability and lawsuits against OMDs will likely be for negligent administrative decision-making, such as poorly designed policies or poor hiring choices/credentialing. In addition to the traditional professional liability insurance discussed in the next section, OMDs, because of their unique role, should inquire whether their policies cover potential liabilities for administrative failings or compliance issues. If not, they should seek coverage for a medical director policy in order to protect themselves from such claims. Even though such claims may be rare, or difficult for a plaintiff to win – especially in a volunteer case – the insurance policy will cover attorney's fees, costs, and other legal expenses that are incurred even in frivolous lawsuits or suits were the OMD is likely to prevail.

Professional Liability Insurance

Perhaps the most fundamental question to ask yourself before undertaking a role as a health care provider, as a medical director, or even as a volunteer, is, "do I have malpractice insurance coverage for this in case something goes wrong?" The best time to ask this question, of course, is *prior* to undertaking the activity. Whether you are covered and what coverage you have will depend upon the capacity in which you are acting as well as the type of malpractice coverage you do have, either claims-made or occurrence.

It is important to first note that medical malpractice insurance coverage (also known as professional liability coverage) typically only covers you for claims for alleged negligence (i.e., medical malpractice) brought against you as a result of clinical or patient care that you provide. This coverage does not typically provide protection to you for injuries resulting from intentional acts, for claims that you defamed or slandered someone, for employment claims (e.g., harassment of a co-employee), or for sexual assault claims against patients. Professional liability coverage also may or may not provide protections for actions taken as a medical director, such as developing

policies and procedures, and for administrative functions. It will depend on the specific wording of your policy.

If you are at the mass-gathering event to provide clinical services as a result of your employment, then in all likelihood the professional liability coverage you already have through your employer will cover you for any claims arising out of that event. Usually your employer will have a contractual arrangement with the entity putting on the event, whereby your employer agrees to provide medical services. The contract will also specify who is responsible for providing professional liability coverage for the clinical care, which in most instances will be your employer. In that instance you will have the same coverage you have when conducting any other sort of clinical activity for your employer. If the other party assumes responsibility for your malpractice coverage, ideally the contract will require them to list you and your employer as additional insureds under their policy. This will protect you in the event the other party's insurer attempted to decline coverage to you at a later point.

If you are engaging in the clinical activity as a paid-for moonlighting activity or as a volunteer, the coverage you have through your regular employer will not likely apply. That said it is always worth first checking with your employer or the carrier directly to see if the activity you are about to engage in will be covered. Getting verification of coverage in writing is best. If they will not cover you, then you will need to explore obtaining coverage from the entity for which you are providing the service. If they are a nonprofit or not otherwise well-funded it is not likely they will purchase coverage for you, and you will need to see a malpractice insurance broker yourself, or ask the carrier who covers you at work if you can purchase additional coverage through them at your own cost. For volunteer work, you should take the same steps, although it is more likely that your employer's insurer will cover you absent the activity being particularly high-risk or outside the scope of your professional competency or specialty.

If you choose to go without verification of malpractice coverage, then you are personally taking on a significant financial risk. This is true even if you are undertaking the work as a volunteer and are confident about getting the protections of the Good Samaritan laws. The reason is the cost of litigation. Even if you are facing what turns out to be a fully frivolous lawsuit, you will still have to defend that suit in court, which will mean hiring an attorney and paying ancillary expenses (attorney travel costs, possibly deposition fees, and possibly expert witness fees), which are not recoverable even if you win or are dismissed from the lawsuit. Most malpractice insurance covers all these costs. To get an idea of the extent of the expense, MPLA data from 2016 to 2018 demonstrate that the average cost a professional liability insurer in the United States spent to defend a case that was dropped, withdrawn, or dismissed, was roughly $28,000 per claim [23]. Without insurance, the provider will personally bear those costs.

If you end up purchasing coverage on your own, it is critical that you understand whether you are purchasing claims-made or occurrence coverage, because you will also be responsible for tail coverage if it is a claims-made policy. The distinction between the two coverages is that for a claims-made policy to apply, both the event that led to the claim and the claim itself must occur within the policy period. If the claim itself is not made until after the policy period then you will not be covered unless you have purchased tail coverage. Occurrence coverage provides protection even if the claim is made after the policy period – and no extra tail needs to be purchased. Occurrence coverage typically costs more than claims-made initially, but when you factor in the cost of tail coverage, the costs tend to even out. Unfortunately, occurrence coverage is getting harder to obtain in the commercial market, and in all likelihood you will only have various claims-made options.

To best protect yourself always look into whether you will have medical malpractice coverage for the particular service you are going to provide at a mass-gathering event. Even if you do not intend to work at such an event it is always worthwhile learning what protection you have from your current coverage for volunteer activities. That will give you peace of mind whenever you feel compelled to assist in a medical emergency outside of your usual job.

Conclusion

Lawsuits for medical negligence and personal injury are an unfortunate "cost of doing business" in the health care profession. Participation as a clinician at a mass gathering event, whether as an independently paid clinician, as an employee of a medical group, as an operational medical director, or as simply a volunteer all create liability risks. Liability risks decrease the

further the provider is removed from direct care of the patient, and in certain situations (e.g., volunteer Good Samaritan, Operational Medical Director) the risks of individual liability are quite low or may be obviated by statutory immunities. That fact notwithstanding it is incumbent upon providers to act reasonably and to be sure to comply with standard risk management practices such as thorough, contemporaneous documentation, obtaining consent when reasonable, and respecting patient privacy as required by HIPAA. Finally, since exercising all reasonable risk management efforts cannot always prevent a lawsuit, liability insurance protection is critical, to cover providers both from lawsuits over direct care and lawsuits over administrative decision-making. Even with a spurious case there are significant legal costs and expenses.

References

1. Va. Code §8.01–20.1.

2. *Data Sharing Project, MPL Closed Claims 2016–2018 Snapshot.*

3. Lyons v. Greither, 239 S.E.2d 103 (Va. 1977).

4. Warren v. Dinter, 926 N.W.2d 370 (Minn. 2019).

5. MINN.STAT.ANN. 604A.01, Rhode Island Chapter 11–56–1, 18 VSA § 4254 (Vermont).

6. Va. Code §8.01–581.20.

7. W.L. Harper Company v. Slusher, 469 S.W.2d 955 (Ky. 1971).

8. Va. Code §8.01–52.

9. W.L. Harper Company v. Slusher, 469 S.W.2d 955 (Ky. 1971).

10. Va. Code §8.01–52.

11. Referring to "medical" boards includes all health care professional boards within a state, e.g., medicine, nursing, and psychology.

12. Va. Code §54.1–2902.

13. WV Code §30–3–13.

14. E.g., wvbom.wv.gov/ InterstateTelehealthRegistration.asp# (accessed April 10, 2022).

15. 15 U.S.C. §8601.

16. WV Code §55–7–15; See Also, Stewart P. H. et al., What Does the Law Say to Good Samaritans?, *CHEST*. 2013;**143**(6):1774–1783.

17. 45 C.F.R. 164.502.

18. 45 C.F.R. 160 Subpart B.

19. 45 C.F.R. §160.404.

20. 45 C.F.R. 164.510(b).

21. See also, Nev. Rev. Stat. Ann. 4.507, N.Y. Public Health Law, Chapter 45, Article 30, §3013 (5).

22. 12VAC5-31–1890.

23. Twenty-eight states recognize "negligent credentialing" in some form as a cause of action, *Rieder* v. *Segal*, 952 N.W.2d 423 (Iowa 2020).

24. *Data Sharing Project, MPL Closed Claims 2016–2018 Snapshot.*

Business Considerations in Mass Gathering Medicine

Andrew Matthews, L. Scott Nichols, and Kevin M. Ryan

Introduction

Special events with more than 10,000 attendees were estimated to number over 24,000 in the United States annually with direct in-event revenues near $40 billion [1]. Medical directors of Emergency Medical Services (EMS) systems are likely to encounter special events and should understand the business considerations of not only the EMS system, but also the considerations that weigh on the minds of local officials, the tourism industry, and event promoters.

Special events for a community can contribute to the local economy through tourism, direct and indirect jobs, and in one study can be viewed favorably by local businesses [2, 3]. Increasing the profile of the city or town can lead to increased tourism, regional/national recognition of the locality, and positive association of the event with the community. Each one of these can prompt further revenue and jobs for residents of the area. As promoters engage with local officials for a planned event, medical directors must also engage early in the planning and preparation phases while understanding the unique interests of each stakeholder, potential revenue streams, and incurred costs for the system. Guiding promoters regarding areas of potential risk and liabilities, as well as medical considerations, will be paramount to ensure a successful event, for a blemish on any one aspect of the event can leave the perception of a poorly planned event.

Having a basic understanding of key business terms will help prepare the medical director to meet with stakeholders and promoters while formulating the anticipated budget based on the event specifics. Though an in-depth review of accounting, finance, and economics is beyond the scope of this chapter, understanding the various costs will prepare the medical director to clearly present a budget for the department. Some of the more common terms used include [4, 5]:

- Fixed costs: costs that do not change with increasing volume or production and can include things such as salary, insurance, and rent, among others.
- Variable costs: costs that change with a change in volume/production and include things such as fuel and medical supplies and will increase with each additional utilization.
- Direct costs: costs that can be specifically linked to a particular service and include things such as labor for the event and materials used for the event.
- Indirect costs: costs that are not easily assignable to a specific product or service and can include things such as support functions and medical direction.
- Shared costs: that portion of event costs not borne by the funding agency.
- Total cost: the sum of direct costs, indirect costs, and shared costs for a particular product or service.
- Marginal cost: the cost to produce one additional unit of a product or service.
- Sunk cost: a cost that cannot be recovered; sunk costs should not factor into decision-making from a business perspective.

In addition to having a better financial comprehension of the current event, measuring the different costs will also give medical directors a better financial understanding planning for future mass gathering events.

Event Promoters and Sponsorship Considerations

In the initial stages of an event proposal, knowing who the promoters are can provide important insight and guide initial meetings between the promoter and EMS medical director. Once the promoter is known, the medical director can learn more about the promoter and determine if they are reliable and have the necessary experience to organize the event or will require additional assistance from the medical director preparing the medical plan. A poorly organized event not only reflects negatively on the event, but also on the community hosting the event and the medical team supporting the event. If possible, ask the promoter for references for past events and reach out to these individuals regarding their experiences working with the promoter, from planning and preparation phases through to conclusion of the event. In addition, determine whether this is an established professional promoter with a history of planning and executing large-scale events or a smaller-scale promoter, potentially new to carrying out special events, or a nonprofit organization. Knowing the type of promoter will help guide decision-making for the medical director as each group will bring different levels of experience planning the medical component for an event, funding the event, and potentially supplying their own medical equipment and staff.

In addition, many events will have sponsorship to support the financing of the event and add to the experience for attendees. Properly vetting the event's sponsors will help identify potential conflicts as well as provide insight into the likely demographics of attendees, expected size of the event, medical resources anticipated, and the presence of liquor and food vendors. Anticipating the types of calls and potential volume based on sponsorship will influence discussions between event promoters and the medical director regarding medical needs and the associated budget to safely manage and mitigate the impact of the event on local area hospitals and resources.

Frequency of the event is another consideration to determine when working with event promoters. Do the promoters envision a repeating event or a onetime event? Promoters seeking repeat events will want to build partnerships with the community and will be open to negotiations with city officials regarding the medical needs for the event. Organizers of repeat events are likely to engage in negotiations with subsequently smaller profit margins as they are interested in a long-term investment with the event and will be open to resources identified as critical by the EMS medical director. On the other hand, a one-off event may see organizers interested in trying to maximize profit margins for the event and decreased flexibility

regarding negotiations with officials and EMS. Regardless of the promoter, size or the frequency of the event, organizers will be interested in securing a profit margin. Though the range of anticipated profit margins for the event organizers will vary anywhere from 10 percent to 30 percent, some factors affecting which end of the spectrum will be influenced by the various factors including frequency of the event and the promoter. As medical director, understanding that organizers are hoping to make a profit will help the medical director understand the promoter's rationale for cost structure, including the medical component, and guide your responses during a potential negotiation regarding medical assets needed to safely care for attendees.

Planning Stage Considerations

Once the promoters obtain local approval for the event, EMS and the medical director must remain engaged throughout the planning stages to ensure a safe event. Though this chapter will not review key considerations for medical planning, considerations for the department during this stage include if their time planning for the event will be sufficient to safely manage it and whether their time will be reimbursed. The invisible workload of meetings to organize an event is real and compensation for attending meetings can be considered. Identifying the key personnel necessary to attend meetings, meeting preparation, the anticipated number of hours each will be present, and maintaining a consistent log of hours with time specifically dedicated to the event will be important for reimbursement purposes. Even if the department does not bill for specific personnel's time planning for the event, ensuring continued access and engagement to key local personnel will be paramount to ensure a safe and successful event. The medical director should also determine early in this phase if they will be the sole provider of medical care at the event or if the organizers will use a contracted party to provide medical care. If the organizers utilize their own medical assets, the extent of local EMS needs required at the event may be smaller; however, the medical director and EMS must remain engaged, providing key insights into local resources and assist with mitigation efforts.

The medical director should also ensure the correct stakeholders are present throughout the planning phases including EMS, public safety, fire marshal, and local healthcare resources among others. Though not part of the scope of this chapter, insurance considerations for the event will be important to review as well as who retains control for stopping an event if deemed unsafe or unable to meet the agreed upon terms established by public safety departments and medical directors. Finally, another item to consider for mitigation is how potential negative publicity such as illicit drug use, injuries sustained during the event, the event being a "super spreader" incident such as during a pandemic, or even event cancellation, might impact the city or town, EMS, tourism, and future events [6]. Such a tragedy occurred on November 5, 2021, when 50,000 people attended a sold-out Astroworld Festival at NRG Park in Houston, Texas. As soon as rapper Travis Scott began the concert, all 50,000 people began to push and surge toward the front of the stage causing the people in the front to be compressed. Within minutes, people began to pass out from asphyxiation. In the end, over 300 people were treated at the field hospital and 8 died in what has been determined to be one of the deadliest live music events in US history.

Medical Component Cost Considerations

Once the risk profile for the event is established and medical needs are known or anticipated based on a thorough medical and security risk assessment, the medical director and the EMS system must begin drafting the cost for providing care and ensuring preparedness for the event. The medical director should have a rough understanding of how many personnel will be needed for various sized events, the level of certification needed to support the event, and anticipated hours of coverage. Given regional variations in hourly rates, the medical director should develop a document of their local hourly rates for various personnel including Emergency Medical Technician-Basic (EMT-B), Advanced Emergency Medical Technician (AEMT), Emergency Medical Technician-Paramedic (EMT-P), physician coverage, advanced practice providers as well as support personnel and determine the number of personnel from each category given the risk profile of the event. After outlining the anticipated medical supplies needed and personnel costs, the medical director can utilize this information to better inform contract negotiations regarding how the event organizers may be billed for

Table 27.1 Cost calculation for EMS to staff the event

	Local Hourly Rate (LR)	Number of Hours	Total
Administrative			
Special Event Coordinator	$LR	X	
Patient Tracking	$LR	X	
Finance	$LR	X	
Incident Commander/ Chief	$LR	X	
Physician/PA/ NP	$LR	X	
Special Operations Support Personnel	$LR	X	
Supervisor	$LR	X	
Other	$LR	X	
Medical			
Med Station Team (Paramedic/ EMT)	$LR(medic) + $LR (EMT)	X	
ALS Ambulance (2 Paramedics)	$LR * 2	X	
BLS Ambulance (2 EMT)	$LR * 2	X	
Bicycle Team with Defib (2 EMT)	$LR * 2	X	
Proceed Out Team (ALS vs BLS)	$LR * 2	X	
Medical Equipment*	**Local Rate**	**Number Utilized**	**Total**
Bandages			
Slings			
IV Fluids			
Medications			
Total:			$

*If reimbursed post event

payroll costs, medical supplies, and overhead for staffing the event. A starting point for calculating costs for EMS are noted in Table 27.1 and will vary based on event characteristics, local resources, geographical variation in the EMS systems such as basic life support (BLS) versus advanced life support (ALS), and whether the use of medical equipment will be reimbursed by the event organizers. Variable costs such as fuel for the various vehicles are not included in the table but are another consideration in a wide area event or for transport. Though not an all-encompassing list of potential costs, this table will serve as a starting point for initial discussions internally at your organization regarding budgets for special events and developing contracts with promoters.

Additional costs for the medical plan may include mobile resources if the event is geographically spread out or transport times to local hospitals prolonged. Costs for staffing additional ambulances, all-terrain vehicles, bicycles, and boats among others will be considerations from the medical director's standpoint. However, in general, the only costs that should be billed to patients should be those that are incurred once the patient is transported from the event to an Emergency Department or other definitive care location. After the transport, the EMS system can direct bill the patient's insurance or if uninsured, may directly bill the patient. Though municipal EMS systems are unlikely to operate with profit margins in mind for special events, the medical director's involvement in drafting the needs for the event as well as the costs for various personnel and resources required will be important when engaging in negotiations with event organizers.

Another consideration regarding medical planning with established promoters is if they will retain their own medical director or consultant that assists with medical preparation. If the promoter/organizer works with their own medical director, meeting with the individual will be important to understand their experience, knowledge of local resources, and the director's role for the event. It is imperative to ascertain where they are licensed to work and if they are licensed in your jurisdiction and if they are operating as an advisor for the event or as a healthcare provider. If they are functioning in an advisor role, you can speak the same language regarding resource typing, potential risks for the event, and your rationale for the proposed medical component for the event and work together to ensure a safe and successful event. Typically, event planners hire medical providers to assume the liability of providing medical care. Make sure that the scope of medical care you will be providing at the event is clearly stated and is covered by your insurance policy as well as ensuring the contract does not extend past your scope of care. A good rule of thumb is to review your insurance policy to see what types of medical care the underwriter *doesn't* cover before making this determination. Finally, it's important that all signed contractual agreements be properly vetted with your legal department.

Summary

Medical directors must have familiarity with various costs and discussing medical needs with promoters as special events occur frequently throughout the United States and are a source of revenue for the host community. Though costs for the medical component will vary depending on the region in the United States, it is important to understand your hourly costs for personnel as well as variable costs. Though municipal systems will likely not operate with profit margins in mind, event organizers will be cognizant of profit margins to varying degrees depending on the size of the promoter as well as frequency of the event. Profit margins may frame their discussions regarding medical assets at the event as they seek to limit certain costs. As medical director, understanding their incentives will help guide discussions while ensuring a safe event as any one blemish can result in the perception of the event being skewed.

References

1. Skolnik J., Stern D., Chami R., Lane A., Kulesza C., Walker M. (2008). Planned Special Events: Cost Management and Cost Recovery Primer. Washington DC: US Department of Transportation; 2009. 75. Report No.: FHWA-HOP-09–028. www.hsdl.org/? view&did=35642

2. Irshad H. Impact of Community Events and Festivals on Rural Places [Internet]. Alberta: Rural Development Division Alberta Agriculture and Rural Development; 2011 [cited 2011 June]. 17 p. www1.agric.gov.ab.ca/$Department/deptdocs.nsf/all/csi13702/$FILE/Community-events-and-festivals.pdf

3. Sroda-Murawska S., Bieganska J. The Impact of Cultural Events on City Development: The (Great?) Expectations of a Small City. In: 5th Central European Conference in Regional Science [Internet]; October 5–8, 2014; Kosice, Slovak Republic. Torun, Poland: ul. Lwowska 1[cited 2015 January]; pp. 87–100. www.researchgate.net/publication/284719781_The_Impact_of_Cultural_Events_on_City_Development_the_Great_Expectations_of_a_Small_City

4. Skolnik J., Stern D., Chami R., Lane A., Kulesza C., Walker M. Planned Special Events: Cost Management and Cost Recovery Primer. Washington DC: US

Department of Transportation; 2009. 75. Report No.: FHWA-HOP-09-028. www.hsdl.org/?view&did=35642

5.   Hinchey P., Goodloe J. Principles of Finance. In: *Emergency Medical Services: Clinical Practice and Systems Oversight*. Cone D., Brice J., Delbridge T., Myers J. (eds). 2nd Edition. West Sussex (UK): John Wiley and Sons, Ltd; 2015; pp. 60–68.

6.   Peric M., Vitezić V. Socio-Economic Impacts of Event Failure: The Case of a Cancelled International Cycling Race. *Sustainability*. 2019 Sept 14;**11**(18):1–15.

Index

1984 Summer Olympics, 126
2019 Pandemic and All-Hazards Preparedness Act, 249
251-NBOMe, 381–382
3,4-methylenedioxymethamphetamine (MDMA), 327, 380–381
9/11, 116
911 response, 112–113

Accidental Death and Disability (National Academy of Sciences), 1
accountability, 86
Acinetobacter baumannii, 375
acute care facilities, transporting patients to, 335
acute mountain sickness (AMS), 237
Administration for Strategic Preparedness and Response, 116
administrative liability, 395
Medical Director, 396–398
Advanced Cardiac Life Support (ACLS), 15, 17, 61
drugs, 57, 58
Advanced Emergency Medical Technician (AEMT), 15, 58
advanced life support (ALS), 12, 69
Advanced Practice Registered Nurse (APRN), 13
aeromedical evacuation, 92
After-Actions Report (AAR), 18
agency partnerships, and crowd management, 268–269
air medical
and helicopter emergency medical service, 113
safety considerations, 113
air quality, 353
air quality index (AQI), 353
air quality index (AQI), local, 46
air traffic control, 99
airport baggage claim area, shooting at, 261
AKI and hyponatremia, prevention of, 235

alcohol, effect of on patient presentation rates (PPRs), 27–28
altitude illness, 354
ambulance transportation, 21
ambulance stand-by, 2
American Association of Critical Care Nurses, 13
American College of Sports Medicine, 226
American College of Surgeons Committee on Trauma, 135
American Heart Association, 392
American Red Cross, 392
Amyl Nitrites (Poppers):, 381
annual cultural events, medical care challenges and, 305
Arba'een Pilgrimage, 253
Area Command, 88–89
artists and crews
maintaining medical standards, 176–177
responding to needs of, 175–176
Astroworld Music Festival (Texas), 100, 128, 133–134, 268, 403
athletes, 156
education before endurance events, 228
minors as, 157
Therapeutic Use Exemptions (TUE), 155–156
triage and management of, 223
with impairments, 228
at-risk categories, planning for, 251–253
at-risk individuals
correct terminology and, 257
displacement of, 249
disproportionate disadvantage and, 248
meeting the special access and functional needs of, 251, 257
mitigating the vulnerabilities of, 254
planning for during disasters, 262
political mass gatherings and, 257
religious events and, 253
at-risk populations
crises and, 261
mass gathering events and, 248–249
needs of, 261, 266

attendees, 6
at community events, 214
at mass gatherings, 3
caring for, 33
crowd size and density, 24
demographics of, 25–26
events revenues from, 401
factors resulting in medical care, 24
medical care at high-profile event, 54–55
medical provider-to-attendee ratios, 13
missing persons protocol and, 102
statistics for care needed by, 6
audiences, 43, 161, 369
confrontation with, 51
mosh pits and, 34–35
profile of, 31
statistics and medical care needs, 22
touring physician and, 363–364
venues and, 25
younger, 24
Australian (Arbon) models, 28–29
automated external defibrillators (AEDs), 36, 45, 61, 64, 68, 175, 364
automobile traffic changes, 216

Baird (Heat Index-Adjusted Prior) Model, 31–32, 35
basic life support (BLS), 12
basilar skull fracture, 181
Bastille Day attack, 287
Bataclan nightclub shootings, 299
Beaver Stadium, 321
Benzodiazepines/Rohypnol (Roofies), 382
bike and cart teams, 69
Black Bloc, the, 289
Black Rock Desert, Nevada, 35, 45, 309, 324
bleeding control kits, 45
bomb attacks
Bomb Response team, 114, 115
Stade de France and Concomitant Paris, 286–287
terrorism and civil unrest, 286–287
Bonnaroo Music and Arts Festival, 72
Boston Baseball Championships, 280–281

Boston Marathon bombing, 48, 54, 97, 218, 269, 272, 285, 322, 324, 329, 335
Boston Marathon map, *275*
Burning Man festivals, 33, 35, 51, 232, 277, 324
  location of, 309
bystanders, 156–157

C.O.L.D. B.R.E.W. acronym, 159, *160*, 165, 167
California AIDS Ride, 26
California Office of Emergency Services (OES), 83
camping-related festivals
  caring for the production teams, 171–172
  risks and medical contingencies at, 169–170
  risks at, 170–171
cannabis/cannabinoids (Marijuana), 382
carbon monoxide exposure/toxicity, 101, 182, 193, 384
cardiac arrest, 36
  administering advanced cardiac life support (ACLS) drugs, 57
  advanced cardiac life support (ACLS) drugs, 58
  cardiac deaths from, 232–233
  marathon running and, 232
cardiopulmonary resuscitation (CPR) certification, 61
care
  continuity of, 363
  delivering, 4
  how the event command center affects, 4
  level of, 22–23
Carnival
  in Rio de Janeiro, Brazil, 259
  in Venice, Italy, 259
cart and bike teams, 69
casualty collection points (CCPs), 64, 91, 95, 102, 325, 330–332
  areas to be used as, 64
  identifying, 274
causation, 391
CDEM Act (2002), 324
celebrations, 259–261
Centers for Disease Control and Prevention, 332
  TBI information on website of the, 183
chemical terrorism/warfare attacks, 384,
children
  as the audience, 24
  heatstroke and, 307
  mass gathering events and, 250

participation in endurance events, 231
  Promenade des Anglais incident and, 287
chronically ill, planning for the, 251
Civil Defense Emergency Management (CDEM) Act, 324
civil unrest and terrorism, 284–286
  coordination and all-services debriefing, 301
  incorporated tactical medical response to, 295–297
  January 6th U.S Capitol Riot, 291–293
  perimeters of care and evacuation, 297
  preparation and planning for, 294–295
  risk assessment of, 293–294
  Yellow Vests Demonstrations, 289–290
climate
  climate change, 3, 103, 249, 302, 305, 312
  climate change and heat-related illnesses, 122
  climate change and mass gathering events, 314
  climate crisis, 314
  effect on mass gatherings, 3
clinical vignette, 193–194
closed head injuries, 193
Coachella, 277
cocaine (coke, blow, crack), 380
CodeRED mobile alert system, 98
cold stress, 236–237
cold-related injuries, 309
  cold stress, 236–237
  predictive modeling tools and, 311–312
  preventive measures, 312
  treatment of, 310–311
Command Staff
  Liaison Officer, 89
  other positions, 89
  Public Information Officer, 89
  Safety Officer, 89
common source outbreak, 373
Commonwealth of Pennsylvania, special events requirements, 200
communication, 97, 98–99, 149–150, 270, 274, 275–276
  at motorsports events, 191–192
  communication devices, 225
  communication plan, 52–54, 218, 237
  during community events, 217
  local ambulance companies and, 222

mass casualty incidents readiness and, 334–335
  media and social media, 276
  planning stage of, 98
  radio, 98
  tools for, 299–300
  use of tables/infographics, 275
Communication, Maintaining Health, Independence, Support/Safety and Transportation (CMIST) Framework, 251, 253, 256, 266
community events, 210, 219
  communication during, 217
  planning for, 210–214
complaints
  chief, *13*
  common presenting, 6
  level of care needed, 22–23
  psychiatric, 23
  types of, 23
Concert for Life in Australia, 26
Concomitant Paris attack, 286–287
concussion, 183
  guidelines for motorsports, *194*
  motorsports and, 193
consent, doctrine, 394–395
contingency planning, 172–173
continuous quality improvement, 18
cost calculation for EMS to Staff the Event, *403*
cost considerations, medical component of, 403–404
COVID-19 pandemic, 3, 135, 136, 154, 264, 266, 270, 275, 355, 378, 395
  India and, 374
  Kingdom of Saudi Arabia and, 376
  PCR screen for, 376
  public health and, 46, 218
  testing requirements, 48
  vaccination requirements and, 137
  vaccinations, 265
crisis management, 274
critical care medicine, 17
critical care nurses, 17
Critical Care Registered Nurses (CCRN), 13
critical illnesses
  risk of, 35, 36–37
  risk of cardiac arrest, 36
Critical Incident Stress Management (CISM), 337–338
crowds
  anticipated volume of the, 222–223
  challenge responding to, 174–175
  characteristics of, 280
  crisis management and, 274
  crowd crush incident, 46, 174, *See also* stampedes
  crowd demographics, 18, 25–26, 42, 67, 80, 126–128, 175, 271

crowd panic, 165
crowd size, 24, 49, 163, 188
crowd size and healthcare demands, 6
crowd size and patient frequency, 127
crowd size estimation, 218, 222–223, 270
crush, 278–280
human stampede in, 278–280
injuries and illnesses, 276–277
management of, 268–269, 277, *278*
management of in mass gathering events, 325–327
management of mass casualty incidents, 323
medical team and team dynamics in managing, 272
problem solving and crowd management, 280
psychosocial considerations and, 277
security and safety plan for, 274
CSCATTT, 334

damages
medical malpractice and, 389
medicolegal concerns and, 392
payment of, 134
DARPA Grand Challenge, 193
data
data plan, 218–219
incorporating, 218–219
Daytona 500, 184
deaths
civil unrests, 291, 292
deaths at, 36
drug-related, 381
endurance sports and, 223
from chemical terrorism, 384
heat-related, 125, 305, 306
heat-related in Chicago, 307
human stampede, 46, 133, 253
in mosh pits, 35
infectious diseases, 375
mass gathering events, 284, 285, 288
motorsports-related, 191
of fellow public safety partners, 285
Oklahoma City bombing, 287
Promenade des Anglais attacks, 287
religious mass gatherings, 326
traumatic, 236
ultra-endurance events and, 231
debriefings, post-events, 219
dehydration, 25, 305
depressants, central nervous system, 382–383
dermatologic, 233
diabetics, 182
dignitaries

at mass gathering events. *See also* VIP care
designating medical support teams, 204
Dignitary Protection Units, 208
inter-agency and community coordination and Collaboration, 205
National Special Security Event (NSSE) and, 202–203
own medical teams and, 205–207
privacy and safety of, 208–209
protective medicine and, 208
special considerations for, 203–204
their entourage, 205–207
threats to, 208
disabilities/disabled
planning for the, 251
statistics for people living with, 248
Disaster Medical Assistance Teams, 118
Disaster Relief Act (1974), 84
disasters, 265–266
disaster planning, 3, 102–103, 226
disaster planning and emergency response to, 4
DNC, 277
documentation
documentation plan, 60
documentation system, 46–49
Documentation Unit Leader, 60
extended events and, 240
medical, 225
driver compartment
driver safety and, 180–181, 183, 184, 189
NASCAR, 184
driver safety, 180
competency to drive and, 182–183
driver compartment and, 180–181, 184, 189
driver physiology and, 181–182
firesuit, 181
head & neck devices and restraints, 181, *182*
drivers
care of, 189–190
driver physiology, 181–182
injuries sustain at NASCAR 2023, *192*
rookie driving tests, 182–183
drug and alcohol use
at electronic dance music (EDM) festivals, 34

Earnhardt, Dale, 184
elderly, the. *See also* at-risk categories
celebrations and the, 260
planning for the, 251
Electric Daisy Carnival, 46, 168

electronic dance music (EDM)
festivals, 29, 34, 72
fans, 173
elevation, 354
Elizabeth II (queen), 257
Emergency Action Plan (EAP), 146
Emergency Alert System (EAS), 98
emergency management cycle, *324*, 324
preparation for recovery, 336
readiness, 327–333
recovery, 336–338
reduction, 324–327
response, 333–336
Emergency Medical Responder (EMR), 15
Emergency Medical Services (EMS)
systems, 1, 2, 14, 96, 107, 112, 168, 284, 290, *See also* staffing
certification of providers, 61
Emergency Medical Responders and, 15
local 911 response, 112–113
mass casualty incidents and, 320
medical direction and, 114
medical directors, 6, 18, 114, 356
municipal, 146
patients access to, 15
personnel, 58
providers, 61
regulations and, 114
reliance on, 67
response leadership, 201
tour medicine and, 345
Emergency Medical Services Act, 1
Emergency Medical Services Venue Assessment, 10
Emergency Medical Technicians (EMTs), 15, 57, 58, 88, 187, 188
emergency medicine, 388
Emergency Medicine physicians, 189
Emergency Operations Center (EOC), 89, 91, 107, 272, 274
local, 292
local and state, 106
Emergency Operations Center (EOC) structures, 105
emergency planning, 102–103
emergency shelters, 92
Emergency System for Advance Registration of Volunteer Health Professionals (ESAR-VHP), 118
emergency vehicles, 51, 138, 271, 320
areas for, 300
types of, 101–102
endemic diseases, 354–355
endurance athletic events
medical facility for, 223–224

pre-event planning and preparation, 221–222
endurance events, 230
  documentation and follow-up and, 240
  medical concerns about athletes in, 232–237
  medical response to, 238–240
  planning for, 237–238
endurance exercise, mental health benefits of, 235
endurance sports events, 47, 221
  athlete education and, 228
  mass participation in, 221
  medical coverage for, 226, 228
  medical operations at, 224–225
  medical planning and team organization and, 223
  predicting crowd size, 222–223
environments, 125, 239, 309, 335, *See also* locations
  cold, 233
  communication and the, 217
  high-risk, 284
  professional sports, 156
  remote and austere, 35
  rural and remote, 212
  standing room, 325
  urban and suburban, 211–212
equipment, *65*, 78
  and supplies, 17
  for category 1 events, 79
  for category 2 events, 79
  for category 3 events, 80
  for category 4 events, 80
  for category 5 events, 81
  personal, 65
Escherichia coli, 375
Esplanade Event, operation plan for, 273
ethanol, 382
ethical challenges, 207–208
evacuations, 51, 299, *See also* transportation
  during wars, 1
  evacuee encampment settings, women in, 250–251
  mass casualty incidents and, 48
  mass gatherings and, 13, 41–42
  plan for EMS response, 103
  rapid, 44, 51
  sequestered, 299
event command structure
  care and, 4
event managers, 167, 211, 215, 216
  communication with, 276
  community event, 214
  permits from municipal agencies, 214–215

event medical care. *See also* mass gathering medical care
  event medical plan, 6, 12, 115
  event medical planners and leaders, 105, 110, 114, 115, 116, 118
  tasks required for, 10
event medical staff
  basic training of, *61*
  Event Medical Director, 6, 10–12, 13, 14, 17, 18, 97, 215
  event medicine (EVM) specialists, 347
event medicine, 51, 57, 97, 118, 177
  event medicine (EVM) physician specialist, 366
  youth and club sports level and, 146
Event or Incident Action Plan, 66
event participants. *See* attendees
event promoters/promotion, 180
  and sponsorship considerations, 401–402
  Astroworld, 133
event security, 99
  external risks, 99,
  internal risks and, 99
  pre-event planning, 99
  uniformed police officers, 99–100
event sites, 51, 377
  camping at the, 33–34
  division of, 94
  location of, 43
  music, 163, 168
  temporary, 45
  transportation within the, 49
event specific conditions, predictive modeling tools for, 308
events
  activities during the, 150–151
  assessment of, 74, *75*
  categories of, 82
  category 2, 79–80
  category 3, 80
  category 4, 80–81
  category 5, 81–82
  category 5 checklist, *82*
  characteristics of, 125–126
  day of, 275
  defining the, 144–146
  duration of, 77
  effect of weather conditions on, 77–78
  equipment and staffing for category 1, 79
  event classification, 230–231
  event features, 29–31, *30*, 33
  features of different types of, 120–121
  large area and mobile, 72
  modifications to, 226
  multi-day, 33–34

nationally syndicated events, 154
  planning of, 149, 237–238
  post event review, 151
  profile of the, 78
  size of the, 74
  the end of, *279*, 281
  themes of, 120–121
  types of, 26, 213–214, 270
  unified command center and, 217–218
  unplanned events vs planned, 212–213
  wilderness, 72
events promoters/promotion
  planning for, 402–403
executive and protectee medicine, 202
executive medicine, training to provide, 202
Exercise Associated Heat Illness, 227
Exercise Associated Hyponatremia (EAH), 227
exertion, prolonged, 232
extended duration events, 126, 230, 240, 309
  documentation for patient care and, 240
  medical needs during, 237
extended events. *See* extended duration events
extraction teams, 69
Extraction Unit, 95
extreme endurance events, medical encounters at, 231–232
extreme mass participation events. *See also* endurance sports events
Exxon Valdez spill, 84

facilities
  optimal receiving medical, 358–359
  used for motorsports event, 187
family reunification, 336
Federal Bureau of Investigation (FBI), 109, 202
Federal Emergency Management Agency (FEMA), 58, 71, 97, 98, 120, 202, 328
  forms and checklists, *8*
  ICS form 205- Incident Radio Communications Plan, 133
  ICS form 208- SAFETY MESSAGE/ PLAN, 129
  Incident Command System and, 84
  training from, 64
Fédération Internationale de Football Association (FIFA) World Cup, 46
Field Intelligence Group (FIG), 100
FIFA World Cup, 154
  Brazil, 376
  Qatar, 309

Finance and Administration Section, 90
fire and hazardous materials, 107
Fire Branch Director, 58
fire departments, 111–112
Firefighting Resources of Southern California Organized for Potential Emergencies task force, 330
FIRESCOPE, 83
Firestone Firehawk 600 race, 185
firesuit, 181
first aid, xiii, 135
    basic, 13, 45
    number of providers, 13
    psychological, 337–338
    stations, 58, 168, 203, 260, 271
    tents and on-site clinics, 47
    training, 45
    training in, 364–365
First Aid and Cardiopulmonary Resuscitation (CPR), 135
fixed treatment locations, 4
flight nurses, 17
foodborne illnesses, *137*, 159
Formula One racing, 46, 146, 181, 184, 193
    driver compartment in, 180
free water, availability of, 25
frostbite, 311
fuel
    driver safety and, 184
    rocket, 193
    type of used in motorsports, 184–185
Fukushima Daiichi tsunami and nuclear disaster, 249
fusion centers, 106

Gamma-hydroxybutyrate, 382
Garissa University College Attack, Kenya, 322
gastrointestinal infections/issues, 46, 233–234, 374–375
Global Citizen Festival (Central Park), 164, 165
global warming, 314, *See also* climate
Good Samaritan laws, 215, 240, 388, 392, 393, 394, 395
    liability and, 390
    medical malpractice and, 389
    protections, 393–394, 398
graduate medical education (GME) physicians, 58
Grande, Ariana, 172
group and division supervisors, 58–60
guest services / customer service, 99

Haemophilus influenzae, 373
Hajj pilgrimage, 36, 124, 125, 128, 248, 253, 321, 373,
    crowd management analysis of, 326
    crowd-related injuries, 278
    heat-related illnesses at, 127
    heat-related injuries, 308
    meningococcal vaccination, 375–376
    public health concerns and, 374, 375
    stampede at, 322
hallucinogens/stimulants, 380–382
HANS device, 184
Happy Land Social Club fire, 325
Hartman, Nicholas, 29
Harvard National Prepared Leadership Initiative, 218
Harvard School of Public Health, 374
hazardous materials (HAZMAT), 100, 328
    hazard assessment, *130*
    response teams, 107, 114–115
hazards
    hazard rating worksheet, *131*
    Hazard Vulnerability Assessment, *130*
    Hazard Vulnerability Assessment Severity Ratings, *131*
    hazard worksheet, *132*
    listing of risks and, *129*
head & neck devices/restraints, 181, *182*, 193
Health and Medical Subcommittee (HMSC), 203
Health and Safety Executive in the United Kingdom (UK), 31
health care
    availability of, 78
    decision-making, 394–395
    psychological and mental well-being of workers, 302
    special teams, 117–118
health care coalitions
    regional, 116, *117*
    support from, 116
Health Information Portability and Accountability Act (HIPAA), 156, 394–395, 399
    forms, 190
Heat Index, 306
heat-related injuries, 305–306
    exertional heat stroke, 307
    factors leading to, *308*
    heat cramps, 306
    heat edema, 306
    heat tetany, 306
    preventive measures and, 307–309
    treatment of, 306–307
helicopters, *117*, 189

Emergency Medical Service (HEMS)
    landing zones, 113
EMS providers, 105, 107
helibase and helispots, 91, 92
helicopter EMS (HEMS), 113, *See also* Emergency Medical Service (EMS)
    rapidly evacuation and, 1
    rescue efforts and, 230
    rotor wash, 51
high profile attendees, specialized plans for medical care of, 54–55
Highland Park Parade, 219
Holy Shroud exhibition, 33
home & visiting medical teams, 149
Homeland Security Presidential Directive 5 (HSPD-5), 105
Hospital Preparedness Program (HPP), 116
hospital-based providers, 58
hospitals, 107
    closest community, 115
    hospital actions, 300
    hospital operations, 335
    prehospital operations, 334,
    regional specialty, 116
    site visits to, 360–363
Houston Fire Department (HFD), 133
HSPD-5, 105
human herpes virus (HHV-2) coinfections, 376
Human Papilloma Virus (HPV), 376
Hurricane Ida, 264
Hurricane Katrina, 248
hygiene issues, 169
hyperthermia, 222, 223, 236, 307, 380, 381, 385
    assessing patient for, 383
    dehydration and, 227
    management of, 224
    rebound, 227
    risk mitigation and, 324
    severe, 383
hypothermia, 3, 125, 159, 163, 214, 227, 233, 236, 310, *See also* hyperthermia
    life-threatening, 237
    mild, 310
    prevention of, 310
    wet, 188

Incident Action Plan (IAP), 86, 146
Incident Command Post, 91
    incident command staff, 58, *59*
Incident Command Structure, 93, 95, *See also* Incident Command System
    Area Command, 88–89
    Command Staff, 89

functional areas of, 87
Safety Officer, 89
unity of command and, 87
Incident Command System (ICS), 14, 83, 96, 149, 238, 330
accountability and, 86
command procedures, 92
communications and, 86
comprehensive resource management, 86
concepts of, 85
establishment and transfer of command, 86
Finance and Administration Section, 90
flexibility of, 95–96
functional areas of the Incident Command Structure of, 84–85
gathering information and intelligence, 87
general staff, 89
groups and divisions, 90
helibase and helispot, 92
history of, 83, 84
implementation and, 93
implementation and application of, 92
Incident Command Structure, 87
Incident Commander, 87–88
Joint Information Center, 92
Logistics Section, 90
management by objective, 85
mass gathering incidents and, 330, 331
Medical Branch Director, 93–94
Medical Branch Groups, 94
Medical Group Supervisor, 93–94
medical services specific positions, 90
missing persons protocol and, 102
modular organization, 85
nationwide adoption of, 84
noncommand functional areas of, 89
Operations Section, 89–90
overview of, 84–85
Planning Section, 90
positions in the Medical Branch, 93
responsibilities of the commander, 92–93
scalability and organization of, 87
span of control, 85
Strike Teams, 91
suggested courses for, 84
terminology used in, 85
training, 64
Unified Command system, 88
unified command/commander, 85, 86
units, 90–91
unity of command, 85

Incident Command System Locations, 91
casualty collection points, 91
Emergency Operations Center, 91
emergency shelters, 92
Incident Command Post, 91
staging area, 91
Incident Commander, 87–88, 89, 92
incident facilities and locations, 86
incident management, 274
Indianapolis Motor Speedway, 182, 185
IndyCar racing, 146, 184
chassis numbers, 183
driver compartment in, 180
Indy Racing League, 181, 193
infectious diseases, 378
gastrointestinal infection, 374–375
mass gathering events and, 372–373
prevention and planning for, 376–378
respiratory illnesses, 373–374
sexually transmitted infections, 376
injuries
and illnesses, 276–277
cold weather and injury patterns, 125
environment-related, 236–237
injury patterns, 18, 63, 239
injury preparation calculus, 288–289
motorsports injury patterns, 192
rock concerts and injury patterns, 126
traumatic, 236
injuries and illnesses, prevention of, 228
Institute of Medicine, Regionalization of Emergency Care, 116
Integrated Public Alert Warning System (IPAWS), 98
Intelligence-Design-Choice-Implementation decision support model, 121
interdisciplinary functions, 107
International Classification of Disease (ICD), 306
International Trauma Life Support (ITLS)
certification, 17
intoxicated patient, generalized approach to management of, 383–384
IPAWS Program Planning Toolkit site, 98

Johnson, Lyndon B., 1
Joint Emergency Services Intra-operability Programme, 334
Joint Information Center (JIC), 92
jump kits, 191

Kaiser Wilhelm Memorial Church, 287
Kentucky Cabinet for Health and Family Services, 392
Ketamine (Special K, Vitamin K, Cat Valium), 381
King-Devick test, 183
Klebsiella pneumoniae, 373, 375,
Korean Conflict, 1
Kumbh Mela, 125, 128, 253, 373, 374, 375, 378

large area and mobile events, 72
Larrey, Dominique Jean, 1
Las Vegas Shooting, 322
law enforcement, 107
federal, 109–111
local, 108–109
overview, 108
role of local, 100
state, 109
Law Enforcement Branch Director, 58
lawsuits
for medical negligence and personal injury, 399
medical negligence, 388–389
legal duty, 390–391
liability, 399
administrative, 395, 396–398
liability insurance, 215
professional, 398–399
liability risks, 388
Liaison Officer, 89
licensees, nonliability of, 392–394
licensure, 395–396
lightning, 52, 159, 253, 305, 306, See also weather/weather conditions
30–30 Rule for Lightning Safety, 125
Lightning Action Plan, 125
lightning-related injuries, 72, 125, 237, 312
preventive measures and, 313–314
treatment of, 312–313
loading dock lifestyle, 369
local resources, preservation of, 3
locations, 121–125, 271–272
coastal. See also venues
of community events, 211
planning and transportation logistics, 271
locked-down and impassable zones, 199
logistics
logistical issues, 261, 282
logistical issues and medical planning and, 9–10
logistics personnel, 60, 71
Logistics Section, 90,
Logistics Section Chief, 60

logistics management, 78
  for category 1 events, 79
  for category 2 events, 79
  for category 3 events, 80
  for category 4 events, 80
  for category 5 events, 81
lone attackers, 287
  obscured, 287–288
Love Parade disaster, Germany, 325

Major Incident Medical Management
    and Support system, 334
Major League Baseball games, 327
management by objective, 85, 87, 92
Manchester (UK) Arena bombing, 172
Manchester Arena concert, 288
marathon running, risk of cardiac
    death from, 232
Mardi Gras activities, New Orleans,
    259, 260
mass casualty events, 272, 300, See also
    mass gathering violence
mass casualty incidents, 113, 320
  analysis of, 337
  assessment of, 333–334
  care of healthcare workers and
    responders, 337–338
  community and, 334–335
  crowd management and, 323
  demobilization and debriefing
    activities, 337
  effect on communities, 334–335
  epidemiology and classification of,
    322–324
  hospital-based response, 335
  management of, 338
  management of resources, 327
  planning, 217
  prehospital management, 336
  prehospital operations and, 334–335
  preparation and scalability of
    resources, 332
  readiness for, 327–333
  readiness through training and
    review, 332–333
  recovery and, 336–338
  special challenges with, 320–322
mass gathering events
  advanced care at, 16–17
  at-risk population, 248–249
  attendees, 3
  categories of, 126
  chemical terrorism at, 384
  climate and environmental
    effect on, 3
  climate change and, 314
  common complaints at, 6
  costs component of medical care, 404
  critical care at, 17
  crowd safety and, 282

definition, 21
economic benefits of, 401
environmental and geographical
    factors and, 324–325
environmental considerations and.
    See also weather conditions
factors affecting, 165
high-risk, 100
impact on local health system,
    215–216
implementation of the Incident
    Command System at, 93
implications of mass casualty
    incidents for, 320–322
infectious risks and, 372–373
inter-agency and community
    coordination and collaboration,
    205
legal considerations and, 388
logistical planning for, 41–42
mass casualty incidents implications
    of, 320
medical care challenges and, 6
medical care planning and, 55
medical component of cost, 403–404
medical plan for, 12
medical plans and resources for, 6
multiple casualties associated with,
    321
planning and contingencies for,
    200–201
planning for, 268, 269–270
planning for children at, 250
planning for vulnerable attendees,
    251
planning for women at, 250–251
post-event debriefing, 18
pre-event briefing and, 65–66
prevention of heat-related injuries
    at, 307–308
psychological and mental well-being
    of medical workers at, 302
reduction of risks at, 324–327
requirements for basic care, 16
respiratory illnesses and, 373–374
size of, 270–271
space and, 3
special planning considerations,
    272–273
statutes and regulations and,
    202–203
the scale and specific need for
    emergency medical services,
    2–3
toxicology issues in, 380
training for managing, 270
type of, 270
VIP attendees at, 200
mass gathering incidents, 302
  Incident Command System, 330, 331

mass gathering infectious diseases,
    372–373, 378
  gastrointestinal infection, 374–375
  Meningococcal disease, 375–376
  prevention and planning, 376–378
  respiratory illnesses, 373–374
mass gathering medical care
  goals of, 6–8
  staffing and, 13
Mass Gathering Medical Care Plan,
    311
mass gathering medicine
  care at events, 4
  goals of, 2
  medical plan for, 6–8
  medicolegal concerns and, 388–389
  origins of, 2
  research and quality improvement
    in, 4
  what it is not, 1
mass gathering medicine specialist
  challenges for, 174, 175–176
  ethical challenges and, 176–177
  professional standards and, 176–177
mass gathering music events
  duration of, 169–170
mass gathering violence.
    See also civil unrest and
    terrorism
  aggravation and escalation of
    violence, 300–301
  communication tools and medical
    care, 299–300
  evacuations and, 299
  hospital actions, 300
  sequestered evacuations, 299
  site security and, 297–299
mass notification systems, 98
mass shooting attack, 288
media and social media, the, 276
medical advance document
  designated point person and the, 360
  strategic plan, 360
medical advance plan, 359
  touring medicine and, 358
medical assistance, tracking requests
    for, 174
Medical Branch, 93
  Deputy Branch Director, 90
  Medical Branch Director, 58, 90,
    93–94
  Medical Branch Groups, 94
  Medical Group Supervisor, 93–94
medical care
  approach to in motorsports,
    186–187
  availability of, 78
  effect of weather conditions on, 65
  logistical issues in planning, 9–10
  personal equipment needed, 65

planning for, 8–10
predicting medical needs, 21
preparing for, 72
preparing for an event, 64
provider mindset and, 64
staffing at mass gathering events, 57
medical care staff, 58
  basic training & credentialling of, 60–61
  during the event, 66
  VIP care and, 203
medical care teams, 58, 64, 68, 149,
    See also medical care staff
  at indoor venues must, 65
  service level agreement and, 78–79
medical concerns, of endurance event athletes, 232–237
medical conditions, atypical, 359
medical coverage, 180
  for endurance events, 221, 226, 228
  for such mass gathering events, 200
medical deployment, goals of, 2
medical direction, 274
Medical Director, 189, 396–398
medical documentation, 72
medical encounters, at extreme endurance events, 231–232
medical equipment, 239
medical facility, 46, 113, 167
  endurance athletic events and, 93–94
  onsite, 10, 168, 187
  outside, 21, 23
  surveillance of the, 169
Medical Group, 90
medical malpractice, 389
  breach of duty of care, 391
  causation and, 391
  duty for, 390
  liability case, 391
medical management, 226–227
medical needs
  prediction models and, 28
  risk assessment and, 165–167
medical negligence, 388–389,
    See also medical malpractice
  and personal injury, 399
medical operations, 274
  law enforcement/security support of, 111
  objective of, 273
medical personnel
  alerting and dispatching, 60
  local, 175
  onsite, 13–14
medical plans
  considerations for special events, 203–204
  cost for the, 404
  endurance sports events and, 223
  for dignitaries and VIPS, 200

for multi-day events, 169
for on-site coverage versus contingency planning, 172–173
medical point person, local, 360
Medical Professional Liability Association (MPLA), 389
medical protocols, 223
medical providers, defining the roles, 146–149
medical provider-to-attendee ratios, 13
Medical Reserve Corps, 117
Medical resource prediction model, *13*
medical response, to civil unrest and terrorism, 295–297
medical risks, and touring medicine, 345–347
medical staff
  conduct of during the event, 66
  medical staffing models, 18–19
  medical support personnel, 58–60
  planning for at motorsports events, 188–189
medical standards
  dignitaries and, 207–208
  touring medicine and, 366–367
medical support teams, designating, 204
medical team
  after the event, 66–67
  and team dynamics, 272
  providing provisions for, 65
Medical Threat Assessment (MTA), 201, 309
medical time out, 150
medical training
  event, 61–64
  event specific, 61–64
  experience for students in, 58
  venue specific training, 64
medical usage rate (MUR), 21, 126, 213
medications, suggested-Infield Medical Center, *195*
medicolegal concerns
  administrative liability, 396–398
  damages, 392
  legal duty and, 390–391
  licensure, 395–396
  nonliability of licensees, 392–394
Meningococcal disease, 375–376
mental preparation, 64
mental status changes, 383
Mephedrone (Diablo, Meow Meow, Eric 3), 381
Methamphetamines (Speed, Ice, Crank, Meth), 381
METHANE system, 333, 334
Methicillin Resistant Staphylococcus aureus, 373
Methylenedioxypyrovalerone (Bath salts), 381

Miami Ultra Music Festival (UMF), 133
Mina Stampede, Mecca, 322
minors, 157
missing persons, 97
  protocols for handling reports of, 102
mobile events, 72
Molly, 381
mosh pits, 34–35
Motor Speedway, 188
motorsports events, 179
  car construction, 183–184
  care of drivers and, 189–190
  clinical vignette, 193–194
  communication at, 191–192
  competency to drive and, 182–183
  concussion guidelines, *194*
  crashes and, 184
  deaths related to, 191
  driver compartment, 180–181, 183
  driver safety and, 180
  firesuit and, 181
  head & neck restraint device, 181, *182*
  importance of driver physiology and, 181–182
  jump kit contents, 191
  medical staffing at, 188–189
  planning issues and, 193
  responses to injuries on the track, 190–191
  vehicle safety and, 183
motorsports medicine, 179–180
Mount Meron, stampede at, 326
Multiagency Coordination Systems (MACS), 84, 105, 106
multiple casualty incidents (MCIs), 57, 94, 165, 288
  training and, 64
multisport events, 232
musculoskeletal injuries, 234
music and cultural festivals, 232
music concerts and festivals, 158
  as mass gathering event, 158–163
  effect of various factors on, 163–165
  population/demographics of, 158
music events. *See also* camping-related festivals
music mass gathering events
  established venues and, 168
  importance of location, 168
  in established venues, 168
  in nonestablished entertainment venues, 168–169
  medical plans, 69–71
  medical plans for, 2
  nonestablished venues and, 168–169
  risks factors at, 170–171

music tours
    day 2 in the work cycle, 349–350
    health challenges and, 352–353
    medical considerations and, 353
    planning for show day events,
        350–352
    risk factors and, 345–347
    work cycle and work duties during,
        348–349
musical events. *See* music concerts and
        festivals
music-related mass gathering events.
        See music mass gathering events
Muslim Pilgrimage to Mecca. *See* Hajj
        pilgrimage
MV Mavi Marmara attack, 325

Nadeau, Jerry, 185
NAEMSP Mass Gathering Medical
        Care Planning documentation,
        210
NAFTA, 103
NASCAR, 11, 181, 193
    2012 medical Verification Form, *196*
    chassis, 183
    Cup teams, 181
    fuel used in vehicles, 184
    impact of crashes on vehicles in, 184
    Season 2023, drivers' injuries at, *192*
National Academy of Sciences,
        Accidental Death and Disability,
        1
National Association of Emergency
        Medical Services Physicians
        (NAEMSP), 13, 32, 298
National Association of State EMS
        Officials, 15
National Basketball Association
        trainers, 202
National EMS Scope of Practice Model,
        13, 58,
National Football League (NFL), 156,
        193, 203, 333, 336
    championship, 46
National Health Service (NHS), 356
National Highway Traffic Safety
        Administration (NHTSA), 15,
        58
National Hockey League (NHL), 156
National Incident Management System
        (NIMS), 58, 64, 84, 85, 105, 238,
        269
    interagency planning and, 105–106
    overview of, *106*
    Unified Command, 106
National Oceanic and Atmospheric
        Administration's weather radio
        system, 98
National Practitioner Data Bank or
        Medical Board, 389

National Preparedness Leadership
        Initiative (NPLI), 275
National Special Security Event (NSSE),
        202–203
National Weather Service, 99
Neisseria meningitides, 376
neurologic psychiatric issues, 234–235
New Orleans, *Mardi Gras*, 259, 260
Nitro Rallycross, 193
Nitrous Oxide (Whippets, Laughing
        gas), 383
NOAA Weather Radio All Hazards, 99
nongovernmental agencies and
        organizations, 118
North American Free Trade
        Agreement regulations, 103
nurse practitioners, 17
nurses, 17, 189

Obama, Barack, 256
Occupational Safety and Health
        Administration (OSHA), 309
Oklahoma City bombing, 287
Olympic Games, 126, 154–155, 373,
        374
    Japan, 376
    Pyeongchang, 155
    Winter Games (1984), 325
onsite medical care, 8, 13–14, 187, 205
    at a motorsports events, 187
    onsite coverage versus contingency
        planning, 172–173
    physician staffing, 58
operational security (OPSEC), 205
operations plan, 273
    communications section of, 274
    crisis management component of,
        274
    flexibility of, 275
    incident management component
        of, 274
    medical direction component of, 274
    medical operations component of,
        274
    medical response at the event, 275
    objective of the medical operations,
        273
    security and safety plan, 274
    tables/infographics component of,
        275
Operations Section, 89–90
    teams within, 91
opioids, 383

P.E.E.R. S.O.P. acronym, 158, *159*, 163,
        165, 167
Pandemic and All-Hazards
        Preparedness Act (2019), 249
Papal visit, to Philadelphia, 254
Papal visits, 253

ParaDocs, 133
paramedic, 15–17
Paris Attacks, 322
patient presentation rates (PPRs), 6,
        13, 21, 22, 24, 67, 68, 213
    effect of age on, 26
    effect of alcohol and recreational
        drugs on, 27–28
    effect of weather conditions on,
        24–25
    football games and, 26
    models for, 32
    prediction of, 25
    prior, 31
    recommendations for model
        selection, 32–33
    seated audience and, 25
    types of events and, 26
patient transportation, 49–52
Patient Transportation Group, 95
patients
    average number of patient contacts,
        30
    estimate of patient contacts, 30
    expected number of patient contacts,
        74
    identification of, 42–46
    multiple patient contacts, 60
    nomenclature for patient
        identification, 48
    number of patient contacts, 75, 80,
        188
    patient care documentation, 12, 14,
        18
    patient contacts, 79
    patient tracking system, 46–49
    protecting the, 175
    severity of patient contacts, 21, 151
    transportation and patients contacts,
        22
    types of patient contacts, 21, 74
Pediatric Advanced Life Support
        (PALS), 17, 61
pediatric patients, 23–24
personal equipment, 65
personnel training, 60–61
Phoenix International Raceway, 188,
        190
    jump kit, 191
physician assistants, 17
physicians, 17, *See also* staffing
    activities of the tour, 360–363
    enlisting trusted physicians on
        show day, 357–358
    on-site, 10–12
    oversight of the Emergency Medical
        System, 114
    role of the touring, 355–357
Plan Risk Manifestation (PRIMA), 32
planning

event organizers philosophy and, 67–68

Planning Section, 90

Planning Section Chief, 60

political mass gatherings, 256–259

prediction models, 28

predictive models

predictive modeling tools, 308

predictive modeling tools, cold-related injuries and, 311–312

pre-event plan, *211*

pre-event briefing, 65–66, 99, 150, 273

pre-event briefing and operations plan, 275

pre-event planning, event security and, 99

prehospital medical care

beginning of, 1–2

prehospital operations, 334–335

prehospital providers, 58, 328

rehospital providers, 12

prehospital registered nurses (PHRNs), 17

Prehospital Trauma Life Support (PHTLS), 17

Presidential Decision Directive 62, 100

Presidential Protection Act of 2000, 202

Primary Care Paramedic (Canada), 58

private security, 111

problem solving plan, 280

Boston Baseball Championships, 280–281

improvements to, 281

production teams, 164, 165, 346, 349, 367

caring for, 171–172

health challenges, 352

music tour events and, 360

music touring events and, 351

on-site, 350

Professional Liability Insurance, 398–399

Promenade des Anglais attack, 287

provider mindset, 64

Pseudomonas aeruginosa, 373

psychiatric complaints, 23

public events. *See* mass gathering events

public health, 135–137, 216–217

Public Information Officer, 89

public safety specialty teams, 114

Pyeongyang Winter Olympiad, 375

racial justice marches, 275

radio communication, 98

rapid sequence induction (RSI) procedures, 58

rate of hospital transports (TTHR). *See* transport-to-hospital rates (TTHRs)

RAVE mobile, 98

readiness, mass casualty incidents, 327–333

real time information, use of, 218–219

recovery, 224, 249, 320, 324, 333, 334

emergency management cycle and, 336–338

incomplete, 235

preparation for, 336

projected duration of, 156

recreational drugs, effect of on patient presentation rates (PPRs), 27–28

Regionalization of Emergency Care (Institute of Medicine), 116

registered nurses, 17

religious gatherings. *See* religious mass gathering events

religious mass gathering events, 126, 253–256, 326

at-risk individuals and, 254

intoxicants used at, 136

remote events, planning for transportation needs, 239

renal issues, 235–236

República Cromañón (Cromagnon Republic) nightclub (Argentina), 134

República Cromañón Nightclub Fire, Argentina, 322

resource management, 13, 86, *See also* staffing

resources

dispatch and deployment of, 87

preparation and scalability of, 332

respiratory arrest, 36

respiratory illnesses, 373–374

mass casualty incidents, 64

response, to mass casualty incidents, 333–336

Richmond International Speedway, 185

risk assessments, 165–167

of civil unrest and terrorism, 293–294

planning for and reducing risks, 167–168

risks

and hazards, *129*

environmental and geographical factors affecting, 324–325

high-risk mass gatherings, 100

internal, 99

reducing, 167–168, 324–327

Route 91 Harvest Festival, 165, 288

rules and regulations, for mass gathering events, 200–201

Running of the Bulls, in Pamplona, Spain, 259

safety, 255, 261

of intellectual disabilities, 265

personnel, 186

political mass gatherings and, 258

security & safety issues, 128–135

Safety Officer, 89

Salmonella typhi, 375

sarin gas attacks, 384

Saudi SALEM, 218

Saudi SALEM tool

factors for risk scoring in the, *132*

risk classification and preparedness of, *133*

Scott, Travis, 403

Astroworld Music Festival, 100

Secondary Assessment of Victim Endpoint (SAVE) algorithm, 331

Secret Service of DSS, 100

security and safety plan

for crowd control, 274

Security Industry Authority (SIA), 135

security teams, 164

service animals, 258

Service d'Aide Médicale Urgente (SAMU) du Paris, 290

sexually transmitted infections (STIs), 376

SFI Foundation in California for their Thermal Protective Performance (TTP), 181

Shia Muslim annual event, 253

show day, 350–352

enlisting additional trusted physicians, 357–358

Sicking, Dean, 184

simple triage and rapid treatment (START) triage system, 330

single incident commander, vs. unified command incident, 87

site security, 297–299

skin conditions, 233

SOAP format, 240

social media, 276

sort–assess–lifesaving interventions–treat/transport (SALT) system, 331

South African model, 31, 33

space, impact on mass gathering medicine, 3

special events, 120, 401

economic benefits of, 401

Special Event Assessment Rating (SEAR) Events, 110, 203

support agencies and, 105

Special Events Contingency Planning Job Aids Manual (FEMA), 137, 214
special weapons and tactics (SWAT) teams, 97, 100, 107, 114, 115, 205, 295–296
  vehicles of, 299
spectators, 53
  cardiac arrest and, 36
  care of at motorsports events, 187–188
  not event, 22, 127
  on-site care and, 384
  PPR at the Olympics, 126
  role of event security and, 100
  sporting events and, 126
sponsor/sponsorship
  community event, 214
  mass gathering events and, 401–402
sporting events, 144–146
  bystanders, 156–157
  communication, 149–150
  coordination with local resources, 149
  environment and, 153–154
  HIPAA, 156
  international venues and, 154
  league and players' association guidelines, 156
  minors at, 157
  multi-team/multi-site events, 153, 154
  nationally syndicated events as, 154
  Olympics, 154–155
  on-site training room facilities, 152–153
  pre-event activities, 149
  venue considerations and, 151–152
  VIP care, 156
Sports Car Club of America, 182
Sports Medicine Licensure Clarity Act, 395
sports, classification of, 145
Stade de France and Concomitant Paris attacks, 286–287
Stade de France bombing site, 299
staffing
  alerting and dispatching medical staff, 60
  bike and cart teams, 69
  Deputy Branch Director, 90
  event medical training and, 61–64
  extraction teams, 69
  for category 1 events, 79
  for category 2 events, 79
  for category 3 events, 80
  for category 4 events, 80
  for category 5 events, 81
  general considerations for.
    See also medical care

group and division supervisors, 58–60
hospital-based providers, 58
incident command staff, 58, 59
incident command training and, 64
logistics personnel, 60
Medical Branch Director, 58, 90, 93–94
medical care personnel, 58
models, 67, 68–71
models of and organizer's philosophy, 67–68
nurses, 17
Operations Section Chief, 90
personnel training and, 60–61
physician assistants, 17
Planning Section Chief, 60
prehospital providers, 58
supervisors, 71
support teams, 71
transport teams, 71
treatment teams, 69–71
triage and multiple casualty incident training, 64
unit and team leaders, 60
venue specific training of, 64
walking teams, 68
stakeholders, identification of, 328–330
stampede, 278–280, 294
  tunnel, 253
standard of care
  breach of, 391
  causation and, 391
standing room environments, 325
Stanley Cup final (2011), 272
state and local regulations, 17
Steel and Foam Energy Reduction (SAFER) barrier, 185
stimulants/hallucinogens, 380–382
stimulants/prescription (Adderall, Ritalin), 381
Stoots v. Marion Life Saving Crew, Inc., 392
Strategic National Stockpile initiative, 332
Streptococcus pneumoniae, 373
Strike Teams, 91
students
  experience for medical training programs, 58
Summer Olympics (Tokyo), 154
Super Bowl, 144
supervisors, 71
support teams, 71
swarm intelligence, 275
SWAT (special weapons and tactics), 100, 107, 114, 115, 205, 295–296
  vehicles of, 299

tactical response teams (TRTs), 295
terminology, definitions of, 21–22
terrorism and civil unrest, 4, 172, 284–286, 295
  9/11, 84, 105
  Boston Marathon bombing, 97
  chemical, 385
  ethical considerations, 301
  lone attackers and, 287
  obscured lone terrorist attacks, 287–288
  perimeters of care and evacuation, 297
  site security and, 297–299
  social and political considerations, 276
  weapons and tactics used in, 288–289
terrorist attacks. See terrorism and civil unrest
Texas Motor Speedway, 185
Therapeutic Use Exemptions (TUE)
  drug use and sports, 155–156
Tokyo subway sarin attack, 324
Toronto food festival, 125
total patient presentations (TPP), 22
tour members, 351, 352, 355, 356, 367
  basic first aid training and, 364–365
  frequency of hospital visits and, 362
  health and safety risks, 343
  medical care of, 369
  optimal medical care and, 359
  triage as priority patients, 351
touring medicine, 342–345
  air quality and, 353
  atypical medical conditions and, 359
  continuity of care, 363
  day 2 work cycle, 349–350
  elevation and, 354
  endemic diseases, 354–355
  enlisting additional trusted physicians, 357–358
  importance of hospital site visits, 360–363
  loading dock lifestyle, 369
  medical risk factors in, 345–347
  medical standards and ethical challenges, 366–367
  preemptive medical considerations, 353
  pretour advisories and preparations, 355
  receiving facilities for various conditions, 358–359
  role of the physician, 367
  role of the touring physician and, 355–357
  show day, 350–352
  tour physician and artists medical needs, 365–366

venue and the touring physician, 363–364

work cycle and work duties in, 348–349

touring physician, 346, 349, 351, 360, 364, 365–366

management of the audience and, 363–364

roles and responsibilities of, 345, 346, 352, 355–357

toxicology, 380, 385

track

responses to injuries on, 190–191

track safety, 185, 190

traffic changes, automobile, 216

training, 270

and review for MCI readiness, 332–333

training room facilities, on-site, 152–153

transportation

emergency, 100–101

of patients to acute-care facilities, 335

planning for emergency, 101

political mass gathering events, 259

pre- and post-disaster plan, 266

strategic planning and, 100–101

transport teams, 71, 78, 212, 239

types of emergency vehicles used for, 101–102

transportation logistics, 271

transport-to-hospital rates (TTHRs), 6, 13, 21, 22, 24, 67, 68, 213

football games and, 26

on-site physician and, 11

types of events and, 26

Trason, Ann, 233

Traumatic Brain Injury (TBI), 183

traveling doctors, 191

treatment teams, 69–71

treatment unit, 95

triage, 48, 95, 334

algorithms, 330–332

and incident management theories, 72

and management of athletes, 223

and multiple casualty incident training, 64

and transport model, 222

establishment of modified, 329

high-quality and care of event goers, 3

provision of on-scene, 165

secondary, 204

tags and the weather, 49

triage unit, 94–95

triathlons, 232

Tropheryma whipplei, 375

U.S Capitol Riot, 291–293

U.S. Americans with Disabilities Act (ADA), 249

U.S. Department of Defense (DOD), 202

U.S. Department of Health and Human Services (HHS), 202

U.S. Department of Homeland Security), 202

U.S. Drug Enforcement Agency (DEA) certifications, 356

Ukraine-Russian war, 248

Ultra Music Festival, 134

ultra-endurance events

elite ultra-runners, 230

participation in, 231

ultra-marathons, 45, 230

ultra-runners, 234

unauthorized demonstration, 295

Unified Command (UC) System, 88, 96, 106

Command Staff, 89

endurance sports events and, 226

Unified Command Center (UCC), 217, 226, 274

unified mission, establishing a, 222

unit and team leaders, 60

Unite the Right rally (Charlottesville), 333–336

United Kingdom (UK)

Health and Safety models, 31

patient prediction guide, 22

United Nations International Strategy for Disaster Reduction (UNISDR), 129

United States Air Shows, 10

United States Secret Service (USSS), 109–110, 202

University of Virginia model, 13, 29–31, 32

Urban Heat Island (UHI), 306

US Department of Health and Human Services (HHS), 116

US Department of Homeland Security, 84, 100, 109, 110, 215, 217

resources of the, 273

Utility vehicles (UTV), 102

vaccinations, availability of, 355

Vancouver Stanley Cup riot, 326

vehicles

speed of, 185

vehicle safety, 183

ventricular fibrillation (VF), 58

ventricular tachycardia (VT), pulseless, 58

venues, 75, 76

bounded or unbounded spaces, 25

established, 168

features of, 25

using venues outside established entertainment, 168–169

Vietnam War, 1

violence, 281

aggravation and escalation of, 300–301

communication tools and, 299–300

inebriated patrons and, 27

medical emergencies from, 217

outbreaks of, 167

persons with disabilities and risk of, 265

political mass gatherings, 256

rival sports team supporters and, 128

terrorism and, 284

VIP care, 156, 176

at mass gathering events, 200

medical standards and ethical challenges, 207–208

planning and considerations for, 201–202

specialized training to provide, 202

volunteer health professionals, registration of, 118

vulnerable populations, 259

walking teams, 68

Weapons of Mass Destruction (WMD), 114

Civil Support Team (CST), 114

weapons, and tactics, 288–289

weather/weather conditions, 23, 24–25, 65, 214

effect of on endurance athletes, 230

effect on events, 77–78

effect on outdoor events, 71–72

endurance sports events and, 226

impact on mass gathering events, 305

mass casualty incidents and, 125

Wertheimer, Paul, 325

Western States Endurance Run, 234

Wet Bulb Globe Temperature (WBGT), 124, 226, 227, 236, 305,

calculator, 309

risk chart, 72

White House Medical Unit, 202

wilderness events, 72

wildfires, 330

Winter Olympics (Pyeongchang), 154

Wireless Emergency Alerts (WEA) system, 98

women
    mass gathering events and, 250–251
    pregnant, 251
Woodstock Festival, 125
work cycle
    day 2, 349–350
    touring medicine and, 348–349

World Anti-Doping Agency (WADA),
    155
World Cup, 144
World Health Organization (WHO),
    21, 306
World Scout Jamboree, Japan,
    376

Yellow River Stone Forest
    Ultramarathon,
    230
Yellow Vests demonstrations,
    289–290, 291

Zeitz method, 129

Printed in the United States
by Baker & Taylor Publisher Services